Fundamentals of

Physiology for Nursing Students

Fundamentals of
Physiology for Nursing Students

Second Edition

RL Bijlani MD SM DSc (Hon) FAMS
Former Professor and Head
Department of Physiology
All India Institute of Medical Sciences
New Delhi, India

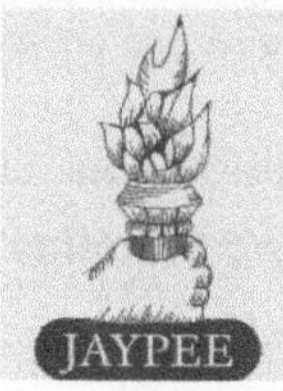

JAYPEE BROTHERS MEDICAL PUBLISHERS
The Health Sciences Publisher
New Delhi | London

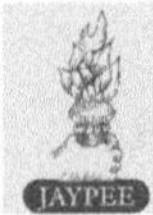

Jaypee Brothers Medical Publishers (P) Ltd.

Headquarters

EMCA House
23/23-B, Ansari Road, Daryaganj
New Delhi 110 002, India
Landline: +91-11-23272143,
+91-11-23272703+91-11-23282021,
+91-11-23245672
E-mail: jaypee@jaypeebrothers.com

Overseas Off ce

JP Medical Ltd.
83, Victoria Street, London
SW1H 0HW (UK)
Phone: +44-20 3170 8910
E-mail: info@jpmedpub.com

Corporate Office

Jaypee Brothers Medical Publishers (P) Ltd.
4838/24, Ansari Road, Daryaganj
New Delhi 110 002, India
Phone: +91-11-43574357
Fax: +91-11-43574314
E-mail: jaypee@jaypeebrothers.com

EU GPSR Authorised Representative
Logos Europe, 9 rue Nicolas Poussin
17000, La Rochelle, France
Phone: +33 (0) 6 67 93 73 78
E-mail: Contact@logoseurope.eu

Website: www.jaypeebrothers.com
Website: www.jaypeedigital.com

Inquiries for bulk sales may be solicited at: jaypee@jaypeebrothers.com

Fundamentals of Physiology for Nursing Students

First Edition: 2001
Reprint: 2005, 2008

Second Edition: 2013, **Reprint: 2025**

ISBN 978-81-8448-752-7

Printed in India

Dedicated to

My Teachers

which includes

My Students

There are three elements necessary to correct reasoning: first, the correctness of the facts or conclusions I start from, secondly, the completeness as well as the accuracy of the data I start from, thirdly the elimination of other possible or impossible conclusions from the same facts.

—Sri Aurobindo

One knows well only what one has understood.

—The Mother
(of Sri Aurobindo Ashram)

Preface to the Second Edition

An author greets the request from his publisher for a second edition with mixed feelings. While he is happy that the book is doing well, he knows too well that preparing the new edition is not even half as interesting as writing the first edition. But life is meant to be useful rather than interesting! Leaving the question of the purpose of life for the moment for the reader to dwell upon at leisure, I have used the opportunity provided by the new edition to rewrite Chapter 1, to add some new information relevant to the book, and to expand the 'question and answer' section at the end of each chapter to provoke thinking as well as to facilitate revision.

The first edition proclaimed itself a textbook for nursing students, but the aspects of physiology relevant to different biomedical courses differ little from one another. Further, the book meets the examination requirements of not only nursing students, but also medical, dental and paramedical students. The broad scope of the book is reflected in the revised subtitle. Those having the time and inclination to read more are advised to get hold of my other book *Understanding Medical Physiology*, which is not only more detailed, but also has more of thought-provoking and amusing digressions.

It is hoped that the second edition, even more than the first one, will be useful to the students in not only learning physiology but also in developing a life-long love for the subject. Suggestions for further improvement of the next edition will be gratefully received: they may preferably be e-mailed to me at *rambij@gmail.com*.

RL Bijlani

Preface to the First Edition

Only he who has observed the internal mechanism of the human body, and is well read in the works bearing on this subject, is qualified to practice the art of healing.

SUSRUTA

A new textbook of physiology especially addressed to nursing students needs no apology. There are very few such books available, and hardly any of them is by an Indian author. The situation does not, however, reflect the lack of need for such a book. Not only do the nursing students need to learn physiology to pass their examinations, knowing physiology makes the practice of nursing both better and more enjoyable. It makes the practice better by making the nurse aware of the rationale behind many of the measures she adopts while taking care of her patients. For example, physiology tells her why an anemic child is being given iron, why a patient having edema may be put on salt-free diet, and why an Rh negative girl is not given Rh positive blood transfusion. Knowing the logic behind a practice improves the confidence and efficiency with which it is implemented. Physiology makes the work of a nurse also more enjoyable because doing something with knowledge of its rationale and significance is far more pleasant than doing it mechanically. It makes the nurse realize her true position as a participant in patient care rather than behave as a passive instrument for carrying out the doctor's orders. However, all these facts still do not explain why a book especially addressed to nursing students is necessary? In other words, why are books on medical physiology unsuitable for the nursing students? One is tempted to say that nursing students need to know a different set of facts as compared to medical students. But that is not true. Having taught nursing students for more than twenty years, and having participated in a workshop in which some leading teachers from nursing colleges in India and Nepal prepared a new curriculum for the BSc course in nursing, I know that the physiology course for nursing students is essentially a shorter version of the course for medical students. The reason for making it shorter is that nursing students have much less time available for studying physiology. With this background, preparing a textbook for nursing students may look like a simple task of preparing an abridged version of a textbook for medical students. That was precisely what I thought when I started working on the present book soon after the publication of my textbook for medical students in 1995. But the work expanded to fill time that was not available, and took all of five years. The reason is that the material had to be condensed with discretion. Some portions had to be simplified, or shortened, or omitted altogether, while others had to be retained as such or even expanded because they were especially relevant to the needs of nursing students. However, one thing which has not been done at all is to compress the contents at the expense of clarity. Cryptic language, even when precise, makes learning difficult and tiresome. Therefore, no undue effort has been made to economize on words. Further, some verbosity has been indulged in deliberately to encourage the student's spirit of enquiry, sense of wonder and use of logic. I consider these words well spent because healthy curiosity and a sharp intellect have much greater and more lasting value than a collection of facts.

The book is not examination-oriented, but if read diligently, will be quite adequate for passing examinations comfortably. Some topics, such as nutrition, which are especially relevant to nursing courses, have been covered in considerable detail. Topics such as environmental physiology and yoga, which are especially relevant to India, have also been included. Although the book has been written primarily with the students of nursing in mind, students of paramedical courses will also find it valuable. Medical students and dental students may also like to use the book for a quick revision near the examinations.

I would be looking for suggestions to make the book more useful, especially for nursing students. Criticism may also be sent on the *Reader Evaluation Form* appended at the end of the book. The reader providing the most valuable comments will receive a complimentary copy of the next edition of the book.

I am grateful to all those who have contributed to the book in some way. Most of the manuscript has been prepared by Mr Satish Sachdeva with his characteristic attention to detail; the first few chapters were typed by Ms Babita Shrestha meticulously and cheerfully.

Ms Promila Kapoor, Dr Nalin Mehta, Dr Ashok Jaryal, Dr Manjunatha and Dr Abhay Shelke were a great help in proofreading. The proposal was initially mooted by M/s Jaypee Brothers Medical Publishers (P) Ltd, New Delhi, India, and promptly okayed and encouraged by Shri Jitendar P Vij (Chairman and Managing Director). To all of them, and other members of the Jaypee family, who have done their bit for the book, my sincere thanks. I am particularly grateful to Shri Jitendar P Vij (Chairman and Managing Director) for tolerating the delay in submission of the manuscript with infinite patience and understanding. Although one tends to take family and friends for granted, their sweetness, sympathies and sacrifices are indispensable for seeing any long-term project through. Finally, my profound gratitude to God; only the readers can judge how far I have been worthy of His love and grace.

RL Bijlani

Contents

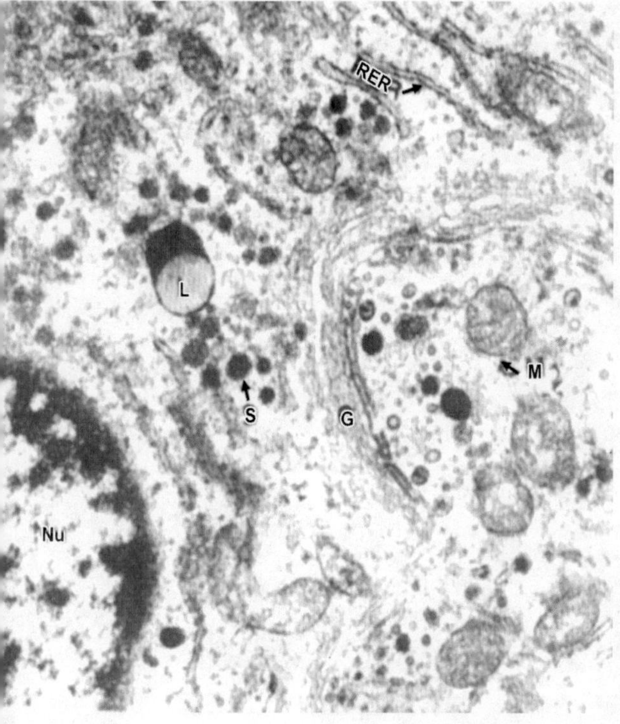

A. Electron micrograph showing part of a cell. Nu, nucleus; L, lysosome; S, secretory vesicle; RER, rough endosplasmic reticulum; M, mitochondria; G, Golgi apparatus. (Courtesy: Prof. Shashi Wadhwa, In-Charge, Electron Microscopy Facility, All India Institute of Medical Sciences (AIIMS), New Delhi).

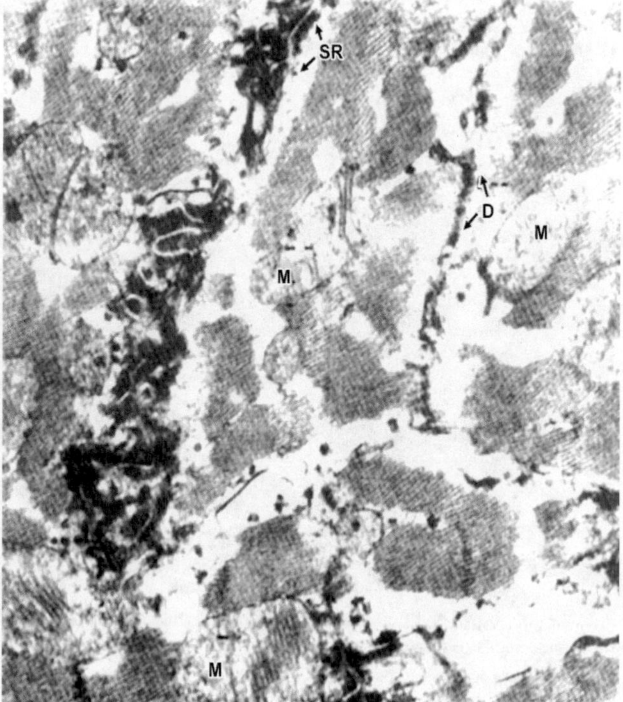

3. Electron micrograph of cardiac nuscle. Note the closely packed parallel ontractile filaments, and high density of nitochondria. SR, sarcoplasmic reticulum, vhich carries the electrical impulse to ne interior of the cardiac muscle; D, ntercalated disc, a low resistance structure vhich carries the electrical impulse rom one muscle fibre to the next; M, nitochondria, which generate the energy equired for contraction. (Courtesy: Prof. hashi Wadhwa, In-Charge, Electron Aicroscopy Facility, All India Institute of Aedical Sciences (AIIMS), New Delhi).

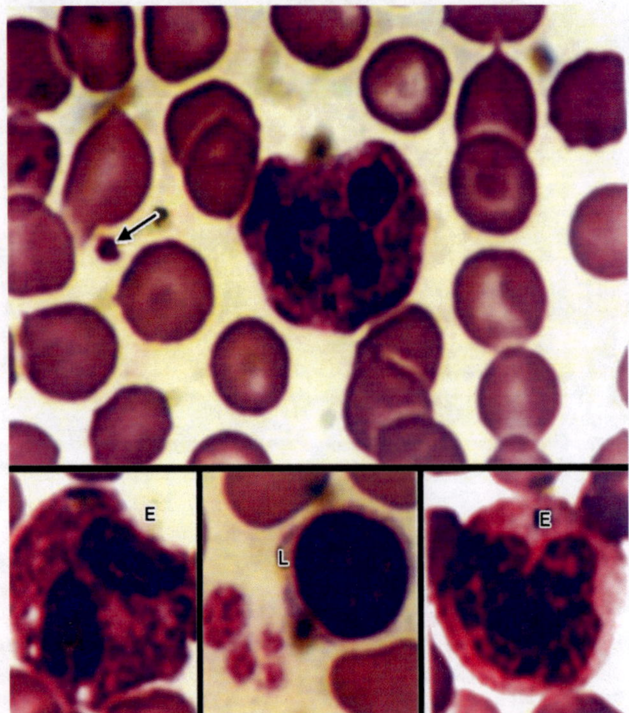

A. Cells seen in a normal peripheral blood smear. N, neutrophil, surrounded by a large number of erythrocytes. The arrov (P) is pointing towards a platelet. E, eosinophil; L, lymphocyte; M, monocyte. Jenner-Giemsa stain. (Courtesy: Prof. Ren Saxena, Department of Haematology, AIIMS).

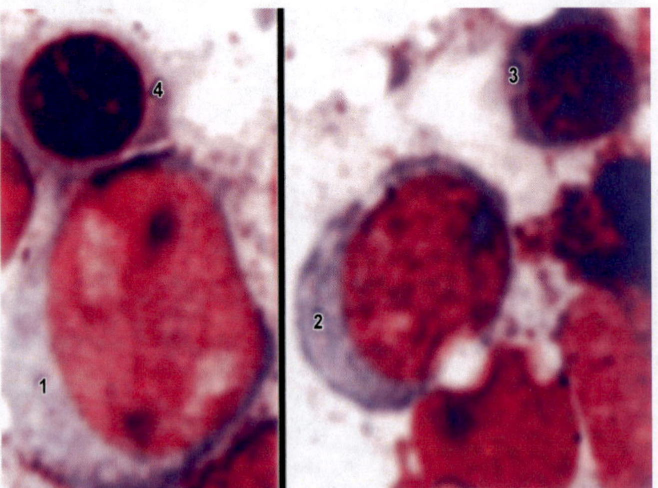

B. Stages of normal erythropoiesis. 1. Proerythroblast: deep blue agranular cytoplasm and large nucleus. 2 and 3. Tw successive stages of intermediate normoblast. 4. Late normoblast: pinkish blue cytoplasm and pyknotic nucleus. Bor marrow smears, Jenner-Giemsa stain. (Courtesy: Prof. Renu Saxena, Department of Haematology, AIIMS).

Plate 3

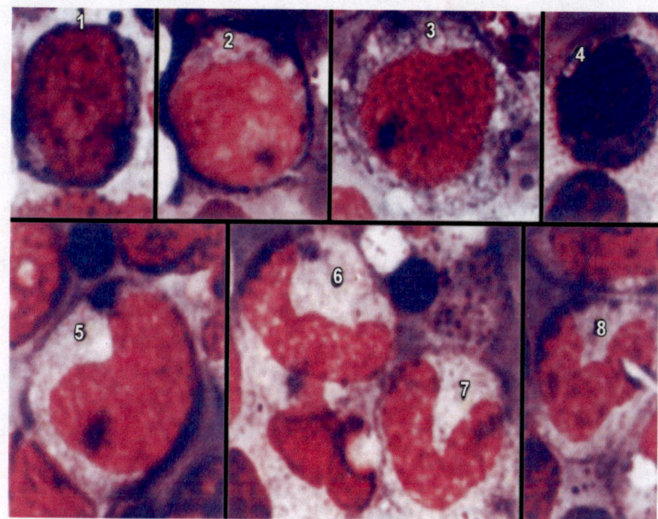

A. Stages in the development of neutrophils. 1. Myeloblast: large cell with deep blue cytoplasm and large nucleus with prominent nuclei. 2. Promyelocyte: larger than myeloblast, with prominent granules in the cytoplasm and nucleoli in the nucleus. 3. Myelocyte: smaller than promyelocyte. Nucleus occupies almost half of the cell cytoplasm and has no nucleolus. Cytoplasm shows fine granules. 4. Basophilic myelocyte. 5. Metamyelocyte: smaller than myelocyte. Cytoplasm shows fine granules. Nucleus is indented in the middle. 6. Stab cell 7. Neutrophil with bilobed nucleus 8. Mature neutrophil with multilobed nucleus. Bone marrow smears, Jenner-Giemsa stain. (Courtesy: Prof. Renu Saxena, Department of Haematology, AIIMS).

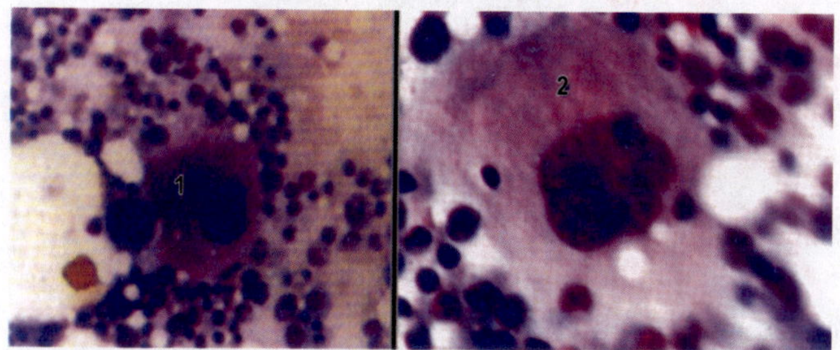

B. Megakaryocytes. 1, lower magnification 2, higher magnification. Note the multilobed nucleus. Jenner-Giemsa stain. (Courtesy: Pof. Renu Saxena, Department of Haematology, AIIMS).

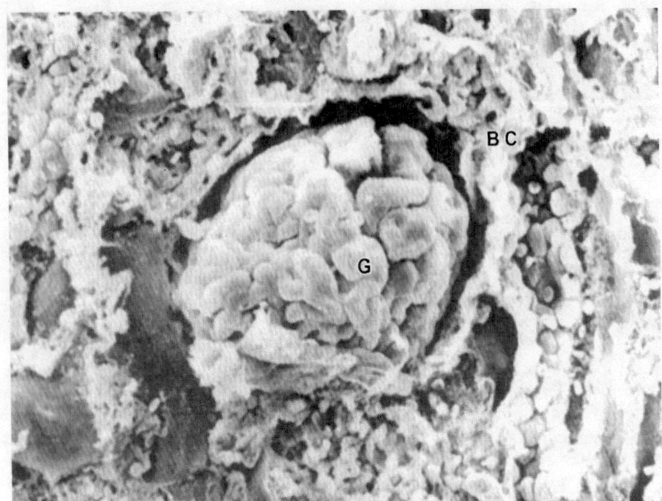

A. A scanning electron micrograph of a bunch of capillaries forming a glomerulus (G) in the kidney. The glomerula capillaries are covered by podocytes. The glomerulus rests in the cup-shaped Bowman's capsule (BC). (Magnification: 432 x (Courtesy: Prof. Shashi Wadhwa, In-Charge, Electron Microscopy Facility, All India Institute of Medical Sciences, New Delhi).

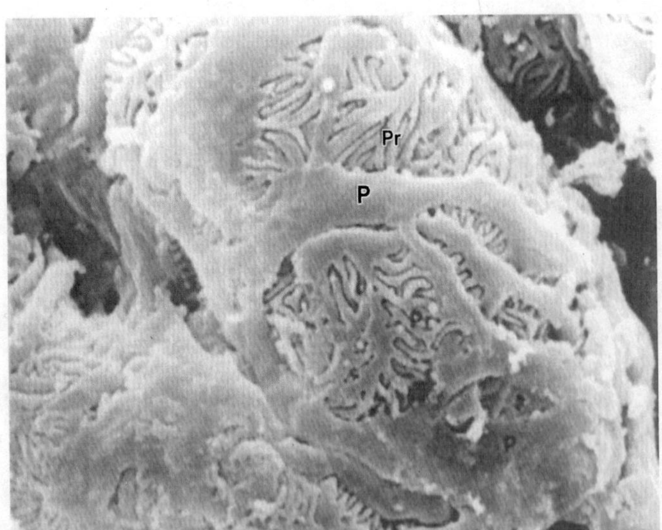

B. A scanning electron micrograph showing glomerular capillaries covered by podocytes (P), the cells whose processes (P interdigitate like a jigsaw puzzle. The result is a sieve through which filtration takes place. (Magnification: 5610 x) (Courtes Prof. Shashi Wadhwa, In-Charge, Electron Microscopy Facility, All India Institute of Medical Sciences, New Delhi).

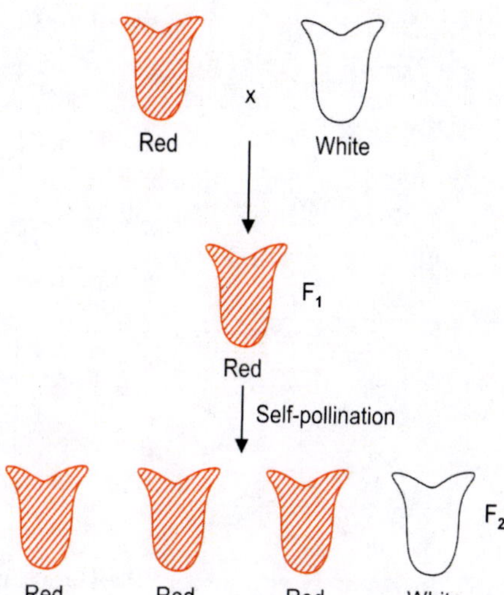

Fig. 2.9 Mendel's simplest experiments with the pea plant. Crossing a pure breeding red flowering plant with a pure breeding white flowering plant gave progeny (first filial generation F_1) bearing red flowers only. Self-pollination of these plants gave progeny (second filial generation F_2) bearing red and white flowers in the ratio 3:1

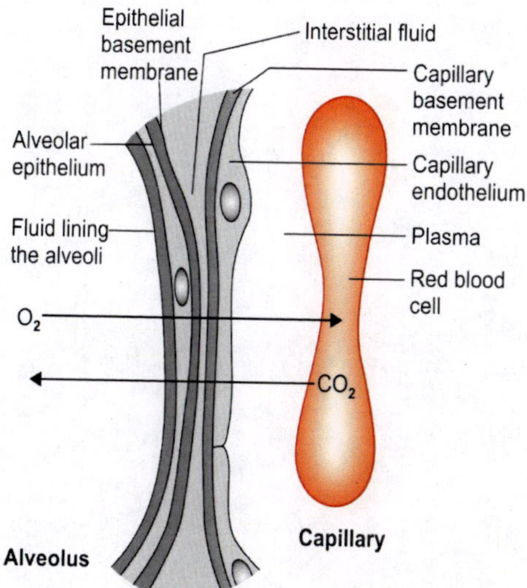

Fig. 6.16B An enlarged version of a small part of the surface where alveolar and capillary membrane are in close contact. The arrows indicate the diffusion of oxygen and carbon dioxide

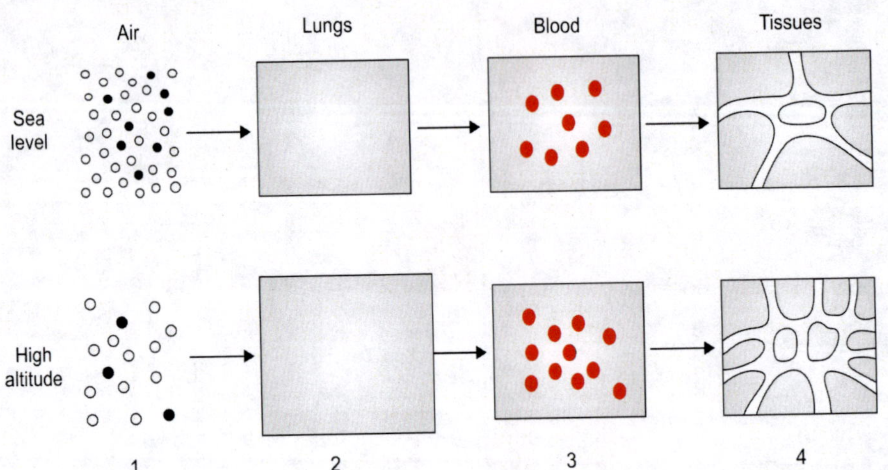

Fig. 7.3 Acclimatization to high altitude. Delivery of oxygen to tissues involves breathing, diffusion of oxygen to the blood across the alveoli, and tissue perfusion with blood. At high altitude, the air has the same proportion of oxygen (indicated by filled circles) to nitrogen (indicated by empty circles) but is less dense. An acclimatized individual compensates for this difference by hyperventilation (1), a larger chest size (2), an increase in RBC count and hence hemoglobin concentration in blood (3), and increased vascularity and improved oxygen utilization in tissues (4)

CHAPTER

1 Getting Introduced to Physiology

"Not in the world of light alone, Where God has built his blazing throne, Nor yet alone in earth below, With belted seas that come and go, And endless isles of sunlit green, Is all thy Maker's glory seen, Look in upon thy wondrous frame, Eternal wisdom still the same."

—OLIVER WENDELL HOLMES

Chapter Outline

- The Unicellular Organism
- Multicellular Organisms
- Principles of Regulation: Control Systems
- Physiology as the Basis of Medicine

Physiology (*physis*, nature; *logos*, discourse) literally means knowledge of nature. The term belongs to an era when physiology and philosophy were not very different from each other. But now physiology means the study of the function of living organisms. This book will concentrate on human physiology, especially from the point of view of health and disease. However, man is unmistakably similar to animals,[1] and a lot of human physiology has been learnt from animals.

The human body is made up of trillions of cells. In other words, human beings are multicellular organisms. They are very complex as compared to unicellular organisms, whose body has just one cell. But human cells have a lot of similarity with unicellular organisms. Therefore we can understand human physiology much better if we understand how a unicellular organism functions.

THE UNICELLULAR ORGANISM

An organism which consists of just one cell, such as an ameba, is a wonderful machine. It burns fuel to get energy for its various functions. When we burn fuel, e.g. wood, we use oxygen from the air. Oxygen oxidizes carbon-containing compounds (organic compounds) in the wood to produce carbon dioxide and water. Combustion produces energy because the organic compounds burnt in the process are high-energy compounds, whereas carbon dioxide and water are low-energy compounds.

$$\text{High–energy organic compounds} + \text{Oxygen} \rightarrow \text{Carbon dioxide} + \text{Water} + \text{Energy}$$

A living cell also burns fuel (we call it food) with the help of oxygen to get energy, and in the process produces carbon dioxide and water. Food also has nitrogenous organic compounds (proteins), the burning of which may produce ammonia in addition to carbon dioxide and water. Carbon dioxide,

[1]This statement is calculated to respect the pride of our species. In fact man is also an animal, although a highly evolved one. Further, he is not the final product of evolution. There is every reason to believe that still more highly evolved creatures will appear on earth in future.

water and ammonia are thrown out of the cell. One wonderful thing about the process of combustion in a cell is that it is carried out with the help of enzymes, which carry out the process in a step-wise fashion, so that the energy obtained from the fuel is not released all at once. That is why the energy can be used for life-processes, and does not burn the cell—it just makes the cell a little warm.

A unicellular organism is totally self-reliant. It lives in sea water. When it finds in the sea a particle which may be used as food, it throws pseudopodia around it, engulfs it into a vacuole, digests it, and burns it to get energy. The oxygen required for the process is obtained from the air dissolved in the sea water. It moves into the cell by diffusion. Waste products such as carbon dioxide and ammonia formed in the cell also move out of the cell by diffusion. Hence the waste products do not accumulate in the cell. The unicellular organism uses the food not only for producing energy but also for growth and repair. In addition, it also reproduces by dividing into two identical cells. Thus the single cell of a unicellular organism is fully equipped to carry out all the functions of life (Fig. 1.1).

A living cell is a wonderful machine. It uses such simple substances from the environment to do so much. It continues to function on its own for so long, it repairs its defects, and it survives through its progeny. A comparable machine is yet to be made by man. But this wonderful machine works only under certain conditions. A few of these conditions are as follows. There should be a regular supply of food and oxygen available. The waste products such as carbon dioxide and ammonia should not accumulate in the cell. The temperature within and around the cell should be neither too cold nor too hot. If it is too cold, enzymatic activity becomes too slow to support life. If it is too hot, proteins, including enzymes, are denatured. The pH within and around the cell should be within narrow limits. The osmolarity of the fluid surrounding the cell should be the same as that within the cell. If the surrounding fluid is hypo-osmolar, water enters the cell, and the cell bursts and obviously dies. If the surrounding fluid is hyperosmolar, water leaves the cell, and the cell shrinks and eventually dies.[2]

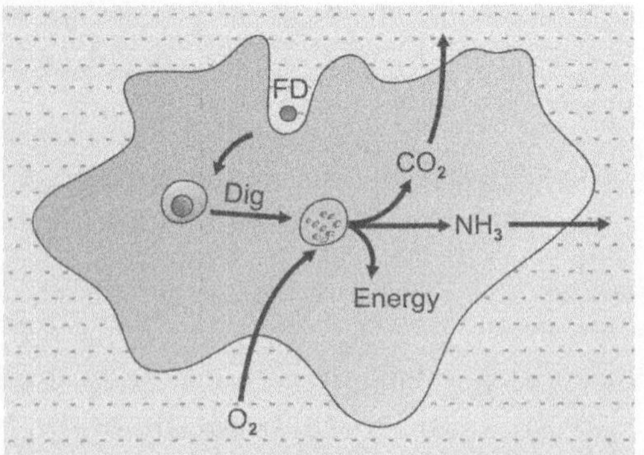

Fig. 1.1 A unicellular organism is self-reliant, and has the luxury of an extensive environment with which it can exchange nutrients and waste products. The nucleus has been omitted for convenience. FD, food; Dig, digestion

For a unicellular organism, these conditions are easy to meet. Food and oxygen are available in the surrounding sea water. A little cell cannot consume much food and oxygen. Therefore the removal of some food and water by these tiny organisms cannot finish the food and oxygen in the sea. Similarly, dumping a little carbon dioxide or ammonia by these tiny organisms in the sea cannot pollute the sea enough to make it too poisonous for the organisms to live in it.[3] The sea water is rather constant in its warmth.[4] The sea water surrounding the unicellular organisms is so huge in quantity that its pH and osmolarity are not materially affected by the life processes of the tiny organisms. You might have observed that the key to the survival of the unicellular organism resides in the sea water, which forms its immediate environment. The environment provides the optimum conditions for its survival.

[2]If you do not understand the consequences of the cell being surrounded by a hypo- or hyperosmolar fluid, revise your knowledge of osmosis (Chapter 3).

[3]These statements are about the short-term situation only. In the long-term, nutrients may be depleted, and waste might accumulate. But that does not happen because of the ecological balance achieved by a variety of organisms, including phytoplankton.

[4]High specific heat minimizes fluctuations in the temperature of a large body of water.

MULTICELLULAR ORGANISMS

Multicellular organisms like man are very complex as compared to unicellular organisms. But they have one fundamental similarity with each other. Each cell of a multicellular organism needs exactly the same conditions for survival as a unicellular organism. Let us see how these conditions are achieved in a complex creature like man who lives not in the sea but on land.

Our cells are not surrounded by sea water, but they do have a thin layer of fluid around them (Fig. 1.2). Thus our cells may not have the luxury of the sea, but each cell at least has a private pond of its own. The fluid surrounding the cells is called the interstitial fluid. The interstitial fluid forms the immediate environment of our cells, just as the sea forms the immediate environment of organisms like the ameba. It is interesting that the composition of the interstitial fluid is very similar to that of sea water. But here we have a problem. The quantity of interstitial fluid is so small that the cell would use up all the nutrients and oxygen in it in a very short time. The waste products would also quickly build up to toxic levels. Therefore it is essential that nutrients in the interstitial fluid be replenished, and waste products removed, continually and promptly. This has been made possible by having a set of tubes, which we call capillaries (Fig. 1.3). The fluid in the capillaries exchanges these substances with the interstitial fluid, and the interstitial fluid exchanges them with the cells. Thus the fluid in the capillaries (blood) acts as an extension of the immediate environment of the cells. But the problem is still not over—now the nutrients can get depleted from the blood, and waste products can accumulate there. This does not happen because blood in the capillaries is in motion. Thus blood can bring a continuous supply of fresh nutrients to the cell, and take waste products away before they accumulate. The motive force behind the movement of blood is the heart (Fig. 1.4). However, you would realize that this 'solution' also merely postpones the problem—it does not actually solve it, because soon a time will come when all the nutrients in the blood have been used up, and waste products have accumulated to toxic levels throughout the blood. The final solution has been found in having a few points in the circulatory system where the capillaries should come in close contact with the external environment. The structure where this happens should be

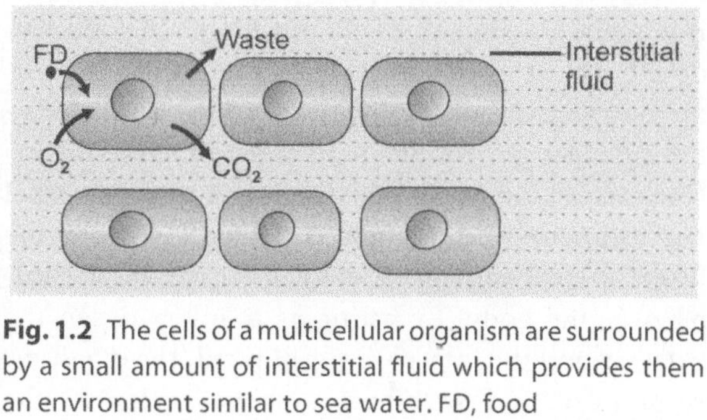

Fig. 1.2 The cells of a multicellular organism are surrounded by a small amount of interstitial fluid which provides them an environment similar to sea water. FD, food

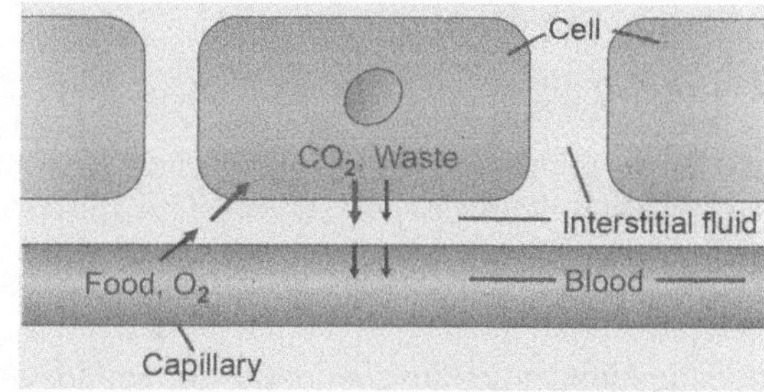

Fig. 1.3 The cells of a multicellular organism exchange nutrients and waste products with the interstitial fluid, and the interstitial fluid exchanges these with blood in the capillaries

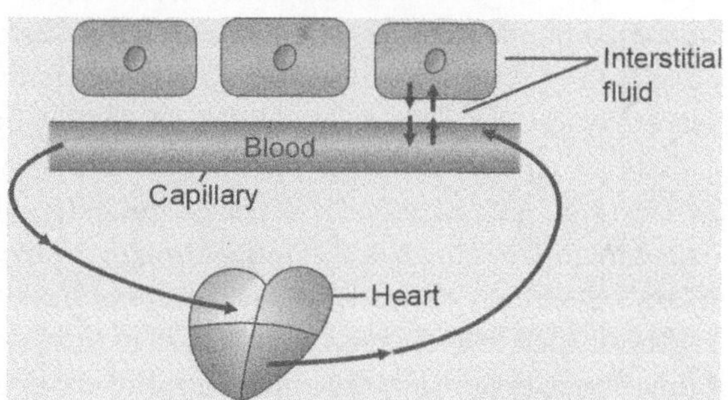

Fig. 1.4 Blood in the capillaries is in motion. As a result, fresh blood is brought in continuously, and 'used' blood taken away. The push for the motion of blood is provided by the heart

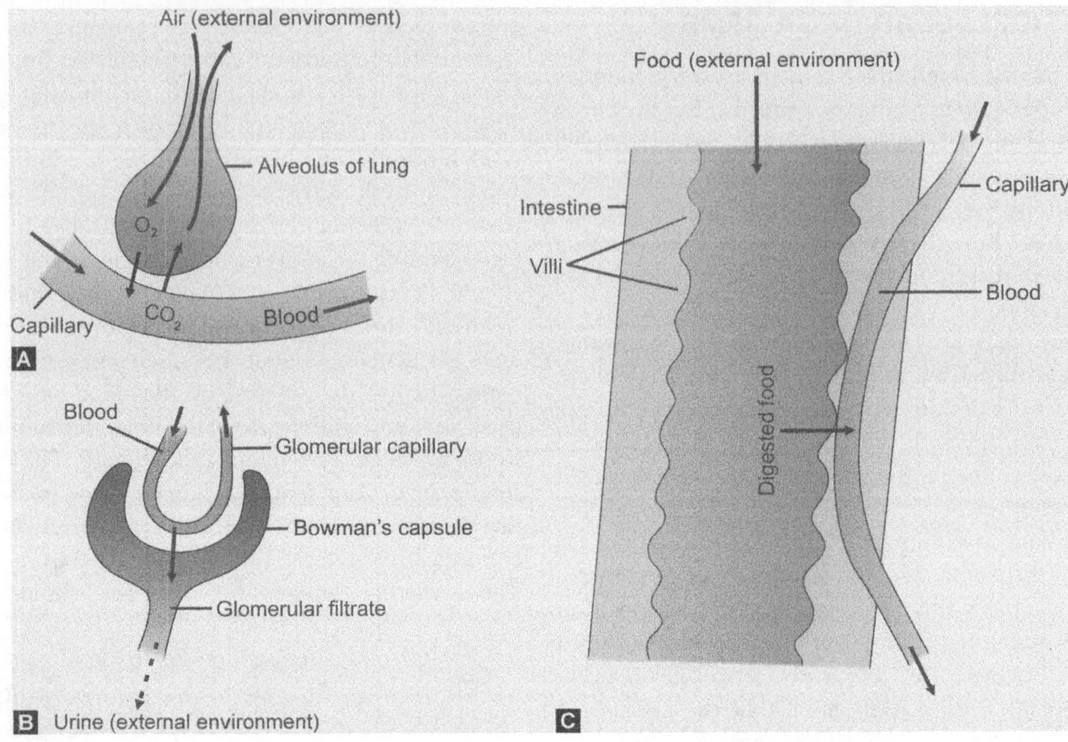

Figs 1.5A to C The ultimate replenishment of nutrients and removal of waste products takes place as the result of an exchange with the external environment. This exchange takes place in specialized organs such as the lungs (A); the kidneys (B); the gastrointestinal tract (C); In these structures the external environment comes in intimate contact with the blood

especially built for picking up some nutrients from the external environment and passing it on to the capillaries, or for picking up some waste product from the capillaries and passing it on to the external environment. Such structures are, principally, the lungs, where oxygen is picked up and carbon dioxide is disposed of, the kidneys, where nitrogenous waste is disposed of, and the gut, where all the nutrients except oxygen are picked up (Figs 1.5A to C). In all these structures, very thin membranes and very few layers of specialized cells separate the external environment from the blood. Thus, although we live on land, eventually the external environment has to bear the burden of keeping us alive, just as in the case of unicellular organisms. Our nutrients and oxygen also come from the external environment, enter the blood, and from the blood enter the 'private pond' of every cell, making the cell 'feel like an ameba in the sea'. The waste products that our cells make also travel from the cell to the 'private pond', and from there to the blood, and are finally discharged into the external environment.

It may be noted that the heart sends blood to all parts of the body. Two important functions that the blood performs everywhere it goes are to supply nutrients and pick up waste products. But while passing through the lungs, the kidneys or the gut, it does something in addition: it picks up nutrients from, or gives up waste products to the external environment. In some of these organs (lungs and kidneys), blood discharges to the external environment waste products picked up from the internal environment of the cells (interstitial fluid) all over the body. By acting as a link between the external and the internal environment, the digestive, respiratory and excretory systems replenish the nutrients used up by the body, and dispose of the waste products formed. The ultimate aim of these systems is to help achieve constancy in the characteristics of the thin layer of fluid surrounding every cell of the body. This fluid, the interstitial fluid, constitutes the immediate environment of the cells, or the internal environment of the body. The importance of the constancy of the internal environment (in French, *milieu interieur*) was first stressed by Claude Bernard in 1857. Claude Bernard was not just an eminent physiologist, but is also considered the father of experimental medicine. The concepts propounded by him were further supported by the extensive experimental work of Walter Cannon in the early twentieth century. Cannon coined the term *homeostasis* to describe the constancy of the internal environment (*homoios*, similar; *stasis*, position).

You might have observed that each system of the body makes a contribution to homeostasis. In turn, it benefits from the contributions which other systems make. For example, the gut replenishes nutrients in the interstitial fluid. In turn, it benefits from the oxygen that has been added to the interstitial fluid by the lungs and also from the removal of waste products by the kidneys. Thus the body is like a society in which there is specialization and division of labor. A health professional specializes in giving health care, and in turn depends for food on the farmer, for clothes on the tailor, and for shelter on the mason. Similarly, in the body each system has specialized in doing one thing for all cells of the body. In turn, cells belonging to other systems of the body fulfill all the remaining needs of this system. Our own body is an excellent example of cooperation and interdependence.

What About the Other Systems?

We have so far seen the contribution of blood, cardiovascular system, respiratory system, gastrointestinal system and kidneys to homeostasis. But there are a few other systems also in the body. Do they also contribute to homeostasis?[5]

[5]You may try answering this question on your own before reading further.

We have seen that the human body is essentially a society of cells. In a society, we also need an organizer or coordinator to see that different members of the society work in such a way that the interests of the society as a whole are well looked after. In the body, the function of co-ordination is performed by the nervous and endocrine systems. To give an example, when we take exercise, our requirement of oxygen goes up. To meet this additional demand, the heart beats faster, and the lungs work harder. How do the lungs know when to step up their activity? This is the job of the coordinating systems. These systems detect the changes resulting from exercise. These changes are contraction of muscles, movement of joints, slight fall in oxygen tension, slight increase in carbon dioxide tension, slight increase in temperature, etc. The coordinating systems process all this information, and then come up with a response. The response is to send messages to the heart and lungs to step-up their activity so that homeostasis is maintained in spite of additional oxygen requirement. Thus coordination has two basic components: communication and information processing (Fig. 1.6). First, there has to be a channel of communication with areas where changes are taking place. In the above example of exercise, the information from muscles, joints, etc. has to reach the coordinator through such a channel of communication. This information-gathering channel is called the sensory limb of the coordinator. Since information is coming from multiple sources, the coordinator has to process this information. Processing means putting together all this information, or synthesizing it, so as to understand what it means in terms of the

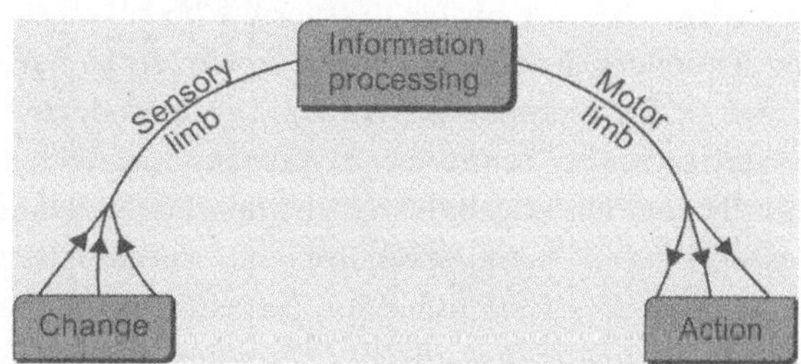

Fig. 1.6 The basic components of coordination

disturbance in homoestasis which it can produce. Further, processing also means deciding what needs to be done. This processing is done in the brain. The result of the information processing is the decision about what needs to be done. This decision is conveyed by the brain to the heart and respiratory muscles. Conveying the decision also needs a channel of communication. This instructional channel is called the motor limb of the coordinator. Thus the coordinator consists of the sensory limb, a processing unit, and a motor limb.

We have seen above that although the coordinating systems, i.e. the nervous and endocrine systems do not contribute directly to homeostasis, they make an indirect contribution to it. Their contribution is to make several other systems work towards homeostasis at the right time at the required level so that homeostasis is maintained in spite of changing circumstances. But there are still a few other systems to be considered. The musculoskeletal system also makes no direct contribution to homeostasis. But apart from giving a shape to the body, it enables the animal to move. Animals need to move to find food, to hunt their prey, and to escape from predators. The gut can replenish nutrients only if the animal finds food in the first place. Hence the musculoskeletal system also makes an essential, although indirect, contribution to homeostasis. Human beings may not find their food the way animals do, but move they also must to earn a living. Even highly civilized societies can support only a few paralyzed individuals and that too rather poorly. How about the skin? Apart from playing a major role in regulation of body temperature, skin is the first line of defense against a wide variety of dangerous microorganisms which our environment is full of. These microorganisms are unable to enter the body because the skin offers an effective barrier. Finally, let us have a look at the reproductive system. The reproductive system seems to contribute to homeostasis neither directly nor indirectly. But it has an important function without which homeostasis becomes meaningless. Reproduction is responsible for perpetuation of the species. No matter how effective the homeostasis, it is not perfect, and therefore every organism dies one day. Therefore, a species which cannot reproduce would soon vanish from the surface of the earth.

We have seen that every part of the body makes some contribution to the survival of the whole organism by doing something to maintain the composition, pH and temperature of the internal environment at an optimal level. The optimal level is that at which the enzyme systems function best, nutrients are available in quantity and quality commensurate with the activity of the tissue in question, and waste products remain well below toxic levels. As you go on to a detailed study of individual systems, keep in mind that the central purpose of all systems is to make a contribution to homeostasis. It is easy to get lost in details and forget this fundamental fact. But keeping this basic fact at the back of your mind will make the study of the details much easier, more interesting and more meaningful.

PRINCIPLES OF REGULATION: CONTROL SYSTEMS

Now we shall study the general mechanisms by which the coordinating systems of the body ensure constancy of the internal environment. The mode of regulation of the internal environment bears a remarkable resemblance to the way an automatic electric iron works. The setting 'cotton' or 'wool' corresponds to a temperature which the iron will maintain. When the temperature rises slightly above the set level, the iron is automatically switched off. On the other hand, when the temperature falls slightly below the set level, the iron is automatically switched on, and stays on till the temperature rises slightly above the set level. In this way, the temperature of the iron always stays close to the set level.

A similar strategy is adopted by the body to maintain homeostasis. For example, if a person loses blood by bleeding, the blood pressure falls. When this happens, the heart starts beating faster and more forcefully, and the blood vessels constrict. This raises the blood pressure towards normal. To take another example, if a person has just taken a meal, her blood glucose level starts rising. In response to the rise in blood glucose, the pancreas releases insulin. Insulin lowers the blood glucose level. As the blood glucose level falls slightly below the desirable level, the secretion of insulin is switched off. If the person now does not eat for the next eight hours, not only will insulin secretion remain off, glucagon secretion will be switched on. Glucagon raises blood glucose. Thus blood glucose will be maintained at a reasonable level in spite of fasting or feasting. The mechanisms which prevent the blood glucose level from rising too high or falling too low are called the control system for regulating blood glucose. The control system for a variable maintains the value of the variable within a narrow range.

A control system (Fig. 1.7) is basically designed to maintain a controlled variable close to a set point. The value of the controlled variable is continuously monitored by a sensor. The current value of the controlled variable is conveyed by the sensor to the controller in the form of a feedback signal. The feedback signal and the set point constitute the inputs for the controller. The feedback signal is naturally affected by any disturbance which alters the value of the controlled variable. The controller compares the feedback signal with the set point; the difference between the two is called the error. The output of the controller is conveyed to an effector. As a result, the effector applies a correction which takes the controlled variable towards the set point. A control system such as this one is called a negative feedback system because the effector response is negative to the initiating stimulus (disturbance). Using the terminology of control systems, the regulation of blood pressure and blood glucose have been illustrated in Figures 1.8 to 1.10.

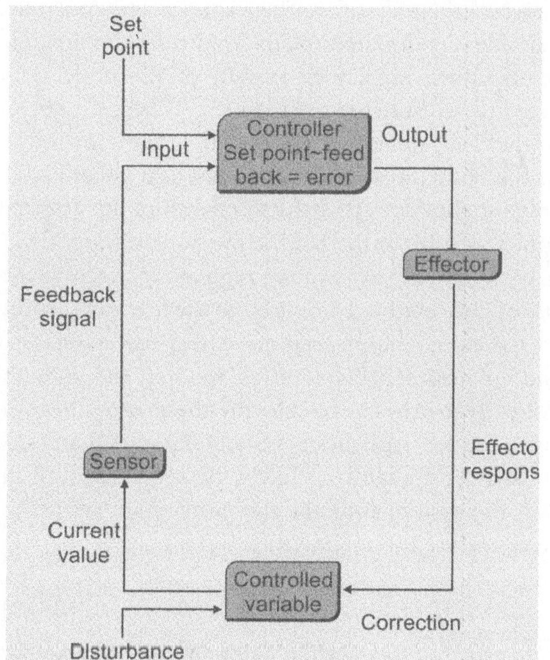

Fig. 1.7 The essential elements of a control system

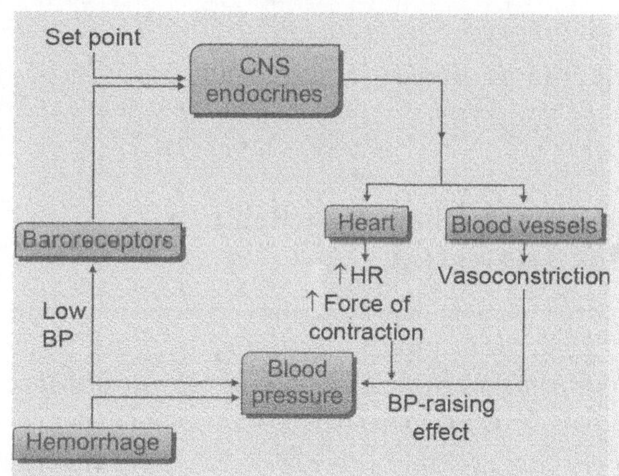

Fig. 1.8 Some basic features of the blood pressure regulatory system. The figure shows how the system responds when the blood pressure falls as a result of blood loss. BP, blood pressure; HR, heart rate; CNS, central nervous system

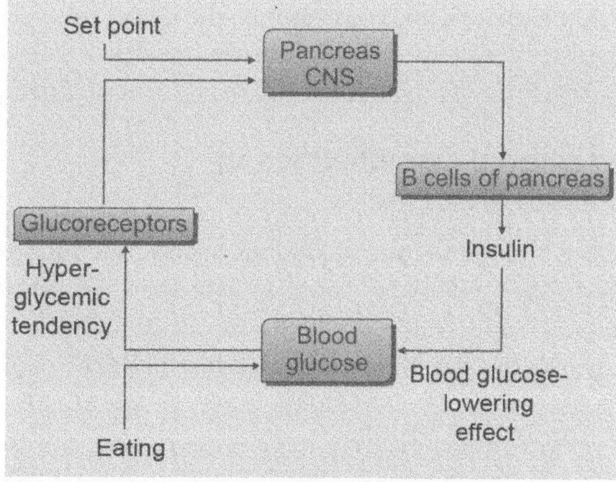

Fig. 1.9 Some basic features of the blood glucose regulatory system. The figure shows how the system responds when the blood glucose rises after a meal

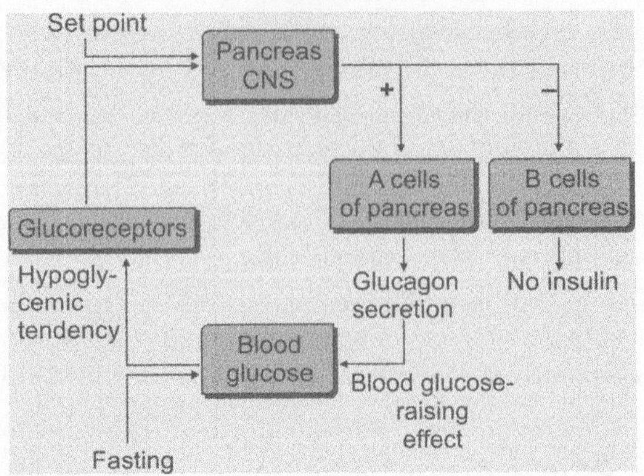

Fig. 1.10 Some basic features of the blood glucose regulatory system. The figure shows how the system responds when the blood glucose falls during fasting

Response Characteristics of a Control System

When we say that a control system maintains a controlled variable constant, we are only approximately right. First, the effect of a disturbance is not corrected immediately; there is a latency, or dead time. Secondly, the effect of a disturbance is not corrected completely; there is a residual change. The response of a control system may be represented graphically. There is a large variety of responses, some of which have been shown in Figures 1.11A and B. The accuracy and promptness of control systems varies a lot. For example, the blood pressure regulatory system is not as accurate as the systems for regulating body temperature or the pH of blood.

Additional Complexities in Control Systems

Many biological control systems are more complex than the relatively simple systems described above. Some features which introduce additional complexities have been discussed briefly below.

Variable Set Point

In some control systems the set point is not fixed. A control system with a variable set point is called a servomechanism. The stretch reflex which regulates muscle length is an example of a servomechanism. The resting muscle length of a skeletal muscle is not fixed–it varies with the posture. Every change of posture needs contraction and relaxation of a few muscles. After the change of posture, the muscle length in the new posture becomes the resting length of the muscles involved. Thus contraction of muscles is required mainly for changing the posture; not much contraction is needed for maintaining the posture. This is helpful. First, it saves the energy required for muscle contraction. Second, it enables us to maintain a posture for a long time without getting tired.

Anticipatory Control

In case of some variables which are regulated very efficiently, the control system starts acting in anticipation of a disturbance. The control system starts working when a disturbance is likely; it does not wait for the disturbance to actually take place. This is possible if the control system also makes use of information about factors which may lead to the disturbance. In this way, the correction can be initiated before the value of the controlled variable has deviated much from the set point. The temperature regulatory system of the body is an example of anticipatory control. When we go out in the cold, shivering begins before the temperature of the body has fallen much. The heat generated by shivering ensures that the temperature does not fall much in spite of the cold. How do you think this is achieved?[6] The temperature regulatory system makes use of information coming from the thermoreceptors in the skin. These receptors detect the coldness of the environment as soon as we step out into the cold. By being in touch with these receptors, the temperature regulatory system 'knows' that a fall in body temperature is likely. In anticipation of the fall, the system initiates shivering. As a result, the temperature is not allowed to fall much.

[6]You may try answering this question on your own before reading further.

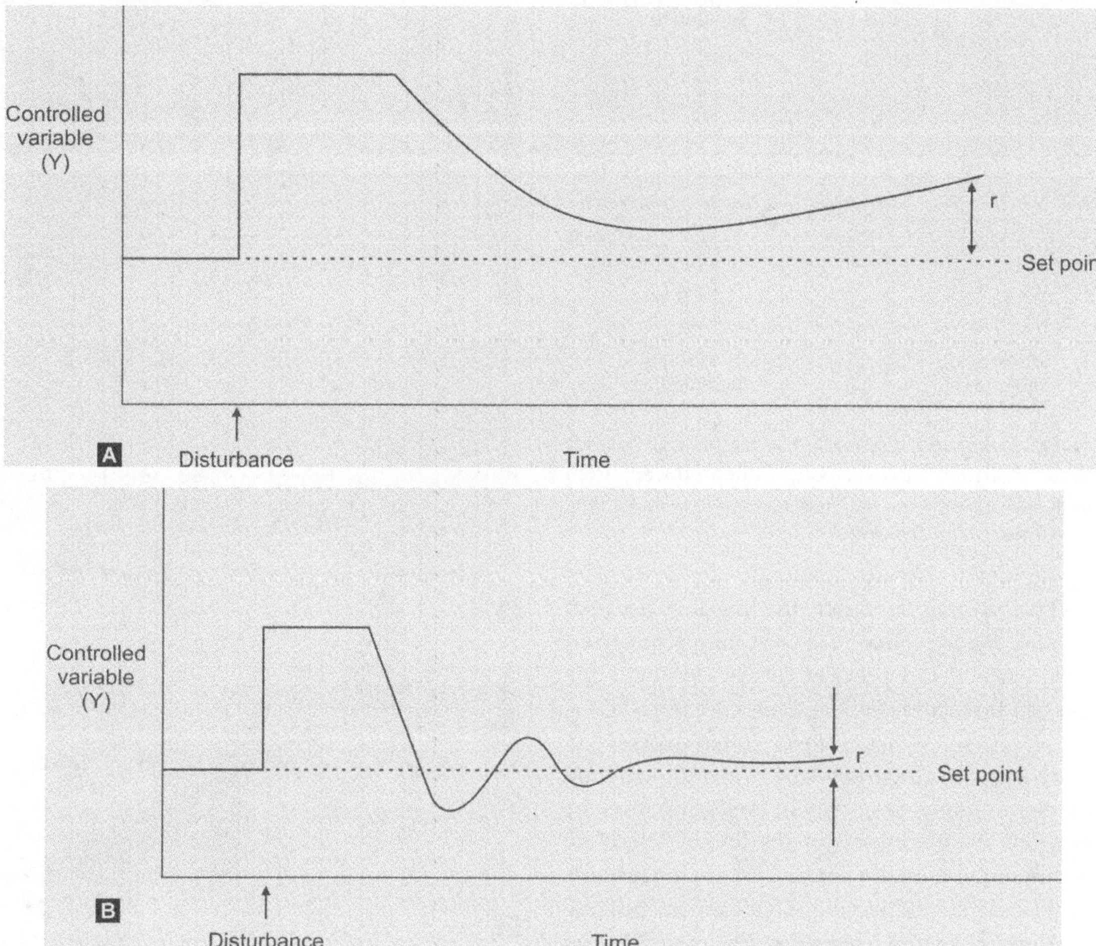

Figs 1.11A and B Response characteristics of a biological control system. The exact characteristics may vary in different systems. Two contrasting patterns of response have been shown in A and B. In B, the response is oscillatory. r, residual change

PHYSIOLOGY AS THE BASIS OF MEDICINE

We have seen above that the aim of all parts of the body is to maintain homeostasis. It may look paradoxical that homeostasis (staying the same) needs so much of continuous activity on the part of so many organ-systems. The paradox results from the fact that life processes (e.g. oxidation of nutrients) are dynamic, and our environment poses physical (e.g. temperature), chemical (e.g. pollutants) and biological (e.g. bacteria and viruses) challenges. 'Staying the same' in spite of dynamic life processes and environmental challenges naturally needs effort. This effort is put in by various systems of the body in the form of responses to challenges arising within the body (e.g. rise in carbon dioxide levels due to oxidation of nutrients), and challenges from outside the body (e.g. hot environment). Health depends on the success of these responses. When the responses are inadequate in relation to the challenge, a person falls ill (Fig. 1.12). If the challenge is overwhelming, even a 'very healthy' person may fall sick. On the other hand, a challenge which can normally be handled quite adequately by most individuals might overwhelm a 'less healthy' person, and make him

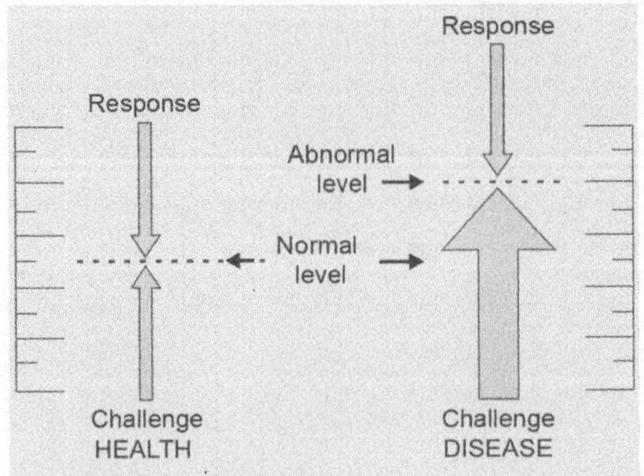

Fig. 1.12 Health and disease are a matter of balance between challenge and response. (Reproduced from Bijlani RL, Manchanda SK. The Human Machine. New Delhi: National Book Trust, 1990, Fig. 1)

sick. Thus, there is no strict dividing line between health and disease. There is a continuous spectrum of health, which can proceed to disease under the impact of a threshold challenge (Figs 1.13A to C).

Once a person is sick, recovery often depends on the same type of responses which operate in good health. For example, fever may be looked upon as the resetting of the thermostat of the body.[7] Therefore when the temperature of a person starts rising towards fever, she may have shivering. This happens because the thermostat is set to a higher level (say, 40°C), and the body temperature is 37°C. Therefore the control system behaves as if the body is cold. It initiates responses which will take the body temperature towards the set point, which is now 40°C. This can be done by shivering, and therefore the person shivers. In the same way, when the person is recovering from fever, she may have sweating. Since the person has recovered, the hypothalamic thermostat is once again set at the normal level of 37°C. But the body temperature is still 40°C. The mismatch between the set point and the body temperature initiates responses for heat loss, such as sweating. As a result of sweating,

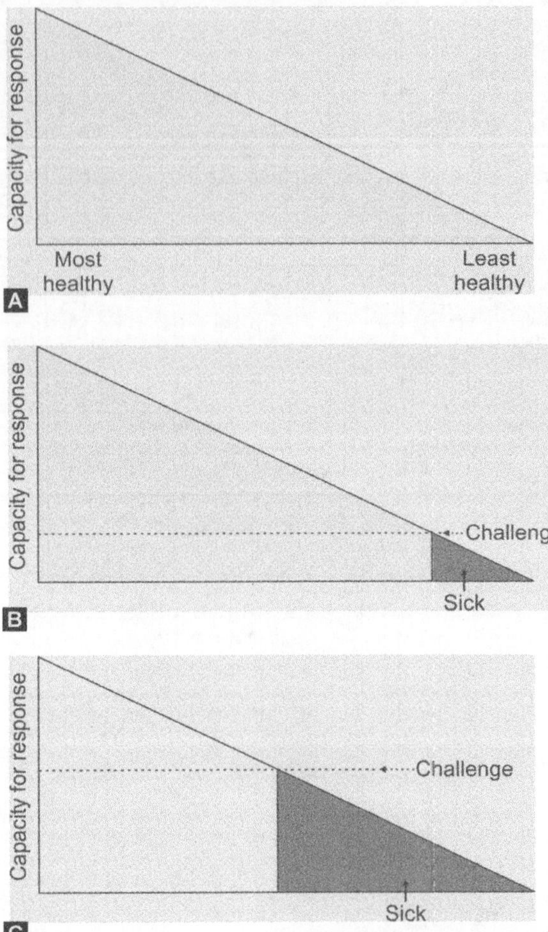

Figs 1.13A to C There is no strict dividing line between health and disease (A); There is a continuous spectrum of health, which can proceed to disease under the impact of a strong enough challenge. How many persons fall sick in the face of a challenge depends on the strength of the challenge. The position of an individual within this spectrum depends on his capacity to mount a response to various challenges. The number of persons falling sick under the impact of a challenge have been shown by the stippled area (B and C). (Adapted from Bijlani RL, Manchanda SK. The Human Machine. New Delhi: National Book Trust, 1990, Fig. 2)

the temperature is brought down to 37°C, and then sweating stops. In short, there is a lot in common between homeostatic mechanisms which operate in health, and the mechanisms which lead to recovery from disease. A variety of self-healing mechanisms

[7]The seat of the thermostat of the body is a tiny part of the brain called the hypothalamus.

are built into the body, and these are adequate for getting well again in most situations. This fact had been recognized by Hippocrates as long ago as 400 BC when he stated that the body possesses the means for its recovery from illness.

In light of the above discussion, we can keep ourselves healthy by adopting a two-pronged strategy. First, we should improve the capacity of our body to meet challenges. Secondly, we should try to minimize the extent to which the body is challenged. Both these measures are not mutually exclusive. However, of the two, the first is more important and practical. Adequate and appropriate nutrition, regular physical exercise, and mental peace are the three most important ingredients of the lifestyle that improves the fighting capacity of the body. Ancient disciplines, such as yoga, promote a healthy lifestyle. The second part of the strategy for staying healthy is to avoid needless challenges to the body. This may be done by avoiding inhalation and ingestion of germs, harmful chemicals and pollutants. Further, one should avoid overuse, misuse or abuse of any part of the body. For example, we should not overuse our back by trying to lift a 100 kg weight, misuse our eyes by spending long hours at the computer, or abuse our lungs by smoking.

Doing all this can keep us fairly healthy but is no guarantee against illness. In case of illness, a doctor or nurse usually takes one of the following four measures. First, she reassures the patient that soon everything will be fine. The reassurance is not hollow: it is based on her knowledge of homeostatic mechanisms. Secondly, she tells the patient not to be impatient. This is because she knows that homeostatic mechanisms take time. Thirdly, she suggests some measures which assist the body in its struggle against the disease. For example, she may suggest hot fomentation of an inflamed area so that the accelerated blood flow through the area may increase further and drain away undesirable substances. Or, she may prescribe antibiotics which may kill some disease-causing germs in addition to those killed by the defence mechanisms of the body. And finally, it may be discovered that the disease was due to a deficiency. It could be a dietary deficiency, or deficiency of some physiological substance produced by the body. In that case the doctor or nurse tries to supply the deficient substance in an effort to restore physiological function. For example, in iron deficiency, she gives iron; in water and salt deficiency (as in diarrhea), she gives water and salt; and in insulin deficiency (diabetes), she gives insulin. It is worth observing that in each of the four approaches outlined above, the doctor or nurse works with nature, not against it. And, each of the four approaches needs knowledge of physiology. Truly, physiology forms the basis of medicine.

QUESTIONS

1. a. What constitutes the internal environment?
   b. Why is it called so?
   c. Why is its constancy important?
   d. List the variables which should be maintained constant in the internal environment.
2. Why is negative feedback called so?
3. Give an example of negative feedback.
4. Why do people get high blood pressure if there is a control system for regulating blood pressure?
5. What is positive feedback? Does it have a place in physiological systems?

ANSWERS

1. a. The internal environment consists of the fluid which surrounds the cells. This fluid is called the interstitial fluid (since the interstitial fluid engages in a constant exchange with the plasma, the plasma is also often considered to be a part of the internal environment).
   b. It is called environment because it surrounds the cells (environment means the surroundings). The interstitial fluid forms the surroundings of the cells. Therefore, this fluid is the environment of the cells.
   It is called internal because it is inside the body.
   A common error made by the students is to say that it is called internal because it is

inside the cells. This is wrong. The internal environment, or the interstitial fluid, is outside the cells, but inside the body. It is an environment because it is outside the cells; it is internal because it is inside the body.

c. Cells get their nutrition from the fluid which surrounds them. Cells also throw their waste products into the fluid which surrounds them. For the cells to function properly, this fluid (the internal environment) should always be able to provide nourishment, and should not have too much of waste products. Further, the temperature, pH and osmolarity of this fluid should also be constantly at a level which is appropriate for the cell. That is why constancy of the internal environment is important.

d. A partial list is as follows:
   - Temperature
   - pH
   - Osmolarity
   - The concentration of glucose, electrolytes, oxygen and carbon dioxide.

2. The product of a control system is its output. The output is ultimately in the form of a certain value for the controlled variable. The value of the controlled variable itself guides the activity of the control system. Thus the output of the control system goes back (feeds back) to the control system to tell it what to do. This feedback results in the control system working in such a way as to negate, or oppose, the disturbance which takes the controlled variable away from the set point. Since the feedback leads to a response from the control system which is opposite (or negative in direction) to the disturbance, it is called a negative feedback system.

   A common error made by the students is to say that it is called negative feedback because it lowers variables, e.g. if the blood glucose rises, the negative feedback system lowers it. This is a wrong answer because the same system also raises blood glucose when it has fallen. When a disturbance raises blood glucose, the system lowers it. When a disturbance lowers blood glucose, the system raises it. The system in both cases is a negative feedback system. 'Negative' only refers to the fact that the response is opposite in direction to the disturbance. Thus the word negative has been used here in an algebraic sense. Fall is negative to a rise; rise is negative to a fall. The negative feedback system can do both—it can lower a variable if it has gone up, and it can raise a variable if it has gone down.

3. The most common example of negative feedback given by students is that of product inhibition. In a chemical reaction,

   $$A + B \rightarrow C,$$

   As the concentration of C rises, the reaction slows down. This is a correct example. But this is not the only example of negative feedback in the body. Regulation of blood glucose, blood pressure, blood pH or body temperature is also achieved by negative feedback mechanisms.

4. The conventional explanation for this phenomenon is as follows:

   In high blood pressure, there is initially a narrowing of blood vessels by fatty deposits. This reduces the lumen of blood vessels. Reduction in lumen raises the peripheral resistance. Rise in peripheral resistance raises the blood pressure. Since the rise in blood pressure takes place gradually over a period of years, the receptors for sensing blood pressure (baroreceptors) adapt to the change, i.e. the receptors do not respond any more by activating the mechanisms for lowering the blood pressure. This is in keeping with the traditional assumption that baroreceptors are equipped for responding to acute changes in blood pressure, not to chronic changes. Hence, the baroreceptors have been generally considered useful for short-term regulation of blood pressure, not for long-term regulation.

   But recent work indicates that:

   a. Baroreceptors do have a role in long-term regulation of blood pressure, and

b. The sensitivity of baroreceptors is reduced in those having high blood pressure.

   Thus while it is true that there is a narrowing of arteriolar lumen in high blood pressure, and possibly contributes to high blood pressure, there may be another factor also involved. The reduced sensitivity of baroreceptors might itself contribute to the hypertension directly, and also indirectly by not responding adequately to the effect of the rise in peripheral resistance. Some support for this explanation is available from studies showing that yogic postures which restore baroreceptor sensitivity also help in bringing down the blood pressure of hypertensive patients.

5. In a positive feedback system, the response is in the same direction as the disturbance. A little reflection would show that the effects of positive feedback could be disastrous (try to answer why before you read further). For example, if a person is exposed to heat, a small increase in body temperature above the set point would raise the temperature still further in a positive feedback system. Now this bigger rise above the set point would have a still stronger effect of raising the body temperature. The result eventually would be a runaway increase in the body temperature which keeps rising till the person is dead. Thus only negative feedback systems can bring a variable back towards the set point after the variable has deviated from it. That is why most physiological systems are of the negative feedback type.

However, there are a few situations in the body where positive feedback operates, and serves a useful purpose. For example, uterine contractions during labor push the fetus down towards the cervix. The downward movement of the fetus stretches the cervix. Stretching of the cervix stimulates uterine contraction. Uterine contraction pushes the fetus down. The fetus going down stretches the cervix. Stretching of the cervix stimulates uterine contraction, and so on. The sequence continues till the baby has been delivered. Here the downward movement of the fetus is a change from a 'set position' which has been brought about by uterine contraction (the disturbance). A negative feedback system would inhibit further uterine contraction, and would try to restore the fetus to the set position. But instead, here the response of the system is to stimulate contraction of the uterus, which in turn moves the fetus further away from its set position in the uterus. Therefore, this is a positive feedback system. But here it serves a purpose. The purpose of labor is to move the fetus towards the vaginal opening so that it can be delivered.

CHAPTER

2 Fundamentals of Cell Biology

"Environment does play an important part, but the original capital on which a child starts in life is inherited from its ancestors."

—MAHATMA GANDHI

Chapter Outline

- The Cell Membrane
- The Organelles
- Inclusions
- Nucleus
- Communication between Cells
- Cell Division
- Genetics

Imagine a child who has just found a piece of colored glass. He enjoys looking at everything around through the glass because he is fascinated by the new colorful look of familiar objects. Probably in the same way, Robert Hooke was trying to see every object around under the new microscope he had just fabricated in the middle of seventeenth century. One of these objects happened to be a piece of cork. Hooke was fascinated by its architecture consisting of neat little compartments. He likened each of these compartments to a room, and therefore called them cells. It took almost another two centuries before Schleiden, a botanist, and Schwann, a zoologist, generalized that the basic unit of every living organism, plant or animal, is a cell similar to the ones in the cork. The cell theory propounded by Schleiden and Schwann has stood the test of time. Now it is an accepted fact in biology that cell is the structural, functional and developmental unit of life. The structure of a 'typical' cell, with which you are already familiar, is shown in Figure 2.1.

Evolution of cells is closely linked to the evolution of life. Evolution of life was probably preceded by a chemical evolution. It seems that about 4 billion years ago conditions on earth favored the formation of a few simple carbohydrates, amino acids and nitrogenous bases from the atmospheric gases. The packaging of these compounds in a membrane resulted in the formation of primitive cells. These cells somehow 'learnt' to oxidize their contents to release energy, and replenished their contents from the surroundings. But gradual depletion of ready-made compounds in the environment compelled the evolution of mechanisms to synthesize at least carbohydrates from the atmospheric carbon dioxide. The crucial step which gave 'life' to these chemical factories was the evolution of mechanisms for self replication accompanied by information transfer. Once the cell could divide, and pass on information so that products of the division would also behave like the parent, the basic features of life had been achieved. Nucleic acids and proteins played a crucial role in this process. Initially, only the cell had a membrane around it and its contents floated freely within. Bacterial cells are still like that, and are called prokaryotic cells. The next step in evolution was the packaging of nucleic acid in a membrane bound structure to form the nucleus, and the appearance of several other membrane bound structures, called organelles, within the cell. This description of the evolution of a cell is extremely brief. But even the most detailed accounts cannot avoid presumptions and flights of imagination because nobody really knows how the micracle called 'life' really happened.

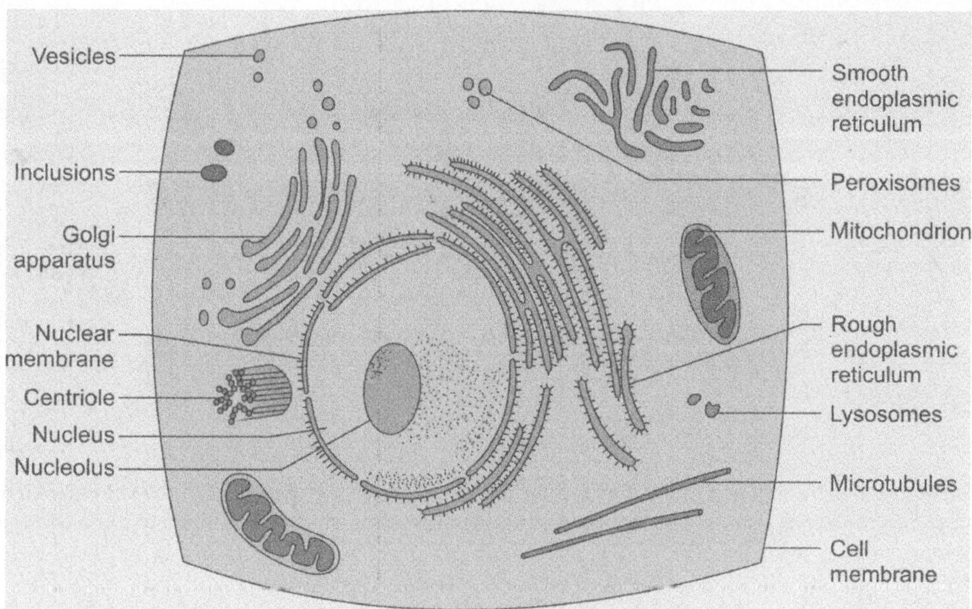

Fig. 2.1 Schematic diagram of a 'typical' cell

THE CELL MEMBRANE

The cell membrane is more than a boundary. It is a vital and dynamic structure responsible for guarding the uniqueness of the contents of the cell as compared to the outside. It is also the first point of contact with any agent that is capable of influencing the cell. The cell membrane is also called the plasma membrane to distinguish it from other cellular membranes which surround the organelles.

Under the electron microscope the cell membrane presents a three-layered structure, 8-10 nm in thickness. The simplest interpretation of the structure is provided by the Danielli-Davson model. According to this model, the membrane consists of a lipid bilayer coated on either side with a layer of proteins. But some observations have prompted several modifications of this model. The currently accepted interpretation is the fluid mosaic model of Singer and Nicolson, first proposed in 1972. The lipid bilayer is intact in this model as well. Its distinguishing features are firstly, the dynamic nature of the membrane, and secondly, the presence of transmembrane proteins which span the entire width of the membrane instead of being confined to the surface (Fig. 2.2).

The physicochemical basis of the lipid bilayer lies in the nature of the lipid molecules. Lipid molecules have hydrophobic nonpolar fatty acyl tails and a hydrophilic polar head. In an aqueous medium, lipid molecules arrange themselves as a bilayer, with the polar heads towards the outside and the non-polar tails towards the inside, facing each other. Phospholipids, cholesterol and glycolipids form the major lipids of the cell membrane. The composition of membrane lipids is affected to some extent by the nature of dietary lipids.

Proteins which span the width of the membrane form hydrophobic linkages with fatty acyl chains. These proteins are known as intrinsic or integral proteins. In addition the membrane also incorporates some surface proteins known as extrinsic or peripheral proteins. These proteins are attached to the polar heads of the lipids through electrical linkages.

The cell membrane, besides acting as a selectively permeable barrier, also acts as a receiver and

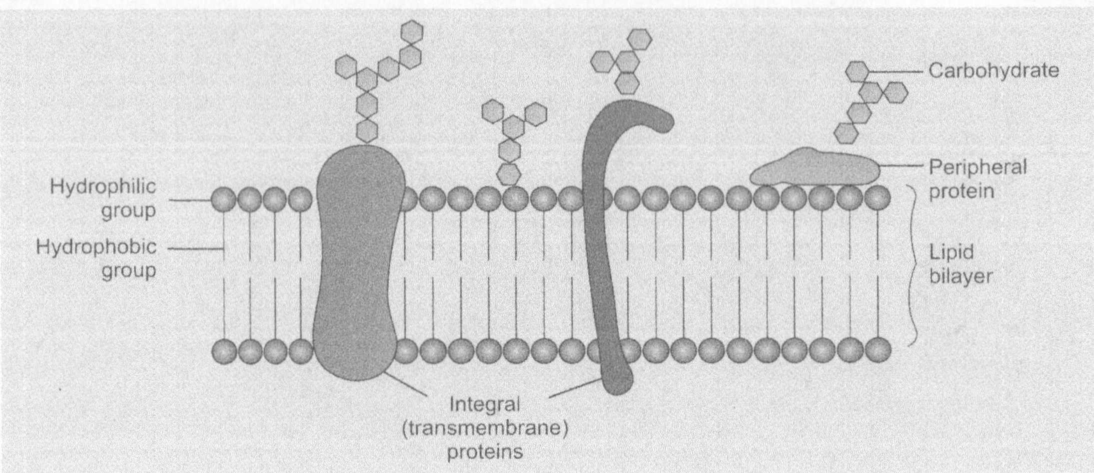

Fig. 2.2 Diagrammatic representation of the fluid mosaic model of the cell membrane. Note the lipid bilayer, the integral proteins which span the entire width of the membrane, peripheral proteins which are confined to the surface, and surface carbohydrates

transducer of information. It incorporates several enzymes, transport proteins, receptors for hormones and neurotransmitters, and antigenic determinants. Since all these functions differ from cell to cell, time to time, and on the inside as compared to the outside surface of the membrane, the cell membrane is a heterogenous, dynamic and asymmetrical structure.

Cell Junctions

In multicellular organisms adjacent cells are joined to each other. At the points of contact the cell membrane shows varying degrees of fusion and specialization depending on the requirements of the tissue. The junctions found in various tissues are classified into three types—tight junctions, gap junctions, and desmosomes.

Tight Junctions

A tight junction is characterized by fusion of adjacent cell membranes so that the junction has a 5-layered appearance under the microscope (Fig. 2.3). The tight junction forms a continuous belt between adjacent cells and prevents or at least reduces transport of substances in the extracellular space between cells. Tight junctions are found in the epithelial lining of the gastrointestinal tract where they prevent the passage of substances from the lumen to the interior of the gut by the intercellular route. Thus the tight junctions ensure that only well digested nutrients are absorbed by specialized mechanisms instead of an indiscriminate flow of materials from the lumen to the gut.

Gap Junctions

At gap junctions there is a 2-nm gap between adjacent cells. The gap is bridged by a few hollow cylindrical structures which allow substances to pass from one cell to another. Gap junctions are thus regions of intercellular communication. They are very widespread in distribution. Even tissues which have tight junctions often have gap junctions deeper down.

Gap junctions are specially important where rapid communication between adjacent cells is a functional requirement, as in smooth muscle and cardiac muscle (Plate 1B). In smooth muscle, a gap junction is called a nexus, and in cardiac muscle it forms a part of the intercalated disc.

Desmosomes

Desmosomes are button-like junctions between adjacent cells involving only small circumscribed spots on the cell membranes. The cell membranes do not

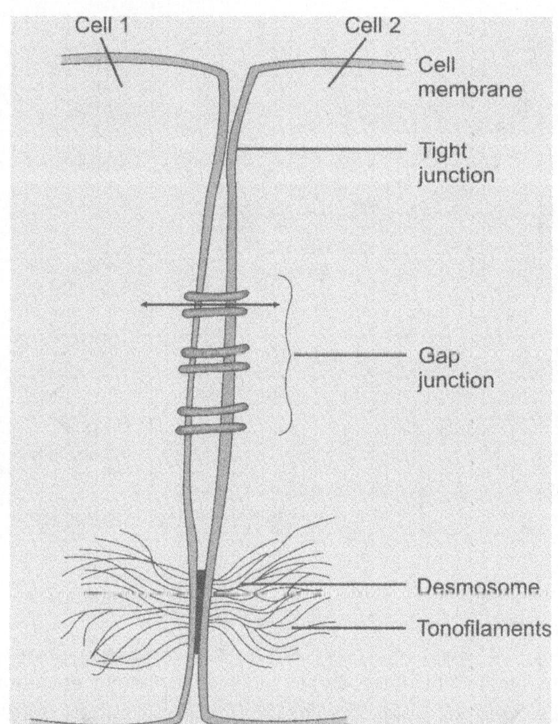

Fig. 2.3 Intercellular junctional complexes. Note that the cell membranes of adjacent cells, which normally have a trilaminar appearance under the microscope, appear 5-layered at tight junctions due to the fusion of outer layers. The gap junction is a region of intercellular communication. Arrows indicate the passage of substances from one cell to another. Desmosomes are especially designed to provide structural support

come in contact with each other at desmosomes but are separated by a gap of 25-30 nm which is filled with a carbohydrate-rich material. On the cytoplasmic sides of the membranes also there are electron-dense plaques in which are embedded fine fibrillar structures called tonofilaments. The function of desmosomes probably is to provide structural support. Desmosomes are most abundant where firm support is essential, as in the epidermis.

The same tissue may have tight junctions near the surface in order to provide an impermeable surface, gap junctions at an intermediate depth to allow intercellular transport and communication, and desmosomes at a still greater depth to keep the cells together (Fig. 2.3).

THE ORGANELLES

The membrane-bound structures within the cell are called organelles (literally, tiny organs). We shall discuss below all of them except the nucleus. The nucleus is so important that we shall discuss it separately a little later. The membranes which enclose organelles are similar to the plasma membrane.

Rough Endoplasmic Reticulum

The cytoplasm shows a network of interconnected flat membranous sac-like structures (cisternae) and tubular structures. The network is known as endoplasmic reticulum (ER). Rough endoplasmic reticulum (RER) is that part of the ER which bears on its cytoplasmic surface granular structures known as ribosomes (Plate 1A). Chemically, ribosomes are made up of ribonucleic acid (RNA) and proteins.

Ribosomes are the site of translation of messenger RNA (mRNA) into proteins. Once a protein has been synthesized on the ribosomes, it may undergo post-translational modification in the cisternal elements of RER.

As is understandable, the highest density of RER is found in cells actively engaged in protein synthesis, e.g. pancreatic acinar cells.

Polyribosomes

mRNA molecules are translated into polypeptide chains by several ribosomes simultaneously. These multi-ribosome-mRNA complexes are called polyribosomes, or simply polysomes. The number of ribosomes in a polysome depends on the length of the mRNA molecule which, in turn, depends on the length of the peptide chain encoded in the mRNA.

Smooth Endoplasmic Reticulum

Smooth endoplasmic reticulum (SER) is that part of the ER which does not have ribosomes. It is more tubular and less vesicular than the RER. SER is primarily a system of intracellular transport. It may be considered the circulatory system of the cell. In addition, it takes on special functions in different parts of the body. For example, in small intestinal epithelium, resynthesis of digested dietary fat into triglycerides takes place in the SER. In adrenal cortex and reproductive system, synthesis of steroid hormones occurs in the SER. In liver, detoxification of several endogenous and exogenous chemicals is carried out in the SER. For these metabolic functions SER carries the necessary enzymes which, being proteins, are synthesized on the RER. In skeletal muscle, SER is modified to form a system, called sarcoplasmic reticulum, for conducting the impulse of excitation and storing calcium ions. SER is best developed in cells which synthesize steroid hormones.

Microsomes

Microsomes are a creation of experimental cell biology. If cellular components are centrifuged in steps at graded speeds, they can be separated into several fractions. One of the 'lightest' fractions contains microsomes, which are derived from the RER and SER.

The Golgi Complex

The Golgi complex (or apparatus) is so called because in the days of light microscopy it could be seen only by the silver impregnation technique, first devised by Camillo Golgi in the nineteenth century. For a long time it was just a mysterious structure close to the nucleus. Electron microscopy has revealed that it consists of a stack of 3-12 flattened saucer like cisternae separated from one another by a distance of 20-30 nm (Fig. 2.4). Each cisternal element has, like a saucer, a convex face and a concave face. A number of vesicular structures can be seen attached to either face. Functionally speaking, vesicles attached to the convex face are those which have detached themselves from the RER and contain the protein products synthesized by the RER. These vesicles are in the process of fusing with the Golgi complex. Vesicles attached to the concave face are those which are in the process of budding off from the Golgi complex. After getting detached from the Golgi complex, these vesicles form secretory granules and other types of vacuolar structures.

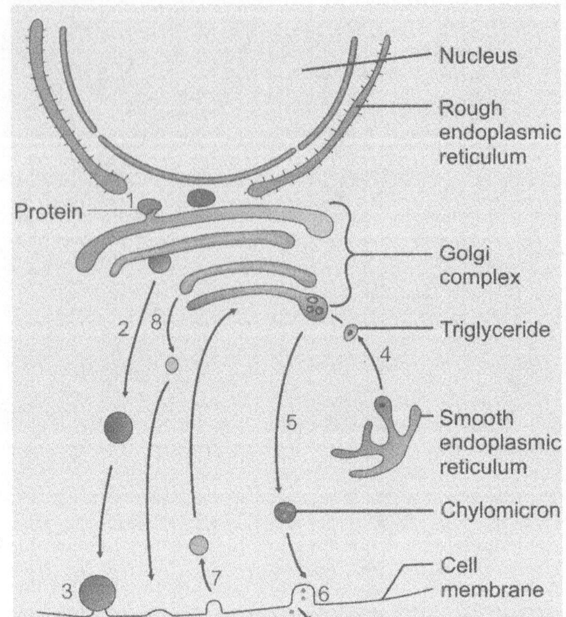

Fig. 2.4 The Golgi complex. Vesicles containing protein secretions synthesized by the rough endoplasmic reticulum fuse with the Golgi complex (1), The Golgi complex stores, concentrates, processes and packs the secretions. The final product detaches itself from the Golgi complex (2), and is finally discharged by exocytosis (3), Similarly triglycerides synthesized in the smooth endoplasmic reticulum may be transported to the Golgi complex (4), processed into chylomicrons, detached from the Golgi complex (5), and discharged by exocytosis (6), The membrane is extensively recycled. The cell membrane may contribute to the membrane of organelles such as the Golgi complex (7), and the organelles may contribute to the cell membrane (8)

Protein and polypeptide secretions of exocrine and endocrine glands are passed on to the Golgi complex after being synthesized by the RER. The secretions are not only stored in the Golgi complex but also concentrated, processed and packed. Concentration is achieved by pumping out water and electrolytes. Processing may include addition of the carbohydrate moiety to proteins to form glycoproteins, sulphation of mucopolysaccharides, or cleavage of the polypeptide chain to form the active product. For example, proinsulin is cleaved by the Golgi complex to form insulin and the C-peptide. The concentrated and processed product is packaged into vesicular structures which detach themselves from the Golgi complex. The fate and nomenclature of these vesicular structures depends on the nature and function of the products. They may form secretory granules or vesicles and be discharged from the cell by exocytosis. Or, they may enclose a variety of hydrolytic enzymes and form lysosomes.

Lysosomes

Lysosomes are vesicular organelles, 200-800 nm in diameter. They are packed with granules which are aggregates of proteins. The proteins packed in lysosomes are hydrolytic enzymes; hence the name lysosomes (lyein, to loosen, to dissolve, to release: soma, body). More than 60 different hydrolytic enzymes have been reported to be present in lysosomes. These enzymes are capable of splitting carbohydrates, proteins, lipids, nucleic acids and mucopolysaccharides[1] into their constituent units such as monosaccharides, amino acids, fatty acids, etc. The lysosomal enzymes are activated by an acidic environment. The lysosomal membrane itself is resistant to the action of lysosomal enzymes.[2] In some cells lysosomes assume a special form and function. For example, the granules of blood granulocytes (a type of white blood cells) are essentially lysosomes. The acrosome of a sperm is also a lysosomal structure and plays a role in penetration of the oocyte.

Lysosomes constitute an intracellular digestive system. They digest unwanted components of the cell itself as well as harmful extracellular substances entering the cell by phagocytosis or pinocytosis. The lysosomes, as pinched off from the Golgi complex, are called primary lysosomes. After a primary lysosome has fused with the vacuole or vesicle containing the material to be digested, it forms the secondary lysosome. After the process of digestion has been completed, a secondary lysosome forms the residual body. The residual body generally discharges its contents by exocytosis. Sometimes, however, residual bodies containing some indigestible substances may be retained in the cell. Such collections of residual bodies gradually increase with age, and are believed to contribute to impairment of physiological function associated with the process of aging.

Peroxisomes

Peroxisomes are ovoid structures, 300-1500 nm in diameter, found in liver cells and in proximal convoluted tubules of the kidney. Their shell possibly arises from the SER. They contain several oxidative enzymes which are synthesized, like other proteins, on the ribosomes. Most of these enzymes produce hydrogen peroxide as a product, and hence, the name peroxisomes. However, one of the peroxisomal enzymes, catalase, breaks down hydrogen peroxide into water and oxygen and thereby prevents cellular damage by hydrogen peroxide. Peroxisomal enzymes are involved in the breakdown of fatty acids and in alcohol metabolism.

Recycling of the Membrane

We have seen that the endoplasmic reticulum gives rise to at least a part of the Golgi complex and peroxisomes, the Golgi complex gives rise to secretory granules and lysosomes, secretory granules fuse with the plasma membrane while discharging their contents by exocytosis, lysosomes fuse with vacuoles the boundary of which originated from the plasma membrane, and the secondary lysosomes again fuse with the plasma membrane while discharging their contents extracellularly by exocytosis. All these processes involve enormous recycling of cellular membrane. The same length of membrane may be present in various organelles, or as plasma membrane at different times.

---

[1]Is there anything left to split!

[2]Unless that is so, lysosomes cannot remain intact. In addition, the cell would die due to destruction of all its components by the enzymes released from lysosomes. This tragedy forms the basis of some diseases.

Mitochondria

Mitochondria (singular, mitochondrion) are the powerhouses of a cell where its energy currency, adenosine triphosphate (ATP), is synthesized. The shape of mitochondria varies from spherical to thin and elongated but is fairly uniform within a given cell type. The number of mitochondria in a cell varies from less than a hundred to three hundred thousand. Their location in a cell is related to the site of maximum energy need.

Mitochondria have a double membrane around them (Figs 2.5A and B). The outer membrane is quite permeable to water and various other substances in the cell, and simply wraps the mitochondrion. The inner membrane, which is highly impermeable, is thrown into folds known as cristae. Hence, the inner membrane has a large surface area.[3] On the inner surface of the inner membrane are closely packed particles, each with a head and a short neck. These particles are known as elementary particles or F^1 particles or inner membrane spheres (IMS). Some of the mitochondrial enzymes are located in the elementary particles while others are present free in the matrix. The matrix also contains DNA, ribosomes and particles, 30-40 nm in diameter. Mitochondria are unique among organelles in containing DNA, ribosomes, and the enzymes required for replication of DNA and protein synthesis. The machinery is utilized for mitochondrial proliferation during cell division and for synthesizing some of the mitochondrial proteins. The partial autonomy of mitochondria, and the fact that their DNA and ribosomes resemble those of prokaryotes,[4] suggest that mitochondria might have originated from symbiotic prokaryotic organisms which got completely incorporated in the structure of eukaryotic cells in the course of evolution.

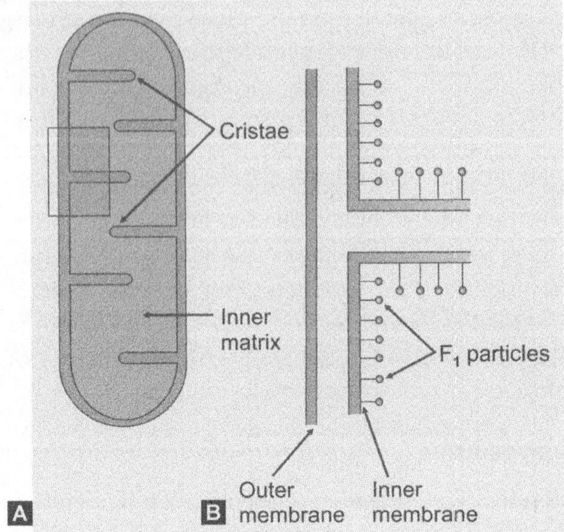

Figs 2.5A and B Diagrammatic representation of ultrastructure of a mitochondrion. The portion enclosed in the rectangle in A has been enlarged in B

The major function of mitochondria is the final oxidation of body fuels and efficient harnessing of the energy released. Final oxidation is accomplished in the Krebs cycle, the enzymes for which are located in the mitochondrial matrix. The energy released is harnessed in the form of high energy bonds of ATP, which is formed by oxidative phosphorylation. The enzymes for oxidative phosphorylation, also known as the electron transport chain, are located in the elementary particles.

The other important function of mitochondria related to energy production is the beta oxidation of fatty acids, some enzymes for which are present in the matrix and others on the inner membrane.

Other functions of mitochondria are to complete the final steps of synthesis of steroid hormones (the initial steps take place in the SER), and to regulate intracellular calcium by concentrating calcium ions in the 30-40 nm particles in the matrix.

---

[3]It may be argued that the large surface area forces it to arrange itself in folds! The fact is that the surface area of the inner membrane is large, and it is thrown into folds: it is difficult to assign a cause and effect relationship.

The surface area is dictated by the metabolic needs of the cell. Cardiac muscle fibers, which need to generate large amounts of ATP, have mitochondria with inner membranes of very large surface area. Hence, the cristae of these mitochondria are very densely packed.

[4]Prokaryotes are cells which lack a nucleus, e.g. the bacterial cells. Cells having a nucleus are called eukaryotic.

In the brown adipose tissue, which is specially rich in mitochondria, mitochondria serve the purpose of heat production as an aid to regulation of body temperature. The mechanism is specially important in some animals and in the human newborn.

Cytoskeletal Elements

These are the cellular elements which lend shape and form to the cell. They also help the cell change its shape. Since change of shape involves bending or folding or some other movement, cytoskeletal elements possess a mechanism for motility. The same or similar elements may also be employed for movement of the entire cell. In fact, motion seems to be a very fundamental biological mechanism. There is a remarkable degree of similarity in the molecular mechanisms of motility from the subcellular through organismal level. The similarity will unfold gradually in subsequent sections of this chapter but before that we shall discuss the structural details of the major cytoskeletal elements.

Microfilaments

Microfilaments are composed of the protein actin organized into fibrillar structures. Actin is a contractile protein present also in skeletal muscle. Microfilaments may not be always present in an organized form in the cell. Actin may be present "dissolved" in the cytoplasm, and may arrange itself into microfilaments only when required.

Microtubules

Microtubules are long tubular elements, about 25 nm in diameter, distributed randomly in all types of cells (Fig. 2.6). They are composed of the protein, tubulin. Detailed structure of a microtubule shows that it is composed of thirteen 'protofilaments', each 5 nm in diameter. Each protofilament is made up of tubulin subunits arranged spirally.

Cilia

Cilia are numerous short projections arising from a cell. In some unicellular organisms, cilia are used for locomotion of the whole organism. But in human beings cilia are used for moving material along the surface of cells that do not themselves move, e.g. in the ciliated epithelium of the respiratory tract.

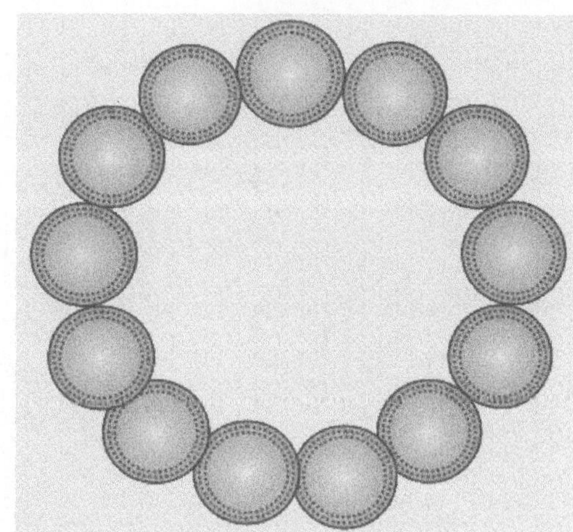

Fig. 2.6 Cross-sectional view of a microtubule showing the thirteen protofilaments

Each cilium arises from a basal body in cytoplasm. The ultrastructure of a cilium shows that it is composed of nine peripheral 'doublets' and two 'singlets' in the center (Fig. 2.7). Each 'singlet' is a microtubule, and has thirteen protofilaments as described above. Each 'doublet' is made up of two closely aligned microtubules A and B. One of them, microtubule A, is complete. But the other one, microtubule B, has only eleven protofilaments and shares a part of its wall with microtubule A. Each doublet also has a long outer arm and a short inner arm made up of the protein dynein.

The basal body has only nine peripheral units, but these are 'triplets', i.e. made up of three microtubules—one complete and two incomplete. It seems the foundation by which the cilium is anchored to the cell is stronger than the cilium, and that is how it should be.

Flagellum

If there are only one or two processes resembling cilia projecting from a cell, and their length is much longer than that of cilia, they are called flagella. In some microorganisms, flagella provide the organism

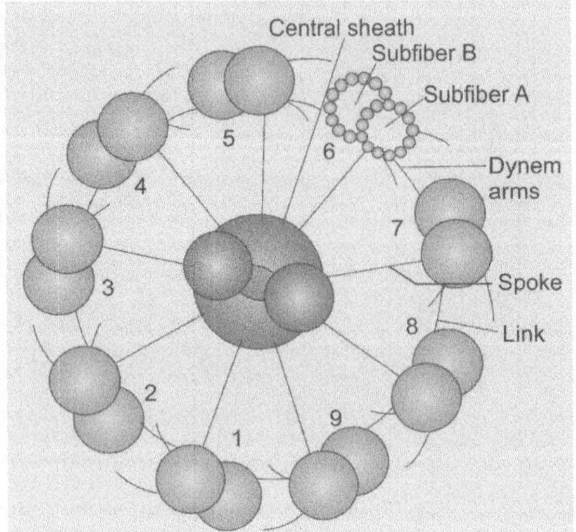

Fig. 2.7 Cross-sectional view of a cilium or a flagellum. (Adapted from Hopkins C. Structure and Function of Cells, 1978. *Courtesy:* WB Saunders Co. Ltd., London)

with a mechanism of locomotion. In human beings, the tail of a sperm is essentially a flagellum.

The ultrastructure of a flagellum is exactly the same as that of a cilium.

Centriole

Centrioles are paired cylindrical structures located near the nucleus. Their structure is very similar to that of the basal body. Centrioles and other microtubular structures of the cell play an important role in formation of the spindle during metaphase of cell division.

Functions of Cytoskeletal Elements

Cytoskeletal elements are responsible for the shape of a cell. But their more fascinating function is to perform some movements. In muscle tissue movement needs (a) an increase in calcium ion concentration in the muscle cell, (b) at least two major contractile proteins: actin and myosin, and (c) energy, which is released by the breakdown of ATP. Breakdown of ATP is catalyzed by myosin which, besides participating in the mechanical aspects of contraction, also acts as an ATPase. Movements engineered by cytoskeletal elements have exactly the same basic features.

In case of microfilaments release of Ca^{2+} triggers the process, myosin present in the cell acts as the ATPase, and also engages mechanically to make actin filaments slide past one another.

In case of microtubules, tubulin plays a role similar to actin, and dynein similar to myosin. The result is that microtubules can slide past each other.

The above mechanisms, employing either microtubules or microfilaments, are used by cells to perform an amazing variety of functions, some of which are listed below:

a. Locomotion by means of pseudopodia,
b. Movement of cilia or flagella,
c. Movement of intestinal microvilli,
d. Changes in cell shape during phagocytosis, pinocytosis, or exocytosis,
e. Transport of neurotransmitters and other substances synthesized in the cell bodies of neurons to the axon terminals,
f. Formation of the mitotic spindle,
g. Cell cleavage during telophase, and
h. Changes in cell shape during organogenesis in embryonic life.

INCLUSIONS

Besides the organelles discussed above, cells may have other structures or chemicals for a specific function. These inclusions sometimes come to dominate the appearance of the cell. Some examples of cell inclusions are the chlorophyll-containing chloroplasts in plant cells, hemoglobin in red blood cells, fat in adipose cells, glycogen in liver cells, mucus in goblet cells, and melanin in pigment cells of the skin and hair.

NUCLEUS

Now we come to the organelle which directs the activities of the rest of cell. Nucleus is the storehouse of genetic information. It also determines what part of the genetic information will be expressed by a given cell, and to what extent it will be expressed at a given moment. The nucleus is enclosed in a nuclear envelope. The nuclear envelope is made up of two membranes separated by the perinuclear space. The outer nuclear membrane is continuous with the endoplasmic reticulum (ER) and the perinuclear space is continuous with the hollow space of the ER. The nuclear envelope is interrupted by large pores, about 100 nm in diameter. The pores have a complex organization so that only an area about 9 nm in diameter is available for passage of materials.

The nucleus contains chromatin material dispersed throughout the nucleoplasm. Chemically, chromatin is deoxyribonucleic acid (DNA). DNA is the basic unit of genes, which determine what a cell does or looks like. Since the characteristics of an organism depend on what its cells do and look like, DNA determines the characteristics of the whole organism. During cell division the chromatin material gets organized into thread like structures known as chromosomes. Chromosomes occur in pairs. The number of chromosome pairs in a given species is fixed. For example, human beings have 23 pairs of chromosomes. Of these, 22 pairs consist of two apparently identical chromosomes each in both males and females. These 22 pairs are called autosomes. The twenty-third pair, called heterosomes, consists of two apparently identical chromosomes (each called an X chromosome) only in females. In males, the twenty-third pair consists of one X chromosome and one much shorter chromosome, called the Y chromosome. Heterosomes are also known as sex chromosomes. Thus the sex chromosomes of a female are XX, and in case of a male they are XY.

The number and chemical configuration of chromosomes is essentially constant from one individual to another. That is why all individuals of a species are so similar. But small differences in the chemistry of chromosomes account for the differences between individuals. The number and quality of chromosomes stay essentially constant through cell division and reproduction, as discussed in greater detail later in the chapter.

Within the nucleus there are also one or more dense collections of granules. Each collection is called a nucleolus. The nucleolus is not surrounded by a membrane. The nucleolar granules are made up of ribonucleoproteins. The function of the nucleolus is to synthesize ribosomes.

COMMUNICATION BETWEEN CELLS

No cell is an island unto itself. Cells influence one another by sending messages. In current terminology, these messages are called signals. The cell which releases signaling molecules is called the signaling cell. The cell which responds to the signaling molecules is called the target cell. The target cell has receptors for the signaling molecules. Cell-to-cell signaling is of many types, depending on the distance between cells (Figs 2.8A to C). The signaling cell and target cell may be in contact with each other. Alternatively, these cells may be separated by a short distance across which the signaling molecules can diffuse from the signaling cell to the target cell: such communication is called paracrine signaling. If the signaling and target cells are separated by a long distance, the signaling molecules (hormones) may be transported by the blood stream: such communication is called

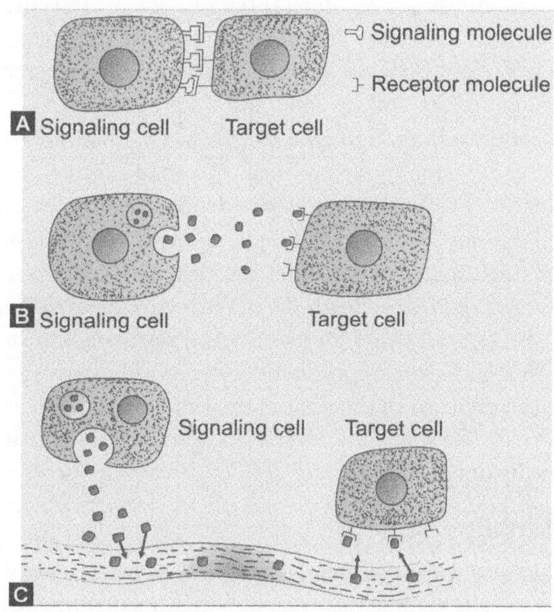

Figs 2.8A to C Different types of cell-to-cell signaling mechanisms. (A and B) Paracrine signaling; (C) Endocrine signaling

endocrine signaling. The nervous system is a special case of cell-to-cell signaling. Here the signaling molecule (neurotransmitter) travels from the signaling cell (a neuron) to the target cell (another neuron, or a muscle cell, or a gland cell) across a junction (synapse).

The process initiated in the target cell by the signal-receptor interaction is called signal transduction. Signal transduction generally consists of a series of enzymatic reactions resulting in a chain of intracellular signaling molecules. Such cascades lead to amplification of the initial signal. The final signaling molecules may influence the rate of metabolic reactions in the cytoplasm or alter genetic transcription in the nucleus. A relatively small group of highly conserved signal transduction mechanisms serves in a wide variety of situations all over the body. These mechanisms will be discussed at appropriate places in the book.

CELL DIVISION

Even a multicellular organism begins its life as a single cell. The transformation of the single cell into a multicellular organism involves the twin processes of cell division and differentiation. Even after the organism is born it continues to grow which again involves cell division and differentiation. Even after growth ceases, cell division and differentiation have to continue, although on a smaller scale, to compensate for normal wear and tear. We shall discuss the process of cell division in some detail. The essence of cell division lies in precise replication and division of the nuclear material so that the daughter cells have exactly the same genes as the parent cell. Cell division of the type required for growth and repair is known as mitosis. Sexual reproduction involves another type of cell division in the sex organs, which is known as meiosis. We shall talk about both mitosis and meiosis one by one.

Mitosis

The need for mitosis varies with the organ or tissue. Some cells such as blood cells, superficial skin cells and cells of the gastrointestinal epithelium have a very rapid turnover, and therefore frequently repeated mitotic division. When a cell is not in the mitotic phase, it is said to be in interphase. The interphase is a variable period of preparation for the mitotic phase and is divided into a G_1 phase during which RNA and protein are synthesized, S phase during which DNA is replicated, and G_2 phase of cytoplasmic growth.

G_1 phase is the first gap phase of extremely variable duration. At some point during G, the critical decision that the cell should undergo division is taken. The duration of G_1 after this decision is likely to be relatively constant. During S phase, an essential part of mitosis has already begun. The DNA is replicated so that at the end of the S phase the cell has exactly double the quantity of DNA of exactly the same quality. This miracle is possible because DNA is a double helical structure. The two strands of the helix have a complementary structure. Prior to replication the two strands separate. Each strand synthesizes its complement. Thus two new double helical structures are produced, identical to the first one. After the S phase there is a second preparatory gap phase, G_2 during which the cell grows so that it has enough cytoplasm for two daughter cells. After the G_2 phase begin the four classical phases of the mitotic, or M phase. The entire process is actually continuous but is divided into apparently well defined phases purely for convenience. Now we shall discuss the four phases of mitosis.

Prophase

The two centrioles move apart to reach the opposite poles of the cell. The two centrioles are connected by a set of spindle fibers.

The chromatin material condenses to form chromosomes. Each chromosome is composed of a pair of chromatids, attached to each other by a centromere. Each chromatid is practically a complete chromosome because DNA has already duplicated during the S phase.

The nuclear membrane "dissolves" and nucleoli may not be seen.

Metaphase

The chromosomes move to the equator of the spindle fibers. The centromeres split, followed by separation of the chromatids.

FROM MULTICELLULAR TO UNICELLULAR

In the course of evolution unicellular organisms possibly evolved into multicellular organisms. Because of the simplicity of unicellular existence, many facts about multicellular organisms have been learnt from studies on primitive life forms. Successful efforts have also been made to grow cells from multicellular organisms in an artificial medium outside the setting of the normal body. At least for some time, the cells can be studied while they grow, divide and function under these simplified artificial conditions. The exercise is known as cell culture.

The basic principle of cell culture is to provide the cells a physical and chemical environment as close to that in the body as possible. In the process what we do achieve is an environment which caters to the minimum essential requirements of the cells. In the absence of circulation, the nutritional and excretory requirements of the cells have to be met by diffusion, as in a unicellular organism. Therefore the tissues are split up into single cells, or at least into small groups of cells, so that at least part of the surface of every cell is available for diffusion. For a short-term culture, it is sometimes enough to divide the tissue into very thin wafers. But for a longer-lasting culture, the tissue is treated with enzymes such as collagenase and trypsin. Collagenase disrupts the collagen fibers which bind cells in connective tissues. Trypsin digests the adhesive components on the cell surface. The medium provides all the major inorganic ions in an appropriate concentration, glucose, amino acids, vitamins, oxygen, physiological pH and a temperature of 37°C. In order to prevent unwanted microorganisms from growing in this nutritious medium, some appropriate antibiotics also might have to be added. Often the cultured cells can survive in this medium but do not divide. They may be stimulated to divide by adding some growth factors, several of which are now known. Or, we may simply add to the medium fetal calf serum or some embryonic tissue because these are rich sources of growth factors.

Even under optimal conditions, human cells have a limited capacity for division, usually limited to fifty mitotic cycles. The older the person from whom the cells have come, less the number of divisions possible. Thus, aging does affect function at cellular level. Under certain conditions some cells can be made to undergo repeated division almost indefinitely. Such cell lines, however, show some loss of differentiation. Tumor cells, which are poorly differentiated, may also divide almost indefinitely in cell culture. This is in keeping with the general principle in biology that differentiation and proliferative capacity are usually inversely related. An ingenious technique achieves fusion of tumor cells and differentiated cells. The product is a cell called hybridoma which has the proliferative capacity of a tumor and functional ability of a differentiated cell. Hybridoma technology is a very useful technique in basic research and also has a lot of applied potential.

The centrioles duplicate so that each pole of the spindle now has two centrioles.

Anaphase

The separated chromatids (now called chromosomes) move towards the opposite poles of the spindle. A constriction appears along the middle of the cell indicating that it is on the way to forming two cells.

Telophase

Telophase essentially reverses the events of prophase. The chromosomes are dismantled to form long, thin strands of DNA which form the chromatin network. The chromatin network gets enclosed in the nuclear membrane. Nucleoli reappear, and spindle fibers disappear. The constriction between the daughter cells deepens. Finally, the two daughter cells separate from each other completely. The process of splitting of the two cells is known as cytokinesis.

Meiosis

Mitosis works very well for maintaining uniformity of cells within an individual, but would be unsuitable for maintaining uniformity in the species which reproduce sexually. Sexual reproduction involves union of a cell from the male and a cell from the female to form the first cell of the progeny. Union of two cells produced by mitosis would result in a cell which would have double the number of chromosomes as compared to the parents. This problem has been solved in biology by modifying the process of mitosis in sex organs. Production of sex cells (called gametes) takes place by means of a special type of cell division known as meiosis. In meiosis the daughter cells have half the number of chromosomes as compared to the parent cell. That is why meiois is also known as reduction division. Union of one male and one female gamete results in the formation of the first cell of the progeny with the right number of chromosomes for the species concerned. After that repeated mitosis coupled with differentiation can serve the purpose of producing a multicellular organism.

GENETICS

Everyday observations must have taught mankind long ago that no two individuals are exactly alike, that children resemble their parents, that some twins are remarkably similar, and that some diseases are familial. What exactly determines the characteristics of an individual, and how parental characteristics are transmitted to children was, however, not known till very recently. The foundations of modern genetics were laid by a monk, Gregor Mendel, in the 1850s. He observed in his monastery garden in Brunn (then in Austria) that there was some definite but confusing relationship between the characteristics of the parents and the progeny among pea plants. He decided to unravel the maze through experiments.

With remarkable research acumen, he chose well defined pairs of contrasting characters, and started with parents which bred true, i.e. if self-pollinated, they always gave progeny exactly like the parents. He studied only one or two traits at a time, obtained a very large number of observations and treated them mathematically. Thus he broke the complex problem of heredity into a few clearly observable features, and handled the data from a statistical angle. The wisdom inherent in the planning and execution of his research has earned him a permanent place of honor in every book on life sciences.

Let us now see some of his experiments (Fig. 2.9). He crossed a pure breeding strain of red-flowered pea plant with a pure breeding white-flowered strain. He observed that the progeny were all red-flowered. Wondering where the white-flowering trait disappeared, he let the progeny self-pollinate. He collected

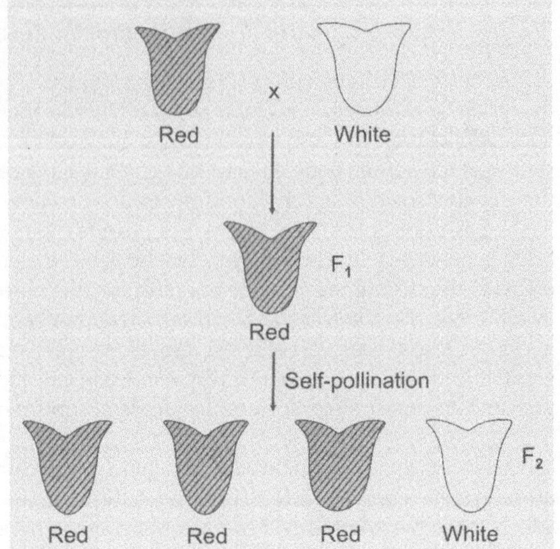

Fig. 2.9 Mendel's simplest experiments with the pea plant. Crossing a pure breeding red flowering plant with a pure breeding white flowering plant gave progeny (first filial generation F_1) bearing red flowers only. Self-pollination of these plants gave progeny (second filial generation F_2) bearing red and white flowers in the ratio 3:1 (For color version see plate 5)

more than 900 seeds from these plants, and planted them. To his delight, the progeny of these red-flowering plants were not all red-flowered. About three-fourths were red-flowered but about one-fourth were white-flowered. From a large number of experiments of this type, he collected enormous amount of data. Without the aid of any computer, he analyzed the data and postulated a scheme of inheritance of characteristics which could explain all his observations. He summarized the essential features of the scheme in terms of a few laws. In broad terms, he proposed that parents have the capacity of passing on a character to the progeny through two alternative 'particles', or genes. In sexual reproduction, the progeny receives two genes for each character, one from the mother and one from the father. The expression of the character in the progeny depends on whether both parents transmit the same types of genes or two different types of genes. If both parents transmit the same type of genes, the progeny is homozygous, and naturally shows the character encoded in the genes. If, however, both parents transmit different type of genes, the progeny is heterozygous for the character concerned. In the heterozygous state, only one trait (the dominant trait) is expressed in the progeny. The other (the recessive trait) remains hidden. However, the heterozygous individual passes on the dominant or the recessive trait with equal probability to its own progeny. Mendel's results have been explained in terms of his theory in Figure 2.10.

Molecular Basis of Genes

When Mendel published his results in 1865, they were greeted with a good deal of scepticism because they were far ahead of time. It took many steps, and nearly a century, before we knew the molecular basis of genes. In 1868 Hackel postulated that hereditary characteristics were transmitted to the progeny

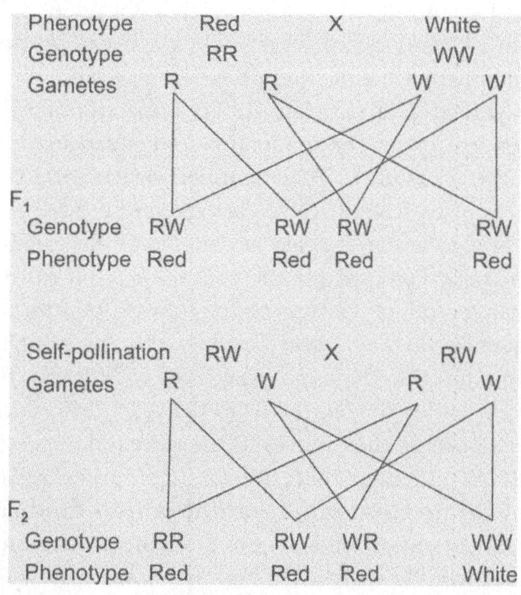

Fig. 2.10 Results of Mendel's experiments illustrated in Figure 2.9. explained. The parents were pure breeding, and hence homozygous. All progeny in F_1 are heterozygous (RW), but since red is the dominant trait, all plants in F_1 bear red flowers. F_1 plants, being heterozygous, give two types of gametes (R and W). Self-pollination of F_1 plants leads to red and white flowering plants in the ratio 3:1 in F_2

through the nucleus. In 1877 Flemming observed that the chromatin material in the nucleus arranged itself into a definite number of chromosomes during some phases of the cell cycle. In 1903 Sutton and Boveri independently observed that the division of chromosomes during the production of gametes (sperm and ovum) followed a pattern similar to that of Mendelian characters. Each individual had chromosomes in pairs, and Mendel had postulated genes to be in pairs. Each gamete carried only one member of the chromosome pair, and Mendel had postulated that a parent transmits only one of the two alternative forms of the gene to its progeny. The progeny acquired a pair of each chromosome—one member from the mother, and one member from the father—exactly as Mendel had proposed for the genes. The similarity was too close to be glossed over! Soon afterwards, chromosomes were shown to be composed of nucleic acids and proteins, but it was not known which of these molecules carried the code for characters. In 1944 Avery, MacLeod and McCarty demonstrated through experiments on the bacteria known as pneumococci that the hereditary material is deoxyribonucleic acid (DNA). In 1953 Watson and Crick proposed the double helical structure of DNA which provided the basis of chemically exact duplication, and hence the suitability of DNA as a molecule for carrying the genetic code. The genetic code was deciphered by Nirenberg in 1961, and the first gene was synthesized under laboratory conditions by Hargobind Khorana in 1970. That, in short, is the more than 100-year journey from hypothetical 'genes' to the molecular basis of genes (Fig. 2.11).

The Basis of Similarity and Variety

The number of chromosomes in every cell of the body is constant for a given species. The portion of a chromosome which codes for a character is called a gene. The position of a gene on a chromosome is called its locus. The loci of genes for different characters are also constant for a given species. The sequence of nitrogenous bases in the DNA constituting a given gene is also very similar in all individuals of a species. Thus a great deal of molecular similarity

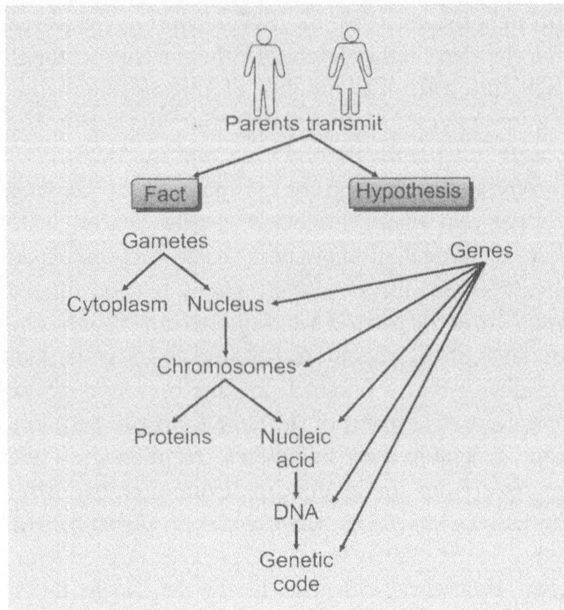

Fig. 2.11 Gradual unfolding of the molecular basis of genes, which were once only a hypothesis

forms the basis of similarity of individuals of a species. However, there are small individual differences in the sequence of nitrogenous bases in the DNA constituting some genes. These differences account for the variety within a species.

The genetic make-up of related species is also quite similar. Greater the phylogenetic distance between species, greater is the difference between their genetic make-ups.

From DNA to Characters

In order to understand how DNA is eventually decoded in terms of a character, it is essential to understand the structure of the DNA molecule. DNA has a double helical structure. Each strand of the helix has repeated units of a nitrogenous base, a sugar (deoxyribose), and a phosphate group. The nitrogenous bases in DNA are adenine (A), guanine (G), thymine (T), and cytosine (C). The nitrogenous bases of the two strands of a DNA molecule are linked by hydrogen bonds. It is found that A is always linked to T, and G always to C. The sequence of nitrogenous bases in a given chromosome in a given individual is fixed. The constancy is possible because during mitosis DNA can replicate itself exactly. Small differences in the sequence account for the differences between individuals. Only one of the two strands of DNA gets decoded into a cha-racter. The code is in terms of the sequence of nitrogenous bases. A set of three bases (triplet) codes for an amino acid. Each triplet coding for an amino acid is also called a codon. A long chain of codons thus codes for a protein.

From DNA to Proteins

DNA is in the nucleus, and proteins are synthesized in the cytoplasm. How does the nuclear code express itself in the cytoplasm? The message is carried from the nucleus to the cytoplasm by the messenger ribonucleic acid (mRNA). A strand of DNA sends the message through a specific strand of mRNA. The specificity is ensured through the complementarity of nitrogenous bases. Each A in DNA codes for a uracil (U) residue in mRNA, each T for an A, each G for a C, and each C for a G. Thus, the mRNA molecule mirrors the portion of the DNA strand which has served as a template for its transcription. The mRNA goes to the cytoplasm and arranges itself on the ribosomes. Then another variety of RNA, the transfer RNA (tRNA), brings amino acids one by one to mRNA, again on the basis of complementarity. For example the codon GUC on mRNA codes for valine. Correspondingly, a tRNA with the sequence CAG will serve as a carrier for bringing valine towards the appropriate site on mRNA. The amino acid is transferred from tRNA to a ribosome. The ribosome then moves to the next codon on the mRNA, and stays there till the appropriate amino acid has been brought there. The process continues till all the amino acids required for the protein have been linked to each other. You may wonder how the amino acid chain knows where to begin and where to stop. There are codes on the mRNA for that also. The codon AUG acts as a start signal, and the codons UAA. UGA and UAG signal termination of the chain. When the chain-terminating codon is reached, the polypeptide chain gets detached from the ribosome and enters the rough endoplasmic reticulum. In the RER some post-translational modification may be induced before the protein is passed on to the Golgi complex.

From Proteins to Characters

What a cell does and what it looks like depends primarily on the proteins which it synthesizes. All enzymes are proteins, and hence alterations in proteins may alter enzymic activities. Several hormones, and vital substances like hemoglobin are also protein. Therefore the characteristics of an organism depend a good deal on its proteins. Although alterations in a few single proteins are known to be linked to diseases such as sickle cell anemia and phenylketonuria. It needs considerable imagination to link characteristics such as shape of the nose to protein molecules. But that is probably partly because of ignorance, and partly because of our unwillingness to go into the complex chain of events responsible for each character and to examine how proteins might influence different links in the chain.

Regulatory Genes

If every cell of the body has exactly the same quantity and quality of genetic material (i.e. genome), why does a liver cell differ from a white blood cell or a muscle cell? The answer lies in the fact that only a small fraction of the genome is expressed by a cell, and the fraction expressed is different for different cells. The portion of the genome to be expressed is determined by regulatory genes. Certain base sequences in the DNA molecule act as promoters of transcription. The activity of promoters is, in turn, influenced by enhancer sequences. The enhancer may be 1000 base pairs away from the promoter but has to be on the same DNA molecule. In addition, the expression of a gene may be induced positively by an exogenous inducer substance. There are also repressor genes which influence gene expression negatively by synthesizing repressor proteins. Gene expression (or lack of it) finally depends on a complex interplay of factors which affect it positively and negatively. Most cells in the body express only 1% of the genome.

Inheritance of Characteristics

Chromosomes are the medium of inheritance. Each gamete has only half the number of chromosomes characteristic of the species (haploid number). During meiosis, not only is the number of chromosomes halved, there is also some exchange of genetic material between the two members of a pair. This phenomenon is called crossing over. The segregation of chromosome pairs at meiosis is a random process, and occurs independently for each pair. Therefore, there are theoretically, 2^{23} combinations that a parent can transmit to a particular child, and 2^{46} genetically distinct children may be born to a single couple. The variety is, actually, even greater, because of the phenomenon of crossing over.

Modes of Inheritance

A trait may be transmitted by a gene (or genes) located on one (or more) of the 22 pairs of autosomes. A given autosomal trait may be dominant or recessive. Accordingly, inheritance of the trait is said to be *autosomal dominant or autosomal recessive*. An autosomal recessive trait will express itself only in the homozygous state (why?).[5] For example, familial hypercholesterolemia is an autosomal dominant trait, and phenylketonuria is an autosomal recessive trait.

Alternative forms of a gene are called *alleles*. Sometimes neither of the alleles present in an individual is clearly dominant or recessive. Such inheritance is called *co-dominant*. A good example of autosomal codominant inheritance is blood group substances A and B. If the gene for group A is present on one chromosome, and that for group B on the other, the person will have blood group AB.

Some traits are transmitted by sex chromosomes. Such traits are called *sex-linked characters*. The only character known to be transmitted by the Y chromosome is the testis-determining factor (TDF), which is responsible for converting the basically female gonad into the testis.

[5] If you do not know why, go back a few paragraphs to find it out.

Diseases with an *X-linked dominant inheritance* are relatively few. Vitamin D resistant rickets is an example of an X-linked dominant trait. But there are several diseases with X-linked recessive inheritance. These diseases usually affect only the males because females are protected by the dominant normal gene on the other X chromosome. Examples of diseases inherited as an X-linked recessive trait are red-green color blindness and hemophilia.

There are many characteristics such as height, or intelligence, and diseases such as diabetes or heart disease, which show influence of heredity but their inheritance cannot be explained in clear terms. These traits follow a continuous distribution, i.e. their range covers a broad spectrum. The behavior of these traits indicates that they are determined by a large number of genes, each of which individually has only a small influence on the trait. Such inheritance is therefore called *multifactorial.* Traits showing multifactorial inheritance show a blending of maternal and paternal features in the progeny. For example a tall father and short mother are most likely to have children of intermediate height. Multifactorial inheritance also results in regression towards the mean. For example, two exceptionally intelligent partners are most likely to bear children who would be intelligent but not exceptionally so. The reason is that exceptional forms of a continuous trait are the result of a rare combination of a large number of heritable factors. Such rare combinations are unlikely to be repeated when one half of genes from two different sources unite to form a new combination.

Examples of continuous traits showing multifactorial inheritance are height, intelligence, body weight, blood pressure, skin color and red cell size. A few discontinuous traits also show multifactorial inheritance, e.g. peptic ulcer.

Appearance of New Characters

It is not uncommon for the child to have characteristics which are not present in either parent. There are several possible mechanisms which can explain this phenomenon.

Homozygosity

Some recessive trait may be manifested in neither parent but they may both be carrying it in their chromosomes. The manifestation is prevented by the dominant gene present at the corresponding point on the other member of the chromosome pair. Half the gametes produced by the parents will have the chromosome with the dominant gene, and half will have the one with the recessive gene. Children born as a result of union of two gametes, both having the recessive gene, will be homozygous with respect to the recessive gene. They will manifest the trait coded by the recessive gene although it was not seen in either parent.

In general, normal characters are the dominant ones. Therefore many abnormalities may be unmasked by homozygosity. Also, the chances of the same abnormal gene being present in more than one member of a family are greater than in the general population. Therefore abnormalities are unmasked more frequently by this mechanism in consanguineous marriages and in small closed communities like Jews or Zoroastrians.

Mutations

Mutations are heritable changes in the genes of an individual during his or her lifetime. These changes are due to an error in the process of DNA replication. Mutations may be 'spontaneous' or may be attributable to some chemicals or ionizing radiations. Keeping in view the complexity of the process and the frequency with which cell division occurs, it is surprising that mutations are relatively rare. The rarity of mutations may be due to the following reasons:[6]

a. Error in DNA replication in somatic cells during mitosis will not have any impact on the next generation. It is only errors in germinal cells during meiosis which may be inherited by the progeny provided the gamete so affected actually participates in fertilization.

[6]Think of the reasons yourself before you read further.

b. There are four nitrogenous bases in DNA and a sequence of three bases codes for an amino acid. Theoretically, four bases can give 43, i.e. 64, different triplets. But there are only 20 different amino acids. Some of the base sequences serve as starting and terminating signals, regulatory genes, etc. But that still leaves many more than 20 triplets to code for amino acids. As a result, most of the amino acids are coded by more than one triplet. Therefore an error in DNA replication does not necessarily alter the amino acid coded by the affected part of the DNA molecule.
c. Only non-lethal mutations manifest in the next generation. If a mutation results in so serious a defect that survival is impossible, the embryo may die in utero or soon after birth. Only neutral mutations and mutations which result in small handicaps are noticeable in the next generation. However, some mutations may even result in a favorable feature which improves the quality of life or has survival value. Such mutations possibly contribute to evolution of new forms of life.

Environment

Environment has a profound effect on genetic expression. For example, the height of an individual is the product of the genetic make-up and environmental factors such as nutrition and exercise. Intelligence quotient is the product of inherited intelligence and environmental factors such as nutrition and environmental stimulation. The genetic make-up of an individual is called genotype. The actual characteristics manifested by the individual are called phenotype. Phenotype is the result of interaction between the two alleles in the genotype and the environment.

The Human Genome Project

We have seen in a general way that characters are coded by genes, and that genes are located on chromosomes. How specific can we get on that point? For example, do we know which part of which chromosome codes for the color of the eyes? Further, do we know in precise detail what part of that chromosome differs in two persons, one of whom has black eyes and the other has blue eyes? Till now we cannot be so specific about all genes, but soon we may be, thanks to the human genome initiative. The initiative, commonly called the 'human genome project', was launched in 1990 by USA. It was completed recently through the participation of several countries around the world, including India. The human genome project is said to be the most ambitious scientific project ever undertaken in human history.

Let us see what has been done under the human genome project. We have twenty-three pairs of chromosomes, of which one pair (sex chromosomes) has dissimilar members in males. Thus there are twenty-four chromosomes (chromosomes 1-22, X and Y) to be studied. The twenty-four chromosomes have an estimated 100,000 genes coded by three billion nucleotides. Each of these nucleotides has one of four nitrogenous bases—adenine (A), thymine (T), guanine (G) or cytosine (C). What we had to do, therefore, were two things. *First*, find the gene on each portion of each chromosome. That is the 'address' of the gene. For example, the address of a particular gene may be D 16 S40. Although it looks complex, the address may be interpreted as chromosome no. 16, block S, house no. 40. Further, the portion of a chromosome constituting one gene may have 10,000 nucleotides. We should know the exact sequence of these nucleotides in terms of A's, T's, G's and C's. That is the *second* thing we had to do. The human genome project was considered complete only when we worked out the nucleotide sequence of every 'house' in each of the twenty-four chromosomes.

Let us first examine the potential uses of the knowledge which human genome project has brought us. We are soon likely to know the precise error in DNA which is responsible for every hereditary disease. That would be the first step towards therapy which might attempt to insert the error-free DNA at the right place. Further, it may make it possible to know in advance who is likely to develop in later life one of the diseases which have a strong hereditary predeliction, such as diabetes, heart disease, Alzheimer's disease or breast cancer. An early warning may help initiate precautions early in life which could prevent or delay the onset of the disease. Here is where some problems also begin. For example, should a woman undergo mastectomy just because she has a high probability of getting breast cancer at a later date? A day might come when any individual may be able to have his entire genetic profile worked out. The data my be fed into a computer to get his potential strengths and weaknesses and to predict illnesses: a sort of modern horoscope. If that becomes possible, it raises the question whether society will tend to classify human beings on the basis of their genes? Will individuals with certain genes be stigmatized or discriminated against? In order to prevent such misuse, can information about individual genomes be kept confidential? These are the types of complex social, ethical and legal issues we are likely to face in the not-too-distant future.

While these fascinating and frightening possibilities belong to the future, the immediate scientific task on hand is to decipher the part of the genome which is expressed in different parts of the body, and the proteins through which it is expressed. This area of work called proteomics, may take even longer than the human genome project. A related issue is to work out the function of these proteins, and in case of enzymes, to work out their role in metabolism: this area of research has been named metabolomics. Gene expression is vulnerable to environmental influences, including nutrition. Nutrient-gene interaction is also a fascinating and rapidly evolving area of research.

CONCLUSION

Cell is the fundamental unit of life, and accordingly cell biology forms the basis of life sciences. This brief chapter can only provide an introduction to this fascinating area in which the frontiers of knowledge are being pushed further every year. If this chapter has succeeded in increasing your appetite for more, and raised some questions in your mind as it is intended to, you will be looking for a more detailed account elsewhere. Some more details on this subject would be available to you in a biochemistry text. If that does not satisfy you, several excellent books on cell biology, genetics and biotechnology should be available in your library.

QUESTIONS

1. Do the two strands of the DNA molecule correspond to the two alternative forms of genes present in an individual?
2. Explain briefly why in spite of all human cells having 46 chromosomes each, all the cells do not look or function alike?
3. Explain why in case of diseases having an X-linked dominant inheritance all sons of the affected males are normal while all daughters suffer.

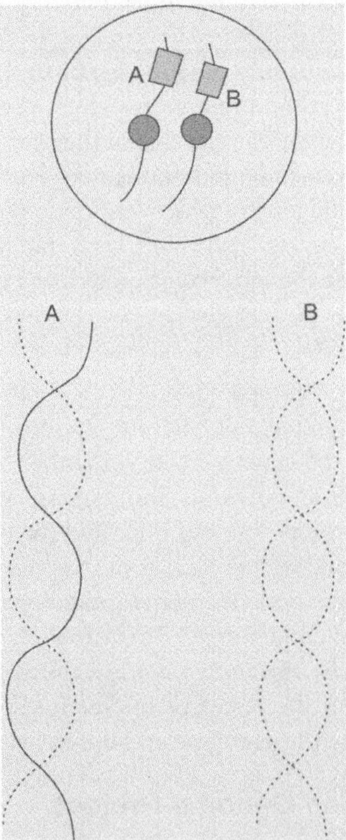

Fig. 2.12 Top. A pair of chromosomes in the nucleus. The rectangles enclose two corresponding loci on each member of the pair. Bottom. The DNA strands constituting the portions of chromosomes enclosed in rectangles in the picture on the top. The character coded by A is dominant; hence B does not express itself. Out of the two DNA strands, only one (shown as a continuous line) is transcribed into mRNA

ANSWERS

1. No. The two genes for each character are present at corresponding loci on each member of a pair of chromosomes. The gene on a given chromosome is made up of DNA, which has two strands. One strand of the DNA that gets expressed is translated into mRNA (Fig. 2.12)
2. It is so because the part of the genome expressed in different cells is different.
3. This is because the affected father transmits only the Y chromosome to his sons. The Y chromosome has no locus for the character responsible for the disease.

   On the other hand, the patient can transmit to his daughters only the abnormal X chromosome because that is the only X chromosome he has. The daughters will get their other X chromosome from the mother, the normalcy of which is not of much use because the abnormal trait carried by the X chromosome from the father is dominant.

CHAPTER

3

Physicochemical Principles of Biological Transport

"To travel hopefully is a better thing than to arrive, and the true success is to labour."

—ROBERT LOUIS STEVENSON

Chapter Outline

- Passive Transport
- Active Transport

The cells in our body utilize nutrients and produce waste products continuously at rates which vary from time to time. The nutrients are picked up from the immediate surroundings, and the waste products dumped into the surroundings, both categories of substances being transported across cell membranes. Besides, the cell guards its internal chemical composition, which is distinctly different from that of its immediate surroundings. Although these processes are unique to living cells, they are governed by physicochemical principles. You are already familiar with these principles but they have been recapitulated here.

Transport across cell membranes may be governed only by physical processes, the membrane acting like any non-living semi-permeable structure. In such cases the transport is called passive. Or, the transport may involve expenditure of biologically produced energy. In such cases the transport is called active.

PASSIVE TRANSPORT

Passive transport across the cell membrane depends on physical factors such as concentration gradient, electrical gradient and pressure gradient. In addition, it depends on the permeability of the membrane. Permeability of the cell membrane to a substance depends on its molecular size, lipid solubility, and whether a special protein (called carrier) is available to shuttle the substance across the membrane. Small molecules or ions are transported faster because they can pass through 'pores' in the cell membrane. Lipid soluble substances are transported faster because such substances can 'dissolve' in the lipid bilayer of the cell membrane and cross it. For some specially important substances, the limitations of particle size and solubility are circumvented by a carrier protein in the cell membrane which shuttles the substance across the membrane.

The major processes by which passive transport is accomplished are simple diffusion, facilitated diffusion and osmosis.

Simple Diffusion

All dissolved substances are in a state of random molecular motion. The molecules, or ions, as a result of this motion, strike the cell membrane. The frequency of collisions depends on the concentration of the dissolved substance. If the substance is present on both sides of the membrane, the frequency of collisions is higher on the side on which the substance is present in a higher concentration (Fig. 3.1). Higher the frequency of collisions, greater is the probability of particles striking a pore through which they can pass to the other side of the membrane. Or, in case of lipid soluble substances, higher the concentration, greater is the probability of the particles striking the membrane and 'dissolving' in it and passing to the other side. Hence, substances diffuse from the side

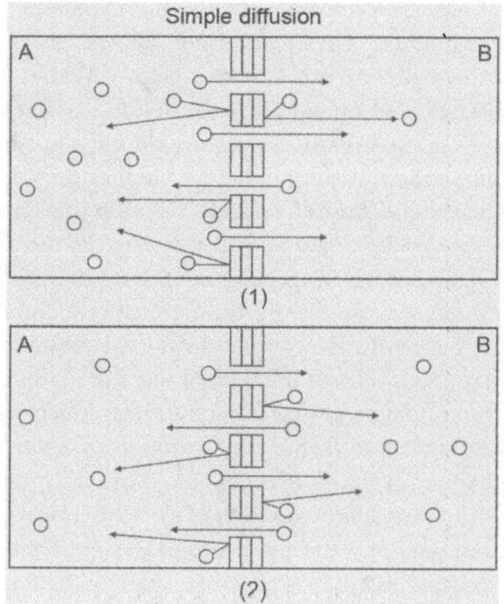

Fig. 3.1 Simple diffusion. (1) The concentration of the solute is higher on side A than on side B. Hence, random molecular motion results in transport from A to B at a rate higher than that from B to A. Thus, the net transport is from A to B. (2) The process initiated in (1) has eventually resulted in equalization of the concentration of the solute on side A and side B. Although random molecular motion continues, the rate of transport now from A to B is the same as that from B to A. Hence, there is no net transport

on which they are present in a higher concentration to one on which the concentration is lower.

If there is an electrical charge across the membrane, a charged particle would have a tendency to diffuse towards the oppositely charged side.

The influence of pressure gradient on diffusion is somewhat nonspecific. Pressure is the result of sum total of the collisions on a given side of the membrane. Pressure has a nonspecific effect of driving substances out. Hence diffusion is increased from the side with the higher pressure to that with a lower pressure.

Besides these factors, molecular size and lipid solubility also affect simple diffusion as discussed earlier.

Respiratory gases are transported across the alveolar membrane in the lungs by simple diffusion.

Facilitated Diffusion

Transport by diffusion may be made faster, and the limitation of molecular size overcome, if a suitable carrier is available in the cell membrane. The carrier helps incorporate even a water soluble substance in the membrane, and makes the transport akin to that of a lipid soluble substance. Since the carrier merely facilitates diffusion, the process is called facilitated diffusion (Fig. 3.2).

That the transport of a substance is carrier-mediated is suggested by the following observations:

1. Minor differences in molecular structure may lead to a substantial difference in the rate of transport. This observation implies that optimal transport depends on a precise fit between the molecule to be transported and the receptor site on the carrier.
2. Substances with a similar molecular structure compete with one another for transport.[1] This observation also indicates a link between molecular configuration and transport, which points to the involvement of a carrier.
3. Transport can be blocked by specific agents. This observation indicates that the blocking agent has a very high affinity for binding with the carrier. If the blocking agent is also transported, the block is competitive, i.e. it can be overcome by high concentrations of the substance whose transport has been blocked. If the blocking agent binds to the carrier but does not get transported, it blocks the carrier irreversibly. Such a block is called non-competitive.
4. The relationship between the concentration of the substance and the rate at which it is transported is linear only up to a certain limit. After that further increase in concentration does not increase the rate of transport (Fig. 3.3).

[1]Competition also occurs between two types of molecules of the same substance, one of which incorporates an isotope. Radioactive isotopes are a valuable tool for the study of transport mechanisms.

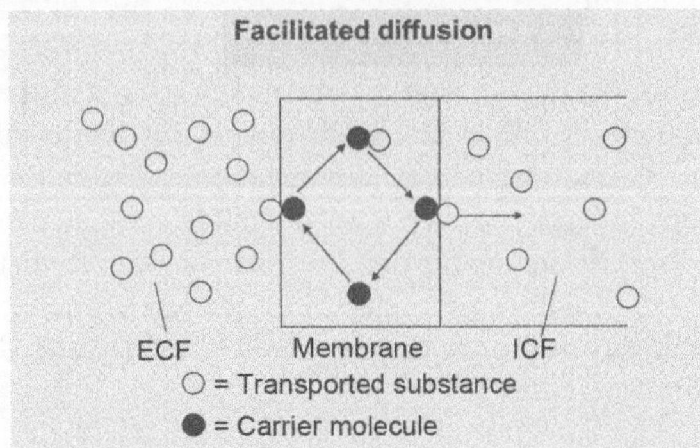

Fig. 3.2 Facilitated diffusion. The substance to be transported is picked up by a carrier (often a membrane protein) which delivers the substance inside the cell. The same mechanism can also transport the substance in the opposite direction if the concentration gradient is reversed. ECF, extracellular fluid; ICF, intracellular fluid

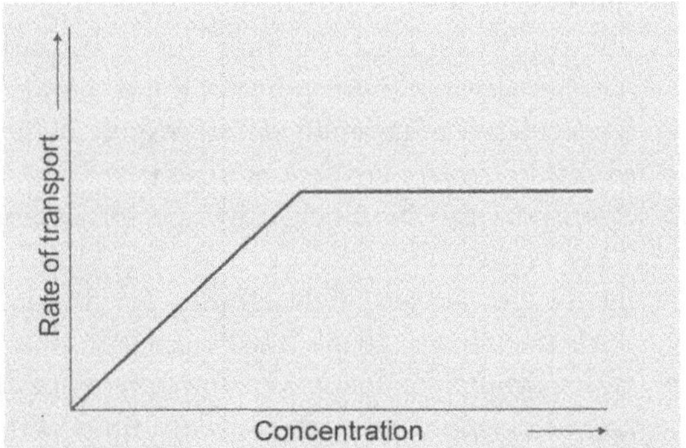

Fig. 3.3 Saturation kinetics, as seen in carrier-mediated transport

Such a relationship is said to follow saturation kinetics. The reason for the relationship is that when all the available carrier molecules are in use, further increase in concentration of the transported substance cannot increase the rate of transport.

In the small intestine, fructose is absorbed by facilitated diffusion.

Osmosis

Osmosis is a special instance of diffusion. Suppose a selectively permeable membrane (often erroneously called a semipermeable membrane) separates two compartments. The membrane allows water to pass through but not a solute (Fig. 3.4). On side A is water, and on side B is the solute dissolved in water. The membrane is permeable only to water, and the concentration of water is higher on side A. Hence, water diffuses from A to B, but in this type of situations water is said to be transported by osmosis. Now let us see why a special term is used in this case.

In ordinary simple diffusion, transport continues till the concentration of the transported substance is equal on both sides of the membrane. But in this case you can understand that no matter how much water moves from A to B, the concentration of water will stay higher on side A because side B can only have a more and more dilute solution of the solute. However, the transport of water by osmosis does not continue indefinitely because osmosis of water increases the hydrostatic pressure on side B. Osmosis is said to stop

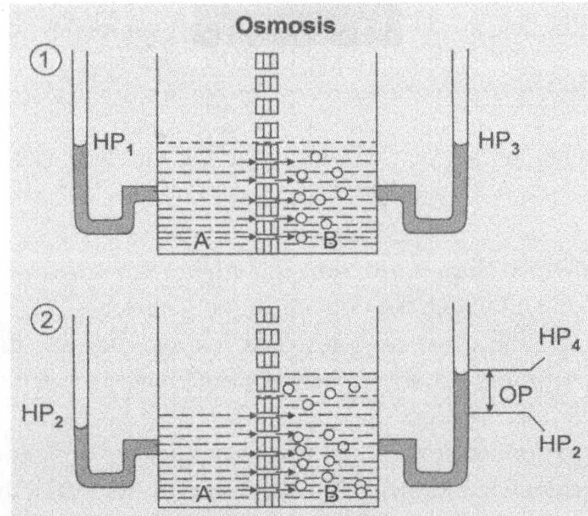

Fig. 3.4 Osmosis. (1) Solvent diffuses from compartment A to B because its concentration is higher on side A than on B. The solute does not diffuse along its concentration gradient because the membrane dividing A and B is semipermeable. (2) The net flow of the solvent stops when the excess hydrostatic pressure on side B just counterbalances the osmotic pull exerted by the solute.

HP_1 and HP_2 hydrostatic pressure in compartment A; HP_3 and HP_4 hydrostatic pressure in compartment B; OP, osmotic pressure when the excess hydrostatic pressure on side B equals the osmotic pressure exerted by the solute. Hydrostatic pressure is a pushing pressure. Hydrostatic pressure on side B tends to push water from side B to A. Osmotic pressure is a pulling pressure. Osmotic pressure exerted by the solute pulls water from A to B. When the pushing and pulling pressures become equal, there is no further net movement of water.

Ultrafiltration

You are familiar with filtration. If we try to pass a solution through a filter, the solvent and other small molecules in the solution pass through while large molecules stay on the filter. Whether a given substance will pass through a filter depends on the relative size of its molecules and that of the pores in the filter. The rate of filtration can be increased by applying pressure. For example, the hydrostatic pressure in renal glomeruli is higher than that in any other capillaries of the body. As a result, water and small molecules filter through the glomeruli rapidly while proteins and blood cells do not. Filtration under pressure is called ultrafiltration (Fig. 3.5).

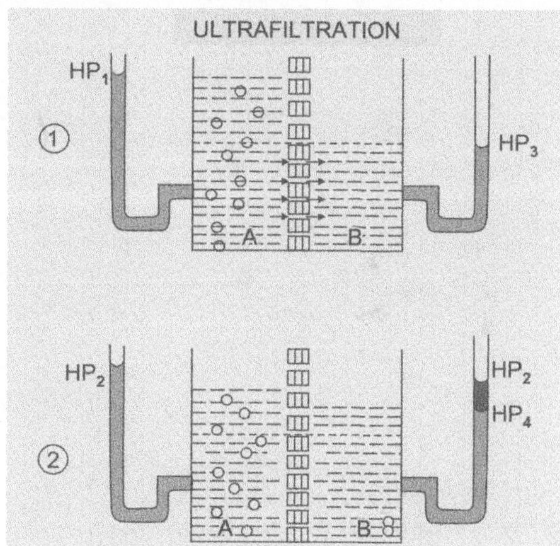

Fig. 3.5 Ultrafiltration. (1) The solvent diffuses from A to B because of the hydrostatic pressure gradient. (2) The net flow of the solvent stops when the osmotic pull exerted by the solute just counterbalances the excess hydrostatic pressure on side A.

HP_1 and HP_2 hydrostatic pressure in compartment A; HP_3 and HP_4 hydrostatic pressure in compartment B. The difference between HP_2 and HP_4 is equal to the osmotic pressure of the solute

Dialysis

Dialysis is a procedure in which the principles of diffusion are applied for the treatment of renal failure. In the patient's blood, nitrogenous waste products accumulate and electrolyte imbalance may occur due to renal failure. A solution is prepared in which the waste products are absent, electrolyte concentration is appropriately adjusted, and nutrients are provided. The solution is separated from the patient's blood by a dialyzing membrane. The process of diffusion tends to normalize the composition of patient's blood.

ACTIVE TRANSPORT

Active transport utilizes biologically produced energy. This makes it possible to transport a substance at a rate faster than can be accounted for by the electrochemical gradient,[2] or even against the gradient. As in case of passive transport, active transport may also be carrier-mediated (Fig. 3.6).

Active transport is required for maintaining the difference in electrolyte composition between the intracellular and extracellular fluids. Inside the cell the sodium ion concentration is much lower than outside; opposite is the situation in case of potassium ions. Active transport is of special significance for transport of several nutrients in the gastrointestinal tract. The absorption of nutrients should obviously continue till the luminal concentration has dropped to negligibly low levels even when sizeable concentrations have built up in the enterocytes. This is possible only through active transport.

Since active transport needs metabolic energy, often a specific ATPase is present in the membrane of actively transporting cells. Active transport may be inhibited by inhibitors of the ATPase, e.g.

[2]The term electrochemical gradient combines electrical and concentration gradients.

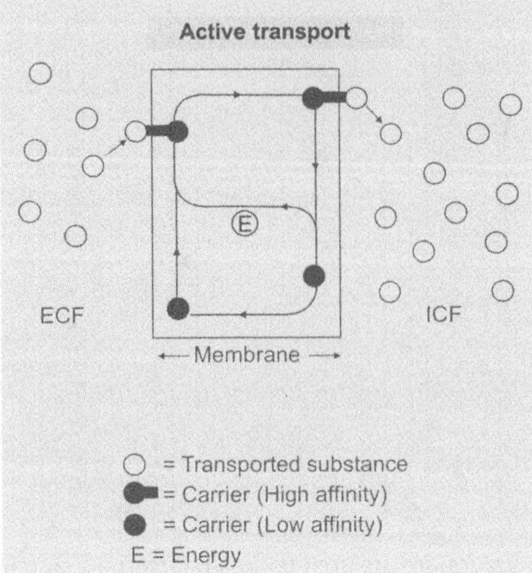

Fig. 3.6 Active transport uses energy. In the model illustrated in the figure, energy is utilized for changing the conformation of the carrier molecule to a high affinity variety, and also for releasing the transported molecule inside the cell. ECF, extracellular fluid; ICF, intracellular fluid

digitalis, which specifically inhibits the Na^+-K^+ ATPase in cardiac muscle and omeprazole which specifically inhibits the H^+-K^+ ATPase in gastric parietal cells.

Active transport may also be non-specifically inhibited by dinitrophenol (DNP) which uncouples oxidation and phosphorylation in biological oxidation, by cyanide which poisons the electron transport chain, and by fluoride or iodoacetate which inhibit anaerobic glycolysis. Active transport in erythrocytes may be inhibited by fluoride or iodoacetate because these cells derive energy only from anaerobic glycolysis.

Secondary Active Transport

Secondary active transport is an ingenious device used by cells to utilize the active transport of one substance to drive the uphill transport of one or more other subtances as well. A few varieties of secondary active transport are as follows:

Coupled Transport

The transport of two substances may be coupled to each other because they bind to the same carrier in the cell membrane.

Co-transport

If the two substances whose transport is coupled move in the same direction, the phenomenon is called co-transport or symport. For example, in the small intestine, absorption of sodium ions is coupled with that of glucose because they bind to the same carrier in the enterocyte membrane.

Counter-transport

If the two substances whose transport is coupled move in opposite directions, the phenomenon is called counter-transport or antiport. For example, in proximal convoluted tubules of the kidneys, sodium is actively reabsorbed. Simultaneously, for each sodium ion reabsorbed, one hydrogen ion is transported by the same carrier into the lumen of the tubule.

Solute-solvent Interaction

Some examples of transport by solute-solvent interaction are secondary to the active transport of some substance.

Osmosis

Entry of a solute into a cell by active transport increases the osmotic pressure within the cell. Hence, water also enters the cell by osmosis. Reabsorption of water from the gut takes place by this mechanism.

Solvent Drag

This is a process which may be further secondary to the osmotic movement of water. Along with water some substances dissolved in water may move in the same direction by bulk flow. This is known as solvent drag.

This chapter by no means exhausts the physico-chemical principles of biological transport. It is merely a recapitulation of a few basic mechanisms which you might have done in greater detail earlier.

FRACTIONS AND MULTIPLES

The implications of several unfamiliar units can be grasped if one is familiar with the meaning of following prefixes:

Mega (M)	=	10^6
Kilo (k)	=	10^3
Hecto (h)	=	10^2
Deca (da)	=	10^1
Deci (d)	=	10^{-1}
Centi (c)	=	10^{-2}
Milli (m)	=	10^{-3}
Micro (mc)	=	10^{-6}
Nano (n)	=	10^{-9}
Pico (p)	=	10^{-12}
Femto (f)	=	10^{-15}
Atto (a)	=	10^{-18}

CONCENTRATIONS

Traditionally the concentrations were expressed in mg/100 mL. This usage is still not completely obsolete. But the molecular weights of different compounds are different. Therefore, although the concentration of substances A and B in blood may be M mg/100 mL each, the number of molecules of each in 100 mL blood will be different. Since substances interact in terms of molecules, expressing the concentration in terms of mass/volume is no longer considered the best mode of expression.

The currently popular modes of expressing concentration are moles/L, equivalents/L and osmoles/L. Usually the concentrations of biological substances are so small that the suitable units usually are millimoles/L, milliequivalents/L and milliosmoles/L, abbreviated as mMol/L, mEq/L and mOsm/L. Often mMol/L is written simply as mM.

One mole of a substance is equal to its molecular weight in grams. Thus one mole of carbon is 12 g of carbon, one mole of oxygen is 32 g of oxygen, and one mole of sodium chloride is 58.5 g of sodium chloride.

Equivalent weight of a substance is in relation to its participation in chemical reactions. For example, one molecule of HCl will completely neutralize one molecule of NaOH. But only half a molecule of H_2SO_4 is enough to neutralize one molecule of NaOH. Therefore the equivalent weight of HCl will be equal to its molecular weight, but the equivalent weight of H_2SO_4 will be half its molecular weight. In case of elements, equivalent weight will be equal to molecular weight/valency for similar reasons. In case of acids and alkalies, when the concentration is 1 gram equivalent weight/L, it is sometimes called a "Normal" or 1 N solution.

Osmolarity of a substance is in relation to the osmotically active entities that its molecule provides. One molecule of NaCl– provides two osmotically active entities, Na+ and Cl–. Thus 180 g/L of glucose (an unionized compound) is equal to 1 mole/L and also 1 osmole/L. But 58.5 g/L of NaCl is equal to 1 mole/L but 2 osmoles/L.

If instead of the volume of the solvent, concentration is expressed in terms of mass of the solvent, the concentration is called the molal or osmolal concentration. Thus the molality of a solution is its concentration in moles/kg and the osmolality is the concentration in osmoles/kg. Since the volume is affected by temperature but the mass is not, molality and osmolality are independent of temperature.

QUESTIONS

1. What is the importance of osmolarity in homeostasis?
2. What concentration of sodium chloride is isosmotic with:
   a. Amphibian extracellular fluids?
   b. Mammalian extracellular fluids?
3. What concentration of glucose is isosmotic with human plasma?
4. What is the relationship between osmolarity and osmotic pressure?

ANSWERS

1. Osmolarity is important for regulation of cell volume. If a cell is surrounded by a solution, the osmolarity of which is lower than that of the intracellular fluid (hypotonic solution), water enters the cell, swelling it up and sometimes rupturing it. On the other hand, if the cell is surrounded by a hypertonic solution, water leaves the cell making it shrunken. Therefore, the cell should always be surrounded by an interstitial fluid the osmolarity of which is the same as that of the intracellular fluid (isotonic solution). The homeostatic mechanisms for regulation of body fluid volume and osmolarity are coupled. But osmolarity is so important for

the body that if the body has to choose between regulation of volume and osmolarity, it may choose to regulate osmolarity even if it means deviation of the volume from normal.

2. a. 0.6%

   b. 0.9%

3. Isotonic sodium chloride solution

$$
\begin{aligned}
&= 0.9\% \\
&= 9.0 \text{ g/L} \\
&= \frac{9.0}{58.5} \text{ moles / L} \\
&= 0.15 \text{ moles/L} \\
&= 0.30 \text{ osmoles/L}
\end{aligned}
$$

Isotonic glucose solution is also

$$
\begin{aligned}
&= 0.30 \text{ osmoles/L} \\
&= 0.30 \text{ moles/L} \\
&= 0.30 \times 180 \text{ g/L} \\
&= 54 \text{ g/L} \\
&= 5.4 \text{ g/100 mL}
\end{aligned}
$$

For simplicity, a 5% solution of glucose is administered, considering it as isosmotic.

Note that in case of sodium chloride. 0.15 moles/L = 0.30 osmoles/L because each molecule provides two osmotically active ions. But since glucose is not ionized, each molecule provides only one osmotically active entity. Hence 0.30 osmoles/L = 0.30 moles/L.

4. At 37°C, 1 milliosmole/L exerts an osmotic pressure of 19.3 mmHg. The osmolarity of body fluids is about 300 milliosmoles/L. Hence, their osmotic pressure = 300 × 19.3 = 5790 mmHg. However, the actual osmotic pressure is about 6% less, i.e. about 5500 mmHg. The reason for the discrepancy is that many oppositely charged ions, e.g. sodium and chloride ions, attract each other. Therefore a sodium chloride molecule actually exerts slightly less than double the osmotic pressure exerted by one molecule of an unionized molecule.

CHAPTER 4

Blood

"Circulating as it does throughout the body and being at the same time that part of ourselves that can be most easily sampled and analyzed, the blood has yielded to research facts of profound significance concerning its components, the blood forming organs, and the so-called blood diseases, and also about the human organism as a whole."

—MAXWELL WINTROBE

Chapter Outline

- Plasma
- Red Blood Cells
- Anemia
- Jaundice
- White Blood Cells
- Immune Mechanisms
- Platelets
- Coagulation
- Hemopoiesis
- Blood Groups

We have all seen blood. It flows from the finger when it gets a cut from a knife. We also know blood is important for life. Therefore, we try to stop bleeding from injuries. A person who loses too much blood in an accident may die. Blood is important because it performs important functions in the body. These functions become possible because blood goes to all parts of the body. Blood carries nutrients such as glucose to every part of the body. Taking substances to or from somewhere is also called transport. Thus blood *transports nutrients* to every cell of the body. Blood also *transports oxygen* to every cell of the body. Blood also *transports waste products* such as carbon dioxide from every cell of the body. Thus blood supplies to cells nutrients and oxygen which give energy. And, blood removes from the cells waste products which are not required by the body. When blood is passing through different parts of the body, it also takes or gives some other substances. For example, while passing through endocrine glands, blood picks up hormones. In this way, blood also *transports hormones*, *antibodies*, *enzymes* and several vital substances.

Although blood appears to be liquid, it is actually a liquid with cells suspended in it. The liquid or fluid part is called plasma. The plasma has three types of cells suspended in it (Plate 2A). The composition of blood is summarized in Table 4.1 and Figure 4.1. Now we shall look at different components of blood in some detail.

PLASMA

Plasma forms about 55 percent of the blood volume. The normal blood volume of an adult is 5 liters. Thus, the normal plasma volume is about 3 liters. If blood is allowed to clot, some plasma proteins are used up in the process of clotting. The fluid left behind after clotting is called serum. Thus,

Serum = Plasma minus some clotting factors.

Table 4.1 Composition of blood

Cells	*Fluid (Plasma)*
1. Red blood cells	1. Water
2. White blood cells	2. Crystalloids
I. Granulocytes	3. Colloids (Plasma proteins)
a. Neutrophils	I. Albumin
b. Eosinophils	II. Globulins
c. Basophils	III. Fibrinogen
II. Agranulocytes	
a. Lymphocytes	
b. Monocytes	
3. Platelets	

Therefore, to get serum, we allow the blood to clot. Then we break the clot to release the serum. And, to get plasma, we prevent clotting by adding an anticoagulant to the blood. Then we allow the blood to stand. The cells settle down, and plasma is left behind at the top. In order to make the cells settle faster, the blood may be centrifuged.

The electrolyte composition of plasma is similar to that of other extracellular fluids, i.e. it has a high concentration of sodium and a low concentration of potassium. In addition, plasma contains a significant concentration of proteins.

Plasma Proteins

The normal plasma protein concentration is about 6.0-8.0 g/100 mL plasma. The major plasma proteins are albumin (4-5 g/100 mL), globulins (2-3 g/100 mL) and fibrinogen (0.3 g/100 mL).

Origin

Albumin, coagulation factors, and alpha and beta globulins are synthesized in the liver. Gamma globulins, which are antibodies, are synthesized by plasma cells in the lymphoid organs.

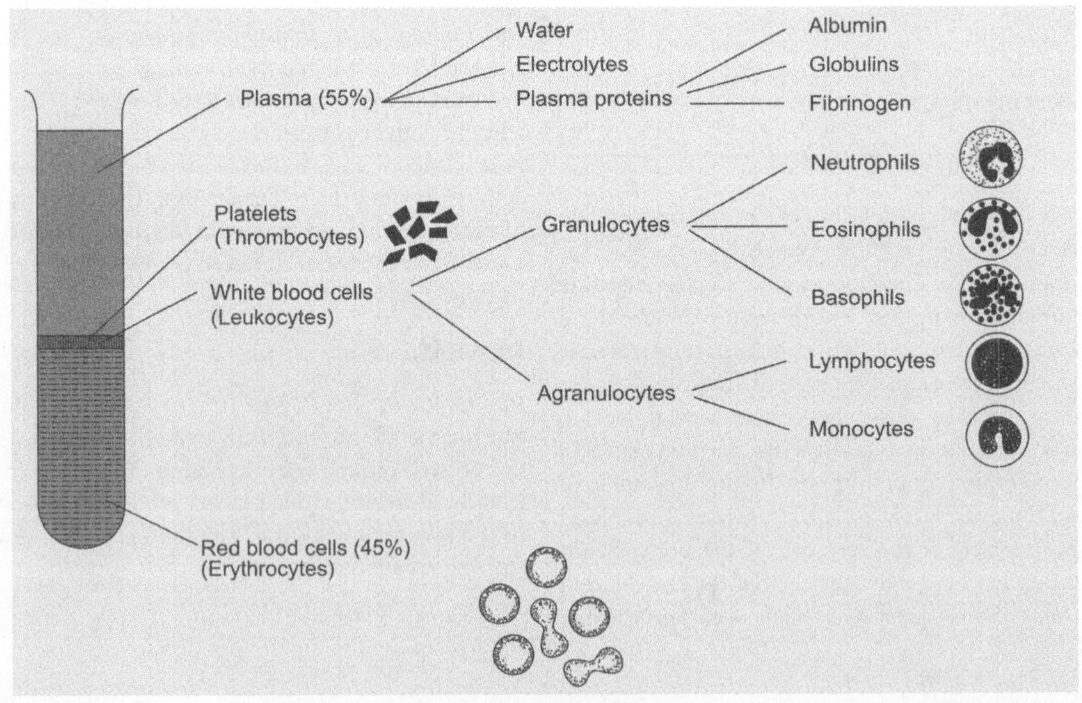

Fig. 4.1 The components of blood

Functions

Some general functions of the major plasma proteins are as follows:

1. Plasma proteins exert an *osmotic pressure* of about 25 mm Hg. This pressure plays an important role in determining the exchange of fluid across capillaries.
2. Plasma proteins contribute significantly to the *viscosity* of blood. Viscosity of blood is an important determinant of the resistance offered by blood vessels to the flow of blood.
3. Plasma proteins are good buffers. Therefore, they contribute to the *maintenance* of pH of the blood.
4. Plasma proteins form a *reserve* which can be used in starvation.
5. Plasma proteins belonging to the gamma globulin fraction are *antibodies* which protect us from infections.
6. Several plasma proteins are involved in the chemical reactions associated with *coagulation (clotting) of blood.*
7. Plasma proteins *transport* hormones and several other small molecules.

WHAT IS A ROUTINE HEMOGRAM?

Hemogram usually refers to a set of commonly performed tests on blood. It is called 'routine' because the hemogram is often ordered on 'every' patient without giving much thought to why it is necessary. The reason for this attitude is that the routine hemogram is simple to do, and frequently turns out to have significance in 'every' patient, sometimes quite unexpectedly. The tests included in the routine hemogram are hemoglobin (Hb), total leukocyte count (TLC), differential leukocyte count (DLC) and erythrocyte sedimentation rate (ESR). For all these tests put together, if done by the conventional inexpensive methods, 5 mL of blood may be collected in a test tube containing EDTA as an anticoagulant. The blood may be drawn from the antecubital vein in a syringe, transferred to the vial or tube, and then shaken to achieve thorough mixing with the anticoagulant. Hb refers to the concentration of hemoglobin in the blood. In healthy adult men it is 155 ± 24 g/L blood.

TLC is normally 7500 ± 3500 per microliter (or cubic mm).

DLC is normally N_{40-75} L_{20-45} M_{2-10} E_{1-6} B_{0-1}. The figures refer to the percentage of neutrophils, lymphocytes, monocytes, eosinophils and basophils respectively.

In the Westergren tube, as well as the Wintrobe tube (which is shorter than the Westergren tube, like its name), the normal rate is 0-10 mm/1st hour for men, and 0-20 mm/1st hour for women. ESR is a nonspecific test in that the ESR is raised in a wide variety of infections and inflammations. Its chief value lies in following the progress of a patient having a chronic disease such as tuberculosis.

RED BLOOD CELLS

Blood is red because it has Red Blood Cells (RBC). RBC are also called erythrocytes. Human RBC are biconcave in shape, and about 7.5 microns in diameter. The number of red blood cells in blood is about 5 million per microliter of blood. One microliter is the same as one cubic millimeter (Fig. 4.2). The RBC count is slightly higher in men than in women. If blood is centrifuged or allowed to stand in a tube, RBC settle down at the bottom of the tube.[1] Then we can see that RBC occupy about 45 percent of the blood volume. We mean the same thing when we say that the packed cell volume (PCV) is 45 percent or the hematocrit is 45 percent.

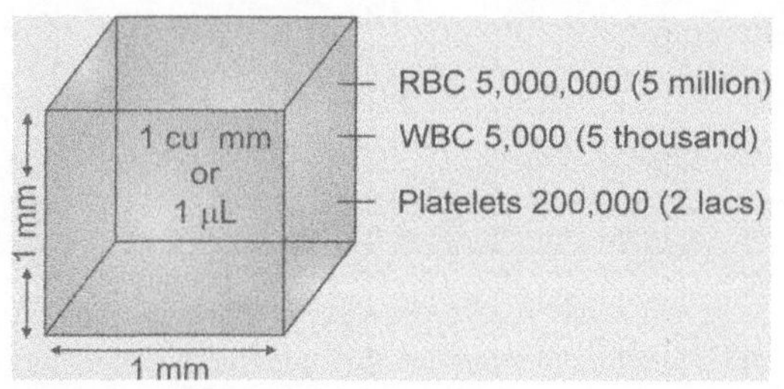

Fig. 4.2 A cube, each side of which is 1 mm, has a volume of 1 cu mm or 1 microliter. This volume of blood has a cell count approximately as indicated

Each RBC is essentially a container having two-thirds water and one-third hemoglobin (Fig. 4.3). Hemoglobin is an iron-containing protein. Hemoglobin

[1]WBC form a thin layer of negligible thickness at the junction of the RBC and plasma. This thin layer is called the buffy coat.

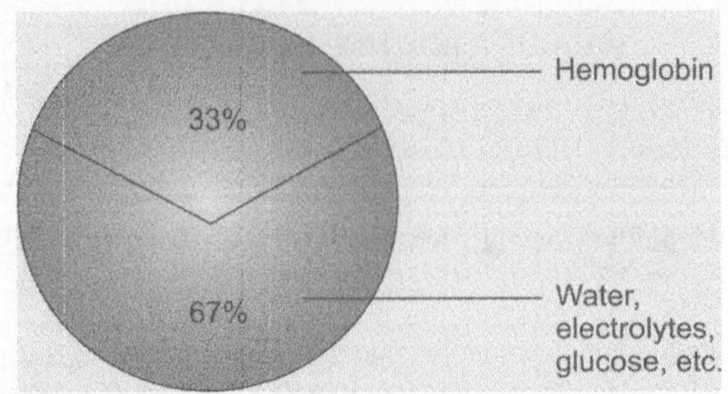

Fig. 4.3 An erythrocyte contains about two-thirds water and one-third hemoglobin. The water has various substances dissolved in it

can bind a large amount of oxygen. Therefore RBC transport oxygen from the lungs to tissues. The concentration of hemoglobin in blood is about 15 g/100 mL blood. From the figures that you already have, it is easy to deduce some more indices (Table 4.2).

The functions of RBC are:

a. To transport oxygen (see above),
b. To transport carbon dioxide (Chapter 6), and
c. To maintain pH of blood. (Chapter 19).

RBC are a dynamic population. Old RBC keep dying and new RBC are produced to replace them. RBC are formed in the bone marrow and are destroyed in the spleen. The average life span of a normal RBC is 120 days. Knowledge of normal physiology of RBC is intimately related to two common abnormal conditions: anemia and jaundice. We shall now discuss these one by one.

ANEMIA

Anemia means a reduction in the concentration of hemoglobin in blood. Since hemoglobin is present in RBC, in anemia usually the RBC count is also low. Since the red cell mass is responsible for the value of the PCV, in anemia usually the PCV is also low.

Hemoglobin transports oxygen to the tissues. Therefore, in anemia, it may not be possible to transport sufficient oxygen to the tissues. This disability becomes particularly prominent during exercise because tissues need more oxygen during exercise. Therefore, an anemic patient gets breathless during exercise. The heart tries to compensate for this handicap by beating more often and more forcefully. Therefore an anemic patient gets palpitation during exercise.

Causes of Anemia

In anemia, the number of RBC is reduced. In order to understand why the RBC population may be reduced, try to think why the population in a village may reduce. It may be because the rate of new additions has gone down, i.e. less children are being born or, it may be because the village is losing people faster. The loss may be because of deaths, or because people from the village have started going to cities. On the same line, anemia may be because less RBC are born, more RBC die, or RBC are lost due to bleeding. The three causes of anemia are discussed briefly below.

Anemia due to Decreased Production of RBC

RBC are produced in the bone marrow. If a person has a nutritional deficiency of some substances required for making RBC, the rate of production of RBC decreases. Common deficiencies of this type are iron deficiency, folic acid deficiency and vitamin B_{12} deficiency.

Table 4.2 Some common hematological indices

Index	*Meaning*	*Value (approx.)*
Mean corpuscular volume (MCV)	Average volume of an RBC	90 cubic microns
Mean corpuscular hemoglobin (MCH)	Average amount of hemoglobin in an RBC	30 picograms*
Mean corpuscular hemoglobin concentration (MCHC)	Amount of hemoglobin per unit volume of RBC mass, expressed as a percentage	33%

*10^{12} picograms = 1 gram

Anemia due to Increased Destruction of RBC

RBC are destroyed in the spleen and a few other organs where macrophages are found. The destruction may be increased if the RBC are defective, as in sickle cell anemia, thalassemia or spherocytosis. The destruction is also increased if the spleen is overactive: the condition is called hypersplenism. The destruction may be increased also if the blood contains antibodies to RBC, certain drugs, or snake venoms.

Anemia due to Abnormal Loss of Blood

Women lose blood regularly during menstrual periods. If the loss is abnormally heavy, it leads to anemia. Other important causes of chronic blood loss are piles, and presence of hookworms in the intestines.

The causes of anemia have been summarized in Figures 4.4A and B. This classification of anemias, based on their causation (etiology), is also called the etiological classification of anemias. A few selected anemias have been discussed in some detail below.

Iron Deficiency Anemia

This is the commonest type of anemia seen in developing countries. It is specially common in pregnant women and children because their iron requirements are high. Anemias resulting from abnormal blood losses are also usually of the iron deficiency type because iron in the diet is unable to replace the losses.

In iron deficiency anemia, RBC are smaller in size than normal. Secondly, these RBC are pale because they contain less hemoglobin. Therefore iron deficiency anemia is microcytic (small cells) and hypochromic (less colored cells).

Iron deficiency anemia should be treated by giving iron tablets. In addition, it is very important to treat the cause of the deficiency, e.g. hookworms, piles or excessive menstrual loss.

Folic Acid and Vitamin B_{12} Deficiency Anemias

Folic acid and vitamin B_{12} are both members of the vitamin B complex group. Both these vitamins are important for maturation of RBC while they are being made in the bone marrow. If there is a deficiency of these vitamins, the 'baby red cells' keep growing but do not divide. Therefore, the red cells are large in size and abnormal looking. Such red cells are called megaloblasts.[2] Therefore folic acid and vitamin B_{12} deficiency anemias are also called megaloblastic anemias. But there are some differences between the two anemias, which have been clarified below.

Folic Acid Deficiency Anemia

Folic acid is found in green vegetables. We usually do not take enough of green vegetables. Therefore folic acid deficiency is quite common, especially in pregnant women. In folic acid deficiency anemia, RBC are large in size and megaloblastic. The anemia can be treated by giving folic acid tablets.

Vitamin B_{12} Deficiency Anemia

Vitamin B_{12} deficiency anemia is also called pernicious anemia.[3] It usually develops because the patient cannot absorb vitamin B_{12} through his intestines. The inability to absorb vitamin B_{12} is because of the absence of a protein called intrinsic factor in the gastric juice. Intrinsic factor is essential for the intestinal absorption of vitamin B_{12}.

Pernicious anemia, or vitamin B_{12} deficiency, is dangerous because of two reasons:

a. It is not only characterized by megaloblastic anemia but also leads to subacute combined degeneration of the spinal cord, which is a serious disorder of the nervous system.
b. If vitamin B_{12} deficiency is treated with folic acid by mistake, the anemia improves but the nervous system continues to deteriorate. Therefore such a mistake is a dangerous mistake.

---

[2] Megaloblast is an RBC which is large in size and abnormally immature in appearance.

[3] Pernicious means dangerous.

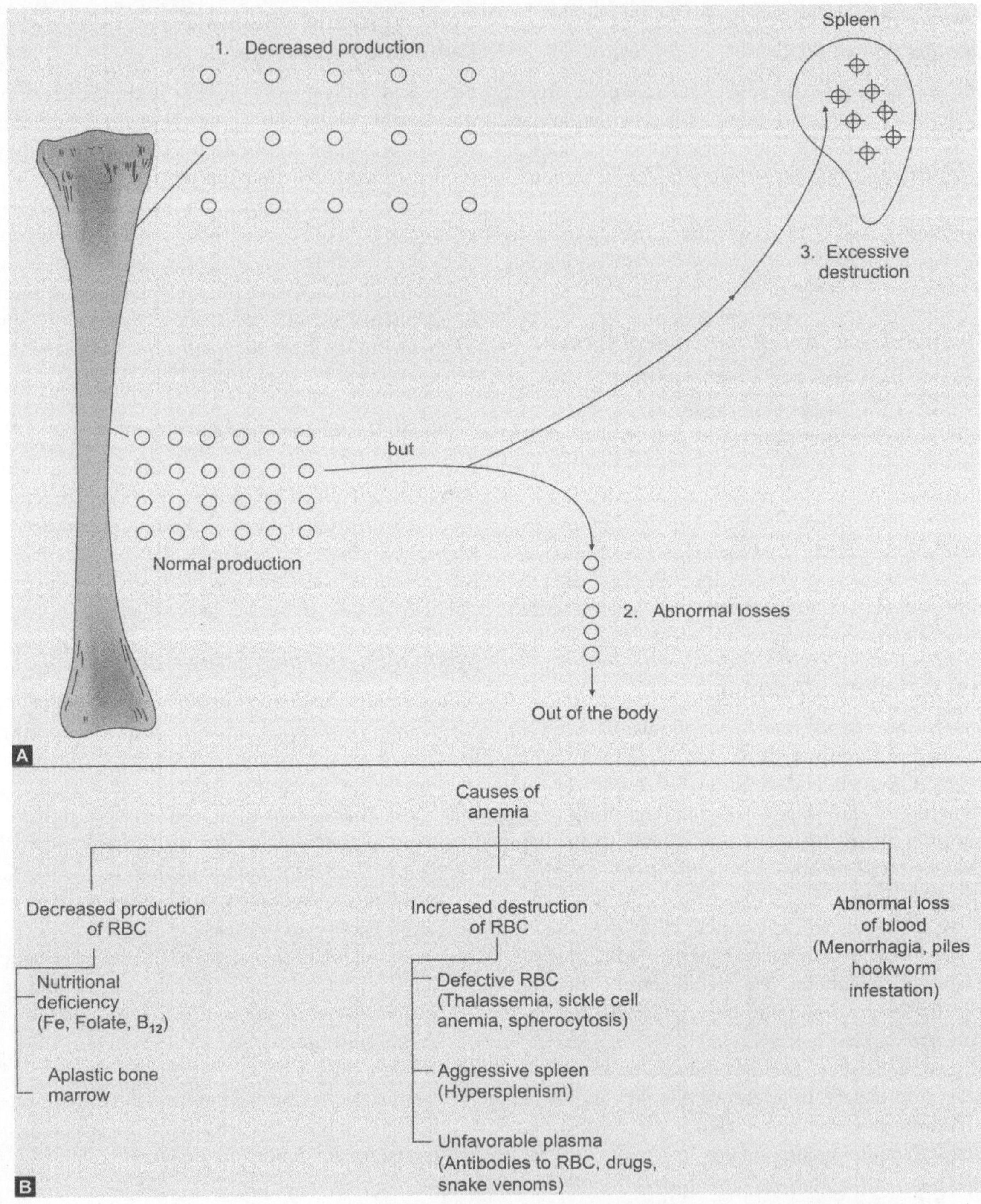

Figs 4.4A and B Causes of anemia. (A) Diagrammatic representation; (B) Etiological classification

Vitamin B_{12} deficiency should be treated by intramuscular injections of vitamin B_{12}. Since vitamin B_{12} can be stored in the liver, one injection of a large enough dose can supply the vitamin for several months.

JAUNDICE

In jaundice, the skin and white portion of the eyes become yellowish. The yellowish color is due to the deposition of bilirubin. Bilirubin is formed as a result of breakdown of RBC.

After the RBC have lived for about 120 days, they grow old and die. They are killed by macrophages in the spleen, liver or lymph nodes. After the RBC die, their hemoglobin is released and chemically decomposed by macrophages (Fig. 4.5). Bilirubin enters the blood and forms a complex with albumin. Albumin is a big molecule, and therefore cannot be filtered by the kidneys. Therefore bilirubin-albumin complex does not pass into the urine. When the bilirubin-albumin complex reaches the liver, the bilirubin part of the complex is taken up by the liver. In the liver, bilirubin combines with glucuronic acid to form bilirubin glucuronide. Bilirubin glucuronide is excreted in the bile. Bile is secreted periodically into the intestine. In the intestine, bilirubin is reduced (opposite of oxidized) by intestinal bacteria. One of the reduced substances is stercobilinogen, which is excreted in the stool. It is responsible for the brownish color of stools. Another reduced substance is urobilinogen, which is excreted into the urine (Fig. 4.6).

The above description applies to normal healthy persons. In some abnormal situations, bilirubin accumulates in the blood, giving rise to jaundice.

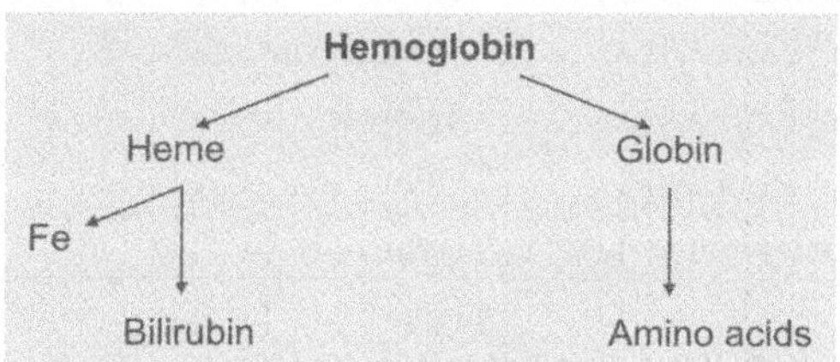

Fig. 4.5 Breakdown of hemoglobin in the macrophages

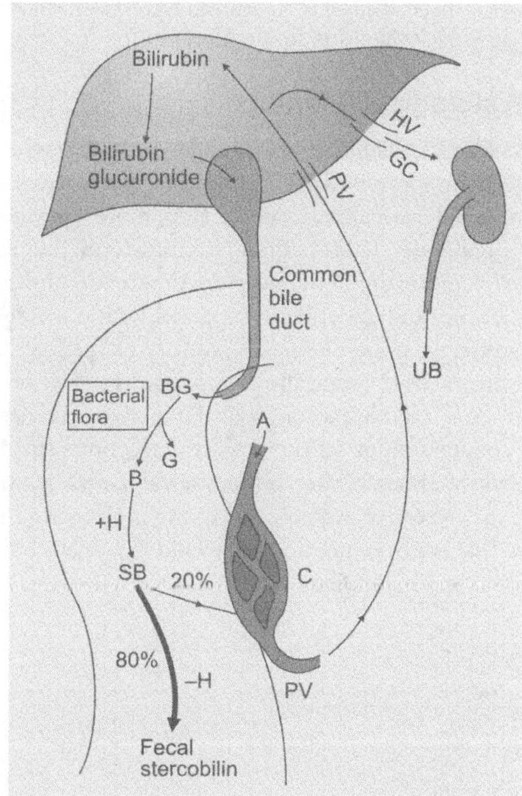

Fig. 4.6 Metabolism and excretion of bilirubin. BG, bilirubin glucuronide; G, glucuronic acid; B, bilirubin; +H, reduction; SB, stercobilinogen; –H, oxidation; A, intestinal artery; C, intestinal mucosal capillary bed; PV, portal veins; HV, hepatic vein; GC, general circulation; UB, urobilinogen

This abnormality can arise in three ways:

a. In hemolytic jaundice, there is excessive destruction of RBC. Excess breakdown of RBC gives rise to excess bilirubin. Excess bilirubin accumulates, and gives rise to jaundice.
b. In hepatic jaundice, the liver cannot conjugate bilirubin adequately. Therefore bilirubin accumulates in the blood, giving rise to jaundice.
c. In obstructive jaundice, bilirubin cannot be excreted into the intestines due to a mechanical block in the common bile duct or some other part of the biliary passages. Therefore it is pushed back from the liver into the blood. Excess bilirubin in the blood gives rise to jaundice.

The three causes of jaundice have been shown diagrammatically in Figure 4.7.

Physiological Jaundice

Physiological jaundice is a mild jaundice which is seen in some newborn children. Therefore, it is also called neonatal jaundice. It is more common in premature babies than in full-term babies. Physiological jaundice appears on the second or third day of life, and generally disappears within a week. It is thought to be due to immaturity of the liver. A newborn's liver, specially a premature newborn's liver, does not have enough of the enzyme required for conjugation of bilirubin with glucuronic acid. It was once thought that physiological jaundice was due to excessive hemolysis in the newborn. But now that is not thought to be a valid explanation for physiological jaundice.

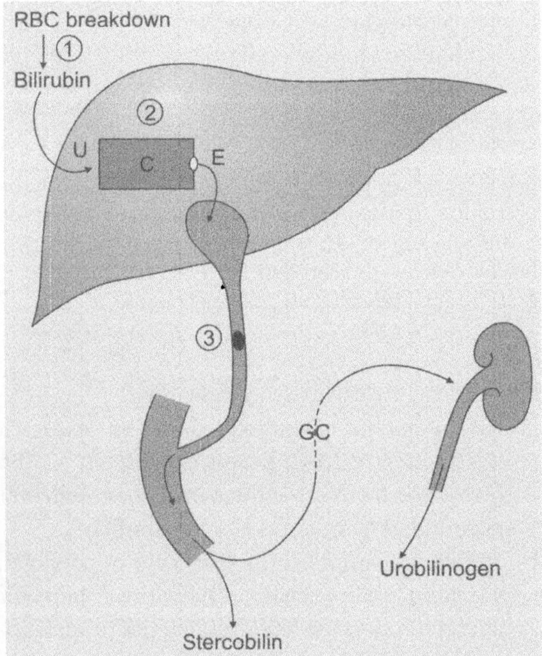

Fig. 4.7 The three causes of jaundice. 1, excessive breakdown of RBC; 2, poor hepatic function; 3, biliary obstruction. U, uptake; C, conjugation; E, excretion; GC, general circulation

WHITE BLOOD CELLS

The white blood cells (WBC) are also called leukocytes. WBC are the soldiers which defend the body against harmful germs and other injurious agents.

Types of WBC

WBC are classified according to their microscopic appearance (Table 4.3). The normal total leukocyte count (TLC) is 4,000-11,000 per microliter of blood. Out of these 50-70 percent are neutrophils (N), 20-40 percent are lymphocytes (L), 2-8 percent are monocytes (M), 1-4 percent are eosinophils (E), and the remaining (less than 1%) are basophils (B). The count expressed in this way is called differential leukocyte count (DLC). A typical normal DLC would be N_{60} L_{30} M_7 E_2 B_1. Clinical hematology laboratories usually refer to neutrophils as polymorphs (P), although strictly speaking, eosinophils and basophils are also polymorphs. Further, these laboratories do not often report the percentage of m onocytes, eosinophils and basophils unless there appears to be something abnormal, or a special request has been made. Therefore the laboratory report of DLC often reads simply somewhat like this: $P_{60}L_{40}$.

Neutrophils

Neutrophils have fine dust-like purple colored granules in the cytoplasm. The nucleus has many

Table 4.3 Types of white blood cells

Cell type	*Features*
I. Granulocytes	Cytoplasm has granules Nucleus is lobed
1. Neutrophils	Granules neutrophilic
2. Eosinophils	Granules eosinophilic
3. Basophils	Granules basophilic
II. Agranulocytes	Cytoplasm has no granules
1. Monocytes	Kidney shaped nucleus
2. Lymphocytes	Large nucleus

lobes, usually three or more. Neutrophils defend us from various infections through the process of phagocytosis.

Neutrophil count increases in infections (specially pyogenic infections) and also in non-infective inflammations. Neutrophil count increases also after tissue destruction, as in burns or myocardial infarction. Immature neutrophils appear in blood in very large numbers in some leukemias.

Neutrophil count may decrease after administration of some drugs which depress the bone marrow.

Eosinophils

Eosinophils have large round red granules in the cytoplasm. The nucleus usually has two or three lobes. Eosinophils help us in killing large parasites which cannot be phagocytosed. Eosinophils also reduce the intensity of allergic reactions. Accordingly, eosinophil count increases in parasitic diseases and allergies. Eosinophil count decreases after administration of adrenal glucocorticoids.

Basophils

Basophils are packed with large purplish black granules in their cytoplasm. The granules are so many that they may hide the nucleus. The nucleus has two or three lobes. Basophils play a role in mediating some allergic reactions. Basophils may also protect us from some parasitic infections, e.g. scabies. Basophil count increases in some allergies and in some leukemias. Basophil count decreases after administration of adrenal glucocorticoids.

Monocytes

Monocytes have a clear cytoplasm and a kidney shaped nucleus. Monocytes migrate out of blood and enter the tissues after staying in blood vessels for about three days. In the tissues, monocytes turn into macrophages. Macrophages protect us from various infections by phagocytosis. Thus monocytes are a part of the mononuclear phagocytic system (MPS), previously called the reticuloendothelial system (RES).

Monocyte count increases in some infections such as tuberculosis and syphilis, and also in some leukemias. Monocyte count decreases after administration of drugs which depress the bone marrow.

Lymphocytes

Lymphocytes have a large round nucleus which occupies almost the entire cell. There is very little cytoplasm, and it is clear, i.e. without any granules.

Lymphocytes defend us against various infections through immune responses. Immune mechanisms have been discussed in some detail below.

Lymphocyte count increases in a variety of viral infections, and in some leukemias. Lymphocyte count decreases whenever the bone marrow is depressed, as by radiation or after administration of some drugs.

IMMUNE MECHANISMS

We have seen above that all types of white blood cells are involved in defending us against infections and other harmful agents. Many of these defence mechanisms are together called the immune mechanisms. Immune mechanisms are of two types: innate and acquired.

Innate Immunity

Innate immunity is always within us because we are born with it. It consists of mechanisms which are useful against a variety of infections but not specific for any particular infection. The most important mechanism of innate immunity is phagocytosis.

Phagocytosis

Phagocytosis, literally, means eating by a cell. A cell, called a phagocyte, eats the germ or injurious agent. The process resembles the way in which an ameba eats.

Blood has two types of phagocytes: neutrophils and monocytes. But phagocytosis takes place in tissues. Neutrophils move out of blood vessels into tissues whenever required for phagocytosis. Monocytes move out of blood vessels into tissues regularly after circulating in the blood stream for about three days. In the tissues, monocytes change into **macrophages** or **histiocytes.** Both these types of cells are tissue phagocytes.

The process of phagocytosis involves several steps (Fig. 4.8). First, the phagocyte throws pseudopodia around the germ or particle to be eaten. Then, the pseudopodia join to enclose the germ in a vacuole. The vacuole is called a phagosome. The phagosome fuses with lysosomes in the cytoplasm. Lysosomes contain various digestive enzymes. Fusion of the phagosome and lysosome results in formation of phagolysosome. In the phagolysosome, the lysosomal digestive enzymes act on the germ or particle which has been eaten. The enzymes break down complex chemicals into simpler compounds. By this process of chemical breakdown, the germ is killed and the particle is disintegrated. The residue is generally thrown out of the phagocyte by a process called exocytosis.

Acquired Immunity

Acquired immunity develops during life as a result of exposure to infectious organisms. This type of immunity acts only against those infectious organisms to which the person has been exposed. For example, the immunity which develops after the measles infection acts only against the measles virus. Therefore this type of immunity is also called specific acquired immunity. Specific acquired immunity is further divided into two types: humoral immunity and cell mediated immunity. Humoral immunity expresses itself by producing antibodies. Cell mediated immunity expresses itself by producing sensitized lymphocytes. Before going into the details of the two types of acquired immunity, it will be better to learn something about the different types of lymphocytes.

T and B Lymphocytes

Like all other blood cells, lymphocytes are also produced in the bone marrow. But the lymphocytes initially produced in the bone marrow are relatively undifferentiated or immature. Further differentiation of lymphocytes takes place either in the bone marrow itself or in the thymus. Differentiation in the bone marrow produces B lymphocytes. Differentiation in the thymus produces T lymphocytes. The two places where differentiation takes place, i.e. bone

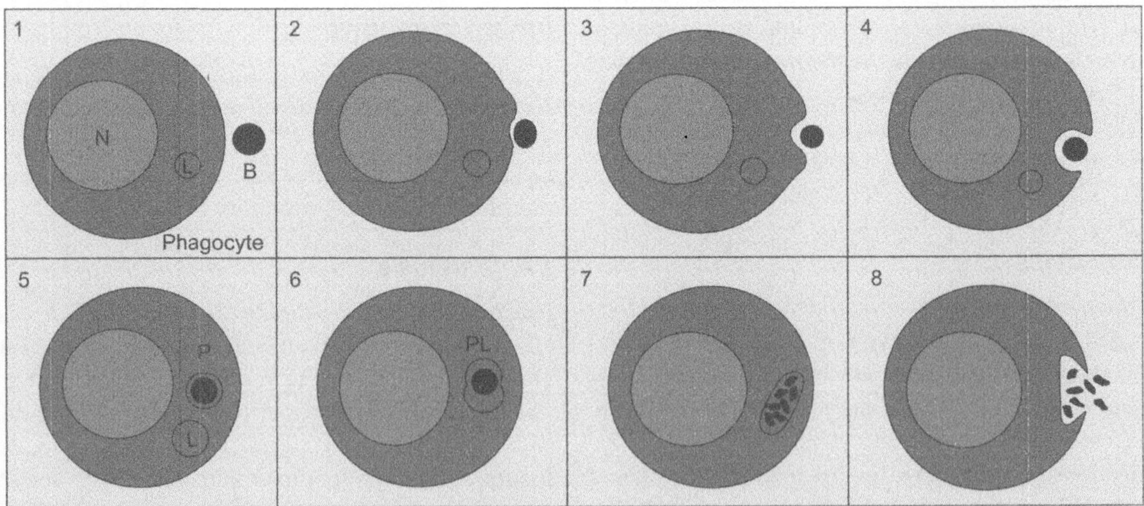

Fig. 4.8 Phagocytosis. 1, Bacterium near the phagocyte; 2-4, Phagocyte throws pseudopodia around the bacterium; 5, Formation of phagosome; 6, Formation of phagolysosome; 7, Digestion of contents of the phagolysosome; 8, Exocytosis. N, nucleus; L, lysosome; B, bacterium; P, phagosome; PL, phagolysosome

marrow and thymus, are called primary lymphoid organs. After undergoing differentiation, T and B cells enter the circulation and settle in lymph nodes, spleen, gastrointestinal tract and respiratory tract. Lymphoid structures of lymph nodes, spleen, gut and respiratory tract are called secondary lymphoid organs. Infectious organisms which enter the body are usually trapped by one of the secondary lymphoid organs. The secondary lymphoid organs respond to the infectious organism by an immune response. The immune response may be of the humoral or cell mediated type.

Humoral Immunity

Humoral immunity is expressed through antibodies. Antibodies are produced in response to antigens. When an infectious organism enters the body, a part of it may act as an antigen. All antigens are proteins. For example, some protein present in the cell wall of bacteria may act as an antigen. The antigen is processed by macrophages, and presented to lymphocytes. After a series of complex steps, a few B lymphocytes get selected (Fig. 4.9). These B lymphocytes are the ones which can manufacture antibodies to the particular antigen which has been presented by macrophages.

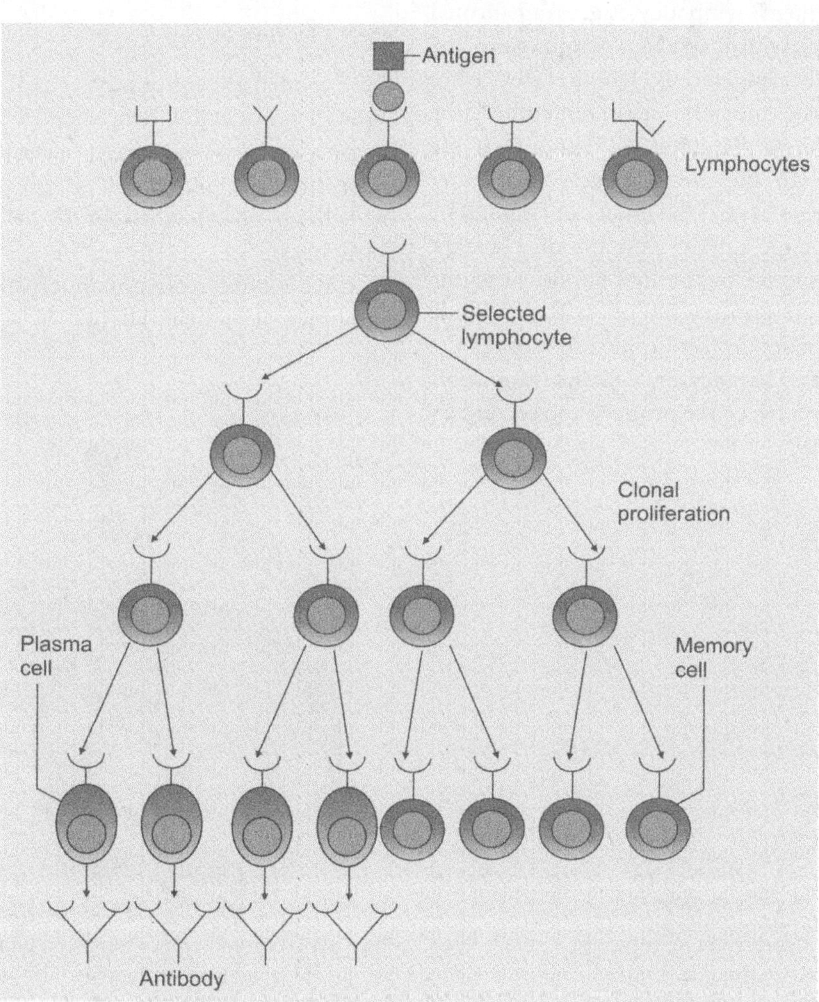

Fig. 4.9 Induction of humoral immunity. For simplicity, the antigen presenting cell has not been shown

Although all B lymphocytes look alike, it seems they differ slightly from each other. Thus there are millions of different types of B lymphocytes in the body. Each type of B lymphocyte can manufacture only a particular antibody. There are only a few B lymphocytes of each type in the body. But when an antigen actually enters the body, the few B lymphocytes which can manufacture an antibody to it get selected. The selected B lymphocytes multiply to produce a large number of daughter cells of exactly the same type which can manufacture the same type of antibody. Thus the capacity of the body to manufacture the antibody of that type increases. Most of the daughter B lymphocytes get transformed into plasma cells, which actually manufacture the antibody. A few daughter B lymphocytes form memory cells. The memory cells 'remember' the previous exposure to the antigen. Therefore if the body is exposed to the same antigen again after some months or even years, the body can respond by manufacturing a large amount of antibodies quickly. The antibody response to the first exposure to the antigen is called the primary response. The antibody response to the second or third exposure is called the secondary response. The memory cells are responsible for the difference between the primary and secondary response (Fig. 4.10).

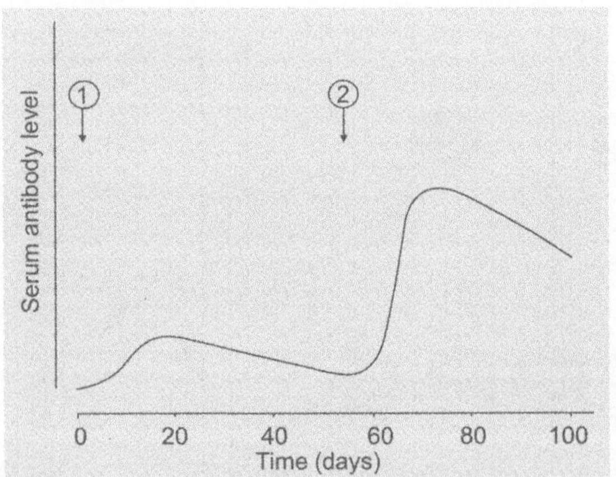

Fig. 4.10 The secondary immune response is much faster and much more intense than the primary response. 1, first exposure to antigen; 2, second exposure

Antibodies help in fighting infections primarily by helping phagocytosis. Infectious organisms get coated by a plasma protein, called complement. Antibodies have three sites of attachment. One of these is specific for some protein (antigen) belonging to the germ. That is why one antibody works against one germ only. The second site of attachment is for the complement. The third site of attachment is for the phagocyte. By using the three sites of attachment, the antibody acts as a bridge between the germ and the phagocyte (Fig. 4.11). In this way the germ and the phagocyte are brought very close to each other. Then the phagocyte can easily eat the germ.

Cell Mediated Immunity

Cell mediated immunity (CMI) is expressed through sensitized T lymphocytes. The sensitized T lymphocytes act specifically against one infectious organism. The sensitized lymphocytes act either by helping phagocytosis or by releasing cytotoxic substances.

CMI is induced in a manner similar to humoral immunity. It is believed that a large variety of T

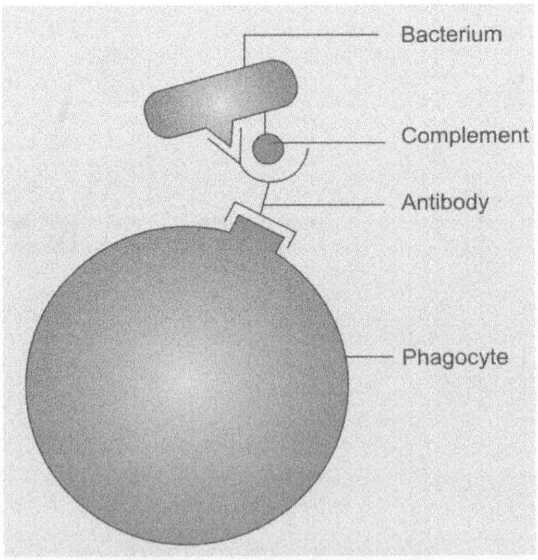

Fig. 4.11 Diagrammatic representation of one of the modes of action of antibodies. The antibody molecule facilitates phagocytosis by acting as a bridge between the germ (bacterium) and the phagocyte

lymphocytes already exist in the body. Exposure to an antigen or the surface of infected cells helps select the appropriate T lymphocytes. The selected T lymphocytes undergo repeated cell division, and finally differentiate into helper T lymphocytes, cytotoxic T lymphocytes and memory cells. Helper T lymphocytes help the phagocytes in digesting the infectious organism. Helper T lymphocytes also release lymphokines which attract phagocytes to the site of infection. Cytotoxic T lymphocytes kill the cells which have the infectious organism within them. In this way the germ is killed, although the infected cell also dies along with the germ. CMI is useful for organisms which produce disease by entering the cells of our body. Memory cells help in making the secondary response better and faster than the primary immune response.

Vaccines

Vaccines protect us from infections by stimulating immune mechanisms. Vaccines are based on the following principles:

1. The secondary immune response is more effective in protecting us from disease than the primary immune response. Therefore, the vaccine is used for inducing the primary immune response without producing disease. When the infectious organism actually enters the body, it gives rise to the secondary immune response. The secondary response is so good that the infectious organism fails to produce disease (Fig. 4.12).
2. It is possible for the vaccine to induce the primary immune response without producing disease because only the antigen is enough for inducing the immune response. The antigen may be introduced into the body without producing disease in one of the following ways:
    a. *Killing the germ and then injecting it:* The dead germ has the antigen but cannot produce disease. Such vaccines are called killed vaccines.
    b. *Attenuating the germ:* An attenuated germ is alive but loses its pathogenicity without losing its antigenicity. Such vaccines are called attenuated vaccines.
    c. *Injecting a related germ:* Some germs similar to the disease-producing germ have the same antigen but do not produce disease. For example, cowpox virus does not produce disease in human beings. But its antigen gives rise to the same antibody in human beings as the samllpox virus. Therefore injecting cowpox virus can protect human beings from smallpox infection later on.
    d. *Injecting a toxoid:* Some germs produce disease by means of a harmful protein called toxin. The body responds to the toxin by producing an antibody called antitoxin. It is sometimes possible to alter the toxin chemically so that it is no longer harmful but is still antigenic. The modified toxin, which is harmless, is called toxoid. The toxoid may be used as a vaccine to produce the primary immune response. After that if the person is exposed to the toxin, the secondary immune response will protect the person against the harmful effects of the toxin. Tetanus toxoid is a good example of this type of vaccine.
    e. *Injecting the purified antigen:* These are vaccines of the future. By modern biotechnology, it is possible to get large quantities of a purified antigen. Injecting only the antigenic protein of a germ gives rise to the immune response without the possibility of ill effects due to other components of the vaccine.

PLATELETS

Platelets are small, irregularly shaped blood cells. They are shiny to look at, and sticky in their behavior. They stick to each other as well as to any rough or injured surface. The normal platelet count is 150,000 to 400,000 per microliter of blood. Platelets are important for prevention of bleeding. Whenever there is an injury which bleeds, platelets collect there. Platelets release serotonin, which constricts blood vessels. Constriction (narrowing) of blood vessels helps in stopping bleeding. Platelets also form a loose

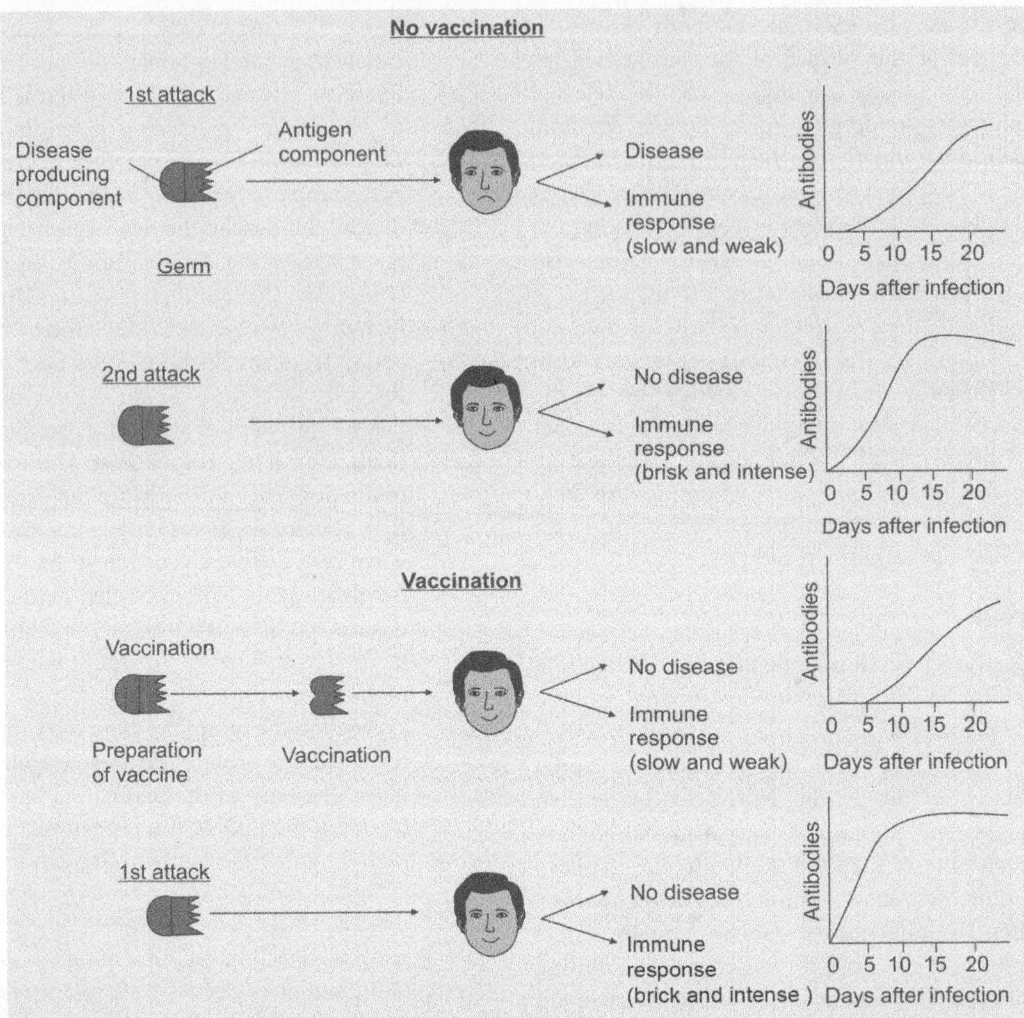

Fig. 4.12 Principle of vaccination. In the absence of vaccination, the first infection produces disease but the second infection does not, because of the efficacy of the secondary immune response. Vaccine acts like the first infection but does not produce disease. After vaccination, the first infection itself evokes the secondary immune response, and therefore fails to produce disease. (Reproduced from Bijlani RL, Manchanda SK. The Human Machine: How to prevent breakdowns. New Delhi: National Book Trust, India, Revised edition, 1999, Fig. 32, p. 96)

plug, which helps in stopping bleeding. Platelets also contribute to clotting (coagulation) of blood. Then platelets bring about retraction of the blood clot. Retraction makes the clot firm. The firm clot prevents bleeding. In this way platelets make many contributions to prevention of bleeding.

COAGULATION

Coagulation is the process by which the blood, which is normally liquid, gets converted into a solid clot. The process of coagulation helps in stopping bleeding from an injury. Coagulation is the end result of a long series of chemical reactions. But the most fundamental reactions are as given below:

$$\text{Prothrombin} \xrightarrow{\text{Prothrombinase}} \text{Thrombin}$$

$$\text{Fibrinogen} \xrightarrow{\text{Thrombin}} \text{Fibrin}$$

Prothrombin and fibrinogen are plasma proteins which are always present in the plasma. Therefore the process of coagulation begins whenever prothrombinase (also called thromboplastin) is produced. Prothrombinase can be produced by two different mechanisms: one requiring only components (called factors) present in the blood (intrinsic system), and the other requiring some components present in the blood and some released from injured tissues (extrinsic system). The reactions involved in the two systems have been shown in Figure 4.13.

Dissolution of the Clot

When healing has progressed to a stage when the clot is no longer necessary, the clot dissolves. Dissolution of the clot is brought about by an enzyme, fibrinolysin (also called plasmin). Fibrinolysin exists in the plasma as a precursor, profibrinolysin (Plasminogen). Activation of profibrinolysin begins at the same time as clotting. But since fibrinolysis is a much slower process than clotting, the clot stays for sufficient time to prevent bleeding.

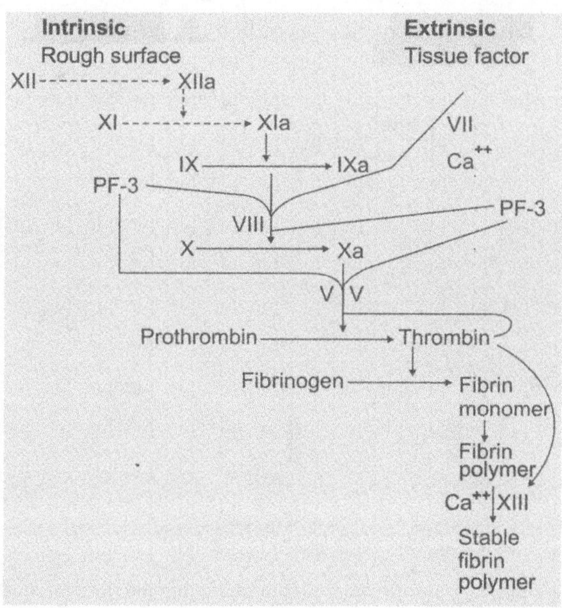

Fig. 4.13 The reactions involved in intrinsic and extrinsic systems of coagulation

Vitamin K and Coagulation

Vitamin K is required as a cofactor for the synthesis of prothrombin in the liver. Therefore deficiency of vitamin K may lead to abnormal bleeding. Vitamin K deficiency may be due to inadequate consumption of green leafy vegetables. But more commonly, vitamin K deficiency is secondary to one of the following:

a. *Malabsorption:* If fat is poorly absorbed, fat soluble vitamins like vitamin K are also poorly absorbed.
b. *Bile duct obstruction:* It also leads to fat malabsorption.
c. *Antibiotics:* They kill the intestinal bacteria which manufacture vitamin K for us.

Anticoagulants

Anticoagulants are substances which prevent coagulation. As seen in Figure 4.13, calcium ions are required at many steps in the process of coagulation. Therefore substances which bind calcium ions act as anticoagulants. Some common anticoagulants, which bind calcium ions, are sodium citrate, potassium oxalate and ethylene diamine tetra-acetate (EDTA). Another common anticoagulant is heparin. Heparin has antithrombin activity, and hence prevents coagulation.

Hemophilia

Hemophilia is an inherited disease in which there is a deficiency of the coagulation factor VIII. The basic abnormality is a defective sex chromosome X. It is a recessive abnormality. Therefore, if a male inherits a defective X chromosome, he suffers from the disease. But if a female inherits a defective X chromosome, the other normal X chromosome protects her from the disease. Therefore such a female acts as a carrier of the disease (Fig. 4.14). Deficiency of coagulation

HOW NOT TO BREAK THE BLOOD

'Sample hemolyzed' is a fairly frequent report from the laboratory. It means wastage of considerable effort and expense, and inconvenience and sometimes even harm to the patient. Hemolysis can be generally avoided by taking the following precautions:

1. The tourniquet around the arm should not be very tight.
2. The puncture should be made only after the spirit used for cleaning the skin has dried up.
3. Blood should be drawn into the syringe slowly and steadily.
4. Blood should be expelled from the syringe after removing the needle. Blood should be expelled slowly, with the nozzle of the syringe touching the side of the tube or vial.
5. Excess of anticoagulant should be avoided. The recommended amounts of anticoagulant are:
   Heparin: 2 mg/10 mL blood
   EDTA: 10-20 mg/10 mL blood
   Potassium oxalate: 20-30 mg/10 mL blood
   Sodium fluoride: 100 mg/10 mL blood
   Potassium oxalate + sodium fluoride: 30 mg/10 mL blood
   (Oxalate/fluoride = 3/1)
   Sodium fluoride + sodium EDTA: 30 mg/10 mL blood
   (Fluoride/EDTA = 2/1)
6. Mix blood with the anticoagulant *gently*.

factor VIII leads to prolonged coagulation time. Therefore if the patient gets an injury, he bleeds much more than a normal person. Minor injuries which go unnoticed in a normal person also lead to bleeding in a patient having hemophilia. The abnormal bleeding may be under the skin or in joints. These patients need repeated blood transfusions for making up the blood lost in bleeding. The blood transfused should be fresh because factor VIII is lost rapidly on storage. A better alternative is to give a factor VIII concentrate, if available.

HEMOPOIESIS

Hemopoiesis means formation of blood cells. Accordingly, erythropoiesis means formation of red blood cells, leukopoiesis means formation of white blood cells, granulopoiesis means formation of granulocytes and thrombopoiesis means formation of platelets. All blood cells are formed in the adult in the bone marrow of a few bones, viz. sternum, ribs, vertebrae, pelvis, and skull. Therefore, if a sample of bone marrow is required for diagnostic purposes, it is usually obtained from either the sternum or the iliac crest (part of the pelvis).

The general principles of hemopoiesis are:

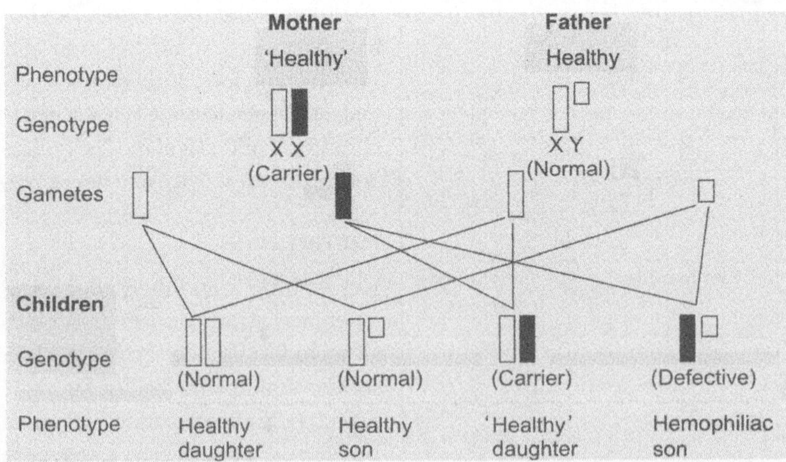

Fig. 4.14 The inheritance of hemophilia. Some females carry the gene for hemophilia. If such a carrier female gets married to a normal male, their child has a 50% chance of being a hemophiliac if it is a son, and a 50% chance of being a carrier if it is a daughter

1. All blood cells arise from a common precursor cell type, called the totipotent hemopoietic stem cell (THSC).
2. Mitotic division of the THSC gives rise to stem cells which are committed to form a particular type of blood cell, e.g. RBC or granulocyte or lymphocyte.
3. The committed stem cells also undergo repeated mitosis. Successive divisions give rise to cells which are better differentiated but poor at cell division.
4. When finally fully differentiated blood cells are formed, they are released into the general circulation.

Some stages in the formation of RBC, WBC and platelets have been shown in Plates 2B, 3A and 3B.

Regulation of Erythropoiesis

Erythropoiesis keeps pace with breakdown of RBC so that the number of RBC in circulation is nearly constant. The rate of erythropoiesis also keeps pace with the requirements. For example, after bleeding, the rate of erythropoiesis is increased. Also, on exposure to hypoxia, the need for blood to carry oxygen is increased, and accordingly erythropoiesis is stimulated. The common factor in all situations in which erythropoiesis is stimulated is tissue hypoxia. Tissue hypoxia stimulates the secretion of erythropoietin from the kidneys. Erythropoietin then stimulates erythropoiesis in the bone marrow.

BLOOD GROUPS

It is common knowledge that blood of one person cannot be transfused into another indiscriminately. Some tests are necessary to determine whether the bloods of the donor and the recipient would 'agree'. The basis of these tests lies in blood groups. The first step in matching the bloods of the donor and the recipient is to type both bloods in terms of the ABO and the Rh systems. The second step is cross matching.

ABO System

ABO system of blood grouping is based on the presence or absence of two antigens, A and B, on the surface of the RBC. If an antigen is present on the surface of RBC, the RBC clump (or agglutinate) in the presence of the corresponding antibody. Antigen-antibody reaction damages the RBC. But this damage does not normally occur because *if an antigen is present on the surface of RBC, the corresponding antibody is absent in the plasma. Conversely, if an antigen is absent from the surface of RBC, the corresponding antibody is present* (Fig. 4.15). These facts are known as Landsteiner's law.

Inheritance of ABO Blood Groups

Blood groups are genetically determined. A person with blood group A may be genetically AA or AO. If he is AA, he can pass on only the gene for group A to his children. If he is AO, he will pass on the gene for group A to some, and for group O to the other children. These genes are passed on to children in this manner by the mother as well as father. Inheritancce of blood groups may be further understood from Tables 4.4 and 4.5.

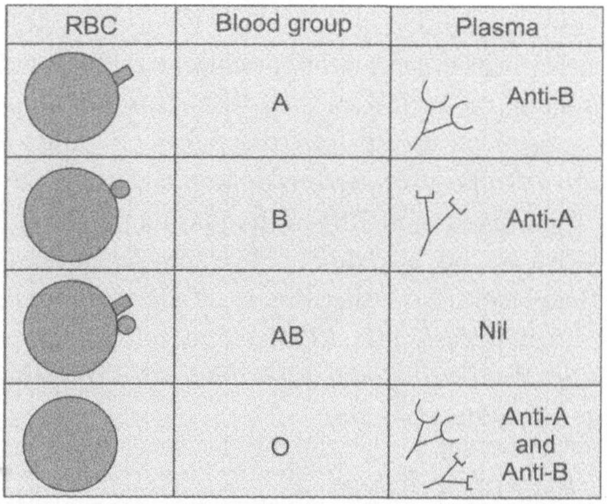

RBC	Blood group	Plasma
	A	Anti-B
	B	Anti-A
	AB	Nil
	O	Anti-A and Anti-B

Fig. 4.15 Blood groups are based on antigenic substances present on the red cell surface. Note that the plasma has antibodies to the antigen (s) which are not present on the individual's red cells

Table 4.4 Blood group phenotypes, corresponding genotypes and types of gametes produced

Blood group (Phenotype)	*Genetic make up (Genotype)*	*Gene passed on to children (Gametes)*
A	AA	All A
A	AO	50% A, 50% O
B	BB	All B
B	BO	50% B, 50% O
AB	AB	50% A, 50% B
O	OO	All O

Table 4.5 Determination of blood group by the genes received from parents

Received from one parent	*Received from the other parent*	*Blood group (Phenotype)*
A	A	A
A	O	A
B	B	B
B	O	B
A	B	AB
O	O	O

Rh System

Rh antigen is different from A or B antigens. About 85 percent of the human population has Rh antigen present on the surface of their RBC. If the RBC have Rh antigen on the surface, the person is called Rh positive. Rh positive persons do not have antibody to the Rh antigen (anti-Rh) in the plasma. Further, Rh negative persons also do not have anti-Rh antibodies in the plasma. Note that this is different from what you learnt in case of the ABO system. But Rh negative persons can develop anti-Rh antibodies if transfused with Rh positive blood.

Rh Incompatibility

If an Rh negative individual is given Rh positive blood, the recipient produces anti-Rh antibodies. But it takes 2-4 months for the antibody concentration to become high. By this time, most of the donor cells die (because the life span of an RBC is only about 4 months). Therefore the antibodies cannot react with donor RBC. And, the antibodies cannot react with recipient RBC because they are Rh negative, i.e. they do not have the Rh antigen. Because the anti-Rh antibodies do not react with RBC in the recipient, there is no outward reaction to the transfusion. But the same person may need a blood transfusion again later in life. If the person is again given Rh positive blood, this time the antibody response is better. (Remember! Because of memory cells, secondary immune response is better than the primary response: Fig. 4.10). Therefore the second Rh positive blood transfusion in an Rh negative recipient leads to a mismatched transfusion reaction. Hence an Rh negative person should never be given Rh positive blood.

Special Risk in Rh Negative Girls

In case of Rh negative girls, giving Rh positive blood carries a special risk. If an Rh negative girl becomes pregnant, the fetus may be Rh positive. Some Rh positive RBC of the fetus may enter the mother's circulation. The mother will then form anti-Rh antibodies to the fetal RBC. These antibodies can enter the fetal circulation and damage fetal RBC. But it takes 2-4 months for the antibody concentration to become high. Therefore, by the time the child is delivered, not much damage has been done. But if this mother had received Rh positive blood any time earlier in life, the fetal Rh positive RBC will give rise to the secondary immune response. As a result, the anti-Rh antibodies will appear earlier during pregnancy, and the antibody concentration will be high. Hence fetal RBC may get damaged to a dangerous extent. Such a fetus may be stillborn, or may have severe jaundice. The condition is known as erythroblastosis fetalis. Therefore an Rh negative girl should never be given Rh positive blood.

Blood Transfusion

Blood transfusion is required for replacing blood loss, if the loss is significant. Before the transfusion, the donor's and recipient's blood are matched for compatibility. The matching has two aspects: grouping and cross matching.

Grouping

As seen earlier, the serum of a person of blood group A has antibodies to the antigen B. Such a serum is called anti-B serum. Anti-B serum agglutinates RBC of group B. For grouping, we take three antisera: anti-A, anti-B and anti-Rh serum. The blood to be grouped is diluted in saline. A drop of the diluted blood is brought in contact with each antiserum separately on a tile or a slide. Naked eye examination after a few minutes is usually sufficient to say whether agglutination of RBC has taken place. If the procedure has been done on slides, presence or absence of agglutination may be confirmed under the microscope. The interpretation is quite simple (Table 4.6).

Cross Matching

In cross matching also, the donor's blood is diluted with saline so that we get a suspension of RBC of the donor. The RBC of the donor are brought in contact with plasma or serum of the recipient on a slide. If the RBC of the donor do not agglutinate, the donor's blood is considered compatible with the recipient's blood. If the RBC agglutinate, the donor is considered unsuitable for that recipient.

Table 4.6 Blood grouping

Reaction with			Blood group
Anti-A	Anti-B	Anti-Rh	
+	–	+	A, Rh positive
+	–	–	A, Rh negative
–	+	+	B, Rh positive
–	+	–	B, Rh negative
+	+	+	AB, Rh positive
+	+	–	AB, Rh negative
–	–	+	O, Rh positive
–	–	–	O, Rh negative

+, agglutination; –, no agglutination

Universal Donor and Recipient

As seen above, it is important that there should be no antigen-antibody reaction between the RBC of the donor and the serum of the recipient.

Suppose the donor's blood group is O. Then the donor's RBC have neither antigen A nor antigen B. Therefore these RBC will agglutinate neither in the presence of anti-A nor anti-B. Therefore group 'O' is sometimes called the universal donor group.

Suppose the recipient's blood group is AB. Then the recipient's serum will have neither anti-A nor anti-B. Therefore this serum will not agglutinate RBC of group A or B or AB or O. Therefore group AB is sometimes called the universal recipient group.

But it is not proper to treat any group as the universal donor or recipient because the possibility of Rh incompatibility and incompatibility due to minor antigens still remains. It is always best if the donor's and recipient's blood group is the same, and cross matching has given no agglutination. But in an emergency, if the ideal donor is not available, the concept of universal donor and universal recipient may be used in conjunction with cross matching.

Reactions to a Mismatched Transfusion

If the donor and recipient's blood are incompatible, there is a mismatch reaction. Antibodies in the recipient's plasma damage the donor's RBC (hemolysis). The damaged RBC release their hemoglobin, which may give rise to jaundice. If the hemolysis is more severe, the patient gets an acute transfusion reaction. It is important to be able to recognize a transfusion reaction. The commonest manifestation of a transfusion reaction is fever, with or without chills. Other warning signals are anxiety, flushing, tachycardia and fall in blood pressure. Some patients may also get pulmonary edema, which may manifest as dyspnea and pain in the chest and back. The immediate management of such a reaction consists of the following:

a. Stop the transfusion.
b. Intravenous saline or glucose-saline to maintain blood pressure.
c. Oxygen, if there is a possibility of pulmonary edema.

Table 4.7 Blood collection for some common tests

Test	*Quantity of blood required*	*Anticoagulant*	*Remarks*
Hemogram (Hb, TLC, DLC, ESR)	5 mL	EDTA	
Blood glucose	2 mL	Potassium oxalate and sodium fluoride	Fluoride stops glycolysis in blood cells. May be done on serum.
Blood urea	2 mL	EDTA	Ammonium oxalate should not be used as anti-ant. May be done on serum. Chill blood after collection. Avoid bacterial contamination.
Liver function tests	10 mL	Not required	Done on serum.
Plasma sodium, potassium and chloride	40 microliters*	Heparin	Sodium or potassium salts of heparin should not be used as anticoagulant. Only the lithium salt of heparin is suitable as anticoagulant. May be done on serum without using any anticoagulant.
Blood pH (arterial)**	40 microliters	Heparin	Whole blood preferable to serum or plasma. Seal and chill sample.
Blood gases (Oxygen and carbon dioxide), arterial	40 microliters	Heparin	Whole blood preferable to serum or plasma. Seal and chill sample.
Blood culture	5-7 mL	Dilute blood in 50 mL medium	Sterile precautions important.

*Autoanalyzers can give the hemogram, blood electrolytes, pH and gases with quantities of blood ranging from 40 to 500 microliters. Up to 200 microliters of blood may be collected in a glass capillary tube. Both plain tubes (for serum) and heparinized tubes (for plasma) are available.

**Arterial blood sample may be obtained from the femoral, brachial or radial artery with due precautions.

BEYOND THE ROUTINE HEMOGRAM

Blood tests are among the commonest tests done on patients. This is because blood can reflect hormonal secretion, metabolic changes, functional state of the liver or the kidneys, nutritional level, respiratory function, etc. through changes in concentration of various substances. However, it may not be possible to collect blood for all these tests together because some tests may require serum (i.e. no anticoagulant), some may require a specific anticoagulant, and some may require a special substance to be added (e.g. sodium fluoride, to inhibit glucose metabolism in RBC, if blood glucose is to be determined). In general, except for the hemogram, most tests can be done on plasma or serum. If rapid separation of RBC is very important for the test, plasma is preferable. Otherwise, for most tests, serum is preferable to plasma because hemolysis is more likely if an anticoagulant has been used. The plasma or serum should be separated promptly after blood collection. Plasma or serum may be stored at 4°C up to 24 hours. If a longer delay in analysis is likely, the sample should be stored in a freezer. The quantity of blood required and the mode of collection for some common tests is given in Table 4.7.

d. Send a post-transfusion blood sample of the patient and the bag containing the remaining blood to the blood bank.
e. Send a call to the attending doctor.

Risks of Blood Transfusion

Besides the risk of mismatched transfusion, blood transfusion carries the risk of transmitting infection from the donor to the recipient. The infections which may be transmitted by transfusion include malaria, viral hepatitis, syphilis, and acquired immunodeficiency syndrome (AIDS). The risk can be reduced by accepting blood only from voluntary donors, and by appropriate screening of the donor's blood.

QUESTIONS

1. Why does removal of the stomach (gastrectomy) lead to pernicious anemia?
2. Why is it dangerous to treat vitamin B_{12} deficiency with folic acid?
3. Why is cross matching essential in addition to grouping before transfusing blood?
4. Why do we match only the RBC of the donor and plasma of the recipient during cross matching? Why not match also the RBC of the recipient and the plasma of the donor?
5. What is psychoneuroimmunology?
6. A person whose blood group is 'A Rh +ve' has on the red blood cells antigens A and Rh, and in the plasma:
   A. No antibodies
   B. Anti-A and anti-Rh antibodies
   C. Anti-B antibodies
   D. Anti-B and anti-O antibodies

ANSWERS

1. Pernicious anemia is due to the deficiency of vitamin B_{12}. For absorption of vitamin B_{12} we need the intrinsic factor. Intrinsic factor is secreted by the stomach. Therefore gastrectomy removes the source of intrinsic factor from the body. In the absence of intrinsic factor, vitamin B_{12} cannot be absorbed. That is how gastrectomy leads to vitamin B_{12} deficiency and hence pernicious anemia.
2. It is dangerous because vitamin B_{12} deficiency gives rise to not only anemia but also neurological deficit. Folic acid corrects the anemia of vitamin B_{12} deficiency and therefore gives a false impression that the patient has been cured. Actually, the neurological deficit continues to worsen.
3. Blood grouping is usually confined to the ABO system and Rh system. But incompatibility may arise also due to antigens belonging to other blood group systems, such as P, MNS, Kell, Duffy, Kidd, Lutheran, etc. Cross matching takes care of incompatibility due to these blood group systems also.
4. When blood is transfused, the small volume of plasma of the donor is diluted in the much larger volume of plasma of the recipient. Therefore the concentration (titer) of donor plasma's antibodies falls to a very low level after transfusion. Therefore they are unlikely to damage the recipient's RBC. But the titer of the antibodies in recipient's plasma remains high. Therefore it is important to ensure that the antibodies in recipient's plasma do not damage the donor's RBC.
5. Psychoneuroimmunology (PNI) is a discipline which has grown and developed at a phenomenal rate during the last twenty-five years. As the term suggests, it deals with the link between the mind, the nervous system and the immune system. It has been shown that prolonged mental stress weakens immunity whereas mental relaxation, peace and joy strengthen immunity The effect is mediated by the nervous and endocrine systems. Thus the popular impression that a child catches a cold easily when the exams are near has a scientific basis. The saying that laughter is the best medicine is also now supported by scientific evidence.
6. C.

CHAPTER

5 Cardiovascular System

"No rest that throbbing slave may ask, Forever quivering o'er his task, While far and wide a crimson jet Leaps forth to fill the woven net Which in unnumbered crossing tides, The flood of burning life divides, Then kindling each decaying part Creeps back to find the throbbing heart."

—OLIVER WENDELL HOLMES

Chapter Outline

- The Route of Circulation
- Cardiac Muscle
- Resting Membrane Potential
- Action Potential
- The Cardiac Impulse
- Properties of Cardiac Muscle
- Electrocardiography
- Cardiac Cycle
- Cardiac Output
- Arteries
- Capillaries
- Lymphatics
- Edema
- Veins
- Regulation of Cardiovascular Function
- Coronary Circulation
- Coronary Artery Disease
- Shock

We have all seen blood but not all of us have seen the heart. However, even a lay person knows the importance of the heart. A person who gets a heart 'attack' may die. Why is the heart so important? In the previous chapter we saw that blood transports nutrients and waste products. For performing this function, blood has to travel from one part of the body to the other. Blood travels in tube-like structures called blood vessels. Arteries, veins and capillaries are different types of blood vessels. Blood travels in blood vessels in a cyclic fashion. It goes round and round throughout the body. In order to keep moving, the blood needs a push. This push is provided by the heart. Heart pushes blood out into blood vessels like a pump. Hence the heart and blood vessels form one functional unit. The unit is called cardiovascular system, in which 'cardio' refers to the heart, and 'vascular' to blood vessels.

THE ROUTE OF CIRCULATION

For understanding the path along which blood circulates, we should know something about the heart. The heart has four chambers (Fig. 5.1). The two right-sided chambers are completely separated from the two left-sided chambers by partitions. Each partition is called a **septum**. The interatrial septum separates the right atrium from the left atrium. The interventricular septum separates the right ventricle from the left ventricle. Each atrium opens into the corresponding ventricle through an opening which is guarded by a valve. The valve allows the blood to flow from the atrium into the ventricle, but not in the opposite direction. The valve between the right atrium and right ventricle is called the **tricuspid valve**. The valve between the left atrium and left ventricle is

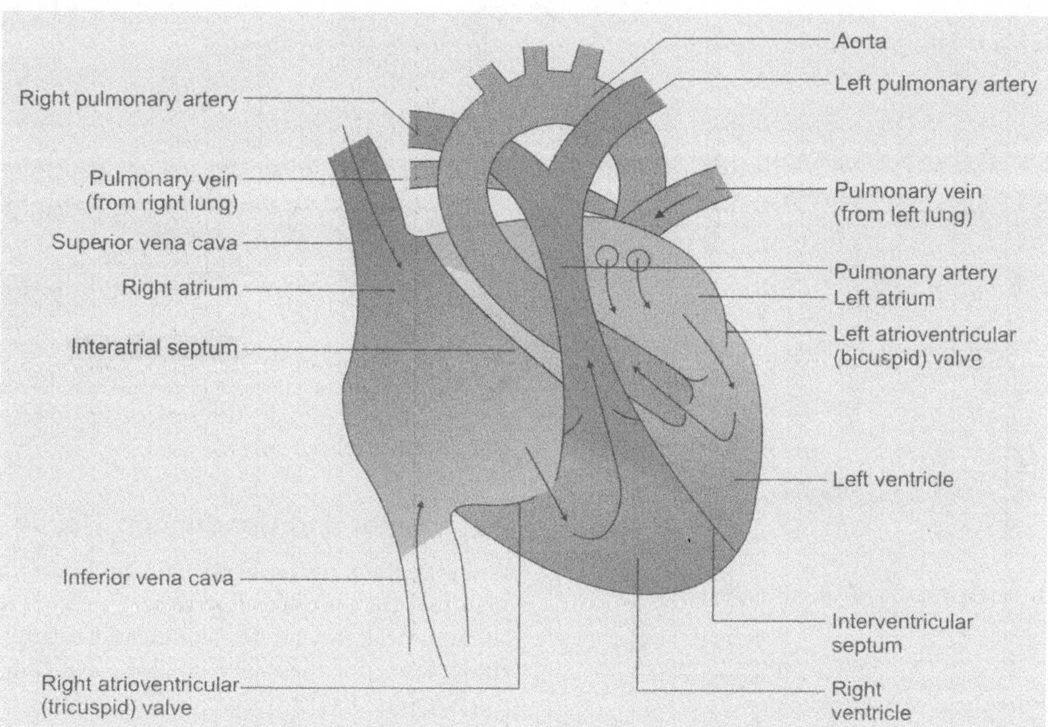

Fig. 5.1 Semi-diagrammatic representation of structure of the heart. Arrows indicate the path of flow of blood. Note the semilunar valves, which have been drawn but not labeled. The right semilunar valve, or pulmonary valve, is between the right ventricle and pulmonary artery. The left semilunar valve, or aortic valve, is between the left ventricle and aorta

called the **mitral valve**. From the right ventricle blood flows into the pulmonary artery. From the left ventricle blood flows into the aorta. These openings are also guarded by valves, called semilunar valves, to prevent blood from flowing in the opposite direction.

We may start with the journey of blood with the right atrium (Fig. 5.2). Blood enters the right atrium from two large veins, the superior vena cava and the inferior vena cava. Superior vena cava brings deoxygenated blood (blood with less oxygen) from upper parts of the body. Inferior vena cava brings deoxygenated blood from lower parts of the body. Thus blood from the whole body (except lungs) returns to the right atrium. This blood has less oxygen because it has given oxygen to the tissues of the body.

From the right atrium, blood goes to the right ventricle. The right ventricle pumps blood into the pulmonary artery.

Pulmonary artery takes blood to the lungs. In lungs oxygen is added to the blood. Oxygenated blood leaves the lungs in pulmonary veins.

Pulmonary veins take blood to the left atrium. From the left atrium, blood goes to the left ventricle. The left ventricle pumps blood into the aorta.

Aorta takes blood to different parts of the body through its branches. The body uses oxygen and nutrients from this blood, and adds to it carbon dioxide and waste products. The deoxygenated blood returns to the right atrium in superior and inferior vena cava. Thus the cycle is completed.

From the above description, note the following:

a. Blood vessels which take blood away from the heart are called **arteries**. Blood vessels which return blood to the heart are called **veins**.
b. The right and left heart act as two distinct but interconnected pumps. The right ventricle

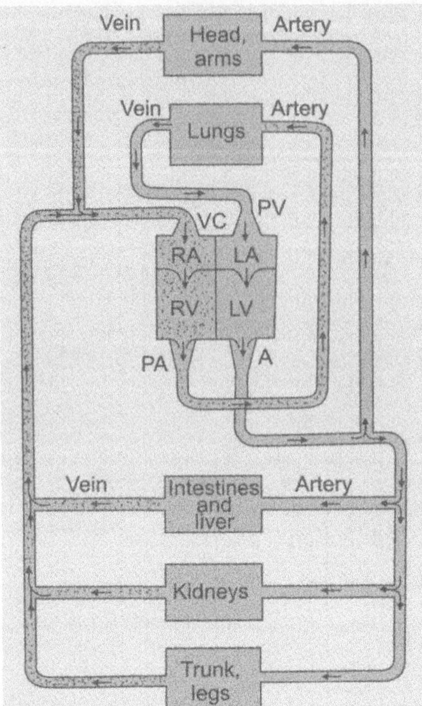

Fig. 5.2 Composite diagram of blood circulation. (Reproduced from Bijlani RL, Manchanda SK. The Human Machine. New Delhi: National Book Trust, India, 1999 Fig. 11, p. 39)

pumps blood to the lungs. The left ventricle pumps blood to all the other parts of the body.

c. Blood pumped by the right ventricle returns to the left atrium. Blood pumped by the left ventricle returns to the right atrium.

CARDIAC MUSCLE

Heart is a muscular organ. Cardiac muscle, when seen under the microscope, shows branched fibers (Fig. 5.3). Cardiac muscle fibers have cross-striations, like the skeletal muscle. At the junction of fibers, there are specialized areas called intercalated discs (Plate 1B). Intercalated discs have an extremely low electrical resistance. Therefore if one cardiac muscle fiber is activated, the activation spreads to the entire muscle mass. This is what we mean when we say that the cardiac muscle is a functional syncytium.

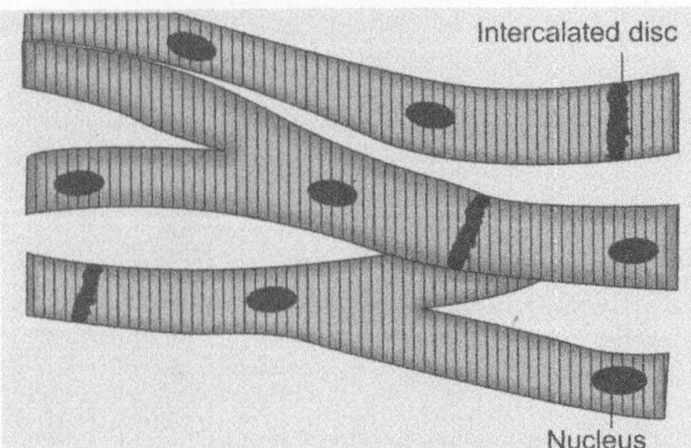

Fig. 5.3 Histological structure of cardiac muscle. Note the cross striations, centrally placed nuclei, branched muscle fibers and intercalated discs

Pacemaker and Conduction Tissue

A few regions of the heart have modified cardiac muscle, which is not well striated. One such region, the sinoatrial (SA) node, is in the right atrium near the opening of the superior vena cava (Fig. 5.4). The SA node has the property of generating regular impulses 'spontaneously' at a rate faster than any other part of the heart. The SA node acts as the pacemaker of the heart, i.e. it determines the rate of the heart. Another similar tissue is situated at the atrioventricular border on the right side of the interatrial septum. It is called the atrioventricular (AV) node. AV node may take over the pacemaker function if SA node fails. AV node continues into the bundle of His. The bundle of His divides into right and left branches in the interventricular septum. The bundle branches divide into a network of Purkinje fibers as they enter the ventricles. The bundle of His and its subdivisions are called the conduction tissue of the heart because they conduct the cardiac impulse (see below).

RESTING MEMBRANE POTENTIAL

Cardiac muscle shows alternate rest and activity. At rest, it shows an electrical potential of about –80 mV across the cell membrane, the outside being positive as compared to the inside (Figs 5.5A and B). This is called resting membrane potential (RMP). RMP is

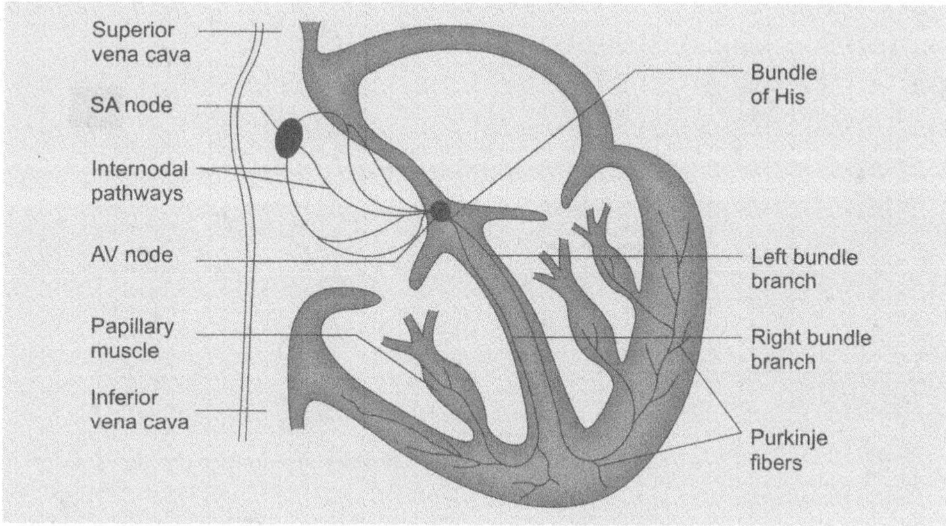

Fig. 5.4 Conduction system of the heart. SA, sinoatrial; AV, atrioventricular

primarily due to the difference in the concentration of certain ions between the inside and the outside of the cell as discussed below.

Potassium

Potassium ion concentration inside the cardiac muscle cell (155 mEq/L) is higher than outside the cell (4 mEq/L). Therefore potassium ions have a tendency to diffuse out of the cell due to the concentration gradient (Fig. 5.6). But potassium is a positively charged ion, and the membrane is positively charged outside as compared to inside the cell. Therefore the tendency of potassium ions to diffuse out of the cell is opposed by the electrical gradient. Finally, an equilibrium is established such that there is no net diffusion of potassium ions. When potassium ions are in equilibrium the membrane potential is called potassium equilibrium potential.

Mathematically, potassium equilibrium potential is given by the Nernst equation as follows:

$$E = -61 \log \frac{[K^+]\text{ inside}}{[K^+]\text{ outside}}$$

$$= -61 \log \frac{155}{4}$$

$$= -61 \log 38.75$$

$$= -61 \times 1.5883$$

$$= -97 \text{ mV}$$

The RMP is very close to the potassium equilibrium potential.

Chloride

Chloride ion concentration outside the cardiac muscle cell (120 mEq/L) is higher than inside the cell (4 mEq/L). Therefore chloride ions have a tendency to diffuse inside the cell due to the concentration gradient (Fig. 5.7). But since chloride ions are negatively charged, their tendency to diffuse inwards is opposed by the electrical gradient. An equilibrium is established at the chloride equilibrium potential, which is also given by the Nernst equation:

$$E = +61 \log \frac{[Cl^-]\text{ inside}}{[Cl^-]\text{ outside}}$$

The equation is slightly different from that for potassium because chloride is a negatively charged ion.

$$E = +61 \log \frac{4}{120}$$

$$= +61 \log 0.033$$

$$= 61 \times (-2 + 0.5185)$$

$$= 61 \times (-1.4815)$$

$$= -90 \text{ mV}$$

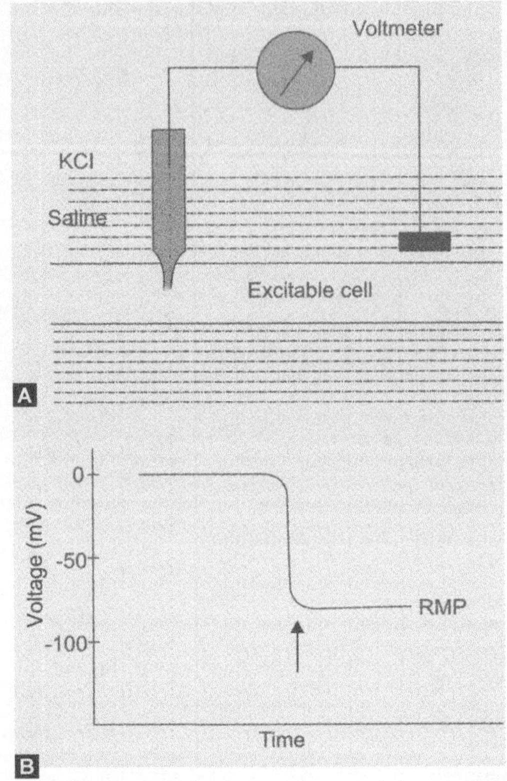

Figs 5.5A and B The resting membrane potential (RMP) may be measured by using an intracellular glass electrode with a tip diameter of less than 1 micron and filled with potassium chloride. (A) Diagrammatic representation of the recording set-up; (B) At the arrow, the intracellular electrode penetrates the cell. The RMP is about –80 mV, being negative on the inside of the excitable cell membrane as compared to the outside

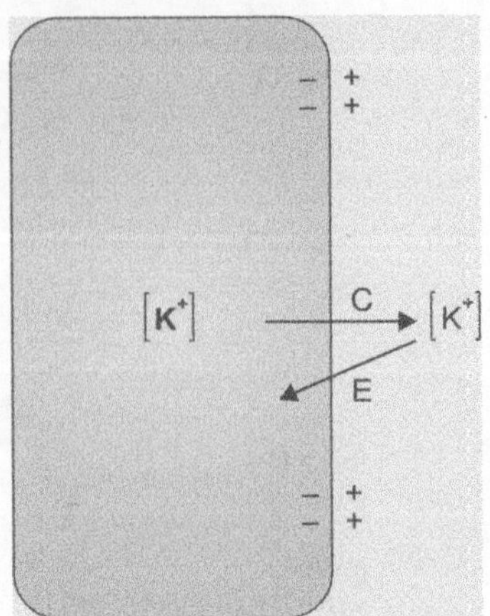

Fig. 5.6 The concentration gradient 'C' favors movement of potassium ions from inside to outside the cell. The electrical gradient 'E' favors movement in the opposite direction. At potassium equilibrium potential, these tendencies are equal

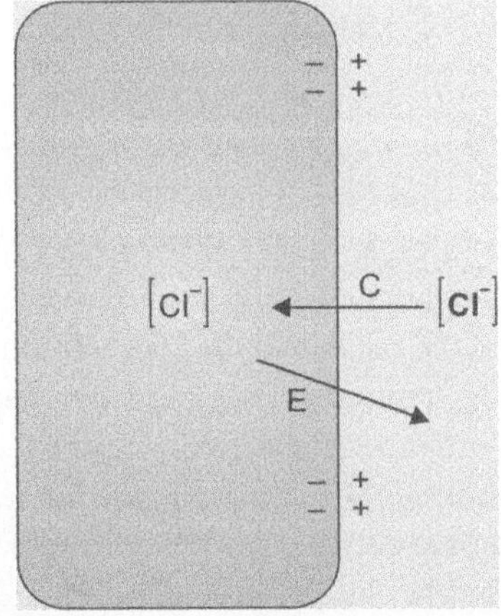

Fig. 5.7 The concentration gradient 'C' favors movement of chloride ions from outside to inside the cell. The electrical gradient 'E' favors movement in the opposite direction. At chloride equilibrium potential, these two tendencies are equal

Thus the RMP is very close also to the chloride equilibrium potential.

Sodium

Sodium ion concentration outside the cardiac muscle cells (145 mEq/L) is higher than inside the cell (12 mEq/L). Therefore sodium ions have a tendency to diffuse inwards due to the concentration *as well as* electrical gradient (Fig. 5.8). This tendency is opposed by an active transport mechanism, called sodium pump, located in the cell membrane. The sodium pump continuously transports sodium ions outwards. However, the sodium pump is successful in maintaining the RMP only because the permeability of the resting cell membrane to sodium ions is low.

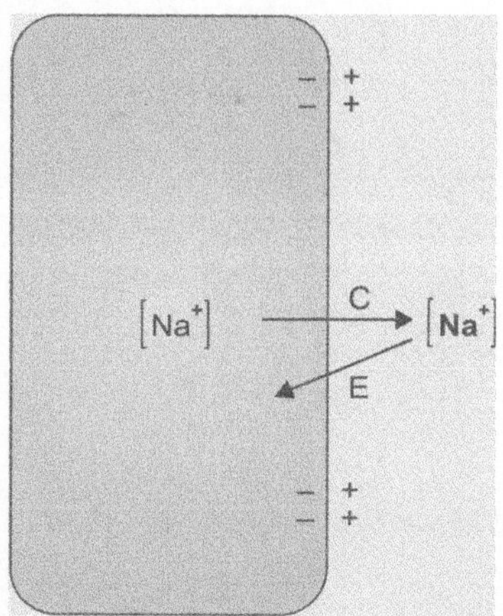

Fig. 5.8 The concentration gradient 'C' as well as the electrical gradient 'E' favor movement of sodium ions from outside to inside the cell. The concentration gradient and electrical potential difference across the membrane are maintained by pumping sodium ions out of the cell by an active (energy-dependent) pump (P)

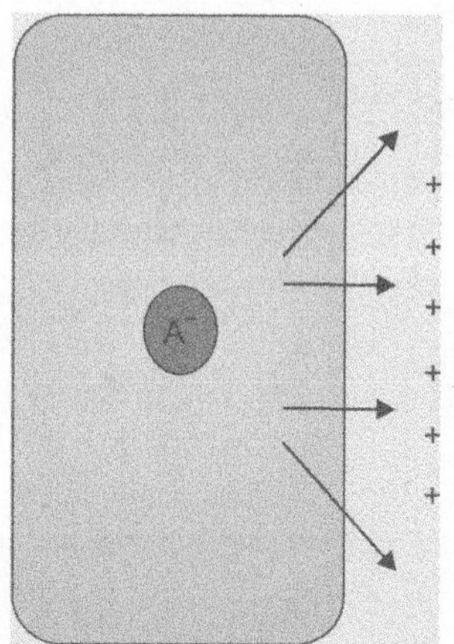

Fig. 5.9 Protein anions are negatively charged and are present only inside the cell. Therefore the concentration as well as electrical gradient favor movement of proteins from inside to outside the cell. But the proteins cannot leave the cell because the cell membrane is impermeable to protein. Hence, protein anions stay inside and maintain the negativity inside the cell

Proteins

Intracellular proteins form negatively charged ions at the intracellular pH. Concentration of proteins is much higher within the cell than outside. In fact, interstitial fluid has only negligible protein. Negatively charged intracellular protein ions play a very crucial role in maintaining the RMP negative on the inside of the membrane. The importance of protein ions lies in that the cell membrane is impermeable to these ions because of their large particle size (Fig. 5.9).

ACTION POTENTIAL

During activity, the membrane potential undergoes a sudden brief change. The change is called action potential. Action potential consists of reversal of polarization, i.e. the cell becomes negative outside and positive inside. But usually the change during action potential is described as depolarization. The terms used in connection with membrane potential have been explained in Figure 5.10.

The genesis of the action potential may be understood in terms of two steps. First the RMP changes towards depolarization. When the depolarization reaches a threshold value, an action potential is fired. An action potential is an all or none change. All or none means that either all the change is there, or none at all. If the change is there, it always has the same duration and magnitude (height).

A few analogies would make the phenomenon clear. Threshold depolarization is like the trigger of a gun. Only when the trigger is pulled beyond a certain point, is a shot fired. The shot is an all or none phenomenon. Every time the shot is fired, it has the same characters. Another analogy: threshold depolarization is like the chain or handle of a water closet. Only when the chain is pulled beyond a certain point, the toilet gets flushed. Flushing of the toilet is an all or none phenomenon.

The action potentials in different parts of the heart have been shown in Figure 5.11.

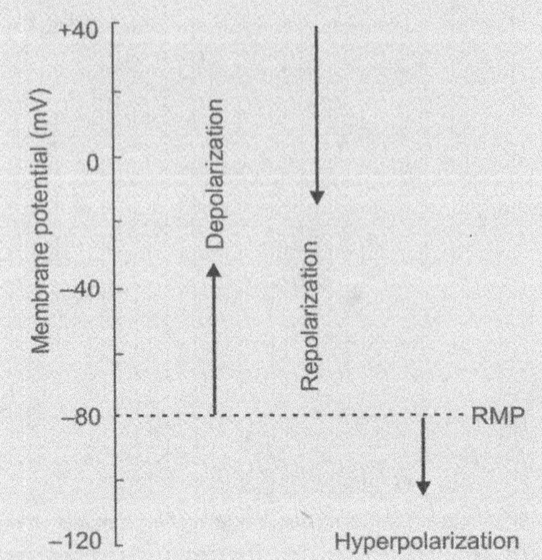

Fig. 5.10 Terms used for describing changes in membrane potential. The charges are named in reference to the resting membrane potential (RMP), indicated here by a dotted line. A change in membrane potential such that the difference between the potential inside and potential outside the cell becomes less is called **depolarization**. In a deplorized cell, the return of membrane potential towards the resting membrane potential is called **repolarization**. A change in membrane potential such that the difference between the potential inside and potential outside the cell becomes greater than at RMP is called **hyperpolarization**

Pacemaker Potential

If you observe the SA node potential in Figure 5.11, you would notice that it has no steady RMP; there is a gradual depolarization during the resting phase. This depolarization is called pacemaker potential or diastolic depolarization. When the depolarization reaches a threshold value, the action potential is fired. The gradual depolarization at rest is apparently spontaneous. Therefore the action potentials are fired rhythmically and spontaneously. That is why the SA node acts as the pacemaker.

Ionic Basis of Action Potential

The sudden depolarization (spike) is due to an increase in the permeability of the cell membrane to sodium ions. Since sodium ions are positively charged, their entry leads to depolarization, and finally reversal of polarization.

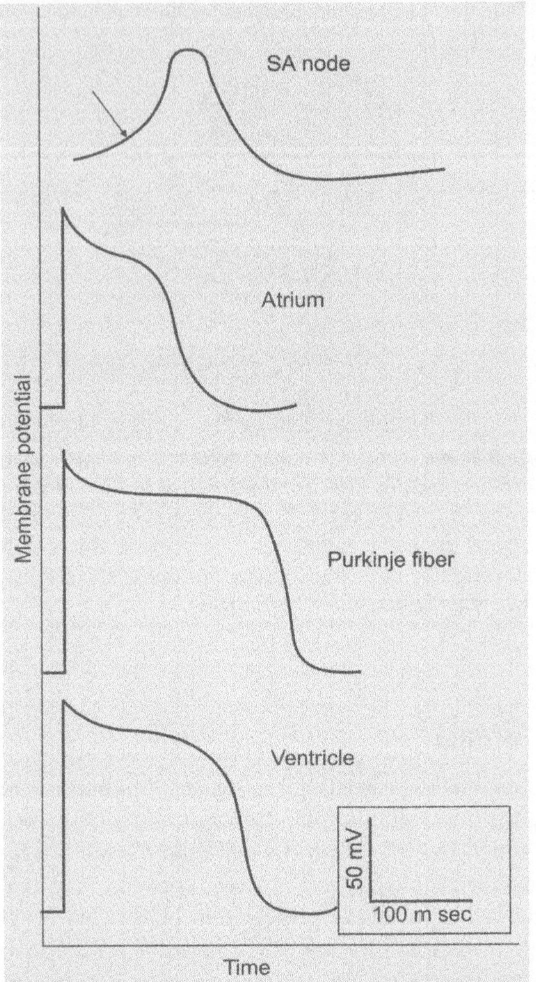

Fig. 5.11 Action potential in different parts of the heart. Note the pacemaker potential (arrow) in the SA node

The sustained depolarization (plateau) is due to increase in the permeability of the membrane to calcium ions. Since calcium ions are positively charged, their effect is similar to that of sodium ions. Thus calcium ions sustain the change which is initiated by sodium ions.

Repolarization is due to an increase in the permeability to potassium. This, together with restoration of sodium and calcium permeability to normal leads to repolarization.

When all permeabilities have returned to resting level, membrane potential stays at the RMP till increase in sodium permeability sparks off the next action potential. But in case of the pacemaker cells, such as SA node cells, the RMP is not steady. As already mentioned, the gradual depolarization in pacemaker cells is called pacemaker potential. Pacemaker potential is correlated with four types of ionic movements, which all contribute to it. First, there is an influx of sodium ions which begins when repolarization has made the membrane potential more negative than −50 mV. This influx is a major contributor to the early part of the pacemaker potential. Second, there is an influx of calcium ions towards the end of pacemaker potential. Besides these two major contributors, two other ionic movements also make some contribution to the pacemaker potential. One is a continuous inward leak of sodium ions. The other is the slowing down of the potassium efflux (outward movement) which brings about repolarization. Slowing down of potassium efflux indirectly helps depolarization during the pacemaker potential.

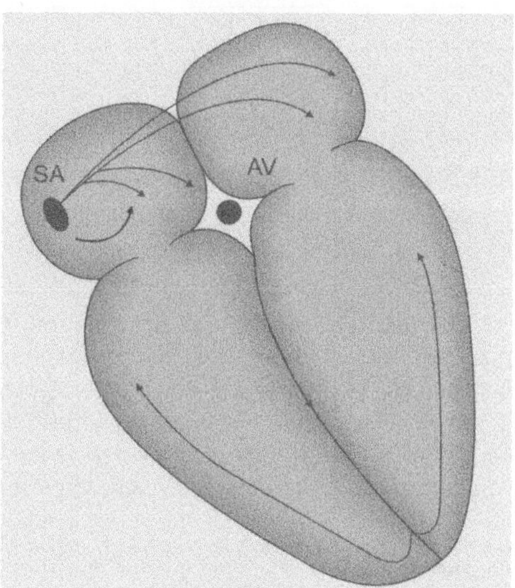

Fig. 5.12 Spread of the cardiac impulse. The impulse is delayed at the AV node by about 0.1 second. SA, sinoatrial node; AV, atrioventricular node

THE CARDIAC IMPULSE

The cardiac impulse originates in the SA node, which generates these impulses rhythmically and 'spontaneously'. The impulse spreads to the atria like 'ripples in a pond'. The spread through the atria is almost 'immediate'. However, when the impulse reaches the AV node, it gets delayed by about 0.1 second. The delay is called AV delay. AV delay is due to very slow conduction through the AV node fibers. After that the impulse is rapidly conducted through the bundle of His, bundle branches, Purkinje fibers, and finally the ventricular muscle fibers (Fig. 5.12).

PROPERTIES OF CARDIAC MUSCLE

Some important properties of cardiac muscle have been summarized below.

Automaticity

The heart does not depend on its nerve supply for its contraction. Nerves only affect the rate and force of contraction of the heart. The ability of the heart to contract even in the absence of activity in its nerves is called automaticity.

Rhythmicity

Some parts of the heart generate rhythmic impulses 'spontaneously'. The ability is best developed in the SA node. The AV node and other parts of the conduction system also have this ability to some extent. But the rate of rhythmic discharge is the highest in the SA node. The rate at which the SA node fires determines the heart rate (pacemaker function). This is so because an impulse originating in the SA node spreads throughout the heart. Before an impulse from the AV node or any other part of the conduction system can initiate cardiac contraction, the next impulse from the SA node is discharged because its rate of firing is the highest (Fig. 5.13).

That is how the rate of firing of the SA node determines the rate at which the heart beats. The SA node is called the pacemaker of the heart because it determines the pace of the heart.

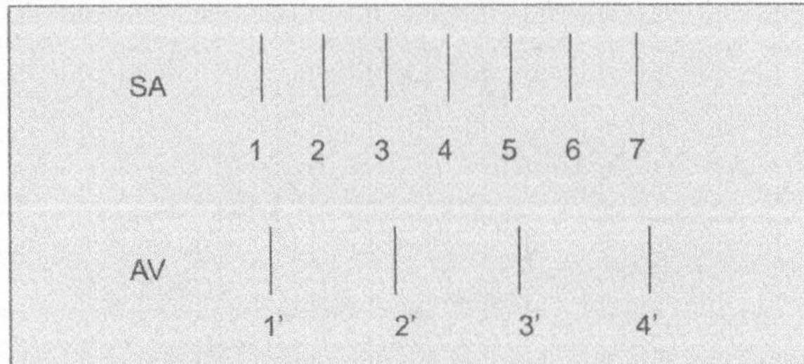

Fig. 5.13 The rate of discharge of impulses is higher in the SA node than in the AV node or any other part of the conduction system. Hence, the SA node impulses precede any potential impulses from other regions. Therefore, only the SA node impulses actually manifest themselves and drive the heart. 1-7, SA node impulses 1'-4', potential AV node impulses

The situation may be understood by imagining a train with two engines. If each of the engines is set for running at different speeds, the speed of the train will be determined by the faster engine. If the faster engine fails, the slower engine will determine the speed of the train (Fig. 5.14). In the same way, if the SA node fails, the heart beats at the slower rate at which the AV node fibers.

Long Refractory Period

Refractory period is the period during which a stimulus fails to give a response. In case of the heart, if a stimulus is given during contraction or first two-thirds of the relaxation period, it gives no response (Figs 5.15A and B). It means that contraction and relaxation of the heart should be over before the next contraction can begin. Therefore cardiac muscle does not give a sustained contraction (tetanus). This is expressed by saying that cardiac muscle cannot be tetanized.

The refractory period of cardiac muscle is much longer than that of skeletal muscle (Chapter 13). The reason is that refractory period is as long as the action potential. The action potential of cardiac muscle is much longer than that of skeletal muscle (Figs 5.16A to C).

All or None Law

All excitable tissues (nerve and muscle) have this property. They require a certain minimum strength of the stimulus to give the response. This strength is called the threshold. Any stimulus stronger than the threshold gives the same response. In other words, either we get all of the response or none at all (Fig. 5.17). However, the response can change if the conditions of the stimulus change. For example, the response increases if the cardiac muscle is exposed to adrenaline.

Length-tension Relationship

The length of a muscle fiber may be increased by stretching it. Within limits, the longer the length of the muscle fibers, stronger is their contraction. This property of cardiac muscle is also called the Starling's law of the heart.

ELECTROCARDIOGRAPHY

We have seen above that contraction of the heart is associated with electrical changes in cardiac muscle cells. The whole heart consists of about 300 g of cardiac muscle tissue. A wave of action potentials moves through the heart with each heart beat. During the passing of this wave, there are phases when a part of the musculature is depolarized, phases when almost the entire musculature is depolarized,

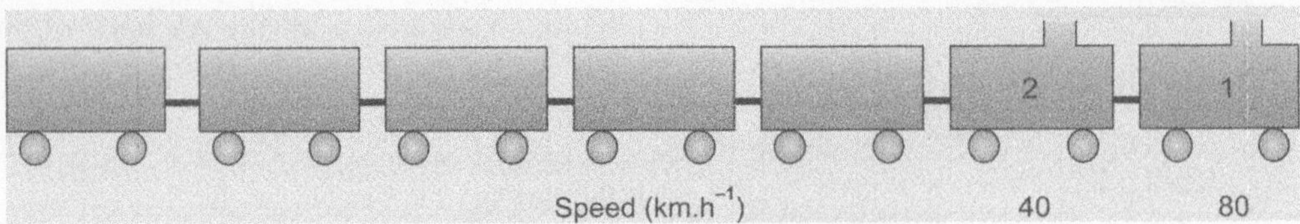

Fig. 5.14 If a train is pulled by two engines (1 and 2) running at different speeds, the speed of the train will be determined by the faster engine (1). The presence of the other engine (2) will become apparent only if the faster engine falls. In the same way, the region with the highest discharge frequency determines the pace of the heart. The ability of the other regions to set the pace of the heart becomes apparent only if the normal pacemaker fails

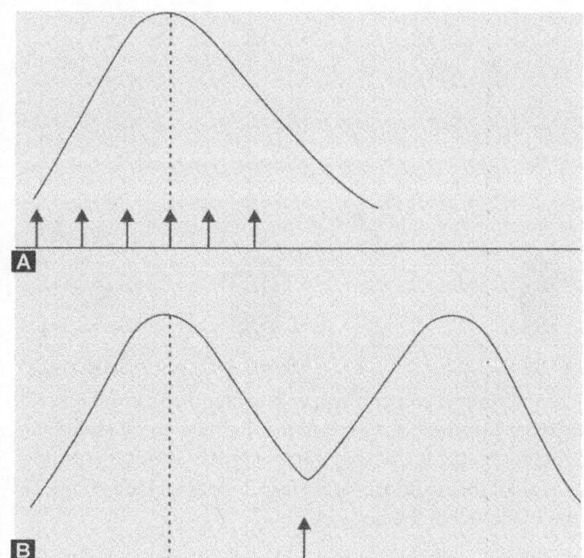

Figs 5.15A and B Refractory period. (A) Curve depicting contraction and relaxation of a chamber of the heart. Electrical stimuli given at points indicated by the arrows do not give any response because they fall during the refractory period of cardiac muscle; (B) A stimulus during the last one-third of the relaxation period gives a response

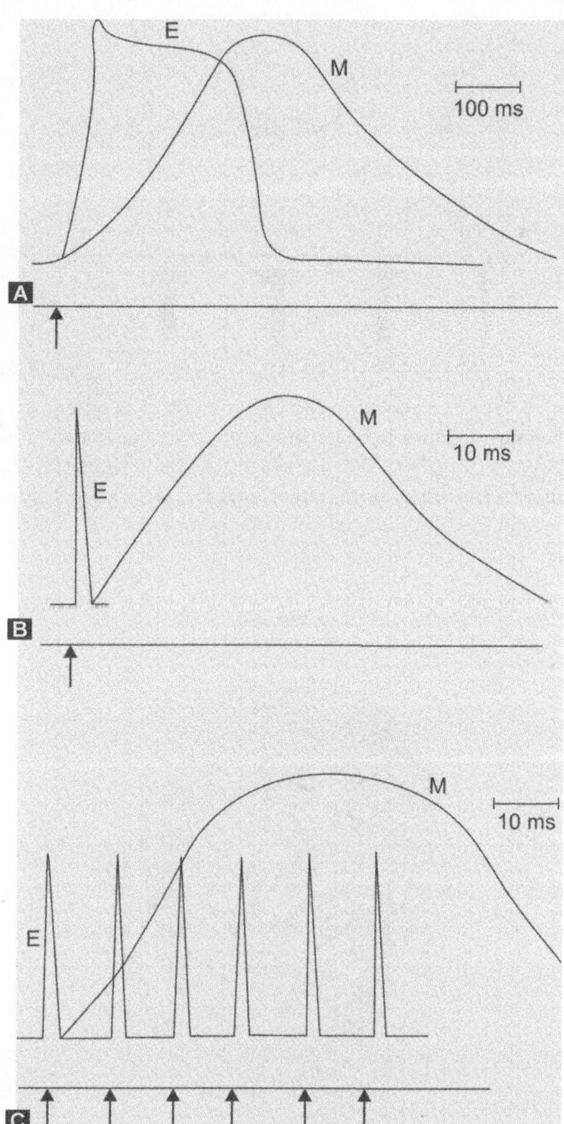

Figs 5.16A to C The duration of refractory period is related to the duration of the action potential. (A) Cardiac muscle. The electrical response 'E', or action potential, is long, 'M' mechanical response, or the contraction relaxation cycle; (B) In skeletal muscle, the action potential is very brief. It is much shorter than the mechanical response; (C) Hence, in skeletal muscle, each stimulus (arrow) gives a separate electrical response. The mechanical responses corresponding to each electrical response fuse together, giving rise to a sustained contraction (tetanus)

and phases when almost the entire musculature is repolarized. The outside of depolarized cardiac muscle cells is negative as compared to that of polarized cells. This results in an electrical current between the depolarized and polarized regions of the heart (Fig. 5.18). Such currents are conducted by body fluids to the surface of the body. The currents can be detected by electrodes placed on the surface of the body. A graphic record of these currents is known as the electrocardiogram (ECG or EKG).

It is important to note that ECG is not the direct result of action potentials. ECG is not due to summation of individual action potentials. ECG results from currents travelling from one part of heart to the another. Obviously, the magnitude of ECG waves is maximum when nearly half the cardiac musculature is polarized, and nearly half depolarized (Fig. 5.19). For the same reason, there is no current flow when the entire musculature is polarized or the

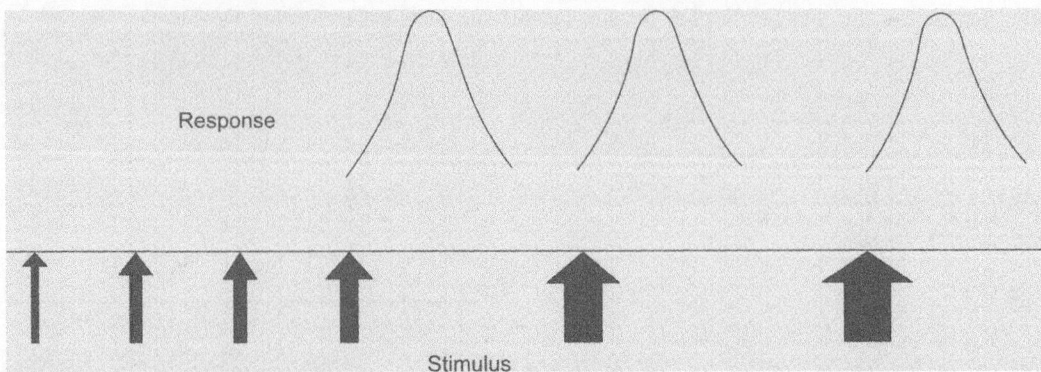

Fig. 5.17 All or none law. Cardiac muscle and all other excitable tissues follow all or none law. The first three stimuli do not give any response because they are too weak, i.e. they are below the threshold for excitation. The next three stimuli are above the threshold and give exactly the same response. Above the threshold, increasing the strength of the stimulus does not alter the response. In other words, a given stimulus either gives all of the response, or no response at all (The change in the strength of stimuli has been diagrammatically indicated by the thickness of the arrows)

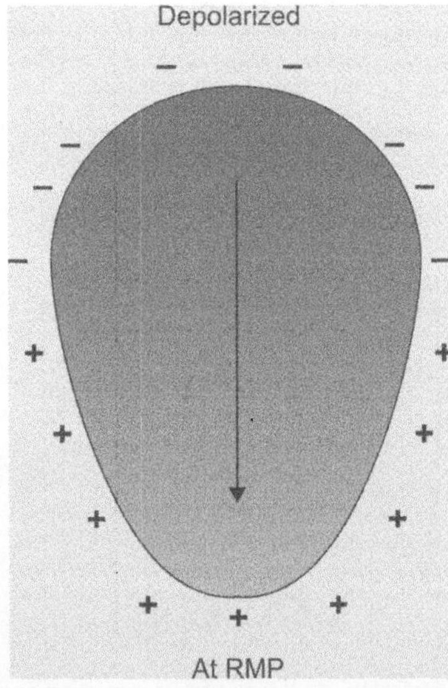

Fig. 5.18 The outside of the cells, and hence the surface of the heart, in the depolarized region is negative as compared to that in the normally polarized region. This results in an electrical current (arrow) from the depolarized to the polarized regions of the heart

entire musculature is depolarized. Therefore, during these phases there is no ECG wave.

Configuration of the ECG

When current travels from one part of heart to another, it has a certain direction known as the axis. The negative and positive electrodes applied to the surface of the body also have a certain axis. The interaction of the two axes determines the magnitude and direction of the ECG wave.

Let us try to understand this interaction by considering the wave of ventricular depolarization, which is the biggest wave in the ECG. The wave travels from the base to the apex. The largest flow of current takes place when the wave has still travelled only half way. At this point the basal half of the ventricles is depolarized, and the apical half is polarized. Considering electronic current, which travels from negative to positive, there is a flow of current from the base towards the apex (Fig. 5.20). The electrodes are also generally arranged in such a way that the positive electrode is towards the direction of the current. That makes the deflection positive. For example, if the negative electrode is on the right arm and positive electrode on the left leg, the deflection will be positive (Fig. 5.21).

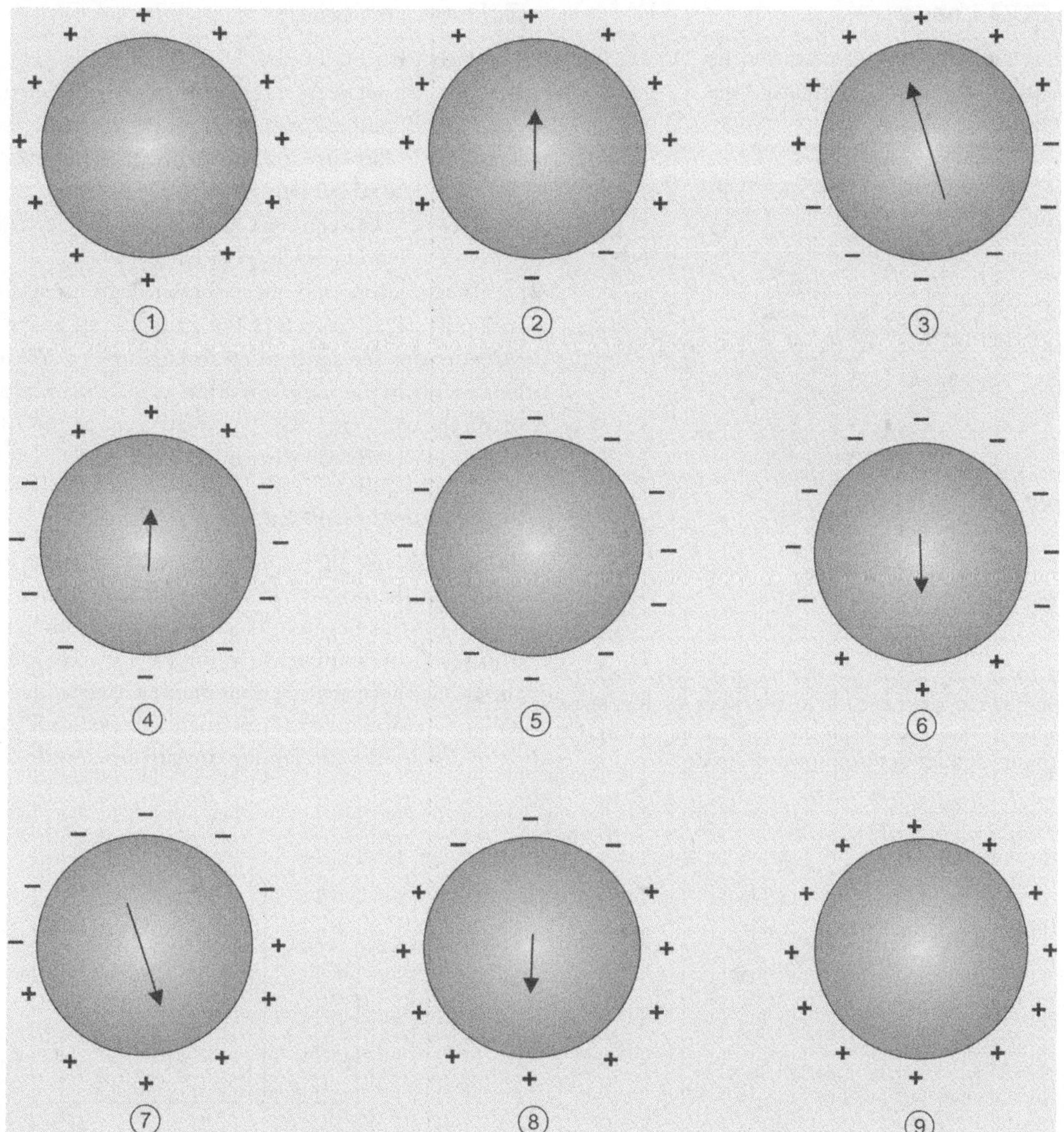

Fig. 5.19 Diagrammatic representation of depolarization and repolarization of a globular mass of cardiac muscle, and the resulting flow of current. 1. Polarized muscle at rest; 2. A small part of the muscle depolarized, associated with flow of a weak current; 3. Approximately half the muscle mass is depolarized, leading to flow of a strong current; 4. Almost the entire muscle is depolarized, leading to flow of a weak current; 5. The entire muscle is depolarized; 6. A small part of the muscle is repolarized, leading to flow of a weak current; 7. Approximately half the muscle mass is repolarized, leading to flow of a strong current; 8. Almost the entire muscle is repolarized, leading to flow of a weak current; 9. The entire muscle is repolarized. Note that no current flows when the whole muscle is polarized (1,9) or depolarized (5). Maximum flow of current takes place when about half the muscle mass is polarized and half depolarized (3, 7). Arrows represent the magnitude and direction of flow of current

The ECG Leads

Three sets of leads are in common use. Using these three sets gives us the 'standard' twelve or thirteen lead electrocardiogram.

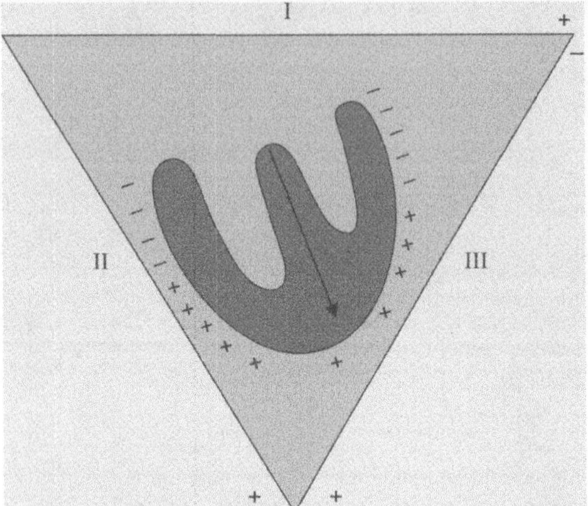

Fig. 5.20 During activation of the ventricles, electrical current flows from the base to the apex of the heart. Electrodes in limb leads I-III are arranged in such a way that the current approaches the positive electrode

Bipolar Limb Leads

These are three in number.

Lead I : Between right arm (negative electrode) and left arm (positive electrode).

Lead II : Between right arm (negative electrode) and left leg (positive electrode).

Lead III : Between left arm (negative electrode) and left leg (positive electrode).

The three leads have been shown diagrammatically in Figure 5.22. Note that the principle of electrode placement is the same in all three leads, i.e. the lead axis points in the same direction as the electrical axis of the heart (Fig. 5.23). The lead axes of the three limb leads have been shown in Figure 5.24.

Augmented Limb Leads

These leads use the same limbs as the bipolar limb leads. But the positive electrode is connected to one limb, and the negative electrode to the other two. This results in an increase in the voltages recorded in the ECG. There are three augmented limb leads.

aVR : Between right arm (positive electrode) and left arm and left leg (negative electrode).

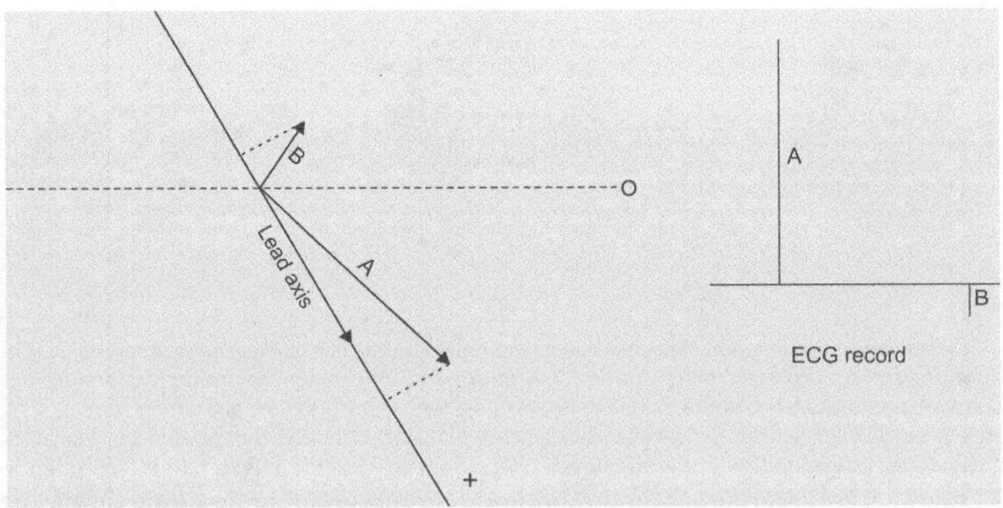

Fig. 5.21 Interaction of the lead axis and the cardiac axis. To know how the ECG record will look, draw a perpendicular from the tip of the cardiac axis on the lead axis. If the perpendicular falls on the positive side of the lead axis, the record will give a positive deflection. Records A and B correspond to cardiac axis at two different points during the cardiac cycle

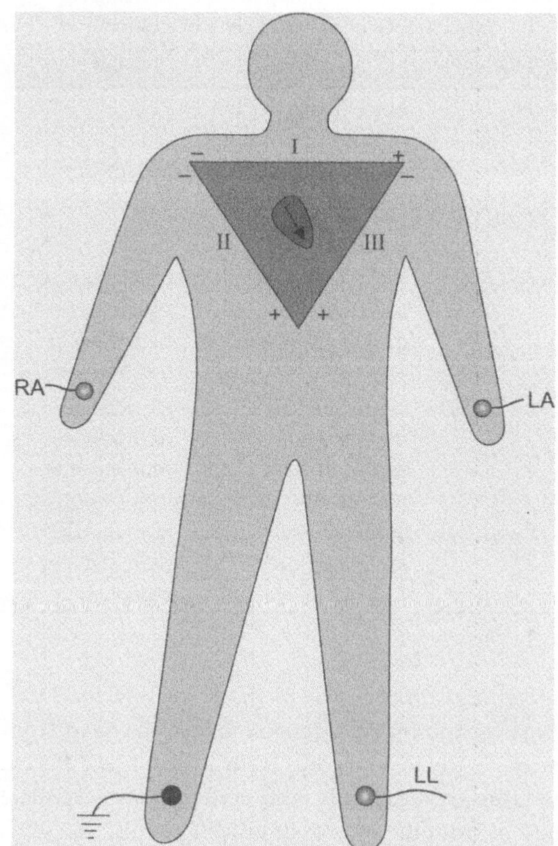

Fig. 5.22 The Einthoven's triangle. RA, right arm; LA, left arm; LL, left leg; I, II, III: limb leads. The insert in the triangle represents the heart and its electrical axis

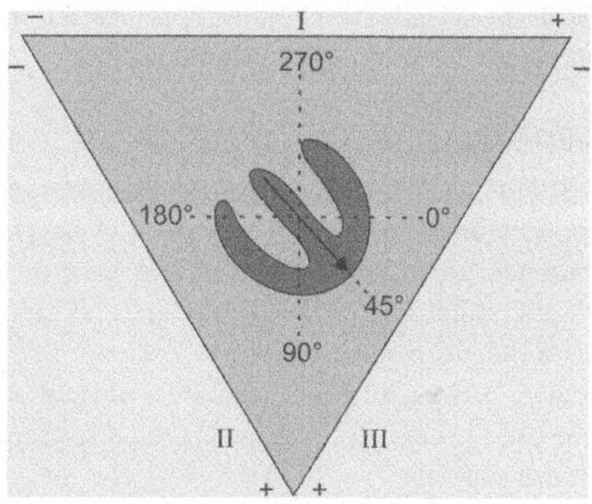

Fig. 5.23 The positions of positive and negative electrodes in bipolar limb leads. The positive electrode is so placed that the lead axis points in the same general direction as the electrical axis of the heart

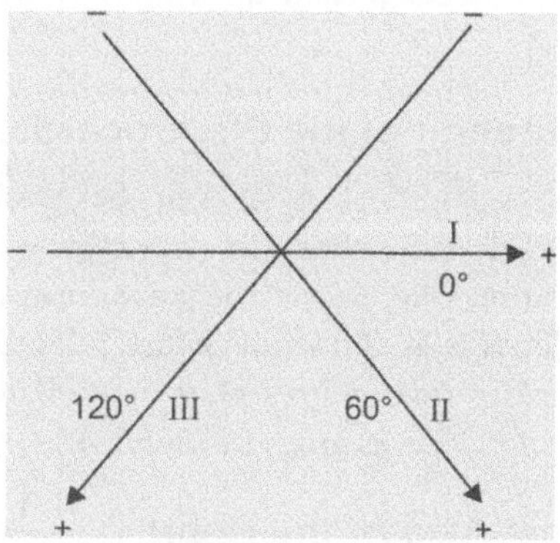

Fig. 5.24 The lead axes of bipolar limb leads I, II and III

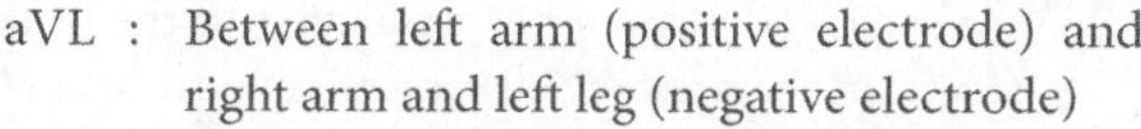

aVL : Between left arm (positive electrode) and right arm and left leg (negative electrode)

aVF : Between left leg (positive electrode) and right arm and left arm (negative electrode).

Unipolar Chest Leads

In these leads the positive electrode is on the chest and negative electrode is connected to the right arm, left arm and left leg through high resistances. The negative electrode is considered to be at zero potential. Thus the chest lead essentially records the potential at the positive electrode. The position of the positive electrode is as follows:

V1 : It is in the right fourth intercostal space at the right border of sternum.

V2 : It is in the left fourth intercostal space at the left border of sternum.

V3 : It is at the midpoint between V2 and V4.

V4 : It is in the left fifth intercostal space in the midclavicular line.

V5 : It is in the left fifth intercostal space at the anterior axillary line.

V6 : It is in the left fifth intercostal space at the midaxillary line.

V7 : It is in the left fifth intercostal space at the posterior axillary line (not always recorded).

In all these leads the right leg is connected to the ground to avoid electrical interference.

Electrodes

Flat metallic electrodes are fastened by straps to the appropriate limb. In case of forearms, the electrodes are fastened above the wrists, and in case of legs, above the ankles. An electrolyte jelly is applied between the electrode and skin to decrease the skin resistance. If the jelly is not available, normal saline may be used instead. But saline has the disadvantage that it dries up fast.

For the chest, we have small inverted cup-like electrodes, which can be fixed firmly over any point on the chest.

The electrodes are connected to the ECG machine, which essentially consists of an amplifier (to amplify the small voltages picked up by electrodes) and a recorder.

Table 5.1 Genesis of the electrocardiogram

Components	*Genesis*	*Remarks*
P wave	Atrial depolarization	
QRS complex	Ventricular depolarization	
T wave	Ventricular repolarization	
P-R interval	Atrial depolarization and conduction through the A-V node	From origin of P wave to the beginning of QRS complex
Q-T interval	Ventricular depolarization and ventricular repolarization	From origin of Q wave to repolarization end T wave
S–T segment	Ventricular repolarization	Q-T interval minus QRS complex

Configuration of the Electrocardiogram

The configuration of ECG can be worked out as explained earlier for the wave of ventricular depolarization (Fig. 5.21). The wave form obtained in most leads is as shown in Figure 5.25. The event in the cardiac cycle represented by each wave and 'interval' of ECG is as given in Table 5.1.

Electrical Axis of the Heart

During ventricular depolarization, the direction of the flow of current when about half the ventricular mass is depolarized and about half is repolarized is called the electrical axis of the heart. This point corresponds to the peak of the R wave in the ECG. For determining the electrical axis of the heart from the ECG, the ECG records from at least two different leads are required. It is most convenient to calculate the axis from the records of Leads I and III. The steps involved are as follows (Fig. 5.26).

1. Measure the net QRS deflection in the two leads. For this purpose, subtract the negative deflection, if any, from the positive deflection.
2. Plot the net deflection on the axes of the two leads.
3. For each lead, draw a perpendicular to the lead axis from the apex of the projected vector. Let the two perpendiculars intersect at a point.
4. Join the point of intersection of the two perpendiculars to the point of intersection of the two lead axes. The joining line is the electrical axis of the heart.

The normal electrical axis of the heart lies between –30° and +110°. If the axis is more negative than –30° it is called left axis deviation, whereas if the axis is more positive than +110°, it is called right axis deviation.

Understanding the normal ECG helps in interpreting abnormal ECGs resulting from abnormalities

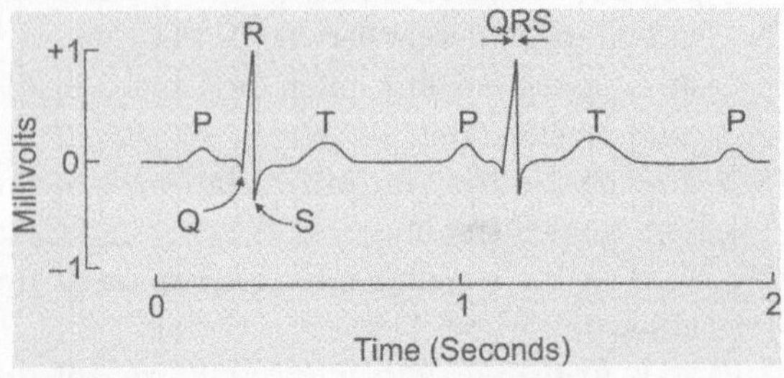

Fig. 5.25 Configuration of the normal electrocardiogram

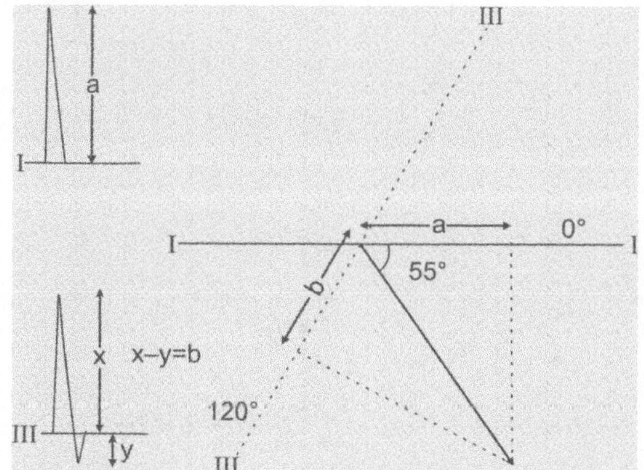

Fig. 5.26 Plotting the electrical axis of the heart. The net deflection in the leads may be plotted as such on the corresponding lead axes as in this diagram. Alternatively, if it is more convenient the plotted length may be a multiple of the length in the actual EKG. For example, if the net height of the QRS complex in leads I and III is 14 and 10 mm respectively, the plotted lengths can be 42 and 30 mm respectively. The electrical axis of the heart in the example illustrated here is +55°

of rhythm, conduction defects, myocardial ischemia or ventricular hypertrophy.

CARDIAC CYCLE

The activity of the heart follows a cyclic pattern. The atria contract first. After a delay, the ventricles contract. The cycle repeats itself about seventy times a minute. One contraction (systole) and one relaxation (diastole) together form a cardiac cycle. Several mechanical, physical and electrical events are associated with the cardiac cycle.

Suppose the heart rate is 75 per min.

If 75 beats take 1 min,

One beat will take $\frac{1}{75}$ min

$= \frac{1}{75} \times 60$ s

= 0.8 s

When the duration of the cardiac cycle is 0.8 s, ventricular systole (generally called just 'the systole') lasts 0.3 s and ventricular diastole (generally called just 'the diastole') lasts 0.5 s. When the heart rate increases, the duration of cardiac cycle decreases. In such a situation, the reduction in duration of diastole is greater than that of systole.

Now the sequence of events during the cardiac cycle will be discussed in some detail. The only way to understand the events is to imagine as if you are actually seeing them. Imagine the chambers of the heart and their valves. Imagine their movements as you read. Use Figure 5.27 to help your imagination. Draw portions of the figure with your own hands as you read along. If you put your eyes (to read), your mind (to imagine) and your hands (to draw) to work together, you will understand it so well that you will never forget it.

In the following description sometimes only the left heart events have been described in detail. But similar events take place simultaneously on the right side.

Let us start with atrial contraction. During atrial contraction, ventricles are relaxed, and atrioventricular (A-V) valves are open (how else can the blood flow from the atria into the ventricles!). The ECG counterpart of atrial contraction is the P wave. The pressure wave of atrial contraction is called the 'a' wave.

After atrial contraction, the cardiac impulse passes slowly through the A-V node and reaches the ventricles. Ventricular depolarization appears as QRS complex in the ECG, and leads to ventricular contraction. Contraction of ventricles raises ventricular pressure. As soon as ventricular pressure rises above the atrial pressure, the A-V valves close. Closure of A-V valves gives rise to the first heart sound. Semilunar valves are already closed at this stage. Since A-V valves and semilunar valves are both closed, ventricles become closed cavities. Contraction of ventricles closed at both ends leads to a steep rise in ventricular pressure. But there is no change in volume because blood stays in the ventricle. Therefore this phase of ventricular contraction is called isovolumetric, or simply isometric contraction. During isometric contraction, the pressure in the left ventricle rises from about 10 mm Hg to about 80 mm Hg. Steep rise of ventricular pressure makes the AV valve rings bulge into the atria, which gives rise to the 'c' wave in the atrial pressure curve.

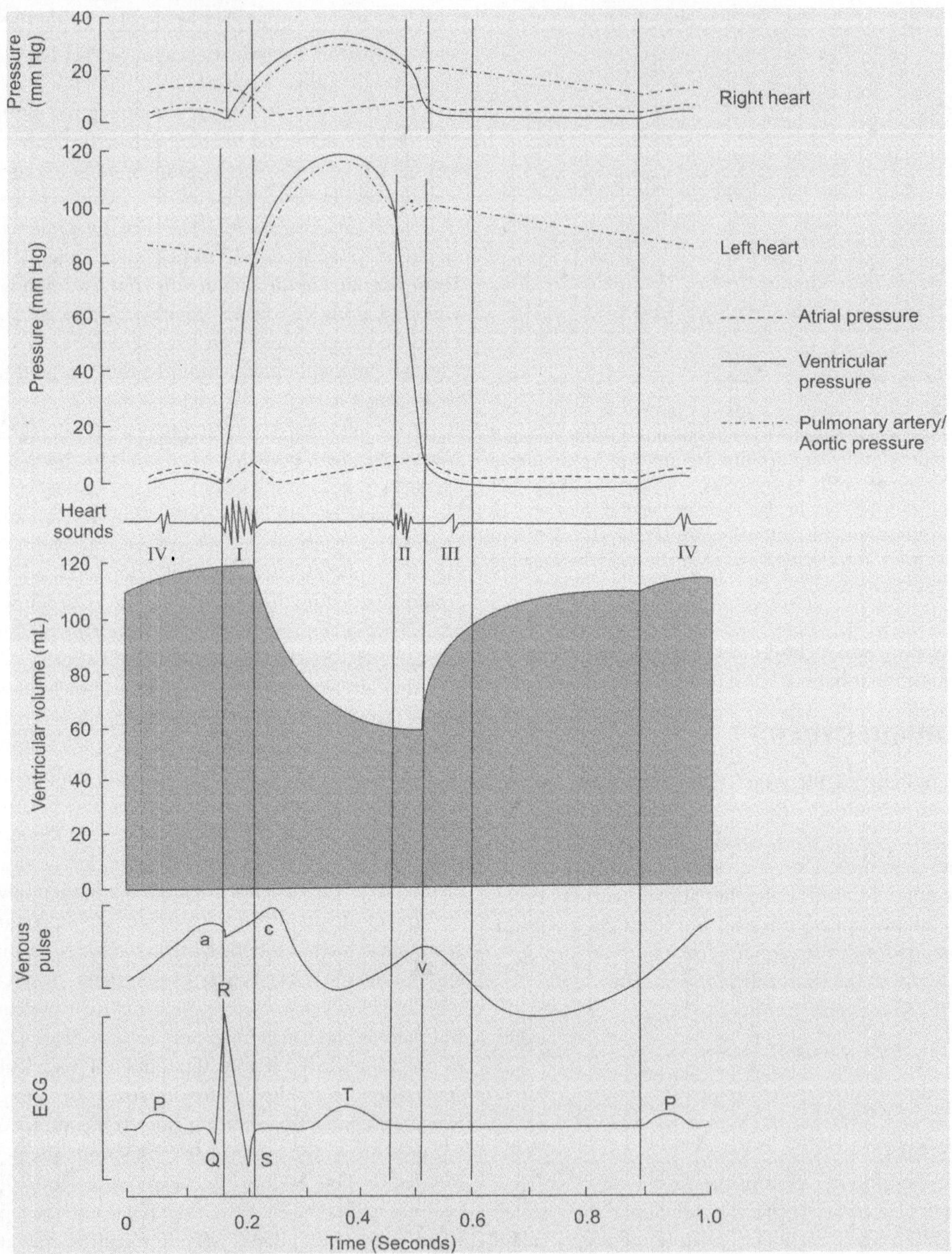

Fig. 5.27 Correlation of different events and aspects of the cardiac cycle

As soon as the left ventricular pressure rises above the aortic pressure, the aortic semilunar valve opens. However, ventricular contraction continues, and blood is pumped out by the left ventricle into the aorta. During this phase, the left ventricular and aortic pressure rises to about 120 mm Hg and then starts falling.

Finally, ventricular contraction comes to an end. The ventricular muscle starts repolarizing, giving rise to the T wave in the ECG. Ventricular pressure falls further. As soon as the left ventricular pressure falls below the aortic pressure, the aortic semilunar valve closes. Closure of the semilunar valves gives rise to the second heart sound. A-V valves are already closed at this stage. Since A-V valves and semilunar valves are both closed, ventricles become closed cavities. Relaxation of ventricles closed at both ends leads to a steep fall in ventricular pressure, without any change in volume. Therefore this phase of ventricular relaxation is called isometric relaxation. During isometric relaxation the pressure in the left ventricle falls from about 100 mm Hg to 20 mm Hg.

In the meantime, while the ventricles were pumping blood, the atria were relaxed and were getting filled with blood returning to them through the veins. Filling of the atria slowly and steadily gives rise to the 'v' wave in the atrial pressure curve. As soon as the ventricular pressure falls below the atrial pressure, the A-V valves open. Blood flows passively from the atria into the ventricles due to the pressure gradient. Initially, the flow of blood is so rapid that it gives rise to a faint sound called the third heart sound. Towards the end of ventricular diastole, atria contract. Contraction of atria pumps some more blood into the ventricles. This flow of blood resulting from atrial contraction gives rise to another 'faint sound' which can only be recorded by phonocardiography. This sound is called the fourth heart sound. Thus we have reached where we started from, and the cardiac cycle starts all over again.

Some of the facts related to the cardiac cycle have been summarized in Tables 5.2 to 5.4.

Table 5.2 Events of the cardiac cycle

Event	*Duration (s)*
Isometric contraction	0.05
Rapid ejection phase	0.10
Slow ejection	0.15
Total (ventricular systole)	**0.30**
Isometric relaxation	0.10
Ventricular filling (passive)	0.30
Ventricular filling (due to atrial contraction)	0.10
Total (ventricular diastole)	**0.50**
Grand total (systole + diastole)	**0.80**

Table 5.3 Pressures in systemic and pulmonary circuits

	Pressure (mm Hg)	
	Systolic	*Diastolic*
Left ventricle	120	20
Right ventricle	25	0
Aorta	120	80
Pulmonary artery	25	15

Table 5.4 Heart sounds

Sound	*Timing*	*Causative/associated event*
First heart sound	Onset of systole	Closure of AV valves
Second heart sound	Onset of diastole	Closure of semilunar valves
Third heart sound	Mid-diastole	Passive flow of blood from atria into ventricles
Fourth heart sound	End-diastole	Active flow of blood from atria into ventricles (due to atrial contraction)

CARDIAC OUTPUT

Cardiac output is the amount of blood pumped by either ventricle in one minute. The amount of blood pumped in one beat is called stoke volume. Therefore,

Cardiac output = Stroke volume × heart rate

The normal resting stroke volume is about 70 mL. The normal heart rate is about 70 per min at rest. Therefore, the cardiac output of a resting healthy adult is about 70 × 70 = 4900 mL/min, or about 5 L/min.

Determination of Cardiac Output

Cardiac output may be determined by using Fick's principle. The method requires the measurement of oxygen consumption and arteriovenous (A-V) oxygen difference. A-V oxygen difference is the difference in the oxygen content of arterial and venous blood. A-V oxygen difference, therefore, represents the amount of oxygen which is picked up by venous blood while passing through the lungs.

In a healthy adult at rest, the oxygen concentration in the venous blood is about 15 mL/100 mL of blood, and in the arterial blood it is about 20 mL/100 mL. Hence the A-V oxygen difference is 5 mL/100 mL of blood. It means that the lungs add 5 mL oxygen to each 100 mL of blood passing through them.

Now, the oxygen consumption is about 250 mL/min. The lungs must be adding these 250 mL of oxygen to venous blood in one minute.

If lungs add 5 mL oxygen to 100 ml blood,
Then lungs add 250 mL oxygen to

$$\frac{100}{5} \times 250 \text{ mL blood}$$

$$= 5000 \text{ mL blood}$$

If lungs add oxygen to 5000 mL of blood every minute, it means that 5000 mL of blood pass through the lungs every minute. The amount of blood passing through the lungs is the amount which is pumped by the right ventricle. Therefore the amount of blood pumped by the right ventricle must be 5000 mL/min. Hence, the cardiac output is 5000 mL/min.

If we put these facts in the form of a formula,

$$\text{Cardiac output} = \frac{\text{Qxygen Consumption}}{\text{A} - \text{V oxygen difference}}$$

In practice, oxygen consumption can be measured by using a spirometer (Chapter 6). The arterial oxygen content may be measured in a blood sample collected from any artery. But the oxygen content of blood in all veins is not the same. Therefore the venous oxygen is best measured in a sample collected from the right ventricle so that we get a mixed venous sample. A blood sample from the right ventricle can be obtained by cardiac catheterization.

Factors Affecting Cardiac Output

Cardiac output is the product of stroke volume and heart rate. Therefore cardiac output is affected by factors which affect the stroke volume, and also by factors which affect the heart rate.

Factors Affecting Stroke Volume

Stroke volume is the amount of blood pumped by either ventricle in one beat (or stroke). It depends on:

a. *Degree of ventricular filling:* If the ventricle fills more during diastole, more blood will be pumped out during systole. This is because cardiac muscle has a property called the length-tension relationship, also known as the **Starling's law of the heart**. If the length of cardiac muscle fibers is more when the contraction begins (the initial length), the contraction is stronger. If the ventricular filling is more, the ventricular musculature gets stretched by blood. Thus the initial length of muscle fiber is increased. Hence the strength of contraction is increased. If the ventricles contract more strongly they pump out more blood. In other words, the stroke volume is increased (Fig. 5.28). Since the degree of ventricular filling depends on the amount of blood returning to them by the veins, we can say that increase in venous return increases the stroke volume.
b. *Contractility of the ventricles:* The same degree of filling of the ventricles may lead to greater pumping of blood if the contractility of the ventricles is increased. Contractility of the ventricles is increased by adrenaline or by sympathetic stimulation. If we show the effect of increased contractility in the graph showing the length-tension relationship, we get curves of the type which were first described by Sarnoff.

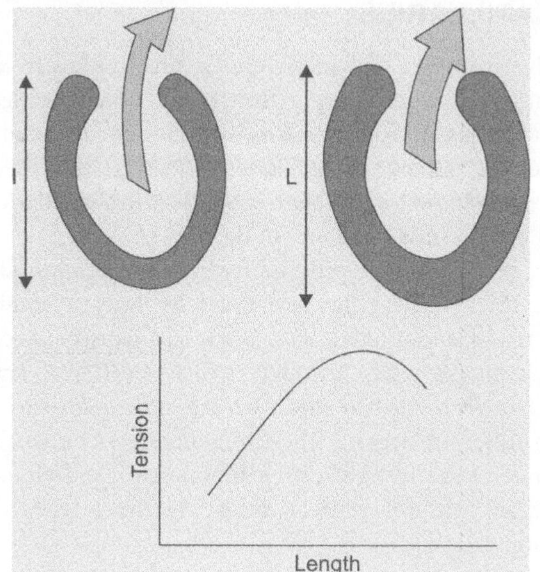

Fig. 5.28 Starling's law of the heart. As the initial length of muscle fibers increases from l to L, the tension developed during contraction increases, resulting in pumping of more blood

c. *Resistance offered to ventricular pumping action:* The left ventricle has to pump blood against aortic resistance. The right ventricle has to pump blood against pulmonary arterial resistance. Increase in these resistances decreases the stroke volume.

Factors Affecting Heart Rate

Heart rate is affected predominantly by the nerves supplying it, and by the adrenal medullary hormones.

a. *Parasympathetic nerve:* The parasympathetic nerve supplying the heart is the vagus nerve. Activation of the vagus nerve decreases the heart rate. The vagus is quite active when a person is physically and mentally relaxed. This 'spontaneous' activity of the vagus is called vagal tone.
b. *Sympathetic nerves:* The sympathetic nerves supplying the heart are derived from the first through fourth thoracic spinal segments (T1-T4). Activation of the sympathetic nerves increases the heart rate. The sympathetic tone at rest is generally low. Sympathetic nerves are activated by physical or mental activity.[1]
c. *Adrenaline:* Adrenaline is a hormone of the adrenal medulla. The effects of adrenaline are similar to those of sympathetic stimulation.

ARTERIES

Arteries are blood vessels into which the heart pumps blood. The left ventricle pumps blood into the aorta. Aorta and its branches are called systemic arteries. The right ventricle pumps blood into the pulmonary artery. Pulmonary artery and its branches are part of the pulmonary circulation. Here we shall discuss some properties of systemic arteries only.

Aorta and large diameter arteries are elastic vessels. Because of their elasticity they can expand when blood is pumped into them, and shrink when blood is not being pumped into them. Therefore arterial blood pressure does not rise too much during systole, and does not fall too much during diastole. Therefore, although the pressure in the left ventricle fluctuates between 0 and 120 mm Hg, in the aorta the fluctuation is only between 80 and 120 mm Hg.

Arteries of smaller diameter, called arterioles and metarterioles, have a thick coat of smooth muscle in their walls, but less elastic tissue. Most of the peripheral resistance is offered by arterioles (Fig. 5.29). Further, because of the thick smooth muscle, the diameter of arterioles and metarterioles can change remarkably. Change in diameter changes the resistance offered by these vessels. Thus, these vessels offer maximum resistance, and the resistance is adjustable.

Smooth muscle extends upto the precapillary sphincters. The contraction of precapillary sphincters plays an important role in regulation of blood flow through organs.

[1]We have already learnt that sympathetic stimulation increases the stroke volume by increasing the contractility of ventricles. Thus sympathetic activity increases the cardiac output by increasing both stroke volume and heart rate

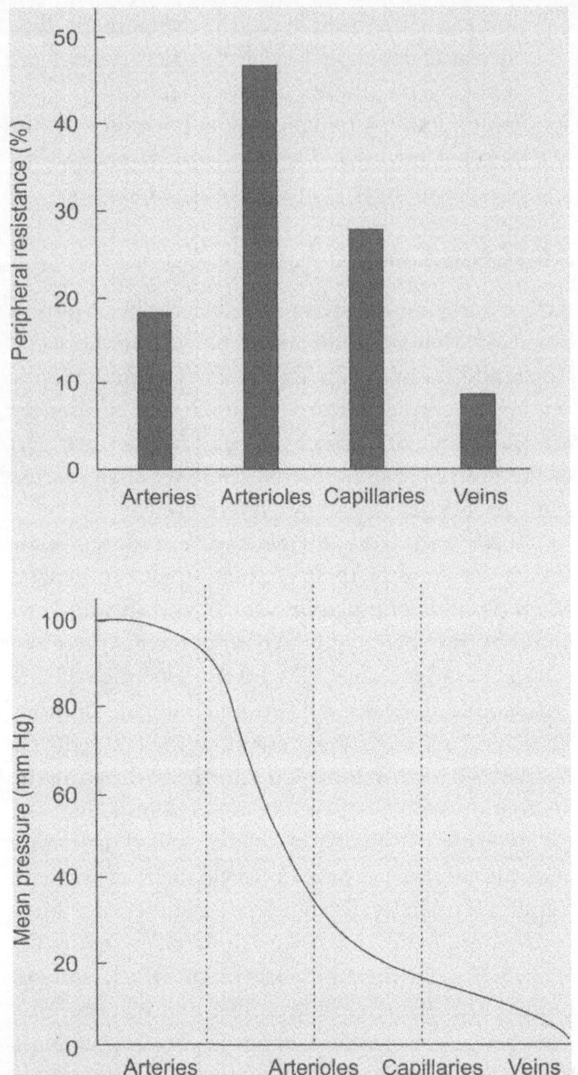

Fig. 5.29 Arterioles account for nearly half the peripheral vascular resistance. Therefore the mean blood pressure falls most steeply as blood passes through the arterioles

There is no blood flow through several capillaries of an organ at rest because their precapillary sphincters are closed. When the organ becomes more active, the sphincters open and the blood flows in. Thus the blood flow can be increased when an organ is active.

CAPILLARIES

The arterioles and metarterioles finally branch off into a network of very thin blood vessels, called capillaries. A capillary is 6 to 10 microns in diameter.[2] But the number of capillaries is so large that their cross sectional area is enormous. Therefore capillaries offer very little resistance to the flow of blood.

Structurally, capillaries have no smooth muscle in their walls. They are lined by only a single layer of endothelial cells. There are gaps between endothelial cells through which nutrients and waste products can pass. The size of the gaps varies in different organs. The differences can be easily understood in light of the functions of individual organs. In this respect, there are three types of capillaries:

a. **Continuous capillaries**, having very small pores for passage of small molecules like those of water, electrolytes, glucose, etc. Such capillaries are the most widespread ones, and are present in muscles, skin, connective tissue, etc.
b. **Fenestrated capillaries**, having large pores which allow even the relatively small protein molecules also to pass through. Fenestrated capillaries are found in glands where it is necessary for protein molecules to escape from capillaries into the secretion of the gland. Such capillaries are also found in kidneys and intestines.
c. **Sinusoidal capillaries**, having large gaps between endothelial cells. These gaps allow not only large molecules but even cells to pass through. Sinusoidal capillaries are found in the bone marrow where it is necessary for blood cells to enter the capillaries to join the circulation. Such capillaries are also found in the liver and spleen.

[2]The diameter of a red blood cell is about 7 microns. Therefore, through some capillaries, the red cells can only squeeze through with difficulty.

Fluid Exchange Across Capillaries: Starling's Hypothesis

Fluid transport across capillaries is evenly balanced so that the circulating blood volume remains constant. At the arterial end of the capillary, along with oxygen and nutrients, some fluid also escapes (Fig. 5.30). At the venous end of the capillary, along with carbon dioxide and other waste products, some fluid also returns to the capillary. The amount of fluid escaping at the arterial end is nearly equal to the fluid returning to the capillary at the venous end.[3] The flow of fluid across the capillary is determined by hydrostatic and osmotic pressures inside and outside the capillary. Hydrostatic pressure tends to push fluid to the other compartment. On the other hand osmotic pressure of a compartment pulls fluid from the other compartment. Let us understand the process through some actual figures (Fig. 5.31). Suppose, at the arterial end the hydrostatic pressure is 35 mm Hg and the colloid osmotic pressure is 25 mm Hg inside the capillary. The osmotic and hydrostatic pressures outside the capillary (in the interstitial fluid) are very small in magnitude. Thus there is a net pressure of 35–25 = 10 mm Hg which tends to filter fluid out of the capillary into the interstitial fluid. At the venous end, the hydrostatic pressure is about 16 mm Hg and the colloid osmotic pressure is 25 mm Hg inside the capillary.

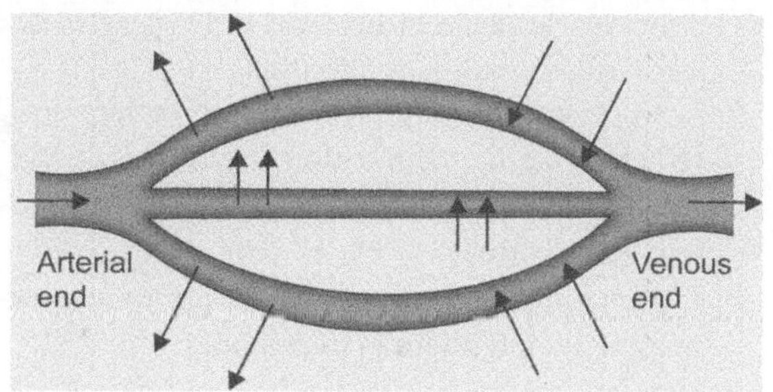

Fig. 5.30 Fluid is filtered out at the arterial end of capillaries. At the venous end, fluid is reabsorbed into the capillaries. Thus the blood volume remains constant

Thus there is a net pressure of 25–16 – 9 mm Hg which tends to reabsorb fluid from the interstitial fluid back into the capillary. Thus, nearly all the fluid filtered at the arterial end is reabsorbed at the venous end of the capillary. Since the pressure favoring

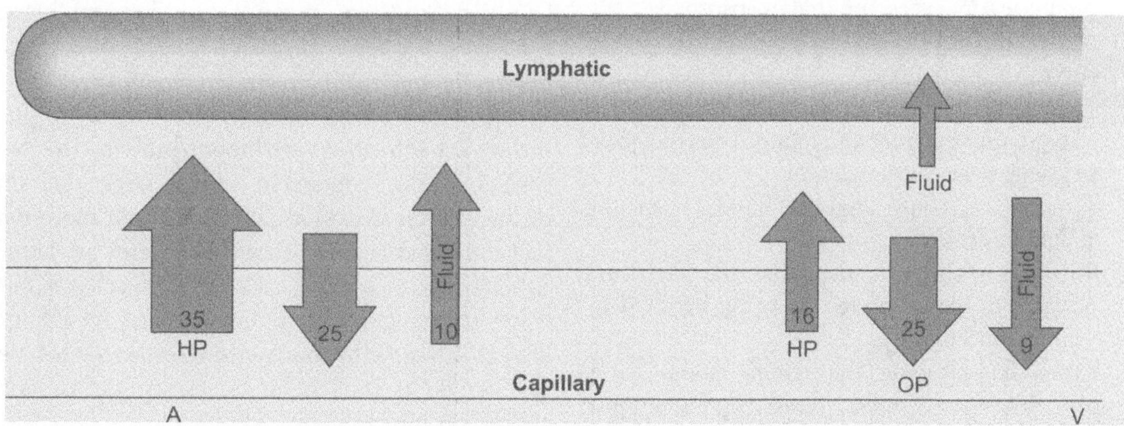

Fig. 5.31 Fluid exchange across capillaries. The balance of hydrostatic and osmotic pressures favors net loss of fluid from the capillaries at the arterial end, and favors net reabsorption at the venous end of capillaries. However, reabsorption at the venous end is slightly less than the filtration at the arterial end. The excess fluid does not accumulate in the interstitial space because it enters the lymphatics. A, arterial end; V, venous end; HP, hydrostatic pressure; OP, osmotic pressure. Figures indicate the pressure in mm Hg

[3]In fact, the amount escaping at the arterial end is slightly more. The excess is absorbed into the lymphatics.

filtration is slightly more than the pressure favoring reabsorption, the amount filtered is slightly more, but it does not accumulate in the interstitial fluid because it is absorbed into the lymphatics.

LYMPHATICS

Lymphatics are also a system of tubes spread all over the body like the blood vessels. But they do not carry blood. Lymphatics carry a clear or milky fluid.[4] Lymphatics are lined with endothelium. The intercellular junctions between endothelial cells allow large molecules such as proteins to pass through. There is no pump comparable to the heart for moving fluid in the lymphatics.

Movement of fluid in the lymphatics takes place by contraction of the smooth muscle lining large lymphatics, and by the squeezing action of skeletal muscle contraction. Lymphatics have valves which ensure one-way flow. All lymphatics eventually open into the venous system. Thus, the lymph is finally returned to the blood. On their way, however, the lymphatics also pass through lymph nodes.

Functions of Lymphatics

1. Lymphatics absorb the fluid filtered through capillaries in excess of that reabsorbed. They return this fluid to the blood. Thus the blood volume is maintained.
2. Lymphatics pick up protein molecules which leak out into the interstitial fluid. Thus they help in saving these substances.[5]
3. Lymphatics absorb digested lipids from the small intestine.
4. They carry large undesirable particles and bacteria to lymph nodes for being handled by immune mechanisms.
5. Lymphatics leaving the lymph nodes carry antibodies and lymphocytes to the circulation.

[4]Lymph gets milky if it contains fat absorbed from the intestines.

[5]Apart from saving proteins, this function also prevents the colloid osmotic pressure of interstitial fluid from rising. If that were to happen, filtration from capillaries could increase so much as to lead to accumulation of fluid in the interstitial space (edema).

EDEMA

Edema is an abnormally large collection of fluid in the interstitial space. The places where it is most prominent are legs and feet (pedal edema), and abdomen (ascites). From the physiology of capillaries and lymphatics, it can be deduced that edema may be due to one or more of the following causes:

1. High capillary hydrostatic pressure, as during late pregnancy due to pressure of uterus on inferior vena cava.
2. High interstitial fluid osmotic pressure due to abnormal leakage of proteins out of capillaries as in inflammation or allergy.
3. Low plasma osmotic pressure, as in hypoproteinemia, e.g. in malnutrition, liver disease (inadequate albumin synthesis), or renal disease (protein loss in urine).
4. Lymphatic obstruction, as in filariasis, or involvement of lymph nodes in malignancy.

VEINS

The capillaries open into small veins called venules. Venules unite to form small veins. Many small veins join to form large veins. By this process, finally we have two large veins, superior vena cava and inferior vena cava. The two vena cavas return the blood to the right atrium.

Veins have a large diameter but a thin wall, which includes a thin layer of smooth muscle. The total capacity of the venous tree is much larger than that of the arterial tree. Normally veins hold more than half the blood volume. That is why veins are known as capacitance vessels. Further, the capacity of veins is subject to regulation. In times of need, for example after bleeding, veins constrict and release some blood for circulation. Thus the large capacity of veins serves a reservoir function.

What Keeps Blood Flowing in the Veins

In veins the hydrostatic pressure is low. The difference between venous pressure and right atrial pressure is small. Further, in leg veins the blood flows against gravity. The factors which still keep blood flowing in veins are (Fig. 5.32):

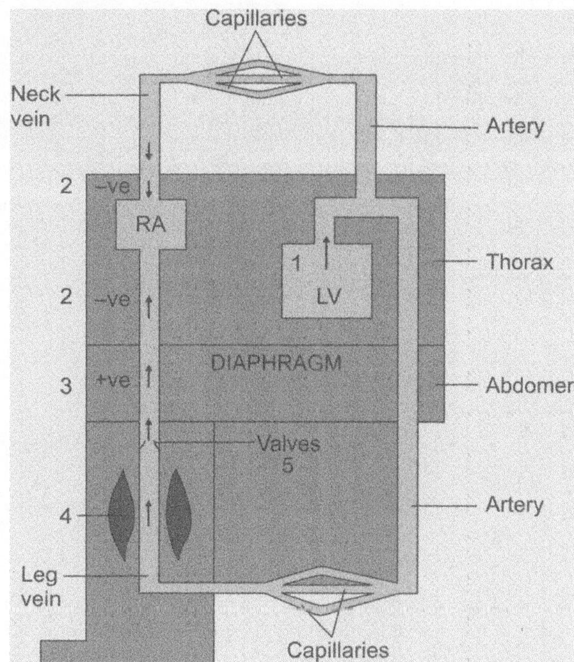

Fig. 5.32 Factors which are responsible for flow of blood through the veins. 1. Left ventricular contraction; 2. Negative intrathoracic pressure; 3. Positive abdominal pressure; 4. Muscle pump; 5. Venous valves; LV, left ventricle; RA, right atrium

1. The push provided by left ventricular contraction. Some effect of it is still present in the veins.
2. The pull created by the negative intrathoracic pressure.
3. The push provided by the positive intra-abdominal pressure.
4. The squeezing action of skeletal muscle contraction, specially in the legs.
5. The valves in the limb veins. These ensure one way flow, i.e. towards the heart.

The situation is comparable to that of a man who leaves home in the morning for work with a good deal of enthusiasm, full of energy. By the evening, he is too tired to make the journey back home, but somehow the push from the office, and the pull of the children and the dinner waiting at home make him return home. In the same way, the blood leaves the heart in the aorta for its journey through the body with great vigor, but by the time it reaches the veins, it is tired. But a few pushes and pulls make it return to the heart.

REGULATION OF CARDIOVASCULAR FUNCTION

Heart beat is essential for life. Therefore nature has provided the heart automaticity, i.e. capacity to function without depending on nerves. But it is necessary for the intensity of heart beat to vary. For example, the heart needs to beat faster during exercise than at rest. The other component of cardiovascular system are the blood vessels. The diameter of blood vessels also needs to vary. For example, blood vessels in skeletal muscles should dilate (i.e. become wider) during exercise so that muscle blood flow can increase. Modulation of function of the heart and blood vessels is brought about by neural and chemical mechanisms. These mechanisms will be discussed briefly here.

Neural Center for Cardiovascular Regulation

Important centers which regulate cardiovascular function are situated in the medulla oblongata (Fig. 5.33). The centers and their respective actions are as follows:

a. *Cardioinhibitory center:* decreases the heart rate.
b. *Cardioacceleratory center:* increases the heart rate.
c. *Pressor area:* increases the blood pressure by constricting blood vessels and increasing the heart rate.
d. *Depressor area:* decreases the blood pressure by dilating blood vessels.

The pressor and depressor area are together known as the vasomotor center. But by common usage, the term vasomotor center is frequently used only for the area which increases the blood pressure by constricting blood vessels.

These cardiovascular centers are under the influence of 'higher' areas of the brain. And, these centers exert their effect through autonomic (sympa-

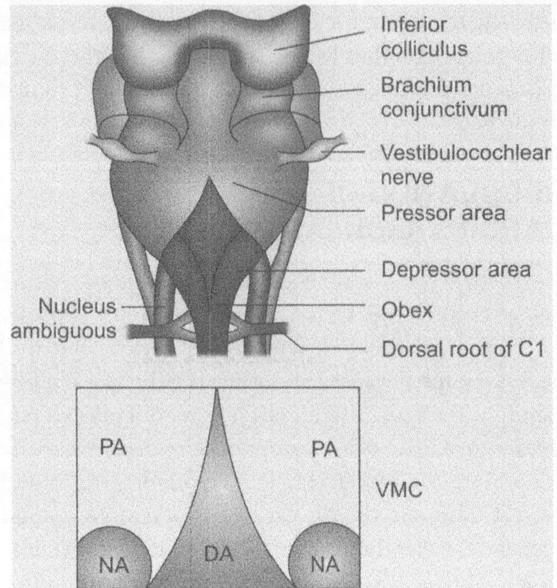

Fig. 5.33 The major areas of the medulla oblongata which regulate cardiovascular function. Although stimulation of the labeled areas produces predominantly the effect suggested by their names, there is no strict demarcation between areas. PA, pressor area; DA, depressor area; NA, nucleus ambiguus; VMC, vasomotor center

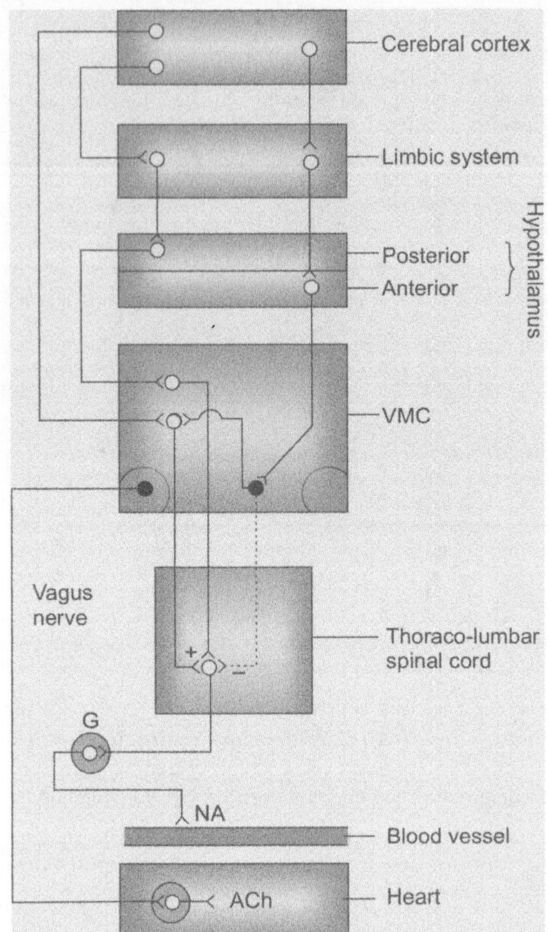

Fig. 5.34 The overall neural control of cardiovascular function. Higher neural control is superimposed on the medullary cardiovascular areas illustrated in Figure 5.33. The influence is ultimately mediated to the target structures by autonomic nerves. The direct inhibitory influence of neurons of the depressor area on the sympathetic outflow from the thoraco-lumbar spinal cord is controversial, and has therefore been shown by a dotted line. VMC, vasomotor center; G, sympathetic ganglion; NA, noradrenaline; ACh, acetylcholine

thetic and parasympathetic) nerves and the adrenal medulla (Fig. 5.34).

Mediation of Effects of Cardiovascular Centers

Decrease in heart rate is mediated by the vagus nerve. Increase in heart rate is mediated by sympathetic nerves supplying the heart. The control of blood vessels is predominantly by sympathetic nerves. The types of nerves supplying blood vessels, and their effects, may be summarized as follows:

a. *Sympathetic adrenergic vasoconstrictor nerves:* These are the predominant variety of nerves

[6]The same substance, adrenaline, can bring about vasoconstriction at some places and vasodilatation at other places because the type of receptors present in the blood vessels are different at these places. Blood vessels having alpha receptors respond by vasoconstriction, and blood vessels having beta receptors respond to adrenaline by vasodilatation.

which regulate the diameter of blood vessels. Increase in their activity constricts blood vessels, and decrease in their activity dilates blood vessels. 'Adrenergic' refers to the fact that these nerves release noradrenaline and adrenaline to bring about their effect.

b. *Sympathetic adrenergic vasodilator nerves:* These nerves supply only the blood vessels in skeletal muscles, salivary glands and liver, and the coronary arteries.[6]
c. *Sympathetic cholinergic vasodilator nerves:* These nerves release acetylcholine to bring about their effect. Such nerves supply only the blood vessels in skeletal muscles.

Further, whenever sympathetic nerves are activated, adrenaline is released into the blood stream from the adrenal medulla. Circulating adrenaline has effects similar to those of sympathetic adrenergic nerves.

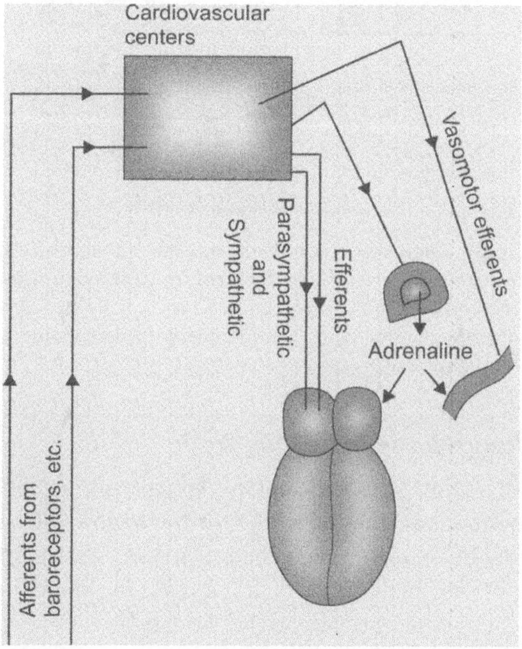

Fig. 5.35 Simplified representation of cardiovascular regulation. Cardiovascular centers in the central nervous system receive information from baroreceptors, chemoreceptors, pressure receptors, volume receptors, etc. at the periphery. They process this information and convey their decision to the heart, blood vessels and adrenal medulla via autonomic (parsympathetic and sympathetic) efferents

The next question that arises is how the cardiovascular centers 'know' when to activate which mechanism, i.e. cardio-acceleratory or cardio-inhibitory, vasoconstrictor or vasodilator. This decision depends on information coming through sensory (afferent) nerves. Based on that information, the centers take a decision. The centers convey the decision through sympathetic nerves, parasympathetic nerves, and adrenal medulla. This chain constitutes a reflex arc (Fig. 5.35). Some important cardiovascular reflexes are described below.

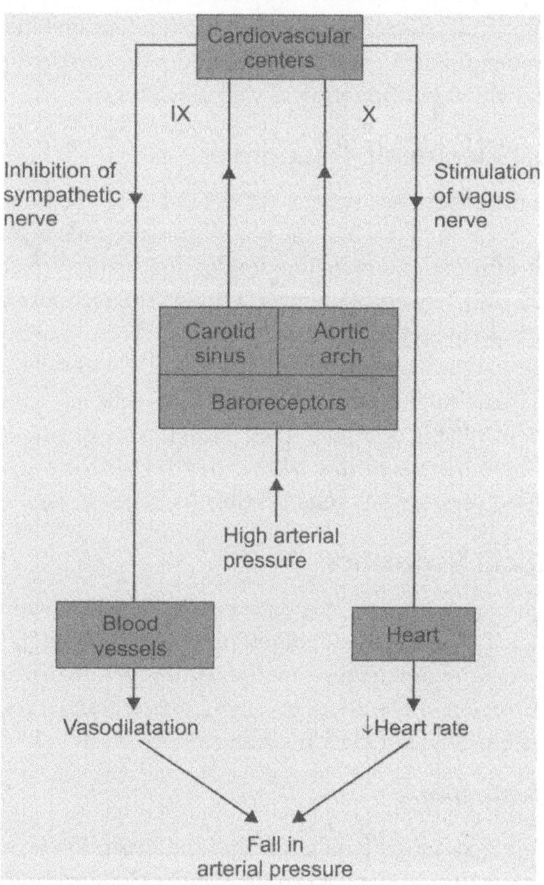

Fig. 5.36 Baroreceptor reflex. An increase in arterial pressure reflexly brings down the pressure, thus regulating it at the normal level. IX, the ninth cranial nerve (glossopharyngeal nerve); X, the tenth cranial nerve (vagus nerve)

Baroreceptor Reflex

As the name indicates, baroreceptors can detect changes in blood pressure. Baroreceptors are situated in the carotid sinus and aortic arch. When the blood pressure increases, baroreceptor reflexes bring about vasodilatation and decrease in heart rate. Both these effects lower the blood pressure towards normal. The opposite happens when the blood pressure falls (Fig. 5.36).

Chemoreceptor Reflex

Chemoreceptors are activated by a fall in PO_2, rise in PCO_2, or a decrease in pH. Chemoreceptors are situated in the carotid body and aortic body. Activation of chemoreceptors leads to a rise in blood pressure (Fig. 5.37). Chemoreceptors are involved in regulation of respiration as well (Chapter 6).

CNS Ischemic Response

Central nervous system (CNS) ischemic response comes into play when the blood pressure falls below 40 mm Hg. At such low levels, CNS suffers from ischemia (effects of low blood flow). The response to CNS ischemia is vasoconstriction, and consequently rise in blood pressure.

You might have observed that reflexes bring about what is 'desirable'. They try to restore normalcy. If blood pressure has fallen, they try to raise it; if blood pressure has gone up, they try to lower it.

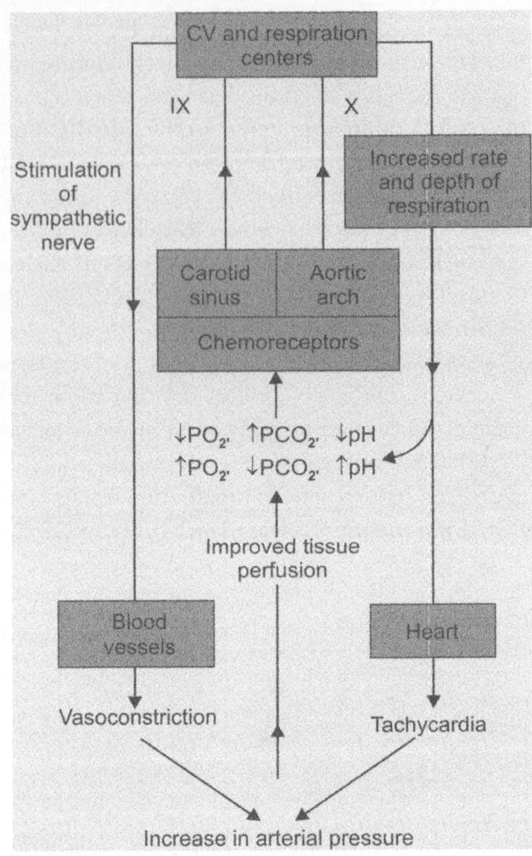

Fig. 5.37 Chemoreceptor reflex. Increase in chemoreceptor activity reflexly raises the blood pressure, which in turn leads to correction of the disturbances which initally stimulated the reflex. IX, the ninth cranial nerve (glossopharyngeal nerve); X, the tenth cranial nerve (vagus nerve)

Local Regulation

There are several regulatory mechanisms which increase or decrease blood flow only through a specific region. These mechanisms operate within the region only without involving the central nervous system. Some of these mechanisms are given below.

Axon Reflex

This is not a true reflex in that the central nervous system is not involved in its pathway. The response is evoked by an injury to the skin, and increases blood flow only in a small area of the skin. The neural pathway of axon reflex is shown in Figure 5.38.

Changes in Gas Tension

If blood flow through a region is less than its metabolic requirements, the tissue PO_2 in the region falls and tissue PCO_2 rises. These changes in gas tension bring about vasodilatation, which improves the blood flow.

Metabolites

If blood flow through a region is less than its metabolic requirements, not only carbon dioxide but also other metabolites such as lactic acid and adenosine accumulate. All these metabolites bring about vasodilatation, which improves the blood flow.

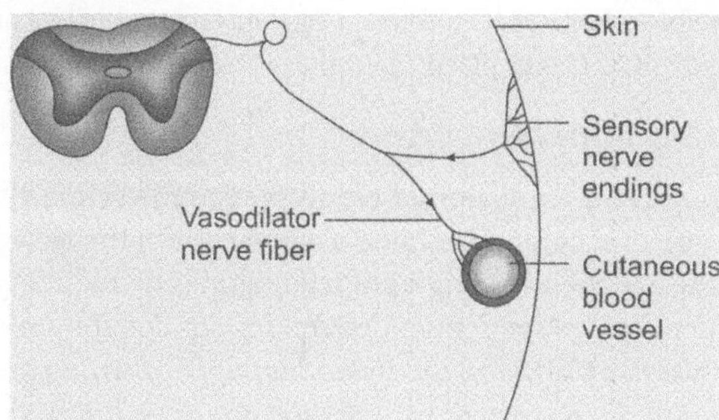

Fig. 5.38 Axon reflex. The neural pathway is indicated by the arrows

Mediators of Inflammatory Response

If a tissue is exposed to a noxious agent, it may respond by an inflammatory response. Inflammation is characterized by local vasodilatation.

Factors Affecting Blood Pressure

In electricity, according to Ohm's law,

Potential = Current flow × Resistance

MEASUREMENT OF BLOOD PRESSURE

Measurement of blood pressure (BP) is an extremely frequent bedside or out patient procedure. It is done using a sphygmomanometer and a stethoscope. Sphygmomanometer may have a mercury manometer or may be of the aneroid type. While the mercury manometer is the reference instrument, it is more bulky, cumbersome and fragile. If, for convenience, an aneroid instrument is used, it should be periodically calibrated against a mercury manometer. Since taking the BP is a common procedure, it is described in some detail below:

Palpatory method:

1. Put the subject at ease. Let him sit quietly for at least 5 minutes.
2. Place the sphygmomanometer cuff around the arm at the level of the heart.
3. Feel the radial pulse.
4. Inflate the pressure cuff. Note the pressure at which the radial pulse just disappears.
5. Deflate the pressure cuff slowly. Note the pressure at which the radial pulse just reappears.
6. The mean of the two readings is taken as the systolic blood pressure.

Auscultatory method:

1. Determination by the auscultatory method is a continuation of the palpatory method.
2. While the deflated sphygmomanometer pressure cuff is still around the arm, feel for the brachial pulse. It is usually palpable in the forearm on the anterior surface of the elbow just medial to the tendon of the biceps brachii muscle. Mark, with a pen, the site where the brachial pulse is best felt.
3. Place the stethoscope over the site of the brachial pulse.
4. Inflate the pressure cuff to a level about 25 mm Hg above the systolic pressure recorded by the palpatory method, or to about 180 mm Hg, whichever is higher.
5. Release the pressure slowly (2-3 mm Hg per second). Be on the look out for the appearance of a series of sounds. The character of sounds, known as Korotkov's sounds, changes as follows:
   Phase I. Clear tapping sound, which is heard while the pressure falls through approximately 10 mm Hg.
   Phase II. A murmurish sound, which lasts while the pressure falls another 10-15 mm Hg.
   Phase III. Clear and loud sounds while the pressure falls another 10-15 mm Hg.
   Phase IV. Muffled sound while the pressure falls through about 5 mm Hg.
   Phase V. The muffled sound disappears.
6. The beginning of phase I (appearance of tapping sound) is taken as systolic pressure. It is, on average, about 10 mm Hg higher than the systolic pressure determined by the palpatory method.
7. The beginning of phase V (disappearance of the muffled sound) is taken as the diastolic pressure.

Precautions

1. Do not skip the palpatory method.
2. Make sure that the site of the brachial pulse has been determined correctly.
3. Release the cuff pressure at the right speed: neither too fast nor too slowly.

In cardiovascular system, potential corresponds to blood pressure, current flow to blood flow (or cardiac output), and resistance to peripheral resistance. Therefore,

Blood pressure = Cardiac output × Peripheral resistance

Therefore, blood pressure is affected by factors which affect cardiac output or peripheral resistance. Factors affecting cardiac output have already been discussed. Peripheral resistance is increased by vasoconstriction and decreased by vasodilatation. Factors which bring about vasoconstriction or vasodilatation have also been discussed already. Cardiac output affects mainly the systolic pressure, and peripheral resistance affects mainly the diastolic pressure.

Regulation of Blood Pressure

Blood pressure regulation may be classified into short-term and long-term regulation.

Short-term Regulation

These mechanisms come into play within seconds or minutes of the occurrence of a disturbance which tends to change the blood pressure. Although these mechanisms prevent any major change in blood pressure, they do not correct the cause of the disturbance.

Baroreceptors and chemoreceptors: Baroreceptor reflexes (p. 88) operate within the range of 70 to 150 mm Hg and correct changes in blood pressure within seconds.

Chemoreceptor reflexes (p. 88) operate within the range of 40 to 70 mm Hg and promptly correct changes in blood pressure.

CNS ischemic response: If the blood pressure falls below 40 mm Hg, the CNS ischemic response (p. 88) may succeed in saving the person by raising the blood pressure to some extent.

Release of adrenaline: Whenever blood pressure tends to fall, adrenaline is released from the adrenal medulla.

Adrenaline raises the blood pressure through its effects on the heart as well as blood vessels.

Capillary fluid shift: When arterial blood pressure increases, capillary hydrostatic pressure also increases. This leads to greater filtration at the arterial end of capillaries and reduced reabsorption at venous end of capillaries (p. 82). Thus some fluid shifts from the blood to the interstitial fluid. This tends to lower the blood pressure. Opposite type of redistribution of body fluids takes place when the arterial pressure falls.

Long-term Regulation

Long-term regulation of blood pressure is primarily regulation of blood volume (Chapter 19). If the blood pressure rises, its long term regulation is by reducing the blood volume. Blood volume is regulated by the kidneys by altering the urine output. In turn, urine output is regulated by the hormones antidiuretic hormone (ADH), aldosterone, angiotensin, and atrial natriuretic peptide. These mechanisms have been discussed at appropriate places in the book. They have been summarized in Figure 5.39 illustrating the sequence of events following an increase in blood volume. If the blood volume is reduced, the same mechanisms work in the opposite direction to restore normalcy.

Hypertension

Hypertension means an abnormally high blood pressure. Some rise in blood pressure with age is

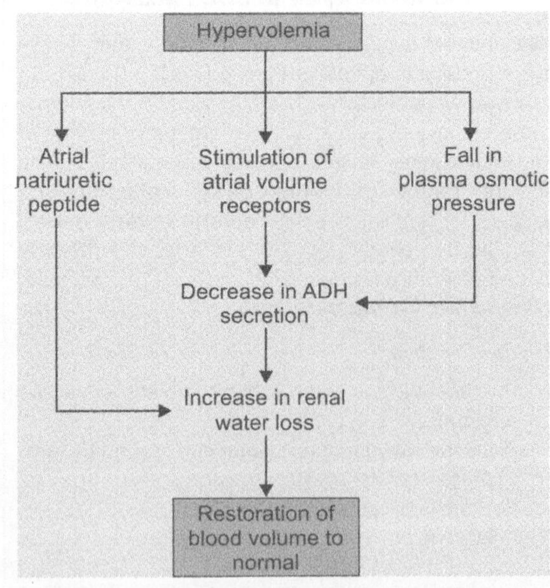

Fig. 5.39 Some of the mechanisms which restore blood volume to normal. Regulation of blood volume is an essential component of regulation of blood pressure

considered normal. Roughly, the normal systolic blood pressure is less than (100+ age in years) mm Hg. If it is higher than that, the person is considered to have hypertension. But systolic pressure is frequently raised temporarily due to mental stress, including the stress created by the atmosphere of the clinic or hospital. Therefore diastolic pressure is a more reliable indicator of normalcy of blood pressure. If the diastolic pressure is above 90 mm Hg, the person is considered to have hypertension. However, a few readings at different visits are necessary before a person is labelled hypertensive and treated for it. As an arbitrary dividing line, if the blood pressure is repeatedly above 150/90 mm Hg on at least three occasions at any age, the person may be considered to have hypertension, once again greater reliance being placed on the diastolic blood pressure.

Classification of Hypertension

There are two main categories of hypertension:

Primary or essential hypertension: In these cases the cause of hypertension is not clearly known. Primary hypertension seems to be the end result of a variety of factors: hereditary tendency, eating too much and eating a bad diet, inadequate physical activity, overweight, smoking and mental stress. Except for heredity, the remaining factors are modifiable, and are collectively referred to as the lifestyle. More than 90% of those who have hypertension have primary hypertension.

Secondary hypertension: In these cases the cause of hypertension is known. The cause may be renal disease, hyperaldosteronism, Cushing's syndrome, pheochromocytoma or long-term use of oral contraceptives.

CORONARY CIRCULATION

Coronary arteries are the blood vessels which supply blood to the heart. Although the chambers of the heart contain so much blood, the blood in the cavities cannot meet the requirements of the heart. Like other parts of the body, the heart also needs specific arteries to carry blood to all its layers. Coronary arteries are of special interest because their partial obstruction is quite common, which is called coronary heart disease. Coronary heart disease may lead to chest pain on exertion (angina), or acute myocardial infarction (heart attack).

Blood flow through the coronary arteries is not uniform throughout the cardiac cycle. During ventricular systole, strong contraction of the ventricular musculature squeezes the blood vessels. Hence coronary blood flow is reduced during systole. This effect is more marked in the left ventricle because it develops a much higher systolic pressure than the right ventricle. During isometric contraction, there is almost no blood flow through the left ventricle (Fig. 5.40).

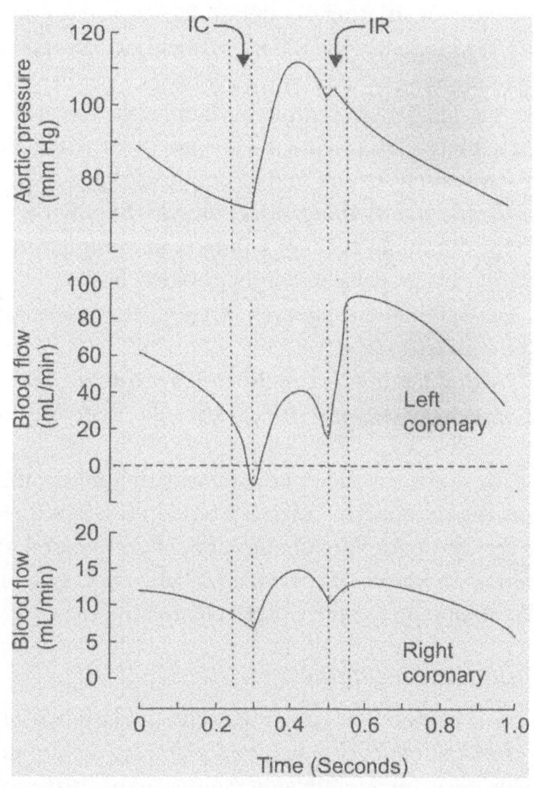

Fig. 5.40 Coronary blood flow during different phases of the cardiac cycle. Note that the blood flow through the left coronary artey is below zero towards the end of isometric contraction. This is to indicate the fact that blood may be sequeezed out of the coronary artery towards the aorta at that point. IC, isometric contraction; IR, isometric relaxation

Regulation of Coronary Blood Flow

Whenever the heart rate or force of contraction of the heart increases, the requirement for coronary blood flow also increases. Accordingly, variations in coronary blood flow are most closely related to variations in cardiac activity. This happens because the most important determinants of coronary blood flow are the metabolites produced by contractile activity.

Neural Regulation

Coronary arteries are supplied by sympathetic and parasympathetic nerves.

Sympathetic nerves act on the coronary arteries in three ways:

1. Vasoconstriction via alpha adrenergic receptors,
2. Vasodilatation via beta adrenergic receptors, and
3. Vasodilatation, indirectly via increase in cardiac activity. Since sympathetic nerves to the heart increase heart rate and force of contraction of the heart, that itself increases coronary blood flow.

The dominant effect of sympathetic stimulation is a significant increase in coronary blood flow.

Parasympathetic nerves act on the coronary arteries in two ways:

1. Vasodilatation via cholinergic receptors, and
2. Vasoconstriction, indirectly, via decrease in cardiac activity.

The dominant effect of parasympathetic stimulations is a decrease in coronary blood flow. But there are very few parasympathetic nerve fibers to coronary arteries. Therefore the parasympathetic effect on coronary blood flow is physiologically not important.

Chemical Regulation

Coronary blood flow is very sensitive to a large variety of chemical changes associated with cardiac activity (Table 5.5). Increase in metabolites associated with activity dilates the coronary arteries. Thus blood flow keeps pace with cardiac activity. This is the dominant mechanism for regulation of coronary blood flow.

Table 5.5 Chemical mediators which dilate coronary arteries

S. No.	*Chemical agent*
1.	Low oxygen tension
2.	High carbon dioxide tension
3.	High hydrogen ion concentration
4.	High lactic acid concentration
5.	High ADP concentration
6.	High adenosine concentration

CORONARY ARTERY DISEASE

In coronary artery disease (CAD) one or more coronary arteries may be partly or almost completely blocked by deposits made up of fats, cellular debris, inflammatory cells and blood cells. These deposits are called atherosclerotic deposits. Atherosclerosis is a generalized process and affects arteries throughout the body. But in some places, such as the heart, atherosclerosis has serious consequences. Atherosclerotic deposits reduce blood flow to the heart. As a result, the blood flow may be adequate at rest, but inadequate during exercise and other situations when the oxygen requirement of the myocardium increases. When the oxygen demand of the myocardium exceeds the supply, the person feels pain in the chest. This pain is called angina pectoris, or just angina. Like essential hypertension, CAD is also a lifestyle disease, and the two are often present together in the same person. Therefore lifestyle modification based on the principles of yoga helps CAD also.

SHOCK

Circulatory shock is a condition in which tissue perfusion is inadequate due to a reduction in circulating blood volume. Circulating blood volume is reduced when the blood volume is reduced. But circulating blood volume may be sometimes reduced also when the blood volume is not reduced. For example, if there is widespread vasodilatation, blood may get pooled in the dilated blood vessels instead of circulating. Or, if the heart cannot pump enough blood, circulating blood volume will be reduced even if the blood volume is normal.

The typical manifestations of shock are low blood pressure, rapid and thready pulse, and cold and clammy skin. The breathing is rapid, and the patient may be very thirsty. Shock is a life-threatening situation, and therefore needs urgent attention.

Depending on the cause, shock may be of several types, some of which have been discussed below briefly.

Hypovolemic Shock

In this type of shock, there is actually a reduction in blood volume. It may be due to bleeding, diarrhea, vomiting or burns.

The immediate response of the body to hypovolemia is activation of baroreceptor reflexes, which may maintain the blood pressure within normal limits. The normal blood pressure is misleading. It does not mean that the patient is out of danger. If a cause for suspecting shock is present, the patient should receive adequate attention even if the blood pressure is normal.

Another early response is stimulation of respiration by the chemoreceptor reflex. This response tends to improve tissue oxygenation. That is why the patient has a high respiratory rate.

The later responses of the body are directed at restoration of the blood volume, such as redistribution of body fluids, reduction in urinary output and increased thirst.

Long-term responses to bleeding are directed at replenishing the loss. They include increased erythropoiesis and increased plasma protein synthesis.

A patient having hypovolemic shock should receive fluids urgently. If the patient is conscious, even oral fluids are better than no fluids at all. Further, the patient should be kept lying down with the foot end of the bed slightly raised to maintain blood flow to the brain. Other specific measures of treatment should also be initiated. If shock is not treated promptly, it may become irreversible and lead to death.

Cardiogenic Shock

Cardiogenic shock is due to a reduction in cardiac output. It may result from coronary artery disease or a disease of heart muscle or compression of the heart by a pericardial effusion.

Neurogenic Shock

Severe pain may produce widespread vasodilatation and thereby lead to shock. This type of shock is called neurogenic.

Anaphylactic Shock

Anaphylactic shock is due to widespread vasodilatation produced by an allergic (hypersensitivity) reaction.

Septic Shock

Septic shock is due to widespread vasodilatation produced by bacterial toxins.

QUESTIONS

1. Comment on the statement that arteries carry pure blood while veins carry impure blood.
2. What is the significance of the delay in conduction of the cardiac impulse through the AV node?
3. What is the significance of the fact that cardiac muscle cannot be tetanized?
4. What is the significance of the length-tension relationship in cardiac muscle?
5. Why is the wave of atrial repolarization not seen in the ECG?
6. What is the osmotic pressure of plasma?
7. What is the significance of determining blood pressure by the palpatory method before going to the auscultatory method?
8. How may burns produce hypovolemic shock?
9. Why does the heart rate increase during inspiration?
10. Atrioventricular (AV) delay:
    A. Is due to slow spread of the cardiac impulse from the SA node to atria
    B. Occurs in the bundle of His

C. Prevents atria and ventricles from contracting simultaneously
D. Is harmful because it delays the spread of cardiac impulse

11. At rest, the human heart pumps the equivalent of the entire blood volume of a person in about:
    A. 1 minute
    B. 2 minutes
    C. 5 minutes
    D. 1 hour
12. For each of the following statements, say whether it is true or false:
    A. Arteries bring blood to the heart whereas veins carry blood away from the heart.
    B. Blood pressure normally refers to the arterial blood pressure.
    C. Parasympathetic stimulation increases the heart rate.
    D. The walls of arteries are more muscular than those of veins.

ANSWERS

1. This is a common statement but it has many errors.
   a. Instead of pure blood, it is better to say oxygenated blood. Similarly 'impure' blood should be called deoxygenated blood.
   b. Pulmonary *arteries* carry deoxygenated blood while pulmonary veins carry oxygenated blood. Therefore the statement is wrong for pulmonary blood vessels.
   c. All arteries (including pulmonary arteries) carry blood away from the heart. All veins (including pulmonary veins) carry blood towards the heart.
2. Because of the AV delay, atria and ventricles do not contract simultaneously. This allows atria to fill up when the ventricles are contracting, and allows atria to contract and send blood into relaxed ventricles. This type of normal smooth functioning would not be possible without AV delay.
3. The function of the heart is to pump blood. This needs alternate contraction (to pump blood) and relaxation (to get filled up with blood to be pumped). A heart which remains contracted for a long period of time would not be of any use.
4. If the blood returning to the heart is more, it stretches the heart. Stretch leads to an increase in the length of the cardiac muscle fibers. Longer length leads to stronger contraction of the heart. As a result, more blood is pumped out. Thus, if the blood returning to the heart is more, the blood pumped out of the heart is more. Conversely, if the blood returning is less, the blood pumped out is less. In this way the length-tension relationship (Starling's law) helps in maintaining a balance between blood returning to the heart and blood pumped out of the heart.
5. The wave of atrial repolarization occurs at the same time as the wave of ventricular depolarization. The wave of ventricular depolarization is so big that it hides the wave of atrial repolarization.
6. The osmotic pressure of plasma is about 5525 mm Hg. Out of this, about 5500 mm Hg is due to electrolytes (crystalloid osmotic pressure). An additional osmotic pressure of 25 mm Hg is due to plasma proteins (colloid osmotic pressure). While considering fluid exchange across capillaries, we have considered only the colloid osmotic pressure because the crystalloid osmotic pressure of plasma is the same as that of the interstitial fluid. The difference between the osmotic pressure of plasma and interstitial fluid is 25 mm Hg, which is entirely due to plasma proteins. This difference does not get equalized because capillaries generally do not allow proteins to leak out into the interstitial fluid. Therefore, it is only the difference in osmotic pressure due to plasma proteins which contributes to the forces determining fluid exchange across capillaries.
7. In some patients having high blood pressure (BP), when the BP is taken by the auscultatory method, there is a silent gap of about 40-50 mm Hg between phase II and phase III Korotkov's

sounds. If the BP is taken by the auscultatory method and the cuff pressure is not raised high enough, one may mistake the phase III sounds for the beginning of Korotkov's sounds. Thus a false low reading may be obtained for the systolic pressure, and the high BP may be missed. One the other hand if the systolic BP has been determined by the palpatory method first, one knows how high to raise the cuff pressure while doing the auscultatory method.

8. In burns, capillary permeability is increased. That leads to loss of fluid as well as plasma proteins from the capillaries into the interstitial fluid. Plasma proteins increase the osmotic pressure of the interstitial fluid. That further increases exudation of fluid from the capillaries. The fluid collecting in the interstitial spaces cannot circulate. Thus, although fluid is not apparently lost from the body, the circulating blood volume is reduced, giving rise to the features of hypovolemic shock.
9. One of the explanations is that during inspiration the negative intrathoracic pressure makes more blood flow from the veins into the right atrium. That stretches the right atrium. Since the SA node is in the right atrium, stretching of the right atrium stimulates the SA node mechanically. As a result, its frequency of discharge increases. Since SA node is the pacemaker of the heart, increased rate of discharge of the SA node increases the heart rate. (Use a similar argument to explain the decrease in heart rate during expiration.)
10. C (see Question 2)
11. A
12. A. False B. True C. False D. True

CHAPTER

6 Respiratory System

"The smooth, soft air with pulse-like waves, Flows murmuring through its hidden caves, Whose streams of brightening purple rush, Fired with a new and livelier blush, While all their burden of decay, The ebbing current steals away, And red with Nature's flame they start, From the warm fountains of the heart."

—OLIVER WENDELL HOLMES

Chapter Outline

- Functional Anatomy
- Volumes and Capacities
- Mechanics of Breathing
- Oxygen Transport
- Carbon Dioxide Transport
- Regulation of Respiration
- Pulmonary Function Tests
- Applied Respiratory Physiology

Like the heart beat, breathing is also a sign of life. The respiratory rate, along with the pulse rate, blood pressure and temperature constitute the clinical vital signs. Pulse rate, respiratory rate and temperature are routinely recorded by the nurse on every in-patient several times a day. Why is respiration such an important function? All cells of the body continually use oxygen to derive energy from nutrients. In this process, carbon dioxide is produced. For life to continue, therefore, oxygen must be supplied to the body, and carbon dioxide must be removed from the body. These functions are performed by respiration.

Respiratory function needs co-operation of lungs, heart and blood. Venous blood, which has lost some of its oxygen to tissues and has picked up some carbon dioxide from tissues, returns to the right atrium of the heart. The right ventricle pumps this blood to the lungs. In the lungs blood is brought in intimate contact with atmospheric air. Oxygen diffuses from air into the venous blood. Carbon dioxide diffuses from venous blood into the air. This blood of 'improved' composition returns to the heart to be pumped again to various tissues (Fig. 6.1).

FUNCTIONAL ANATOMY

The respiratory system consists mainly of a series of tubes (airways) which branch out like a tree. The airways lead to the lungs (Fig. 6.2). Before reaching the airways, air passes through the nose. The inner lining of the nose (nasal mucosa) is warm and moist, and has ciliated epithelial cells. Therefore, the air passing through the nose becomes warm and moist. Dust particles in the air get trapped in the moisture, and get swept by the cilia. The process of making air warm, moist and clean continues in the airways (trachea and bronchi). The bronchi finally form alveoli. Alveoli have very thin walls made up of extremely flattened epithelial cells. Blood capillaries come very close to the alveolar walls. This structure is ideal for exchange of gases between the alveolar air and blood (Fig. 6.3).

Volumes and Capacities

Respiratory function is frequently measured in terms of volume of air moved by the lungs under

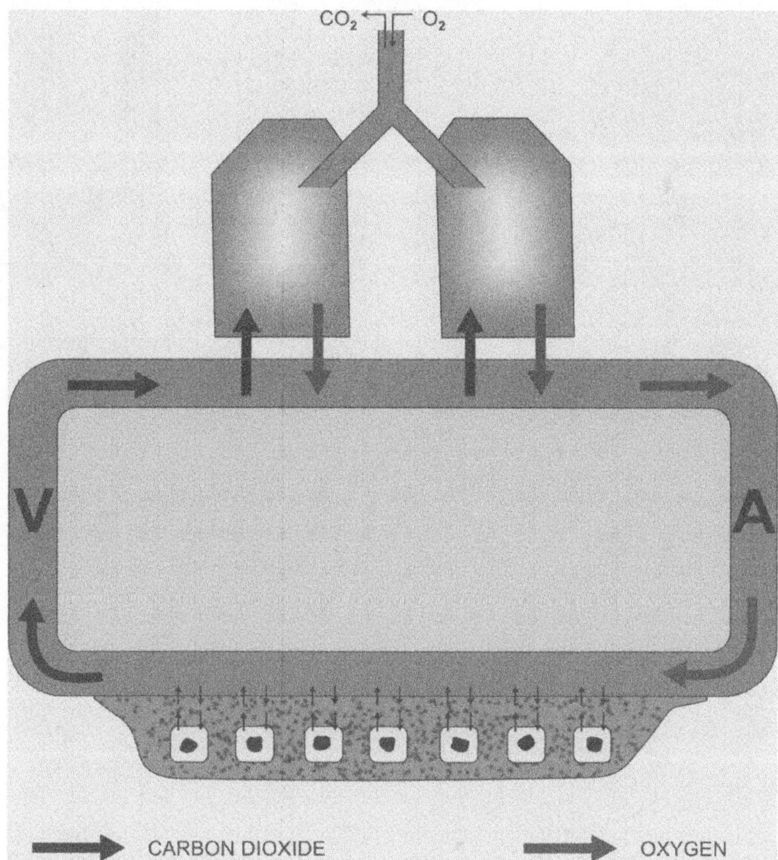

Fig. 6.1 The purpose of respiration is on one hand to collect oxygen from the external environment and to deliver it to the tissues, and on the other to collect carbon dioxide from the tissue and to release it into the external environment. The lungs, blood and interstitial fluid act as intermediaries in the process. A, arterial side; and V, venous side of the circulation

specific conditions. Volumes are basic values while capacities are derived from volumes. Each **capacity** is the sum of two or more **volumes**. As you read the description of each volume and capacity below, try to form its mental picture by breathing according to the description, and looking at Figure 6.4. There are four fundamental volumes and four capacities.

Tidal Volume

It is the volume of air breathed in or out in one breath.

Inspiratory Reserve Volume

It is the maximum volume of air that can be inspired over and above the volume normally breathed in at rest.

Expiratory Reserve Volume

It is the maximum volume of air that can be expired over and above the volume normally breathed out at rest.

Residual Volume

It is the volume of air remaining in the lungs at the end of a maximal expiration. This is a volume which you can imagine but cannot breathe in or out.

Total Lung Capacity

It is the volume of air in the lungs at the end of a maximal inspiration. Thus total lung capacity (TLC) includes tidal volume (TV), inspiratory reserve volume

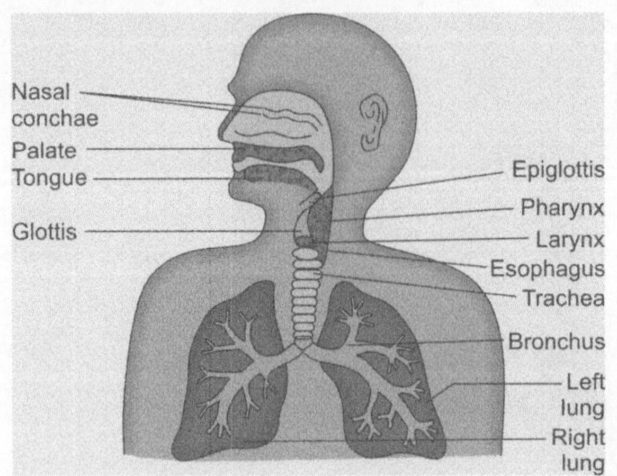

Fig. 6.2 Diagrammatic representation of structure of the respiratory system

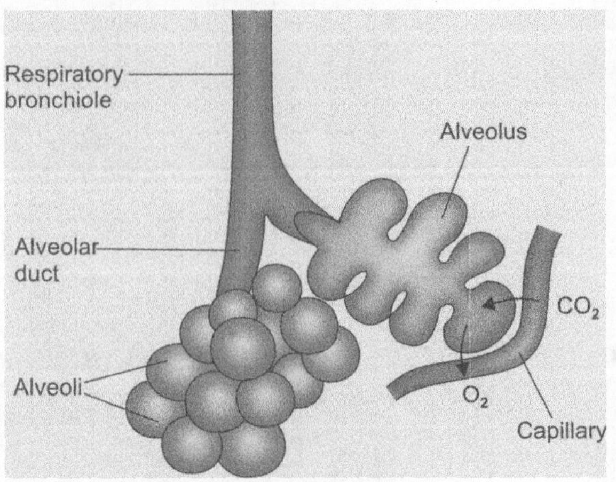

Fig. 6.3 Schematic diagram of the alveolo-capillary gas-exchange unit. (Reproduced from Bijlani RL, Manchanda SK. The Human Machine: How to prevent breakdowns. New Delhi: National Book Trust, 1990)

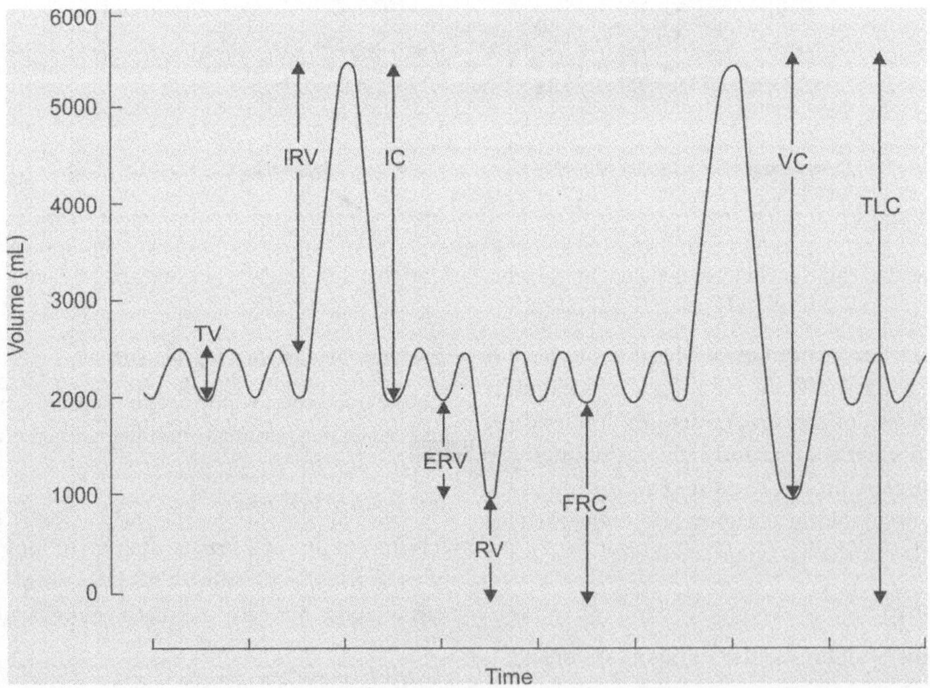

Fig. 6.4 Lung volumes and capacities. Diagrammatic representation of a spirographic tracing: inspiration upwards, expiration downwards. TV, tidal volume; IRV, inspiratory reserve volume; IC, inspiratory capacity; ERV, expiratory reserve volume; RV, residual volume; FRC, functional residual capacity; VC, vital capacity; TLC, total lung capacity

(IRV), expiratory reserve volume (ERV) and residual volume (RV). Or, TLC = TV + IRV + ERV + RV.

Inspiratory Capacity

It is the maximum volume of air that can be inspired starting with the resting end-expiratory position. Thus, inspiratory capacity (IC) = TV + IRV.

Functional Residual Capacity

It is the volume of air remaining in the lungs at the end of a normal expiration. Thus, functional residual capacity (FRC) = ERV + RV.

Vital Capacity

It is the maximum volume of air that can be expired after a maximal inspiration. Thus, vital capacity (VC) = IC + ERV = IRV + TV + ERV.

Sometimes while measuring VC the subject is asked to breathe out not only as much air as possible but also as fast as possible. VC measured in this way is called timed vital capacity. Normally, about 80 percent of the VC is breathed out in the first second of expiration. This fraction is called FEV_1 which stands for forced expiratory volume in one second. FEV_1 is reduced in obstructive lung diseases (Fig. 6.5).

The normal values of lung volumes and capacities have been given in Table 6.1.

Some More Volumes Relevant to Pulmonary Physiology

Minute Volume

Minute volume (MV) is the volume of air breathed in or out in one minute. Thus, MV = TV × Respiratory rate per minute.

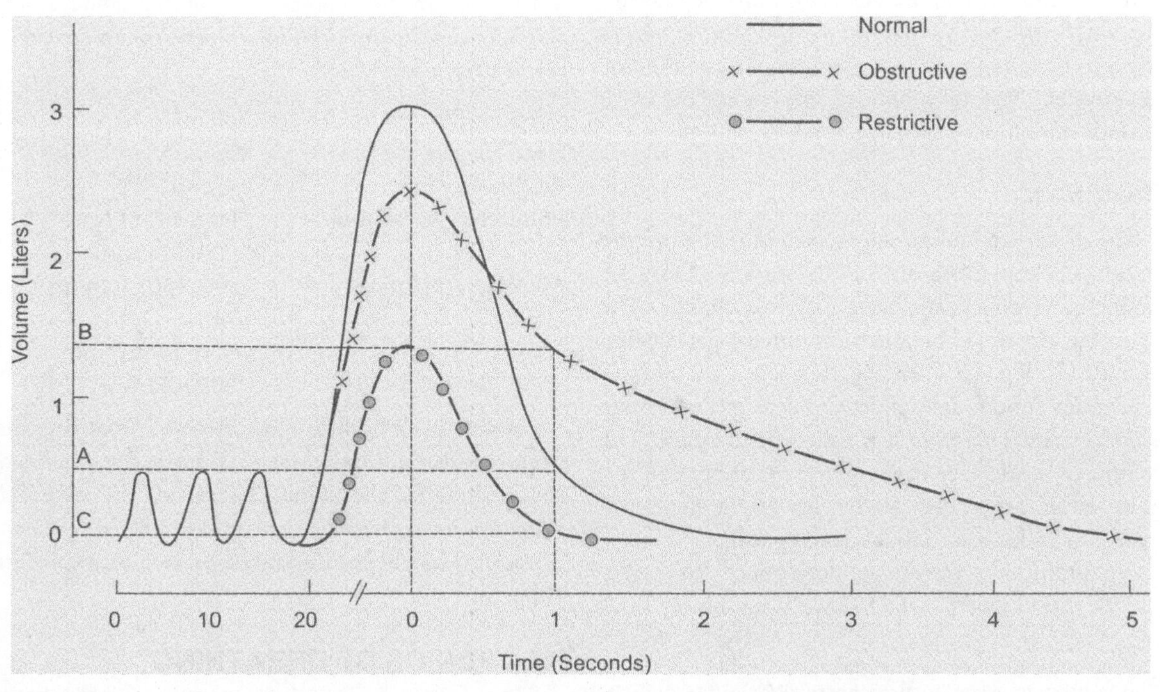

Fig. 6.5 Timed vital capacity. The vital capacity in this diagram is 3 liters in normal, 2.5 liters in obstructive lung disease, and 1.3 liters in restrictive lung disease. Out of this, the volume expired in the first second is 2.5 liters, 1.2 liters and 1.2 liters respectively. Hence the .FEV_1 is 2.5/3 = 83%, 1.2/2.5 = 48% and 1.2/1.3 = 92% respectively. Thus in obstructive lung disease, the FEV_1 is markedly reduced although the total vital capacity is not that much affected. In contrast, in restrictive lung disease, the total vital capacity is markedly reduced but FEV_1 is normal. A, B, C are lines corresponding to FEV^1 for normal, obstructive lung disease and restrictive lung disease respectively

Table 6.1 Lung volumes and capacities in healthy adult males*

Volume or capacity	Value (L)
Tidal volume	0.5
Inspiratory reserve volume	3.0
Expiratory reserve volume	1.0
Residual volume	1.0
Total lung capacity	5.5
Inspiratory capacity	3.5
Functional residual capacity	2.0
Vital capacity	4.5

*Approximate values, rounded off to the nearest half liter.

Maximum Voluntary Ventilation

Maximum voluntary ventilation (MVV) is the volume of air that can be breathed out by the lungs in one minute by maximal effort, increasing both the rate and depth of breathing. To determine MVV, the subject is asked to breathe as fast and as deeply as possible **for 15 seconds**. The total volume of air breathed out in 15 seconds is multiplied by 4 to get MVV.[1]

Dead Space

When air is breathed in, only a part of it reaches the alveoli. The remaining air is in the airways. Only the air in the alveoli participates in gas exchange. The air in the airways is breathed out unchanged during expiration (Fig. 6.6). Hence the space in airways behaves as functionally dead so far as gas exchange is concerned. Therefore it is called **dead space**. The volume of dead space in the airways is about 150 mL in an adult. Since this dead space has a structural basis, it is called **anatomical dead space**.

In addition to anatomical dead space, there may also be some alveoli which have poor blood flow. Poor blood flow leads to poor gas exchange in these alveoli. Thus these alveoli also behave like dead space (Fig. 6.7). Physiological dead space includes anatomical dead space and dead space due to alveoli with poor blood flow.

Pulmonary Ventilation and Alveolar Ventilation

Pulmonary ventilation is the amount of air breathed in and out. It is quantitatively indicated by the minute volume, i.e. tidal volume × respiratory rate. But all the pulmonary ventilation is not useful for gas exchange. The amount going to the dead space does not participate in gas exchange. Only the amount going to the alveoli participates in gas exchange. Therefore useful ventilation is measured as alveolar ventilation. Out of the tidal volume air, the part which goes to alveoli is the part which does not remain in the dead space (Fig. 6.6). Therefore, alveolar ventilation is (tidal volume–dead space) × respiratory rate.

Suppose TV = 500 mL
Dead space = 150 mL
Respiratory rate = 14/min
Pulmonary ventilation = 500 × 14 mL/min
= 7000 mL/min
Alveolar ventilation = (500–150) × 14 mL/min
= 350 × 14 mL/min
= 4900 mL/min

Hence deep breathing is efficient breathing. In deep breathing, tidal volume is more, but the dead space remains the same. Therefore the alveolar ventilation achieved is proportionately greater. The point has been illustrated by two examples in Table 6.2.

MECHANICS OF BREATHING

Air enters the lungs during inspiration and moves out of the lungs during expiration. The movement of air follows a simple principle: it moves from a higher pressure to a lower pressure. The change in pressure follows Boyle's law, i.e. if a given amount of gas is

[1]The subject is asked to breathe maximally for only 15 seconds because it is dangerous to do so for a longer period. Breathing like that removes (washes off) carbon dioxide from the body. Fall in carbon dioxide level in the blood causes constriction of cerebral blood vessels. Cerebral vasoconstriction may lead to unconsciousness.

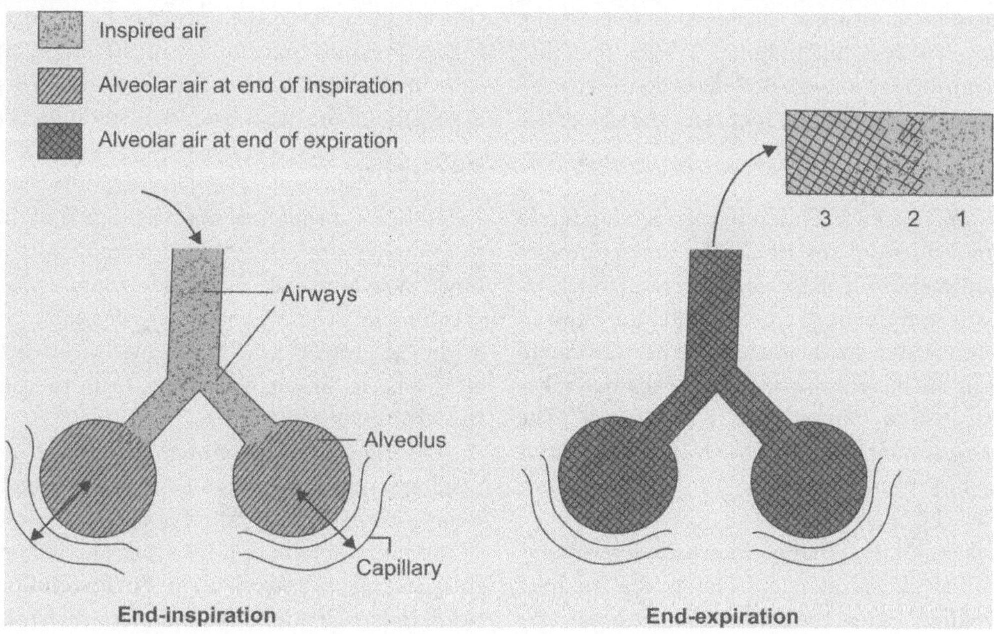

Fig. 6.6 Dead space. At the end of inspiration, airways have inspired air (atmospheric air) whereas alveoli have a mixture of inspired air and the air already present in alveoli. The composition of alveolar air keeps changing as a result of gas exchange. During expiration, the first air to come out is the 'inspired air' from the airways (1). Then comes out a mixture of 'inspired air' and alveolar air (2). The last part of expired air is the alveolar air (3)

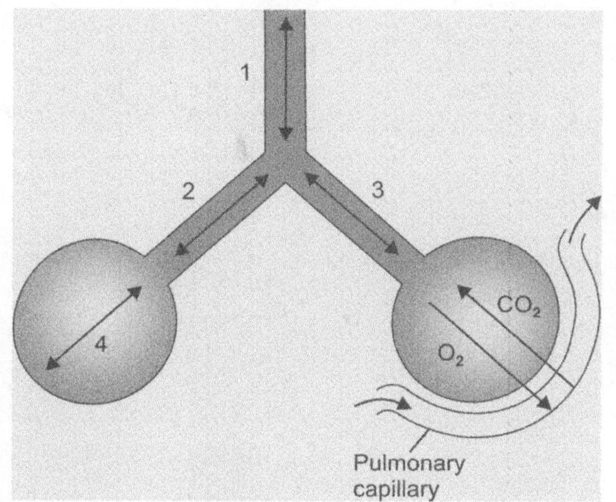

Fig. 6.7 Dead space. Airways (1, 2, 3) constitute the anatomical dead space. An alveolus which is not perfused with blood (4) is also functionally like the airways and forms a part of the physiological dead space. A normally perfused alveolus has been shown for comparison. Although total absence of perfusion is an extreme situation, inadequately perfused alveoli also contribute to the dead space

Table 6.2 Effect of tidal volume on alveolar ventilation

	Low tidal volume	*High tidal volume*
Tidal volume	300 mL	600 mL
Respiratory rate	20 per min	10 per min
Pulmonary ventilation	6000 mL/min	6000 mL/min
Dead space	150 mL	150 mL
Alveolar ventilation	3000 mL/min	4500 mL/min

made to occupy a larger volume, its pressure falls; and if the gas is made to occupy a smaller volume, its pressure rises.[2]

Inspiration

Inspiration is brought about by an expansion of the chest. The chest (thorax) expands on all sides.

[2]Provided, of course, the temperature remains constant.

It expands *from above downwards* due to the contraction of the diaphragm.[3] When the diaphragm contracts, it moves downwards. Downward movement of the diaphragm increases the size of the thorax from above downwards.

The thorax expands *from side to side (transversely)* and *from front-backwards (antero-posteriorly)* due to upward movement of the ribs. Ribs move upwards due to contraction of external intercostal muscles. The upward movement of ribs expands the chest in two directions due to their shape. The movement resulting in an increase in transverse diameter has been compared to "bucket handle movement". The movement resulting in an increase in anteroposterior diameter has been compared to "pump handle movement" (Fig. 6.8).

Expansion of the thorax increases its volume. Thus the air already present in the lungs now occupies a larger volume. Hence the pressure in the lungs falls (Boyle's law). Since the atmospheric air is now at a higher pressure than the air in the lungs, air moves in from the atmosphere into the lungs. This is how expansion of the lungs leads to inspiration (Fig. 6.9).

Expiration

Expiration is brought about by a return of the thorax to a smaller size. Thus the air already present in the lungs now occupies a smaller volume. Hence the pressure in the lungs rises (Boyle's law). Since the air in the lungs is now at a higher pressure than the atmospheric air, air moves out from the lungs into the atmosphere (Fig. 6.10).

During quiet breathing, expiration does not need any muscular effort, i.e. it is a passive process. Relaxation of the inspiratory muscles and elastic recoil of the lungs are enough to return the volume of the thoracic cage to a smaller size. But forceful expiration needs muscular effort. The muscles which bring about

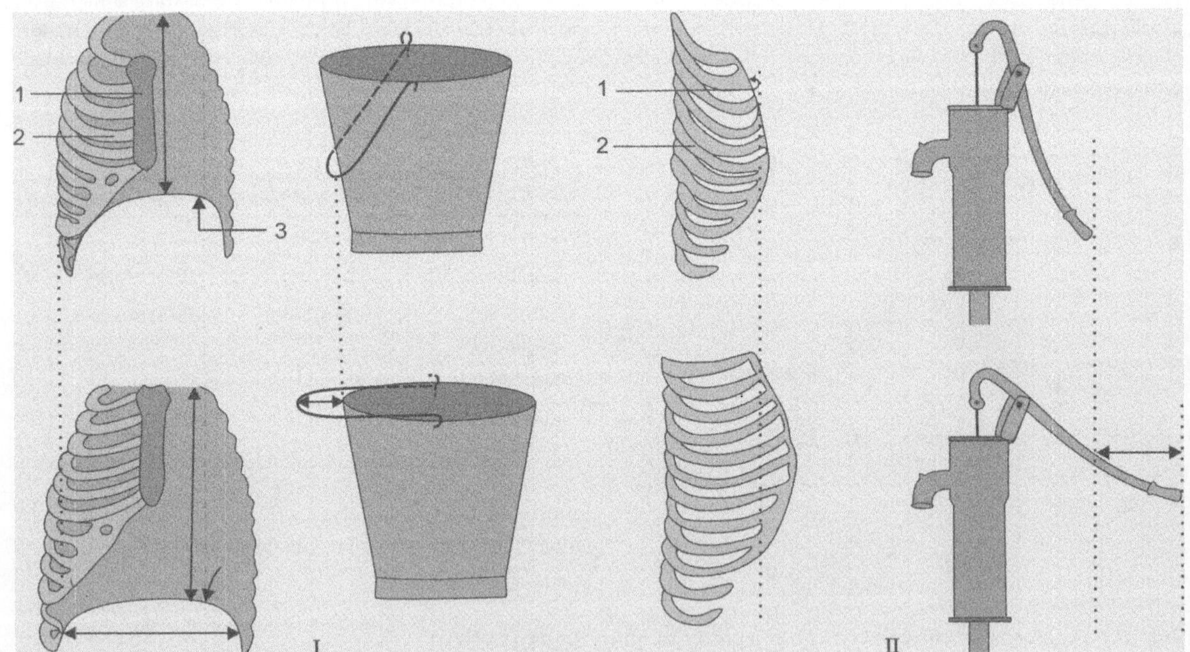

Fig. 6.8 Expansion of the chest during inspiration. I. 'Bucket handle movement'. II. 'Pump handle' movement. (1) Sternum; (2) Rib; (3) Diaphragm (Reproduced from Bijlani RL, Manchanda SK. The Human Machine: How to prevent breakdowns. New Delhi: National Book Trust, India, 1990)

[3]Diaphragm is the muscular partition between the thorax and the abdomen.

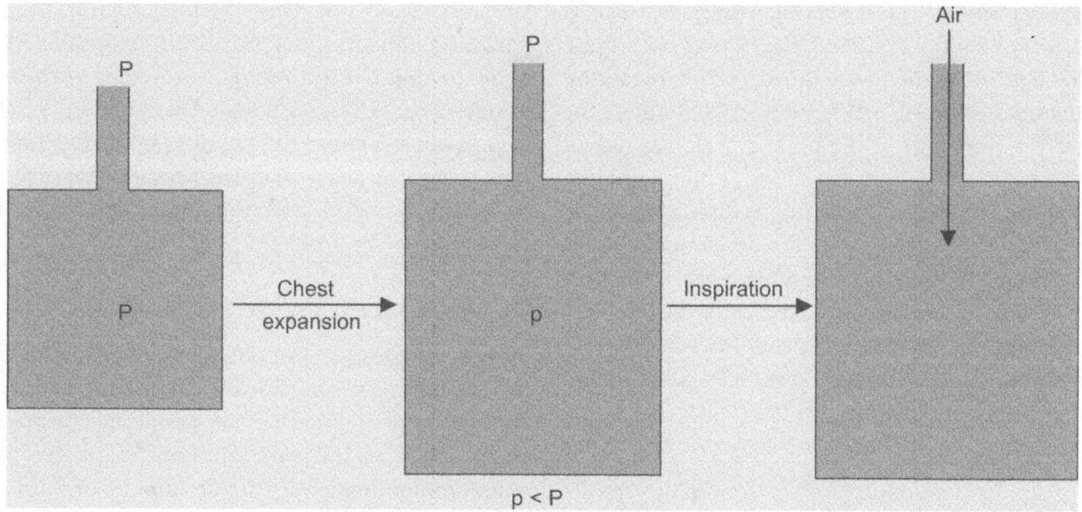

Fig. 6.9 Chest expansion leads to a fall in the pressure within the chest. Since air moves from a higher pressure towards a lower pressure, chest expansion leads to inspiration

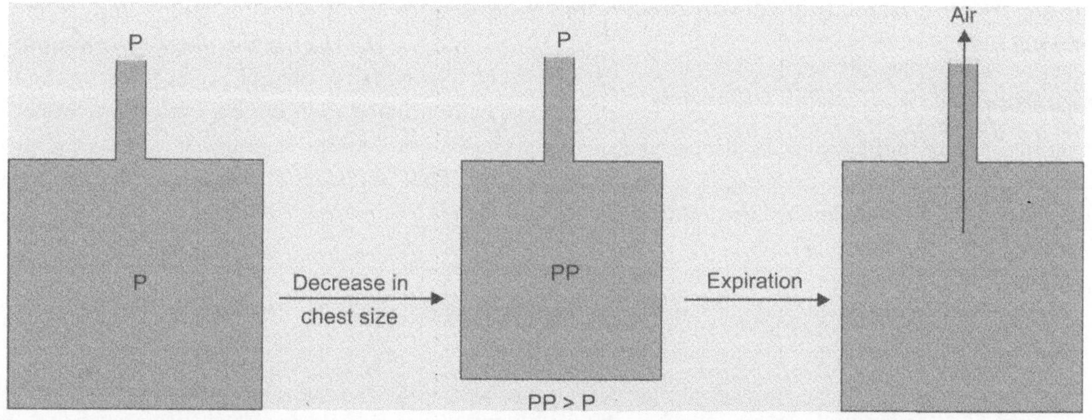

Fig. 6.10 Decrease in the dimensions of the chest leads to an increase in the pressure within the chest. Since air moves from a higher pressure towards a lower pressure, return of the chest to a smaller size leads to expiration

forceful expiration are the abdominal muscles and the internal intercostal muscles.

Thoracic, Abdominal and Clavicular Breathing

We have seen above that we may breathe in using the intercostal muscles (thoracic breathing) or the diaphragm (abdominal breathing). Diaphragmatic breathing is called abdominal breathing because the downward movement of the diaphragm during inspiration presses on the abdominal contents, thereby making the abdomen bulge out. Most of us tend to be thoracic breathers, which is unfortunate because abdominal breathing is more efficient. Pure abdominal breathing is, however, possible only when we are lying down supine. In the sitting or standing posture, we should try to breathe using a mixture of thoracic and abdominal breathing. Using both these mechanisms also increases the depth of breathing (i.e. the tidal volume), making it possible to meet the oxygen requirements of the body at a slower rate of breathing. Slow and deep breathing is more efficient than rapid and shallow breathing, as discussed above.

Clavicular breathing uses the accessory muscles of breathing among the shoulder, neck and back muscles. These muscles are used only during very deep breathing, or if there is an obstruction in the respiratory tract. In any case, it is good to use them off and on to keep the clavicular breathing mechanism in good shape, and to aerate the upper zones of the lungs. Healthy breathing patterns can be inculcated by practicing a few yogic breathing exercises regularly.

Respiratory Pressures

There are two important respiratory pressures to understand.

Intrapulmonary or Alveolar Pressure

This is the pressure in the lungs. As discussed above, it is below the atmospheric pressure (i.e. negative) during inspiration and above the atmospheric pressure (i.e. positive) during expiration. The variation during quiet breathing is small. At the peak of quiet inspiration the alveolar pressure is about –1 cm H_2O, and at the peak of quiet expiration it is about +1 cm H_2O (Fig. 6.11). During forceful breathing, the maximum inspiratory pressure may be –100 cm H_2O and the maximum expiratory pressure may be +100 cm H_2O.

Interpleural Pressure or Pleural Pressure

This is the pressure just outside the lungs. The lungs are covered on the outside by the visceral pleura. The thoracic wall is lined on the inside by the parietal pleura. Between the two pleural surfaces is a very thin space containing a very small amount of fluid. The thin space is called the pleural cavity (Fig. 6.12A). The pressure in the pleural cavity is the interpleural or pleural pressure. The pleural pressure is negative during both inspiration and expiration. During quiet breathing, it is –8 cm H_2O at the end of inspiration, and –4 cm H_2O at the end of expiration (Fig. 6.11). The negative pleural pressure keeps the lungs partially inflated even during expiration. Sometimes a chest injury results in entry of air into the pleural cavity. That abolishes the negative pleural pressure and leads to collapse of the lungs (Fig. 6.12B).

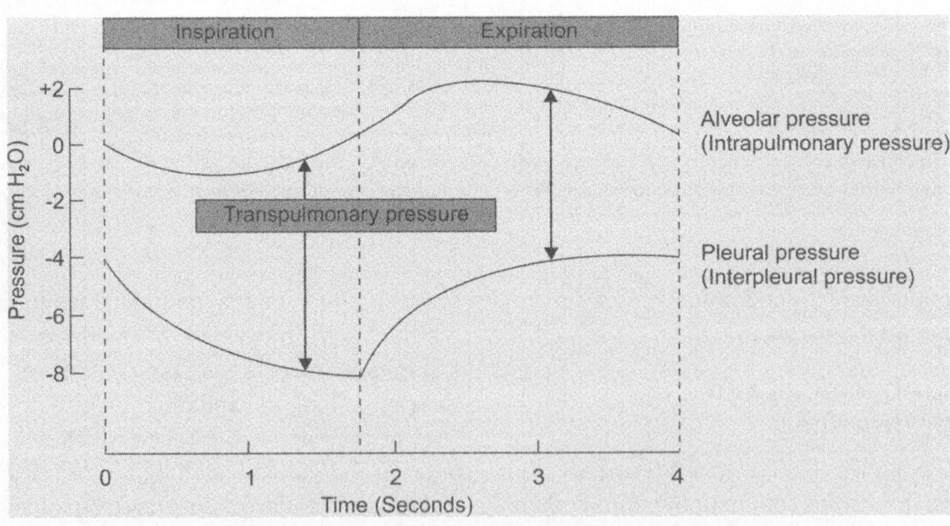

Fig. 6.11 Alveolar pressure and interpleural pressure during the respiratory cycle

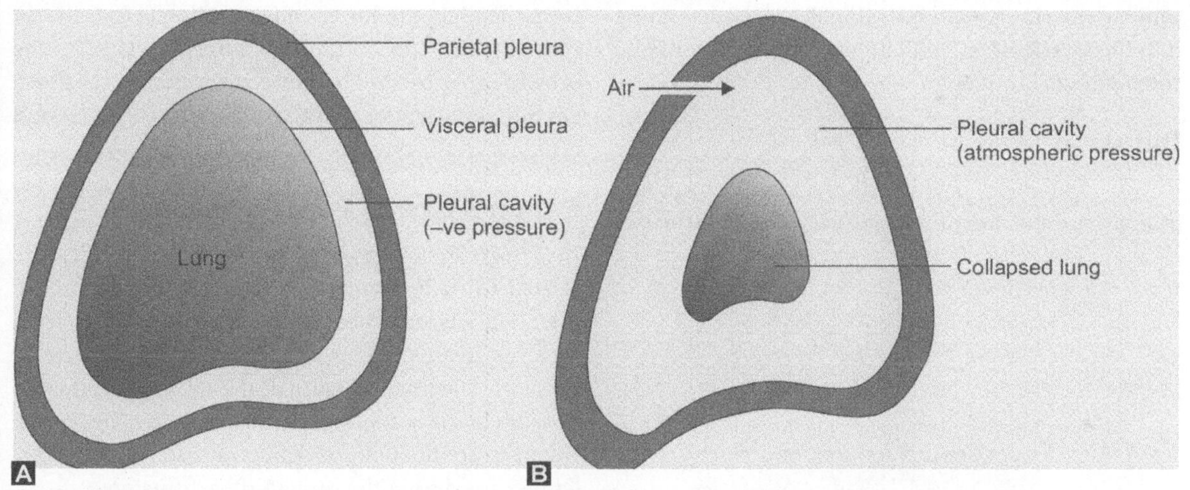

Figs 6.12A and B The pleural pressure is normally negative. An injury to the chest wall leads to abolition of the negative pressure, leading to collapse of the lung

Compliance

The lungs and thoracic cage are both elastic structures. Hence they show a mathematical relationship between distending pressure and change in volume. The compliance of lungs is 0.2 L/cm H_2O. What it means is that if the pressure within the lungs is increased by 1 cm H_2O, their volume increases by 0.2 L. The compliance of the thoracic cage is also 0.2 L/cm H_2O. But the compliance of lungs and thoracic cage together. (i.e. whole respiratory system) is 0.1 L/cm H_2O. Compliance is a measure of distensibility of lungs. In some diseases, e.g. fibrosis, the lungs become stiff. In these cases, their compliance is reduced.

Surfactant

Surfactant is a surface tension reducing agent. A surfactant lines the alveolar surface. Chemically, the surfactant in the lungs is dipalmitoyl lecithin. By reducing surface tension, surfactant makes it easier to inflate the lungs, i.e. it increases the compliance. In cystic fibrosis, difficulty in breathing is due to lack of the surfactant.

Airway Resistance

Like all tubes, airways offer resistance to the flow of air. As in case of blood vessels, maximum airway resistance is offered by medium sized airways. The large airways have a low resistance due to their large diameter. The small airways have a low resistance due to their high *total cross-sectional* area. But medium sized airways offer the maximum resistance. The resistance increases further if there is a decrease in the diameter of airways (broncho-constriction), as in bronchial asthma. Increased airway resistance produces difficulty in breathing. The difficulty is experienced more during expiration than inspiration. This happens because during expiration the alveolar pressue is positive. The positive pressure compresses the airways. Compression decreases the diameter further, thereby increasing the airway resistance still more. That is why a patient of bronchial asthma is more uncomfortable during expiration, and may have expiratory wheezing. Wheezing is a whistling sound produced by the air as it forces its way through narrow airways.

OXYGEN TRANSPORT

Tissues get oxygen from the air in three steps. First, oxygen is transferred from the lungs to pulmonary capillaries. Second, oxygen travels from pulmonary capillaries to the tissue, i.e. oxygen is transported by the blood. Third, oxygen is transferred from tissue capillaries to individual cells (Fig. 6.13). Before going into these processes, it will be relevant to recapitulate some physical principles.

Diffusion

If two containers having different concentrations of a gas are put in communication, the gas diffuses from the higher to lower concentration (Fig. 6.14). In case of gases, concentration is directly related to the pressure they exert. Therefore, one can also say that a gas diffuses from the compartment where its pressure is higher to the one where its pressure is lower.

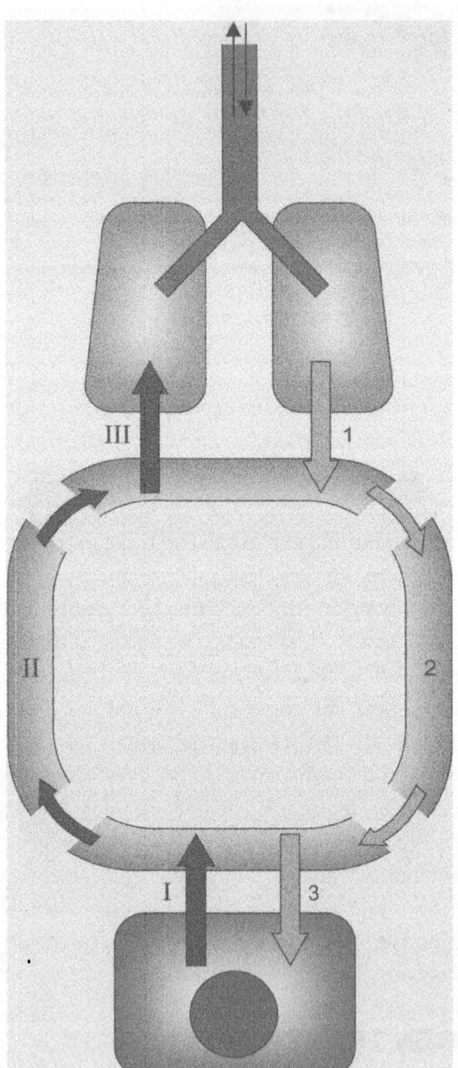

Fig. 6.13 The three components of the mechanism by which atmospheric oxygen is provided to tissues (1, 2 and 3). The corresponding steps in elimination of carbon dioxide have also been indicated (I, II and III). Empty arrows, oxygen; filled arrows; carbon dioxide

Dalton's Law of Partial Pressures

In a mixture of gases, each gas exerts a pressure related to its concentration, quite independently of the other gases in the mixture. The pressure exerted by an individual gas is called its partial pressure or 'tension'. The total pressure of the mixture is equal to the sum of the individual partial pressures (Fig. 6.15). Because of the independence of partial pressures, while considering the direction of diffusion of a gas, we have to consider only the partial pressure of that gas in the two compartments. We do not have to consider for that purpose, the pressure of other gases present.

Oxygen Transfer in the Lungs

Oxygen is transferred from the alveoli to the pulmonary capillaries by the process of diffusion. Diffusion takes place due to the difference bet-

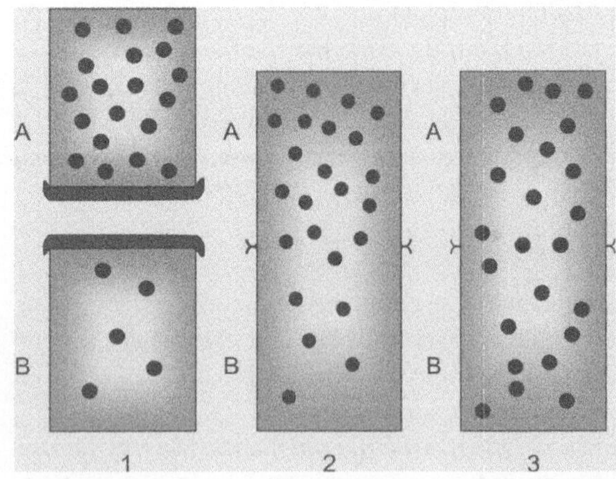

Fig. 6.14 Diffusion. 1. Two sealed containers A and B. Both contain the same gas but its concentration is higher in A than B. 2. The seals are removed and A and B are joined to form a single chamber. 3. The end result of diffusion

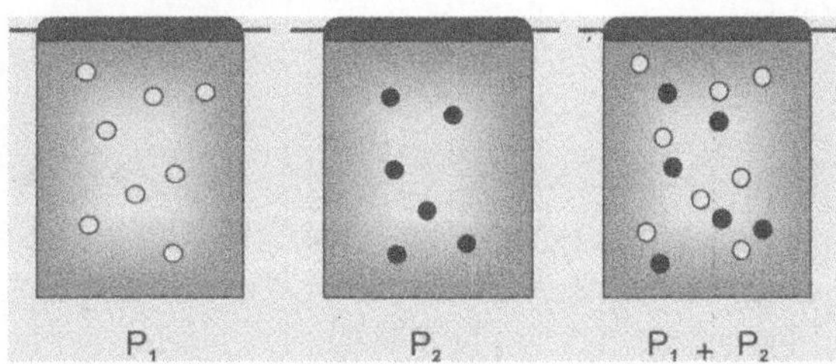

Fig. 6.15 Dalton's law of partial pressure. Two gases, when alone, exert pressures P_1 and P_2 respectively. When the same quantities of the two gases are present together in the same volume, they exert pressure $P_1 + P_2$

ween the partial pressures of oxygen in these two compartments. At sea level, the alveolar PO_2 is about 100 mm Hg. The pulmonary capillary PO_2 at the point of entry is about 40 mm Hg. The difference is adequate for rapid diffusion of oxygen to pulmonary capillaries. As a result of diffusion, the pulmonary capillary PO_2 also rises to about 100 mm Hg at the point of leaving the alveolus.[4]

Although the barrier between alveoli and pulmonary capillaries is extremely thin, it can be resolved into the following layers (Figs 6.16A and B).

1. Fluid lining the alveoli
2. Alveolar epithelium
3. Epithelial basement membrane
4. Interstitial fluid
5. Capillary basement membrane
6. Capillary endothelium
7. Plasma
8. RBC membrane

Oxygen Transport in Blood

After crossing the RBC membrane, oxygen combines with hemoglobin. Hemoglobin has a very high affinity for oxygen. As the PO_2 increases, the amount of oxygen carried by hemoglobin increases. However, when 1 g of hemoglobin has combined with 1.34 mL oxygen, 100 percent saturation is reached. Increasing the PO_2 further cannot make more oxygen combine with hemoglobin (Fig. 6.17). The curve shown in Figure 6.17 is called the oxyhemoglobin dissociation curve. It can be conveniently drawn if you simply

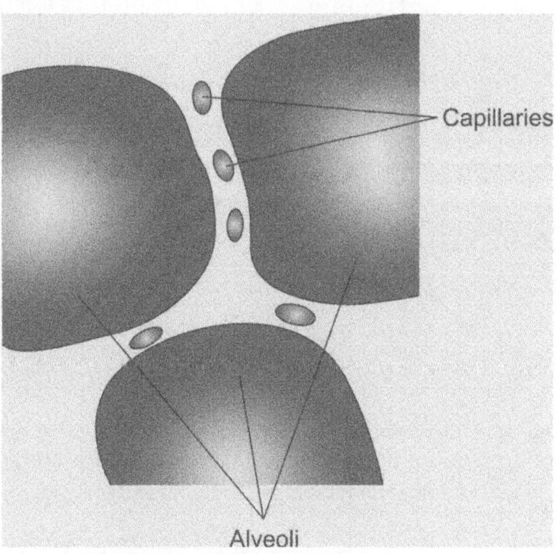

Fig. 6.16A Diagrammatic representation of alveoli and pulmonary capillaries where they come in relation to each other

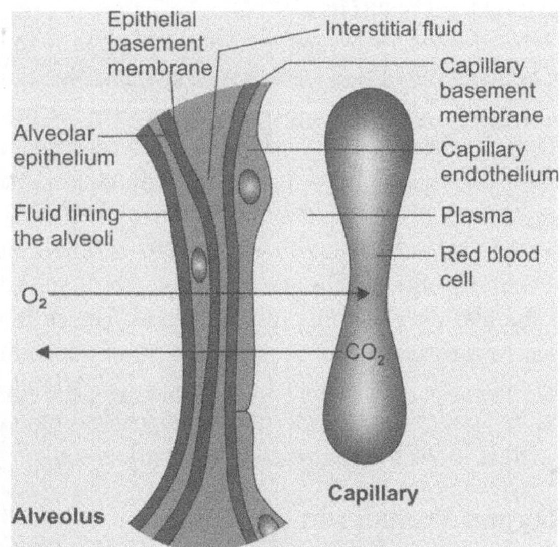

Fig. 6.16B An enlarged version of a small part of the surface where alveolar and capillary membrane are in close contact. The arrows indicate the diffusion of oxygen and carbon dioxide (For color version see Plate 5)

[4]In fact, equalization of PO_2 occurs by the time blood has travelled about one-third the length of the pulmonary capillary. This leaves considerable physiological reserve.

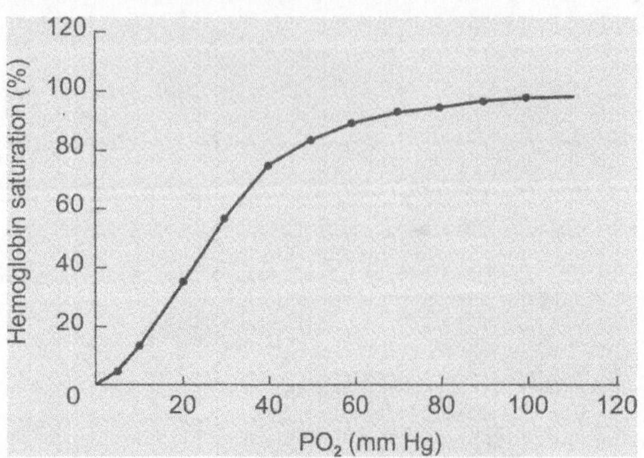

Fig. 6.17 Oxyhemoglobin dissociation curve at 37°C and pH 7.4 showing the relationship between oxygen tension and percentage saturation of hemoglobin with oxygen

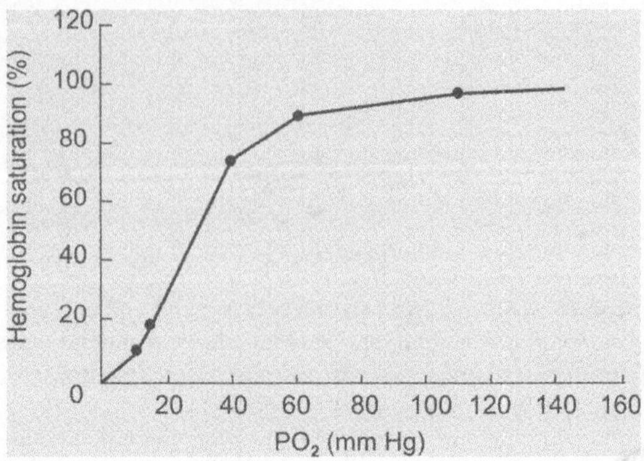

Fig. 6.18 Oxyhemoglobin dissociation curve drawn on the basis of very few plotted points

remember that the approximate saturation at a PO_2 of 10 mm Hg is 10 percent, at 15 mm Hg it is 20 percent, at 40 mm Hg it is 75 percent, and at 60 mm Hg it is 90 percent (Fig. 6.18).

In addition to oxygen transported in the blood by hemoglobin, a small quantity is also dissolved in the plasma. Suppose the PO_2 is 100 mm Hg. At this PO_2 hemoglobin is 100 percent saturated and carries 1.34 mL oxygen/gram. Suppose the hemoglobin of a person is 15 g/100 mL blood. This person will carry 15×1.34 mL = 20.1 mL oxygen per 100 mL blood. At a PO_2 of 100 mm Hg, the amount of oxygen dissolved in the plasma is 0.3 mL/100 mL blood. Hence the total oxygen content of blood at a PO_2 of 100 mm Hg will be 20.1 + 0.3 = 20.4 mL oxygen per 100 mL blood. Now you can understand why arterial blood contains about 20 mL oxygen per 100 mL blood.

Oxygen Transfer in the Tissues

One important aim of respiration is to deliver oxygen to the tissues.[5] Oxygen transported in the blood reaches the tissues in the capillaries. The transfer of oxygen from capillary blood to tissues also takes place by diffusion, which is due to the difference in PO_2. The PO_2 at the arterial end of capillaries is about 100 mm Hg. The PO_2 in the interstitial fluid is about 40 mm Hg, and in the cells it is still lower. The large PO_2 gradient results in rapid transfer of oxygen to tissues (Fig. 6.19).

The amount of oxygen transferred to tissues is, to some extent, determined by tissue requirements. A very active tissue has a low PO_2. That increases the difference between blood PO_2 and tissue PO_2. Hence, the amount of oxygen transferred is more. Further, a very active tissue also has a high PCO_2, a low pH, and a higher temperature. All these three factors shift the oxyhemoglobin dissociation curve to the right (Fig. 6.20). The shift to the right means that for a given fall in PO_2, the amount of oxygen released by hemoglobin is greater. Thus, a more active tissue gets more oxygen. The effect of PCO_2, temperature and pH on the oxyhemoglobin dissociation curve is called **Bohr effect.**

Another factor which shifts the oxyhemoglobin dissociation curve to the right is an increase in the concentration of 2, 3-diphosphoglycerate (DPG) in the red blood cells. The 2, 3-DPG concentration in RBC increases when the tissue demand of oxygen exceeds the supply, as during exercise, at high altitude, and in anemia.

CARBON DIOXIDE TRANSPORT

Tissues get rid of carbon dioxide in three steps. These steps follow a sequence opposite that involved in

[5]Which is the other important aim?

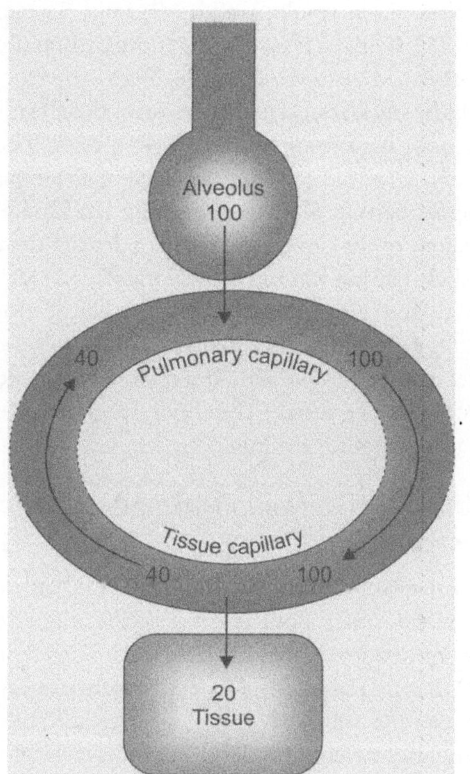

Fig. 6.19 Transfer of oxygen from lungs to tissues is based on diffusion driven by the pressure gradient

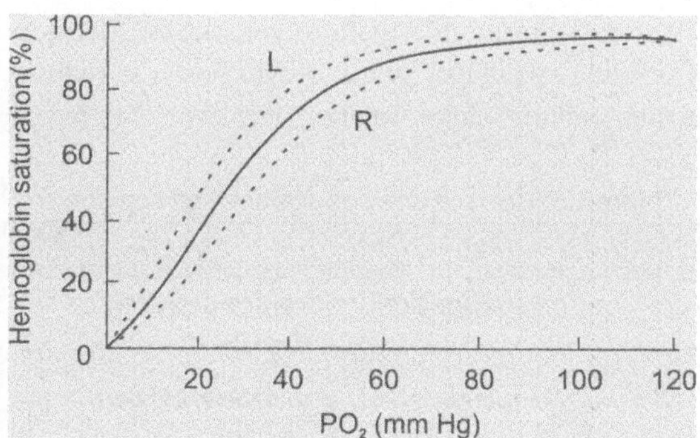

Fig. 6.20 Various factors may affect the oxyhemoglobin dissociation curve. Shift to the right (R) is brought about by fall in pH, increase in PCO_2, increase in temperature and increase in concentration of 2,3-DPG in red blood cells. Changes in the opposite direction bring about shift to the left (L)

oxygen delivery. First, carbon dioxide is transferred from the tissues to tissue capillaries. Second, carbon dioxide travels from tissue capillaries to pulmonary capillaries, i.e. carbon dioxide is transported in the blood. Third, carbon dioxide is transferred from pulmonary capillaries to the lungs, from where it is breathed out into the air (Fig. 6.13).

Carbon Dioxide Transfer in the Tissues

The transfer takes place by diffusion. The PCO_2 in cells is about 46 mm Hg, in the interstitial fluid about 45 mm Hg, and at the arterial end of capillaries about 40 mm Hg (Fig. 6.21). You might have observed that these pressure differences are much less than in case of oxygen. These small differences are enough to remove the necessary amount of carbon dioxide because carbon dioxide is much more soluble than oxygen.

Carbon Dioxide Transport in Blood

Carbon dioxide transferred from the tissues to the blood is transported in the blood in three forms: as dissolved gas, as bicarbonate, and as carbamino compounds.

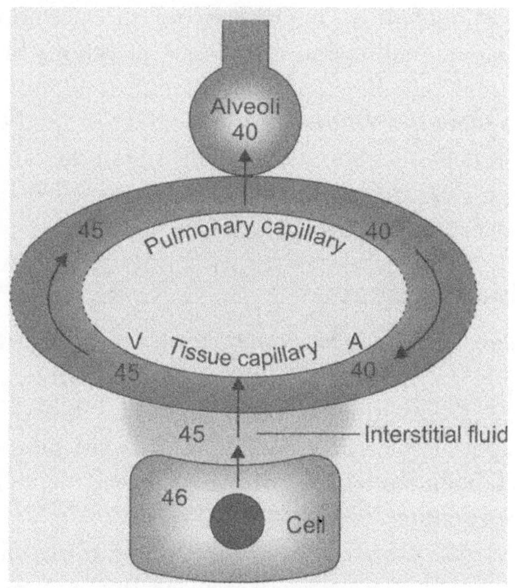

Fig. 6.21 Transfer of carbon dioxide from tissues to lungs takes place by diffusion, driven by the pressure gradient

Dissolved Carbon Dioxide

A small part of the carbon dioxide carried in the blood is in the dissolved form. Dissolved carbon dioxide accounts for about 7 percent of the carbon dioxide transported.

Bicarbonate

This is the form in which the largest fraction of carbon dioxide is transported. Bicarbonate is generated by dissolving carbon dioxide to form carbonic acid. Carbonic acid dissociates to form hydrogen ions and bicarbonate. Red blood cells (RBC) play an important part in this process because they contain carbonic anhydrase, an enzyme which can catalyze the formation of carbonic acid. Transport in the form of bicarbonate accounts for about 70 percent of carbon dioxide transport.

Carbamino Compounds

Carbon dioxide combines chemically with hemoglobin and several plasma proteins to form carbamino compounds. Transport in this form accounts for only 20 percent of carbon dioxide transported.

Carbon Dioxide Transfer in the Lungs

Carbon dioxide is removed from the pulmonary capillaries by diffusion. The PCO_2 of venous blood is 45 mm Hg while that of alveolar air is 40 mm Hg. Thus there is a difference of 5 mm Hg in the PCO_2 which makes carbon dioxide diffuse into the alveoli (Fig. 6.21). Carbon dioxide is finally expelled from the alveoli during expiration.

Haldane Effect

Haldane effect describes the effect of PO_2 on carbon dioxide transport. At a low PO_2, blood can transport more carbon dioxide. At a high PO_2 blood can transport less carbon dioxide. Let us see how this effect facilitates transfer of carbon dioxide in tissues as well as lungs.

In the tissues, carbon dioxide diffuses from cells into the tissue capillaries. As this is happening, simultaneously oxygen diffuses in the opposite direction. As a result, blood PO_2 falls. The fall in blood PO_2 helps in transporting more carbon dioxide in the blood due to the Haldane effect.

In the lungs, oxygen diffuses from the alveoli into the blood. As a result, the blood PO_2 rises. The rise in blood PO_2 reduces the capacity of the blood to transport carbon dioxide due to the Haldane effect. Therefore more carbon dioxide is released from the blood for getting expired in the lungs.

Haldane effect is so effective that it doubles the quantity of carbon dioxide picked up from the tissues and makes possible the release of this double quantity in the lungs. Therefore Haldane effect is very important for the body.

Relationship between Haldane Effect and Bohr Effect

Haldane effect describes the effect of PO_2 on carbon dioxide transport. Bohr effect describes the effect of PCO_2 on oxygen transport. Both are similar in the sense that increase in the partial pressure of one gas decreases the transport of the other gas (Table 6.3). But quantitatively, Haldane effect is much more effective than Bohr effect.

REGULATION OF RESPIRATION

Respiration is an involuntary activity. We breathe without being aware of it. But at the same time, we can alter the respiratory pattern voluntarily. Alteration of respiratory control by use of will power is required during talking and singing. Further, the oxygen

Table 6.3 Haldane effect and Bohr effect compared

	Cause	*Effect*
Bohr effect	Increase in PCO_2	Reduced oxygen carriage
	Reduction in PCO_2	Increased oxygen carriage
Haldane effect	Increase in PO_2	Reduced carbon dioxide carriage
	Reduction in PO_2	Increased carbon dioxide carriage

requirement and carbon dioxide production in the body are not constant. Their rate increases during physical activity. The rate and depth of respiration increase involuntarily to meet the increased requirement.

Respiratory function is also a bridge between the body and the mind. When we are anxious, angry or agitated, breathing becomes rapid and shallow. The relationship works also in the opposite direction: if we make a voluntary effort to breathe slowly and deeply, we feel relaxed and peaceful. That is why anger may be controlled by taking a few deep breaths. Similarly, several yogic breathing exercises which involve slow and deep breathing also have a relaxing effect.

The mixture of voluntary and involuntary regulation, and the two-way relationship between breathing and the mind, make respiratory regulation fairly complex. For simplicity, we may divide the regulation into neural and chemical regulation.

Neural Regulation of Respiration

The best understood (but not necessarily the most important) neural centers of respiratory regulation are situated in the medulla oblongata and pons.

Medullary Respiratory Centers

The medulla has the basic mechanism for generation of respiratory rhythm, i.e. alteration of inspiration and expiration.

There are two groups of respiratory neurons in the medulla (Fig. 6.22).

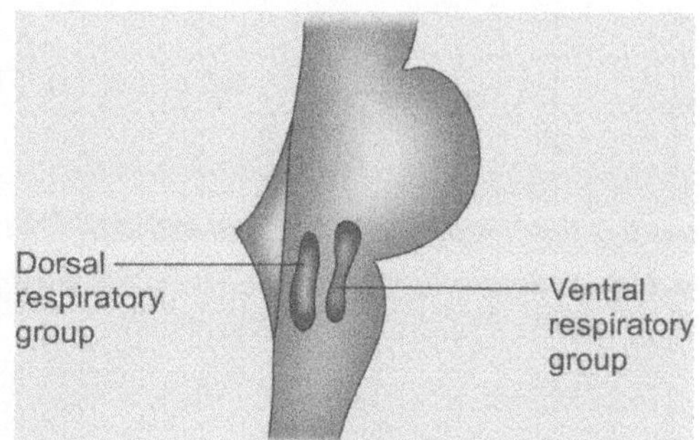

Fig. 6.22 The dorsal and ventral respiratory groups of neurons. The dorsal group has predominantly inspiratory neurons while the ventral group has predominantly expiratory neurons

The **dorsal respiratory group** shows neuronal activity during inspiration. It is believed that this brings about inspiration while absence of activity brings about expiration passively.

The **ventral respiratory group** of neurons are silent during quiet breathing. During forceful breathing, majority of the neurons of this group show activity during expiration. Therefore, it is believed that the principal role of these neurons is to bring about active expiration during forceful breathing.

Pontine Respiratory Centers

The pontine centers act by influencing the medullary respiratory centers. Pons also has two respiratory centers (Fig. 6.23).

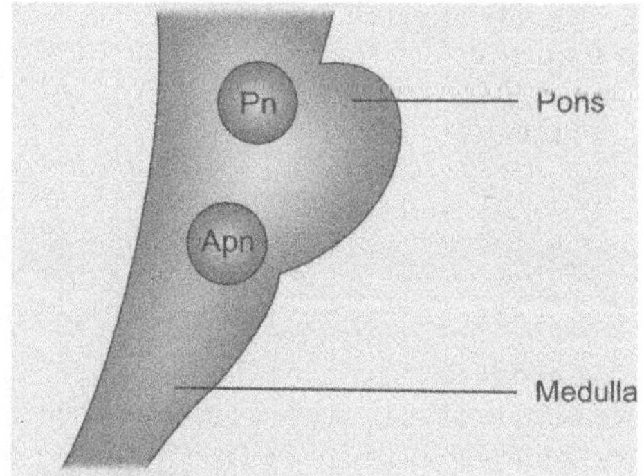

Fig. 6.23 The pontine respiratory centers. Pn, pneumotaxic center; Apn, apneustic center

The apneustic center exerts a strong stimulatory influence on the inspiratory center. If the apneustic center is not held in check, as can be done experimentally, breathing consists of inspiratory spasms which are only briefly interrupted by expiration (Fig. 6.24). Such breathing is called apneustic breathing.

But normally the apneustic center is held in check by the vagus nerves and the pneumotaxic center.

Pneumotaxic center is the other pontine respiratory center. It is situated above the apneustic center. It exerts a strong inhibitory influence on the apneustic center.

The interaction of the two medullary centers, the two pontine centers and the vagi has been shown in

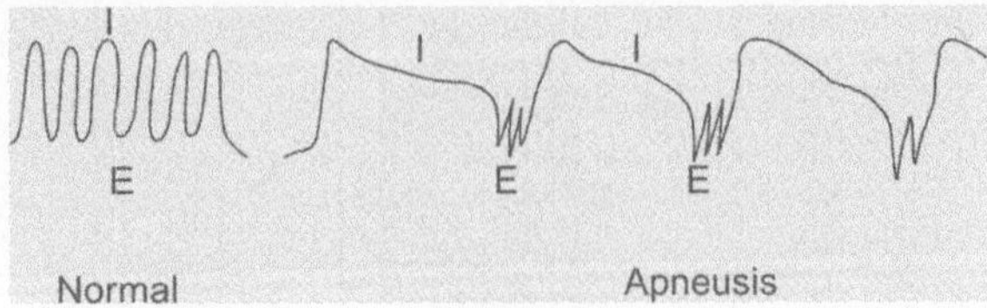

Fig. 6.24 Normal breathing and apneustic breathing compared. I, inspiration; E, expiration

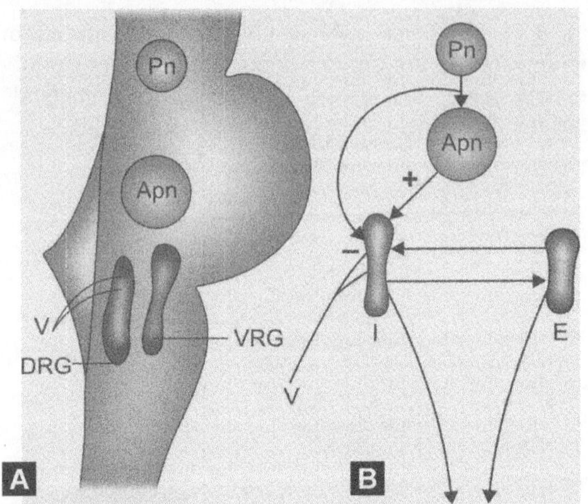

Figs 6.25A and B (A) Approximate location of the pontine and medullary respiratory centers; (B) Interaction of the respiratory centers and vagus nerve. Pn, pneumotaxic center; Apn, apneustic center; V, vagus; DRG, dorsal respiratory group; VRG, ventral respiratory group; I, inspiratory neurons; E, expiratory neurons; +, stimulatory effect; –, inhibitory effect

Figures 6.25A and B. Note that the basic respiratory rhythm is generated by the two medullary groups, which may be called the inspiratory and expiratory center respectively. The apneustic center threatens to 'spoil' this rhythm by stimulating the inspiratory center. But the rhythm is maintained because the apneustic center is inhibited by the pneumotaxic center and the vagi. We shall discuss the role of vagi in respiration again a little later.

Higher Neural Influences

The medullary and pontine respiratory centers are further influenced by higher regions of the nervous system such as cerebral cortex and the limbic system. The cerebral cortical influence makes possible voluntary control of breathing. The limbic influence is responsible for alterations in breathing associated with emotional changes.

Respiratory Reflexes

Some of the better known respiratory reflexes have been discussed below:

1. *Hering-Breuer reflex:* This reflex was discovered by Hering and Breuer in 1868. This reflex operates on the basis of information about the degree of inflation of lungs. When lungs are full, inspiration is inhibited. When lungs are empty, inspiration is stimulated. That make sense. Lungs are full at the end of inspiration. That is the time when inspiration must come to an end so that expiration can begin. Lungs are empty at the end of expiration. That is the time when inspiration must begin. The degree of fullness of lungs is detected by pulmonary stretch receptors. The information collected by pulmonary stretch receptors is conveyed to the central nervous system by the vagus nerve. Vagal fibers carrying this information inhibit the inspiratory center in the medulla oblongata (Fig. 6.26).

   In human beings, Hering-Breuer reflex is functional only in infants; in adults it operates only when the tidal volume exceeds 1 liter.
2. *Head's paradoxical reflex:* This reflex was discovered by Head in 1889. If the vagi are cooled to 5° C, conduction in the fibers which mediate Hering-Breuer reflex is blocked. Under these conditions, inflation of lungs stimulates inspiration, i.e. further inflation. The reflex does not make sense: therefore it is called paradoxical. The reflex possibly plays a role in the newborn. The newborn is delivered with empty lungs. The first breath cannot fill up the lungs completely, but if every inflation produces more inflation, it would facilitate filling up of the lungs.
3. *J reflexes:* These reflexes are due to stimulation of J receptors, discovered in 1954 by A.S. Paintal, an eminent Indian physiologist. 'J receptors' stands for juxtapulmonary capillary

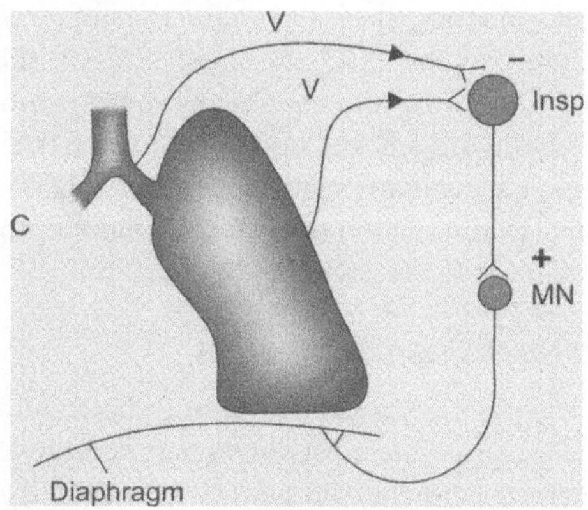

Fig. 6.26 Diagrammatic representation of the mechanism underlying Hering-Breuer reflex. Information about the degree of inflation of lungs is conveyed from the pulmonary stretch receptors by afferent fibers of the vagus nerve (V). Activation of the vagal fibers leads to inhibition of inspiratory neurons (Insp) in the dorsal group of medullary respiratory neurons. The inspiratory neurons act by stimulating the motor neurons (MN) which supply inspiratory muscles such as the diaphragm. –, inhibitory influence; +, excitatory influence

receptors. The name tells us that these receptors are located very near the pulmonary capillaries (Fig. 6.27). These receptors are stimulated by pulmonary congestion. J receptors convey their message to the central nervous system by fibers in the vagus nerves.

The reflex effects of experimental stimulation of J receptors are apnea, hypotension, brady- cardia and reduction in muscle tone. It is believed that J receptors may get stimulated in severe exercise, specially at high altitude. Their reflex effects would discourage exercise, and thereby force the person to stop exercising before he gets a complication like pulmonary edema.

4. *Cough reflex:* Cough is initiated by irritant rece-ptors located in the larynx and other airways which are also supplied by vagal fibers. The reflex prevents foreign bodies from entering the airways.

   Cough reflex may be absent in an unconscious patient. Therefore suction is required to keep such a person's airways clear from secretions.

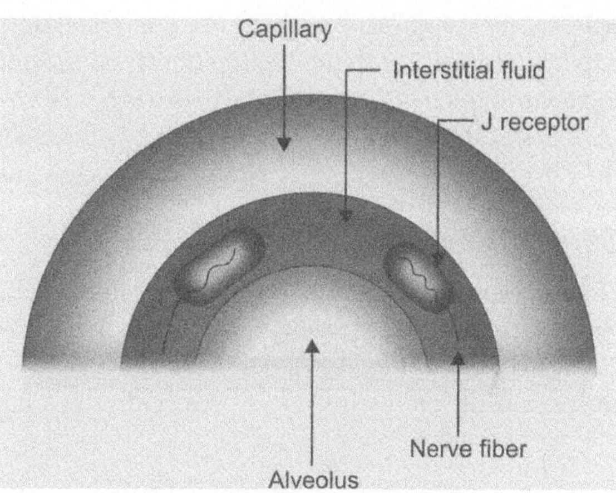

Fig. 6.27 J receptors are located in the interstitial space between alveoli and pulmonary capillaries

   If secretions collect in his mouth, they may enter the airways and make it difficult for him to breathe, which may even lead to his death. An unconscious person may die even due to his own tongue falling back and blocking his airways. This is important to keep in mind while administering artificial respiration to an unconscious person.

Chemical Regulation of Respiration

Chemical regulation of respiration also involves the nervous system. But it is called chemical regulation because the signals which activate the regulatory system are chemical, i.e. PCO_2, PO_2 and pH. It is easy to understand that if respiratory activity is not sufficient to meet the demands of the body, carbon dioxide will accumulate, and oxygen will be used up. Hence, PCO_2 will rise and PO_2 will fall. Along with rise in PCO_2 hydrogen ion concentration will increase because carbon dioxide is an acidic substance. Hence the pH will fall. In the chemical regulation of respiration you would observe that an increase in PCO_2, a fall in PO_2 or a fall in pH stimulate respiration. Stimulation of respiration means an increase in the rate and depth of respiration. Stimulation of respiration tends to reverse the changes in PCO_2, PO_2 and pH. That is, the PCO_2 falls, PO_2 rises and pH rises. Hence the chemical stimuli for respiration are reduced. In this way the normal level of PCO_2, PO_2 and pH is maintained, and respiratory activity keeps pace with production of carbon dioxide and consumption of oxygen by the body (Fig. 6.28).

Chemical regulation of respiration is brought about by two sets of receptors: central and peripheral.

Central Chemoreceptors

These receptors are located in the medulla oblongata but are different from the medullary respiratory groups discussed earlier (Fig. 6.29). They are stimulated by an increase in the hydrogen ion concentration. But in actual practice, they are indirectly stimulated by an increase in the PCO_2 of blood. Carbon dioxide diffuses easily into the central nervous system and raises the hydrogen ion concentration of the fluid bathing the chemosensitive neurons. The body responds to stimulation of central chemoreceptors by an increase in the rate and depth of breathing.

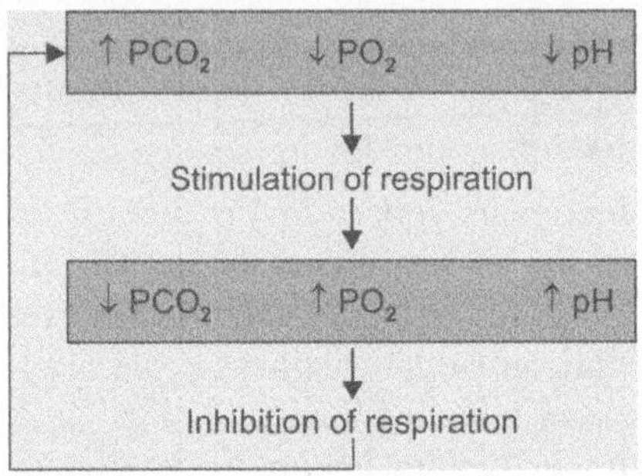

Fig. 6.28 Chemical regulation of respiration. Stimulation of respiration reverses the changes which stimulate respiration. In this way the partial pressure of CO_2 is neither allowed to rise much nor allowed to fall much—it is maintained nearly constant at the normal level

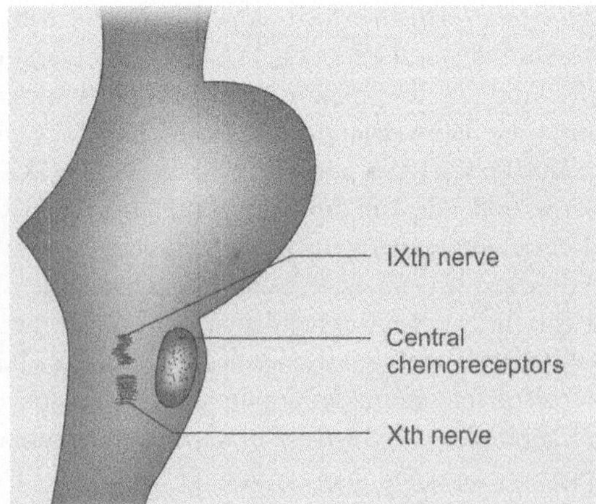

Fig. 6.29 Anatomical location of the central chemoreceptors which regulate respiration

Peripheral Chemoreceptors

These receptors are located in the carotid body and aortic body (Fig. 6.30). The most potent natural stimulus for peripheral chemoreceptors is low arterial PO_2. To some extent they are also stimulated by rise in arterial PCO_2 or hydrogen ion concentration. The information about the degree of stimulation of peripheral chemoreceptors is conveyed to the central nervous system by IXth and Xth cranial nerves. The body responds to stimulation of peripheral chemoreceptors also by an increase in the rate and depth of breathing.

What we know about neural and chemical regulation of respiration is only a part of the story. It leaves many observations unexplained or poorly explained. But knowing more has proved difficult

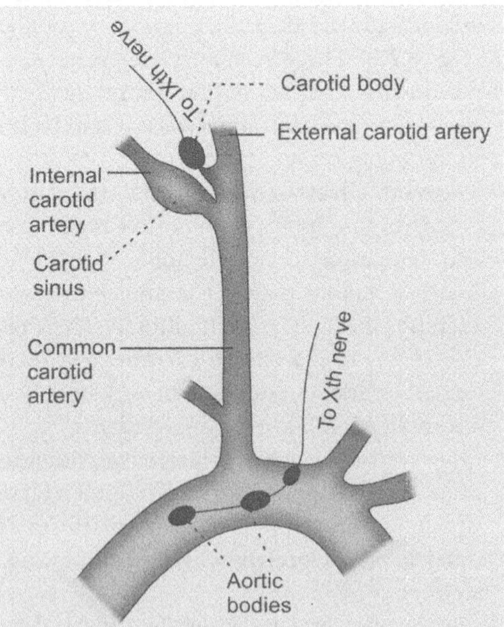

Fig. 6.30 Diagrammatic representation of peripheral chemoreceptors and their innervation

because there are limitations to the studies that can be done on conscious animals. And, an animal under anesthesia does not have a normally regulated respiration. Further, what we learn from animals may not be entirely applicable to human beings.

PULMONARY FUNCTION TESTS

Pulmonary function tests (PFT) are of very limited value for diagnosis of lung disease. The value of PFT lies in:

a. Giving the functional nature of the disease (e.g. obstructive or restrictive), and
b. Telling the anesthetist whether lung function is adequate for tolerating anesthesia.

Some of the more important PFT have been discussed below.

Tests of Ventilation

The main aim of these tests is to distinguish between restrictive and obstructive diseases. **Restrictive diseases** are characterized by reduced expansion of the lungs. The restriction on expansion may be because of a decrease in elasticity of the lungs (as in fibrosis). It may also be due to a bone deformity in the thorax which prevents the lungs from expanding sufficiently (e.g. scoliosis). **Obstructive diseases** are characterized by increased airway resistance. Airway resistance may be increased by bronchospasm (as in asthma), secretions (as in bronchitis), or a tumor, within the airways or pressing them from outside. The single most important test of ventilation which helps in distinguishing between restrictive and obstructive lung diseases is timed vital capacity. If the total vital capacity is reduced but FEV_1 is normal, the disease is restrictive. If the total vital capacity is normal or nearly normal, but FEV_1 is low, the disease is obstructive (Fig. 6.5). If total vital capacity and FEV_1 are both reduced, the disease has both restrictive and obstructive elements (Fig. 6.31).

Another important measurement which can be calculated from the FEV_1 curve is peak expiratory

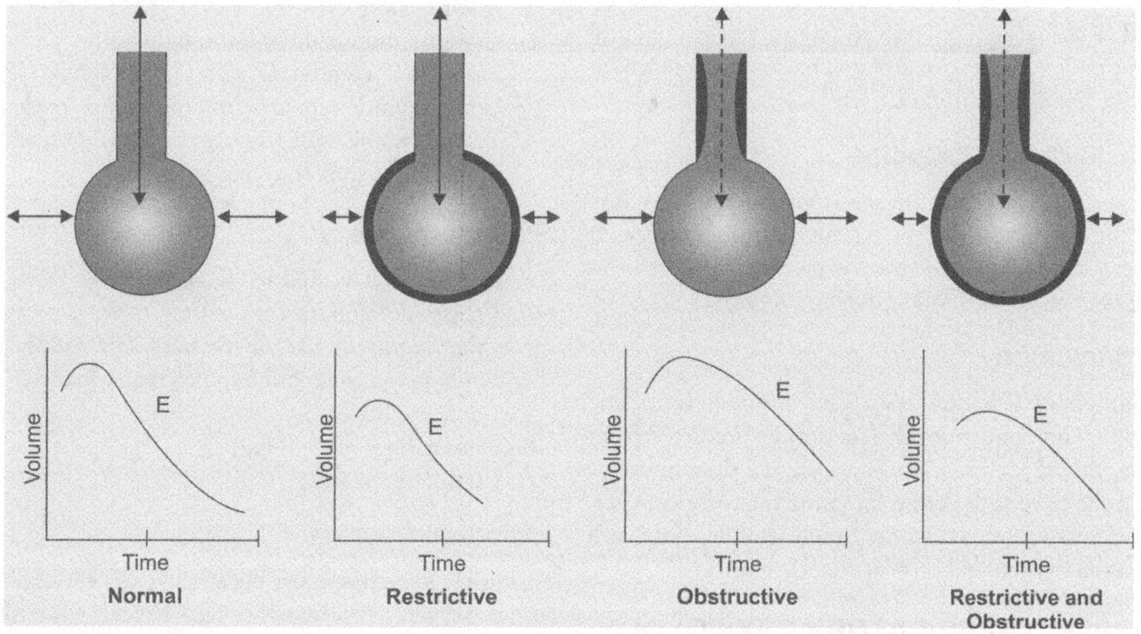

Fig. 6.31 Timed vital capacity as a diagnostic test for restrictive and obstructive lung disease. In restrictive lung disease, the vital capacity is reduced but can be breathed out at the normal rate. In obstructive lung disease, the vital capacity may not be much reduced but is breathed out slowly in spite of the effort. E, forced expiration of the vital capacity

flow rate (PEFR). PEFR is reduced in obstructive lung disease.

Tests of Diffusion

The diffusion capacity of lungs is usually assessed from the carbon monoxide diffusion capacity. Assuming that the diffusion capacity for oxygen is 1.0, the diffusion capacity for carbon monoxide is 0.8 and that for carbon dioxide is 20.3. Thus if the diffusion capacity for carbon monoxide is known, that for oxygen and carbon dioxide can be calculated.

Tests of the End-result of Respiration

The ultimate purpose of respiration is to supply adequate oxygen to the tissues and to get rid of carbon dioxide. These functions can be assessed by measuring PO_2, PCO_2 and pH of arterial blood.

Test of Response to Respiratory Stimulants

Sometimes it is useful to measure the respiratory response to stimulants such as low PO_2 or high PCO_2. The response to these stimulants may be reduced either because of reduced sensitivity of neural mechanisms, or because of mechanical factors which make breathing difficult.

Tests during Exercise

In order to improve the sensitivity of the tests, any of the above tests may be repeated during exercise. If the defect is mild, the test may give a normal value at rest but an abnormal one during exercise.

Conclusion

Pulmonary function tests have limited diagnostic value. Their outcome can generally be predicted from the clinical presentation. However, if a small number of tests have to be done for confirmatory purposes, the most valuable tests are timed vital capacity, and arterial oxygen and carbon dioxide tension.

APPLIED RESPIRATORY PHYSIOLOGY

In this section we shall discuss some common phenomena associated with respiratory disease which can be understood better in the light of respiratory physiology.

Hypoxia

Hypoxia is a state in which tissues suffer from the effects of oxygen deficiency. Depending on the cause of hypoxia, it is generally divided into four categories: hypoxic, anemic, stagnant and histotoxic (Fig. 6.32).

Hypoxic Hypoxia

If hypoxia is due to a decrease in oxygen supply, it is called hypoxic hypoxia. It may be due to:

a. Decrease in PO_2 of inspired air, as at high altitude, or
b. Decrease in transfer of oxygen from lungs to blood, as in lung diseases.

Anemic Hypoxia

If hypoxia is due to a decrease in the oxygen carrying capacity of blood, it is called anemic hypoxia. Anemic hypoxia is seen in:

a. Anemia, and
b. Carbon monoxide poisoning. Since carbon monoxide combines with hemoglobin, less hemoglobin is left for combining with oxygen. Therefore the situation in carbon monoxide poisoning is similar to that in anemia.

Stagnant Hypoxia

Stagnant hypoxia is due to sluggish blood flow. If blood stays in capillaries for a long time, it cannot meet the requirements of tissues. The result is stagnant hypoxia. Stagnant hypoxia may be seen in:

a. Cardiac failure,
b. Hemorrhage, or
c. Circulatory shock.

Histotoxic Hypoxia

Histotoxic hypoxia occurs because tissues are unable to use oxygen. Histotoxic hypoxia is seen when the cytochrome system is poisoned, as in:

a. Cyanide poisoning, or
b. Diphtheria.

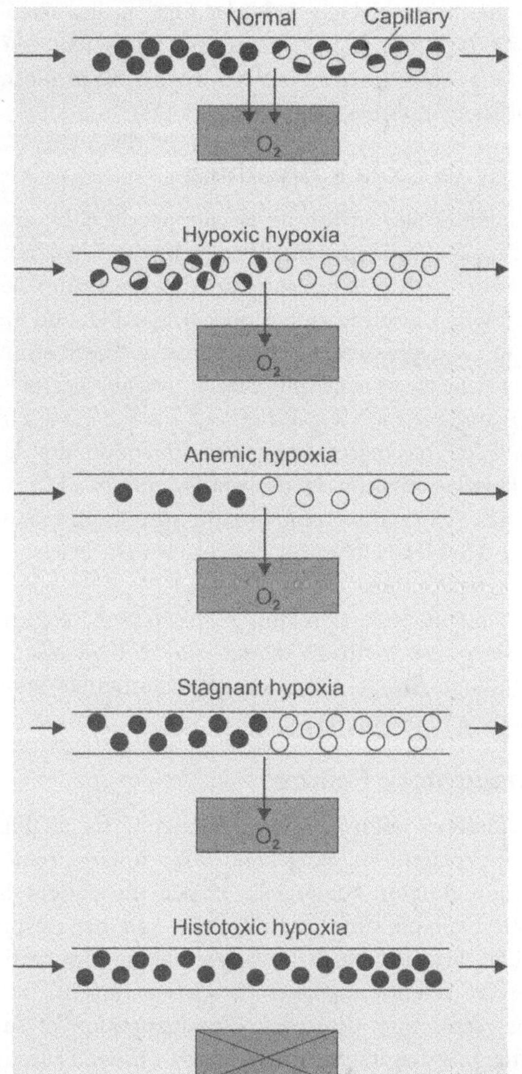

Fig. 6.32 Different types of hypoxia. Normal oxygen supply to tissues depends on normal oxygenation of blood and normal blood flow. In hypoxic hypoxia, oxygenation of blood is impaired due to a reduction in oxygen tension. In anemic hypoxia, oxygenation of blood is impaired due to a reduction in oxygen carrying capacity of blood. In stagnant hypoxia, blood flow is impaired. In histotoxic hypoxia, tissues are unable to utilize oxygen normally. The circles represent red blood cells (RBC). Filled circles represent RBC carrying hemoglobin fully saturated with oxygen. Half filled circles represent RBC carrying hemoglobin partially saturated with oxygen. Empty circles represent RBC carrying deoxygenated hemoglobin

Cyanosis

Cyanosis is bluish discoloration of skin due to the presence of more than 5 g/100 mL of deoxygenated hemoglobin in blood. This is because deoxygenated hemoglobin is bluish in color while oxygenated hemoglobin is reddish. The common sites where cyanosis is observed are lips, nail beds, ear lobes, cheeks, and mucous membrane of the mouth.

Cyanosis is classified into central and peripheral.

Central Cyanosis

Here all arterial blood in the body is poorly oxygenated. It is due to hypoxic hypoxia, and may therefore occur at high altitude or in lung disease.

Peripheral Cyanosis

Here only the capillary blood in the extremes of the body is poorly oxygenated. Therefore the nails and the tips of the nose show bluish discoloration.

This occurs due to cutaneous vasoconstriction, as after exposure to cold.

Dyspnea

Dyspnea means difficulty in breathing. Physiologically dyspnea indicates that the breathing reserve is less than normal, or the work of breathing is more than normal.

Breathing Reserve

It is calculated as follows:

Suppose minute volume at rest	= 6 L/min
Maximum voluntary ventilation (MVV)	= 120 L/min
Breathing reserve (BR)	= 120 – 6
	= 114 L/min
BR (%) or dyspneic index	$= \frac{114}{120} \times 100$
	= 95%

If the BR (%) falls below 60 percent the patient generally feels dyspneic. That is why this ratio is also called dyspneic index.

For example, if MVV of a patient is 10 L/min, and his resting minute volume is 6 L/min, his

$$\text{BR}(\%) \text{ will be } \frac{10-6}{10} \times 100 = 40\%$$

Hence this patient will be dyspneic at rest.

Increased Work of Breathing

The work of breathing is increased during hyperventilation associated with exercise. That also reduces the BR (%), and leads to dyspnea. For example, if the minute volume during heavy exercise increases to 72 L/min, in a normal person with an MVV of 120 L/min,

$$\text{BR}(\%) \text{ will be } \frac{120-72}{120} \times 100 = 40\%$$

Hence this person will also feel dyspneic during exercise.

Orthopnea

Orthopnea means dyspnea which is worse on lying down and improves on sitting or standing up. This type of dyspnea is seen in left ventricular failure. In left ventricular failure, lungs are congested (Why?).[6] Orthopnea occurs because the lungs are much more congested in the lying down posture. In the erect posture, gravity clears the congestion except at the bases of the lungs.

Breath Holding

When we hold our breath, gas exchange with the atmosphere stops but the tissues continue to use oxygen and produce carbon dioxide. Therefore during breath holding arterial PO_2 falls and PCO_2 rises. Both these factors are powerful respiratory stimulants. Therefore a point is reached where the respiratory drive becomes so strong that the person cannot hold the breath any longer. This point is called the breaking point. The breaking point is generally reached when alveolar PO_2 is 56 mm Hg and alveolar PCO_2 is 49 mm Hg (What are the normal values?).[7] Because of this mechanism it is impossible to commit suicide by holding the breath.

Cheyne-Stokes Breathing

Cheyne-Stokes breathing is characterized by alternating apnea (stoppage of breathing) and hyperventilation (high rate and/or depth of breathing). It is seen when respiratory response to low PO_2 and high PCO_2 is depressed. Poor response to these stimuli may lead to apnea. Apnea leads to a further fall in PO_2 and rise in PCO_2. When PO_2 has fallen very low and PCO_2 has increased to a very high level, they lead to hyperventilation. Hyperventilation raises PO_2 and lowers PCO_2, thus removing the stimuli for respiration. That leads to apnea. Thus apnea alternates with hyperventilation.

Cheyne-Stokes breathing is seen physiologically in sleep, especially in infants and at high altitude. Pathologically, it occurs in left ventricular failure (leading to pulmonary edema) or brain damage.

Respiratory Failure

Respiratory failure is characterized by the inability of the patient to oxygenate blood and to remove carbon dioxide adequately. Hence the patient has both hypoxia (low arterial PO_2) and hypercapnia (high arterial PCO_2). Hypercapnia, or carbon dioxide retention, makes the patient insensitive to this respiratory stimulant. The respiration of such patients is maintained by the hypoxic drive. Therefore giving them 100 percent oxygen may raise their arterial PO_2 but removes the only stimulus they have for respiration. Hence 100 percent oxygen depresses respiration in such patients. It is better to give them a mixture of air and oxygen to breathe. Often leaky masks achieve this end automatically; they waste oxygen but save the patient!

The symptoms of both hypoxia and hypercapnia are predominantly cerebral. Hypoxia may

---

[6]In left ventricular failure (LVF), the left ventricular pumping action is inadequate. Therefore blood collects in the left atrium, raising left atrial pressure. From the left atrium, the rise in pressure gets reflected in the pulmonary veins and pulmonary capillaries. That is why in LVF the lungs are congested (with blood).

[7]The normal alveolar PO_2 is about 100 mm Hg and alveolar PCO_2 is about 40 mm Hg.

lead to mental confusion or impaired conciousness. Hypercapnia leads to cerebral vasodilatation (Chapter 5). That may give rise to headache, slurred speech, and a special variety of tremors known as flapping tremors.

Oxygen Toxicity

Excess of everything is bad, even if the excess is that of life-giving oxygen. Excess of oxygen (high PO_2) at cellular level can damage many intracellular enzymes and the unsaturated fatty acids in cell membranes. Oxygen toxicity is also due to its forming hydrogen peroxide and free radicals.

Clinically, the tissues most susceptible to oxygen toxicity seem to be the central nervous system (probably because nerve cells are the most sensitive in the body) and lungs (probably because they are the first to be exposed). The most prominent neurological symptom of oxygen toxicity is convulsions. Prolonged exposure to high concentrations of oxygen produces pulmonary fibrosis leading to a diffusion defect and consequent hypoxia. The hypoxia can be corrected by a still higher concentration of oxygen which may produce more fibrosis, thus leading to a vicious cycle. In premature infants, prolonged stay in an oxygen tent has been associated with the development of a cataract due to retrolental fibroplasia.

Artificial Respiration

Respiratory arrest may occur as a result of drowning, poisoning, suffocation, electrocution, myocardial infarction or cerebrovascular accident. The cause may be reversible, temporary or curable but the body cannot wait much for the oxygen supply to be restored. Unless vital organs like the brain and heart are supplied with oxygen within 2-3 minutes, respiratory arrest leads to death. Therefore, it is important to restore respiration, artificially if necessary, as a lifesaving measure. Since respiratory arrest could occur in an emergency situation, no equipment may be available. In such cases, manual methods of artificial respiration prove valuable. In the meantime, the patient may be transported to a hospital where a mechanical method of artificial respiration may be used, if required. A mechanical ventilator is essential if artificial respiration has to be maintained for a prolonged period of time.

Manual Methods

Before starting with the artificial respiration, the patency of airways should be checked, and restored if necessary. Airways may be blocked by water or secretions, or by the tongue. During unconsciousness, the tongue is relaxed, and may fall backwards to block the airway. As soon as one is faced with a situation requiring artificial respiration, the clothing around the neck and chest of the victim should be loosened, secretions or water should be wiped from the mouth and throat, and the neck should be extended to get the tongue out of the way.

The simplest manual method is the mouth to mouth method. In this method, while maintaining the head tilt to keep the tongue out of the way, air is blown into the victim's chest through an airtight mouth to mouth contact. If the effort meets an undue resistance, the airways are again checked for any obstruction. While blowing air into the lungs, the nostrils of the victim are pinched with the fingers to prevent air escaping through the nose. After a reasonable amount of air has been blown in, the rescuer removes his mouth from that of the victim and watches the chest deflate itself. The procedure is repeated 12 to 20 times per minute.

Many other manual methods of artificial respiration have been devised but they all require more training, and are probably less effective, than the mouth to mouth method. The search for other methods is motivated primarily by esthetic and hygienic reasons.

Mechanical Methods

Mechanical methods are a must if artificial respiration has to be continued for prolonged periods of time. Most ventilators require an endotracheal or tracheostomy tube. The tube is not only useful for connecting the patient to the ventilator but also for removal of secretions from the airways. There are two broad categories of mechanical ventilators: Positive pressure and negative pressure type. In positive pressure ventilators, inspiration is achieved by forcing air into the lungs at positive pressure. In negative pressure ventilators, chest expands as a result of negative pressure applied around it. Expiration is a passive process in both types of ventilators, and is achieved by the elastic recoil of lungs and thorax.

In positive pressure ventilators, air may be pumped into the lungs at constant volume or at constant pressure. The constant pressure type of ventilators can sometimes be operated in the assisted ventilation mode. The patient triggers the inspiration himself, but adequate pressure is generated only with the help of the ventilator. Assisted ventilation becomes useful when a patient's respiration has started recovering.

In negative pressure ventilators, the whole body (except the head), or only the chest and abdomen, are enclosed in a rigid airtight chamber (iron lung). Negative pressure is generated intermittently in the chamber mechanically. Negative pressure ventilators are not much used these days because of being very bulky and inconvenient.

If appropriate nursing care is available, a patient can be maintained on a mechanical ventilator for several months.

QUESTIONS

1. Calculate the oxygen content of the venous blood in a person whose hemoglobin level is 15 g/ 100 mL and venous PO_2 is 40 mm Hg.
2. Why may it be sometimes dangerous to give 100 percent oxygen to a patient with chronic respiratory disease?
3. Why is a poisonous gas like carbon monoxide used for detemination of diffusion capacity of lungs?
4. Why is the diffusion capacity of lungs for carbon dioxide about 20 times greater than that for oxygen?
5. In lung diseases with a diffusion defect, which is the diffusion that suffers more: that of oxygen or of carbon dioxide?
6. How is carbon monoxide poisoning treated?
7. Why is it better to breathe through the nose than through the mouth?

ANSWERS

1. a. *Oxygen carried by hemoglobin*
   At a PO_2 of 40 mm Hg, the saturation of hemoglobin with oxygen is 75 percent.
   Hence oxygen content in combination with hemoglobin
   = 1.34 × 15 × 0.75 mL/100 mL blood
   = 15.075 mL/100 mL blood

   b. *Oxygen is dissolved form*
   Dissolved oxygen is proportional to PO_2.
   At 100 mm Hg, dissolved oxygen = 0.3 mL/100 mL
   Therefore at 40 mm Hg, dissolved oxygen
   $= 0.3 \times \frac{40}{100}$ mL / 100 mL boold
   = 0.12 mL/100 mL blood

   c. Total oxygen content
   Hence total oxygen content of venous blood
   = 15.075 + 0.12
   = 15.195 mL/100 mL blood
   = 15.2 mL/100 mL blood (approx)
2. In some patients with chronic respiratory disease, the PO_2 is low and the PCO_2 is high due to poor respiratory function. The kidneys respond to high PCO_2 by retaining bicarbonate in the body. This renal mechanism is designed to regulate the pH of body fluids (Chapter 19). If the pH is normal, high PCO_2 is not an important stimulus for central chemoreceptors. Therefore such patients depend only on low PO_2 to continue their respiration through the peripheral chemoreceptor mechanism. Therefore, if such a patient is given 100 percent oxygen to breathe, correction of the low PO_2 may remove the sole stimulus for respiration. Therefore giving 100 percent oxygen may lead to dangerous depression of respiration in these patients and may even cause death.
3. The rate of diffusion depends on the pressure gradient. Therefore, in order to measure diffusion capacity of lungs for any gas we should know the partial pressure of the gas in (a) the alveoli, and (b) pulmonary capillaries.
   The difference between these two pressures gives the pressure gradient. But it is very difficult to

measure the partial pressure of a gas in pulmonary capillaries. The problem gets simplified if we use carbon monoxide. Carbon monoxide has a very high affinity for hemoglobin. Therefore at very low concentrations of carbon monoxide, almost all the carbon monoxide in blood is in combination with hemoglobin, and its partial pressure in pulmonary capillary blood can be considered zero.

Therefore in case of carbon monoxide the pressure gradient can be considered to be equal to the partial pressure of carbon monoxide in the alveoli. That is why carbon monoxide is a suitable gas for measuring diffusion capacity of lungs.

Although it is poisonous, the concentration of carbon monoxide used is so low as to be harmless.

4. The rate of diffusion is directly proportional to the solubility of the gas. Since carbon dioxide is much more soluble than oxygen, for a given pressure gradient, its diffusion is about 20 times faster than that of oxygen.
5. The diffusion of oxygen suffers more because the diffusion capacity for carbon dioxide is much greater.
6. Carbon monoxide poisoning is best treated with hyperbaric oxygen (Oxygen at high pressure). If oxygen is given at 2000 mm Hg, it results in 6 mL/100 mL of dissolved oxygen in the blood. This quantity is enough for resting metabolic requirements and can keep a person alive till carbon monoxide gradually dissociates from hemoglobin.
7. As the air passes through the nose, it is cleansed, warmed and humidified. The mouth is not equipped to bring about these useful changes in the air before it enters the larynx.

CHAPTER

7 Adaptation to Environment

"The word normal, as applied to human body temperature, is a splendidly misleading description ... ... Normally the majority of us do not have a 'normal' temperature."

—ANTHONY SMITH

Chapter Outline

- Regulation of Body Temperature
- Acclimatization to Hot Environment
- Heat Syndromes
- Acclimatization to Cold Environment
- Life at High Altitude

Man is affected by his environment in several ways. Generally, the effects of changes in environment are such that they help in adaptation to the change. Conversely, environment is also affected by human activity. For example, human beings have introduced considerable pollution in the environment. The pollution, in turn, affects human health. But in this chapter we shall concentrate on adaptive responses of the human body to extremes of environment.

It is necessary right in the b eginning to clarify the meaning of some apparently similar terms commonly used in environmental physiology.

Acclimatization refers to all the changes in physiological function which help in adjusting to a specific environment. The changes included in acclimatization are as follows:

a. changes acquired during the life time of the individual by long-term exposure to the environment, and
b. inherited characteristics which have developed over generations as a result of living in a specific environment.

Acclimation refers to the responses of an individual to alterations in only one environmental variable. This generally happens in experimental rather than natural situations.

Adaptation is a general term which refers to any characteristic of an organism which favors survival in a specific environment. Thus adaptation could include acclimatization as well as acclimation. Hence the term adaptation may be used loosely while describing any favorable responses to one or more environmental variables.

REGULATION OF BODY TEMPERATURE

Regulation of body temperature is remarkably good in human beings. The environmental temperature may be –20°C or +50°C, but the mouth temperature is about 37°C in both cases. Living tissues can function only within a narrow range of temperature. Therefore regulation of body temperature enables us to survive in different seasons and in different geographical areas.

The purpose of temperature regulation is to provide the right temperature to tissues. Therefore, it is enough if the immediate environment of the tissues (internal environment of the body) is at the right temperature. Hence, only the temperature of the internal environment (e.g. blood) is maintained constant by the regulatory mechanisms. The temperature of internal organs is nearly the same as that of blood. This temperature, called the core temperature, is about 37°C and remains constant in healthy persons. But the skin temperature, called the shell temperature, is not constant. The skin temperature changes in the same direction as the environmental tempe–rature, i.e. skin temperature is low in cold weather and high in warm weather. Clinically, the core temperature is measured from the following sites:

a. Oral temperature.
b. Axillary temperature, which is about 0.3°C lower than the oral temperature.
c. Rectal temperature, which is about 0.5-1.5°C higher than the oral temperature.

What is Normal Temperature

Saying that the normal temperature is 37°C is only approximately true. There are small fluctuations which are considered normal. For example, the temperature is higher during the day than at night. In women, the basal body temperature shows a rise of about 0.5°C at the time of ovulation and stays at the higher level till the onset of menstruation. There is also a rise in temperature after meals, physical exercise and emotional outbursts. At the end of heavy physical exercise the temperature may rise by as much as 4°C. A child's temperature may rise after playing or crying, and the parents may mistake it for fever.

Heat Balance

Regulation of body temperature is the result of heat gain being balanced by heat loss. The major factors which affect the heat balance of the body have been discussed briefly below.

Factors Promoting Heat Gain

There are two ways of gaining heat. One, by increasing heat production; and two, by reducing heat loss.

Heat production is increased by:

a. Shivering, which increases heat production by skeletal muscles.
b. Sympathetic stimulation, which releases adrenalin, which in turn increases the metabolic rate and hence heat production.
c. Exercise, which increases heat production by skeletal muscles.
d. Eating a meal, due to the thermic effect of feeding.

Heat loss from the body is reduced by:

a. Cutaneous vasoconstriction, which leads to reduced heat loss from the skin by radiation.
b. Increased insulation, which is achieved in animals by the fur becoming more fluffy, and in human beings by appropriate clothing.
c. Reduced air movement, which is achieved by staying indoors with the fans switched off.
d. Warming up the environment, which is achieved by seeking warmth, e.g. by sitting in the sun or by using fire or a heater.
e. Reducing the surface area exposed to cold, by sitting close to one another or by assuming a curled up posture.

Factors Promoting Heat Loss

Heat loss may be promoted directly by increasing the dissipation of heat. It may also be promoted indirectly by reducing the conservation of heat.

Heat dissipation is increased by:

a. Cutaneous vasodilatation, which increases heat loss from the skin by radiation.
b. Sweating, which increases heat loss from the skin by evaporation. Sweating wets the surface of the body and evaporates. As it evaporates, it takes heat from the body. It is well to keep in mind that it is evaporation and not just sweating, which produces cooling. When the humidity is high, evaporation is very slow. Therefore one feels very uncomfortable in high humidity in spite of sweating. In other words, it is the sweat which dries, not the sweat which drips, that helps in losing heat.
   Sweat glands are distributed all over the body. Their nerve supply is unique in that it is sympathetic but cholinergic. Human beings can tolerate heat very well due to a powerful sweating mechanism. In fact, very few species of animals sweat in response to heat, and none of them as efficiently as human beings.

c. Panting, which also increases evaporative heat loss. Panting is seen only in dogs, horses and cattle. Panting involves rapid and shallow breathing. As air passes over the warm and moist nasal turbinates and tongue, it hastens evaporative heat loss from these surfaces.
d. Increasing air movement, as by the use of fans.
e. Cooling the immediate environment.
f. Increasing the surface area of the body by postural adjustment.

Heat conservation may be reduced by reducing clothing, specially clothing which may trap heat. Animals with fur and feathers reduce heat conservation by assuming a less fluffy look.

Temperature Regulatory Mechanisms

Temperature regulatory mechanisms involve three steps: *detection* of change in temperature, *processing* of information about change in temperature, and eliciting an appropriate *response.*

Change in body temperature is detected by skin receptors and also by temperature-sensitive neurons in the hypothalamus. Hypothalamic neurons detect small changes in the temperature of blood flowing through the brain.

Hypothalamic temperature-sensitive neurons as well as skin receptors finally convey information about changes in temperature to the hypothalamus for processing. After appropriate processing, anterior hypothalamus activates heat dissipation mechanisms if the body needs to lose heat. Alternatively, posterior hypothalamus activates mechanisms for heat conservation and production if the body needs to raise the temperature.

The principal responses which result in heat dissipation are cutaneous vasodilatation and sweating. The principal responses which result in heat conservation or production are cutaneous vasoconstriction, shivering and enhanced sympathoadrenal activity.

The Classical Model of Thermoregulation

If the environmental temperature is 25-27°C, the body temperature stays normal without any active regulatory mechanisms coming into play. Therefore the range 25-27°C is called the thermoneutral zone. This environmental temperature is the most comfortable one.

When the environmental temperature rises above this comfortable temperature, the temperature of blood circulating through the brain also rises above 37°C. The hypothalamus is normally set to maintain the temperature of this blood at 37°C. Therefore 37°C is called the normal set point of the hypothalamus. If the temperature of the blood circulating through the hypothalamus is above 37°C, the anterior hypothalamus activates the mechanisms for heat dissipation, i.e. cutaneous vasodilatation and sweating. As a result, the body loses heat and the temperature of blood as well as the core temperature fall. When the temperature becomes normal, the mechanisms for heat dissipation are switched off.

When the environmental temperature falls below the thermoneutral zone, the skin receptors sense it. The information is conveyed to the hypothalamus. The hypothalamus may also sense directly a fall in the temperature of the blood circulating through it. As a result, the posterior hypothalamus brings about cutaneous vasoconstriction and shivering till the core temperature matches the set point of the hypothalamus.

Fever

Fever is an abnormal increase in core temperature. A normal rise in temperature due to exercise, is not fever. Fever is generally associated with an inflammatory response, which may or may not be due to an infection. In the inflammatory response, white blood cells release endogenous pyrogens (e.g. interleukin-1) which lead to fever.

Pyrogens reset the hypothalamic set point at a higher level so that the body now aims at a temperature which is higher than normal. This can explain some symptoms associated with fever. At the beginning of the disease, the hypothalamus is reset at a higher level but the body temperature is still normal. Since the body is cold as compared to the set point, the hypothalamus initiates the shivering response. Therefore shivering is often seen during the rising phase of fever. When the body temperature has come up to the new set point, shivering stops. On the other hand, when the disease responsible for the fever is cured, the hypothalamic thermostat is again reset at the normal level. But the person still has fever. Since the body is now warm as compared to the set point, the hypothalamus initiates the sweating response. Therefore sweating is often seen during the falling phase of fever.

Antipyretics such as aspirin are believed to reset the hypothalamic set point to the normal level if it is set at an abnormally high level. That is how they bring down the body temperature in fever. Since antipyretics do not affect heat production or dissipation mechanisms directly, these drugs do not affect the body temperature if it is already normal.

ACCLIMATIZATION TO HOT ENVIRONMENT

Long-term exposure to hot environment leads to the development of physiological characteristics which make stay in that environment more convenient and comfortable. Daily exposure to heat for 10-14 days leads to reasonably good adaptation. The adaptive changes are concerned primarily with sweat secretion. An acclimatized individual:

a. Has an enhanced capacity to sweat, i.e. he can sweat more,
b. Has a lower threshold for sweating, i.e. he starts sweating at a lower temperature,
c. Has a better distribution of sweat, i.e. he sweats all over the body, and
d. Has sweat with a lower salt concentration, i.e. he loses less salt during sweating.

As can be easily understood, the first three changes make sweating more efficient. The fourth change makes it easier to replace losses due to sweating because it is easier to replace water than salt.

The consequences of these changes are that an acclimatized individual can tolerate heat better, can survive higher environmental temperatures, and can perform more physical work in hot environment.

HEAT SYNDROMES

Acute exposure to heat leads to sweating and consequent thirst. However, if the heat is too much for the individual to cope up with, or water and salt are not adequately replaced in response to thirst, it may lead to various heat syndromes. It takes less heat to produce a heat syndrome in a non-acclimatized individual. Heat syndromes of increasing degree of severity are heat cramps, heat exhaustion and heat stroke.

Heat Cramps

This is a painful condition of limb muscles. It follows excessive sweating, which can be due to heat or exercise. Heat cramps are primarily due to water and salt depletion, and can therefore be treated with water and sodium chloride.

Heat Exhaustion

This is a condition of cardiovascular failure. Water and electrolyte loss coupled with widespread vasodilatation leads to a picture resembling cardiovascular shock (cold, moist skin; rapid, thready pulse; sometimes low blood pressure).

Loss of consciousness may occur, but is uncommon. The body temperature is normal or low.

Treatment consists of making the patient lie down in a cool area. Intravenous fluids may sometimes be necessary.

Heat Stroke

This is a condition of failure of temperature regulation. The patient's core temperature may be 41°C or even higher. The patient has no sweating, but is often unconscious, and may be in delirium. Kidney damage is common, leading to acute renal failure. Mortality is high: hence treatment should be started promptly.

The treatment consists of energetic measures to cool the patient. Immersing the patient in a tub of ice cold water is the best way to cool him. If that is not possible, the body should be covered with wet ice cold towels and sheets. Cooling should be continued till the body temperature has fallen to 38°C (101°F).

ACCLIMATIZATION TO COLD ENVIRONMENT

Human beings exposed to cold environment for long periods of time may adapt to it in different ways. However, one of the commonest ways is by increasing heat production. We have already learnt that acute exposure to a low environmental temperature leads to heat production by shivering. But long term exposure triggers other mechanisms of heat production. These mechanisms are collectively called non-shivering thermogenesis (NST). NST is due to increased metabolic rate in liver, other abdominal viscera and skeletal muscles. The NST response to cold is possibly mediated by sympathetic nervous system and thyroid hormones.

Hypothermia

The metabolic requirements of tissues are reduced at low temperatures. At a body temperature of 25°C, the oxygen requirements are 40-45 percent of those at normal body temperature (Figs 7.1A and B). This fact is made use of in cardiac surgery and neurosurgery. Several operations on the heart or brain require temporary suspension of circulation. This is made possible by using a cardiopulmonary bypass machine. In this machine, a pump takes over the function of the heart, and an oxygenator takes over the function of the lungs. However, it is still helpful if the oxygen requirement of the body can be reduced during surgery. The reduction is achieved by cooling the body, i.e. by inducing hypothermia. The reduced metabolic requirements can be easily satisfied with the help of the bypass machine.

Sudden exposure to very low temperatures may make the tissues inactive but the tissues may stay alive for quite a long time due to reduced metabolic requirements. Therefore, a patient who has been exposed to a very low temperature for a few hours or days may appear dead when brought to the hospital, but may be actually alive. Such a patient should be rewarmed and efforts should be made to resuscitate him. Resuscitation should not be stopped unless rewarming also fails to revive the patient. In short, a cold patient is not dead unless warm and dead.

LIFE AT HIGH ALTITUDE

The primary problem at high altitude is low atmospheric pressure (Fig. 7.2). It is important to note that the composition of air does not change at

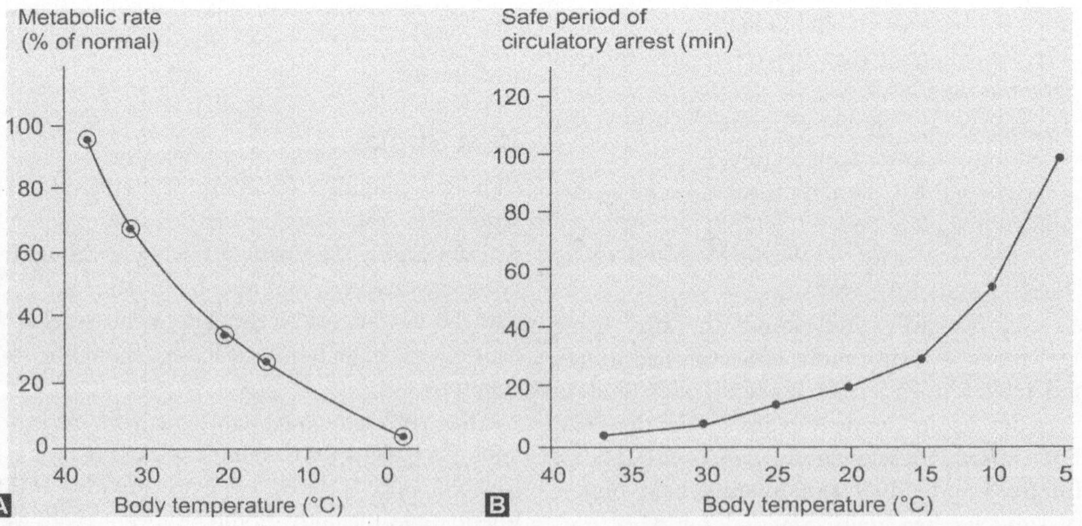

Figs 7.1A and B Since the metabolic rate falls with the body temperature (A) the maximum safe period of circulatory arrest increases as the body temperature falls (B)

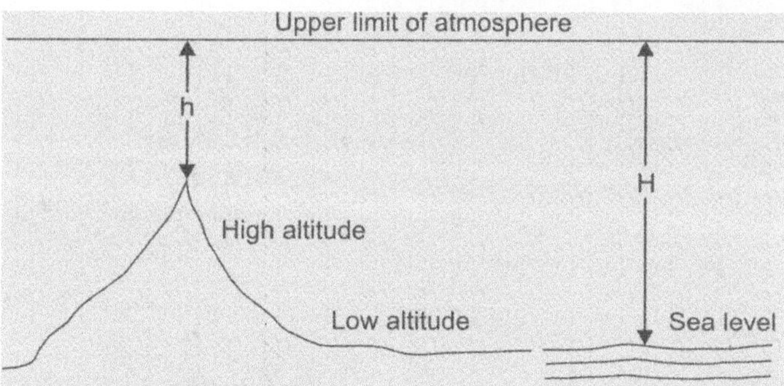

Fig. 7.2 At high altitude the atmospheric pressure is low because the column of air above the surface of the earth (h) is smaller than the corresponding column at sea level (H). Therefore, although the air at both places has 20 percent oxygen, the PO_2 is much lower at high altitude. At an altitude of 18000 feet, the atmospheric pressure is half that at sea level

high altitude. Oxygen forms 20 percent of the air at high altitude just as at low altitude. Hence the partial pressure of oxygen (PO_2) is low at high altitude.

Thus, at sea level, atmospheric pressure = 760 mmHg, and PO_2 = 20 percent of 760 = 152 mmHg. At an altitude of 5.5 km (18,000 ft), atmospheric pressure = 380 mmHg, and PO_2 = 20 percent of 380 = 76 mmHg.

Effects of Acute Exposure to High Altitude

Appreciable effects occur only on exposure to altitudes above 7000 feet.

Hyperventilation

The low atmospheric PO_2 at high altitude leads to fall in the PO_2 of blood (hypoxic hypoxia). That leads to stimulation of carotid body chemoreceptors. The response to the stimulation is hyperventilation. Acute exposure to high altitude may increase pulmonary ventilation by up to 65 percent.

Work Capacity

The acute effect of high altitude is a reduction in work capacity. The capacity improves gradually as a result of acclimatization but still does not match the work capacity of the natives.

2,3-diphosphoglycerate Concentration

Within hours of exposure to high altitude, the diphosphoglycerate (DPG) concentration of red blood cells increases. This response follows hypoxia due to other causes as well. Increase in the concentration of DPG reduces the affinity of hemoglobin for oxygen. The phenomenon is advantageous at tissue level because it increases the delivery of oxygen. But the same phenomenon can be disadvantageous in the lungs where less oxygen would be picked up by hemoglobin at a given PO_2.

Central Nervous System Effects

The central nervous system (CNS) is very sensitive to hypoxia. Hypoxia depresses the CNS. Therefore at an altitude of about 12,000 feet, a person feels lazy and sleepy, and may get a headache. Depression of cortical neurons, which normally inhibit primitive aggressive behavior, results in a release phenomenon. This may lead to loss of self-control. The phenomenon resembles both in its mechanism and manifestation, the effect of alcohol. At higher altitudes, there may be loss of judgement, twitchings, convulsions and finally unconsciousness. Consciousness is lost at an altitude of 23,000 feet when breathing air, and at an altitude of 47,000 feet when breathing oxygen.

Acclimatization to High Altitude

Delivery of atmospheric oxygen to the tissues involves three major steps (Fig. 7.3). Each step involves a drop in PO_2. If the starting PO_2 is low, the body undergoes acclimatization so as to:

a. Reduce the pressure drop during transfer,

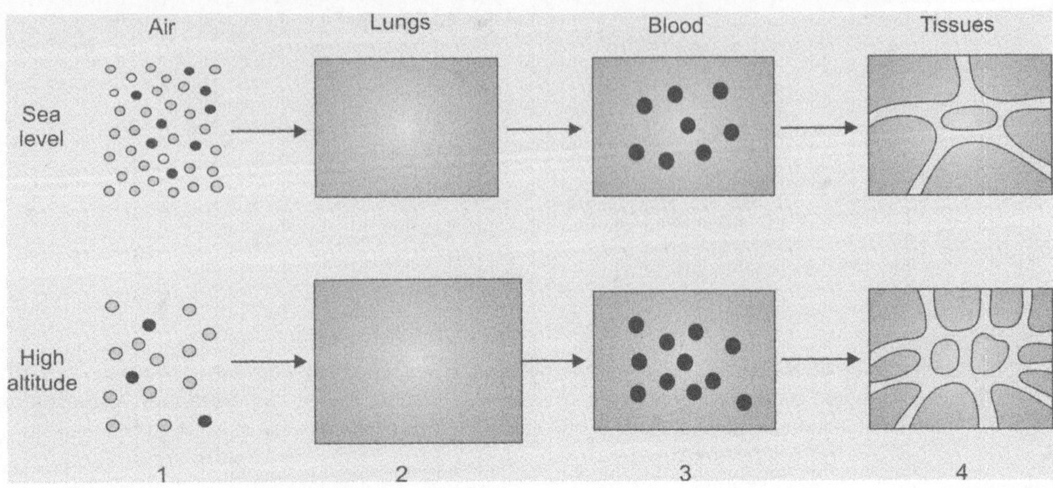

Fig. 7.3 Acclimatization to high altitude. Delivery of oxygen to tissues involves breathing, diffusion of oxygen to the blood across the alveoli, and tissue perfusion with blood. At high altitude, the air has the same proportion of oxygen (indicated by filled circles) to nitrogen (indicated by empty circles) but is less dense. An acclimatized individual compensates for this difference by hyperventilation (1), a larger chest size (2), an increase in RBC count and hence hemoglobin concentration in blood (3), and increased vascularity and improved oxygen utilization in tissues (4) (For color version see Plate 6)

b. Increase the oxygen carrying capacity of blood, and
c. Improve the ability of the tissues to utilize oxygen.

Given enough time, acclimatization can be so good that a highlander is not only comfortable at high altitude, his work capacity is also comparable to that of lowlanders. Now we shall examine in some detail the adaptive changes which make such excellent acclimatization possible.

Hyperventilation

It was mentioned earlier that acute exposure may increase pulmonary ventilation up to 65 percent. But within 3-4 days of stay at high altitude, there is a further increase in ventilation. The minute volume may increase by 500 percent primarily as a result of increase in the tidal volume. An acclimatized individual may achieve a tidal volume of as much as 5 liters.

Some of the mechanisms underlying the hyperventilation are an enhanced sensitivity of respiratory chemoreceptor mechanisms, and the 'thinness' of the atmosphere which makes hyperventilation easier and less tiring.

Hyperventilation is very useful in reducing the degree of hypoxia at high altitude.

Large Chest

Hyperventilation, as described above, is seen in lowlanders upon acclimatization within a few days. Highlanders who have been living at high altitude for many generations do not show so much hyperventilation. Instead, they have a large chest size while the rest of their body size is smaller. In this way their ventilatory capacity is increased in relation to their body mass.

Polycythemia

Hypoxia is a potent stimulus for erythropoiesis. Hence, within a few weeks of stay at high altitude, the hemoglobin (Hb) concentration of blood rises. Increase in Hb concentration increases the oxygen carrying capacity of blood. The increased capacity is helpful in fighting the effects of hypoxia due to high altitude.

Increased Vascularity of Tissues

Normally, only a few capillaries in a tissue are open. The rest of the capillaries are closed and constitute a reserve. At high altitude some of these reserve capillaries also open up. More open capillaries means more blood flow. More blood flow brings more oxygen to the tissues. Thus at least part of the effect of lower PO_2 is overcome.

Improved Ability of Tissues to Use Oxygen

There is some evidence that staying at high altitude for several generations induces characteristics which facilitate oxygen utilization, such as increased number of mitochondria and higher activity of oxidative enzymes.

Exercise at High Altitude

Exercise increases oxygen requirement while at high altitude the availability of oxygen is low. Therefore exercise further aggravates the effects of high altitude. Hence work capacity is impaired at high altitude except in those who have been living there for several generations.

Further, the challenge posed by exercise as well as high altitude is basically that of oxygen deficiency. Because of this similarity, exercise performed at high altitude hastens the process of acclimatization.

Maladaptation to High Altitude

Some individuals find it particularly difficult to adapt to high altitude. Even those who adapt well may show some undesirable effects if stationed above 16,000 feet for more than 3-4 weeks. Some relatively common forms of maladaptation to high altitude have been discussed briefly below.

High Altitude Pulmonary Edema

It is a serious condition usually seen only in unacclimatized individuals. It is precipitated by exercise. The underlying mechanism is not well understood but pulmonary vascular hypertension is a major contributory factor. The condition may be treated with oxygen, rest, and return to low altitude, if possible.

Acute Mountain Sickness

High altitude pulmonary edema described above is one form of acute mountain sickness. Another serious form which it can take is cerebral edema, giving rise to disorientation, hallucinations and other related symptoms. Cerebral edema is due to the normal response of cerebral blood vessels to hypoxia, i.e. vasodilation.

Chronic Mountain Sickness

Chronic mountain sickness develops slowly and is closely related to the process of adaptation. The hemoglobin level keeps rising till it becomes so high that the increased viscosity of blood seriously impairs blood flow through the tissues. The result is that in spite of the high hemoglobin level, tissue oxygen supply is poor. Poor tissue oxygenation gives rise to excessive tiredness, mental fatigue and headache. The high hemoglobin level gives the person a pink color but poor oxygenation makes it quickly turn blue on slight physical exertion. Pulmonary vasoconstriction in response to hypoxia may give rise to pulmonary hypertension. The condition is also known as Monge's disease. Treatment basically consists of return to sea level.

CONCLUSION

The human organism is sufficiently flexible and adaptable to be able to live in a wide range of environments. Further, using science and technology, man has expanded his reach even to inhospitable environments. Man can fly at very high altitudes in pressurised planes and has even invaded space.

QUESTION

1. Why is sweating ineffective if the humidity is high?

ANSWER

1. The reason is that evaporation is extremely slow when the humidity is high. If the sweat does not evaporate, it does not take any heat from the body. That is why, when the humidity is high, the sweat drips from the body but does not dry. It is sweat which dries that cools the body, not the sweat that drips.

CHAPTER

8 Gastrointestinal System

"To eat is human; to digest, divine."

—MARK TWAIN

Chapter Outline

In case of unicellular organisms, food is acquired directly from the immediate environment by simple processes such as phagocytosis or pinocytosis. In multicellular organisms, the route is indirect. Food enters the gastrointestinal tract, where it is digested. After digestion, it is absorbed into the blood. Blood transports the nutrients to the neighborhood of every cell. Depending on the needs of the cells, nutrients diffuse from the blood into the interstitial fluid, and from the interstitial fluid into the cells (Figs 8.1A and B). The cells may use the nutrients to obtain energy, or to make new molecules, which may finally build new tissues for growth and repair.

Essentially the same chemical units which constitute our food are also the nutrients which give energy, and the nutrients which build new tissues. But the form in which these chemical units are arranged is different in each case. The situation is comparable to the building blocks with which children play. A child may arrange the blocks in so many different ways to get vastly different looking structures. In order to achieve rearrangement of the building blocks of our food, it is first necessary to break the food into its blocks. Then the body can utilize or rearrange the blocks as it likes. The process of breaking down complex food molecules into simple molecules is known as **digestion**. The next event in the gut is the transfer of these simple molecules to the blood stream. This process is called **absorption**. Absorption is a very important step. The gastrointestinal tract may be considered a hollow tube running through the body. Whatever is in this tube is essentially outside the body, although it appears to be inside it (Fig. 8.2). The contents of the tube may be considered truly inside the body only after absorption (Fig. 8.3). The next step after absorption is the utilization or **assimilation** of absorbed food. It may be used for providing energy, or may be stored as an energy rich compound depending upon the nature of the nutrient and the requirements of the body (Fig. 8.4).

Digestion is brought about by enzymes. Digestive enzymes are either secreted by the gastrointestinal cells, or brought to the gut from the pancreas. Digestion and absorption proceed as the food travels along the gut. In the next few pages, food will be followed as it travels from the mouth to the anal canal, and the events in each region will be discussed. But before that, it is important to learn something about the structure of the gastrointestinal tract.

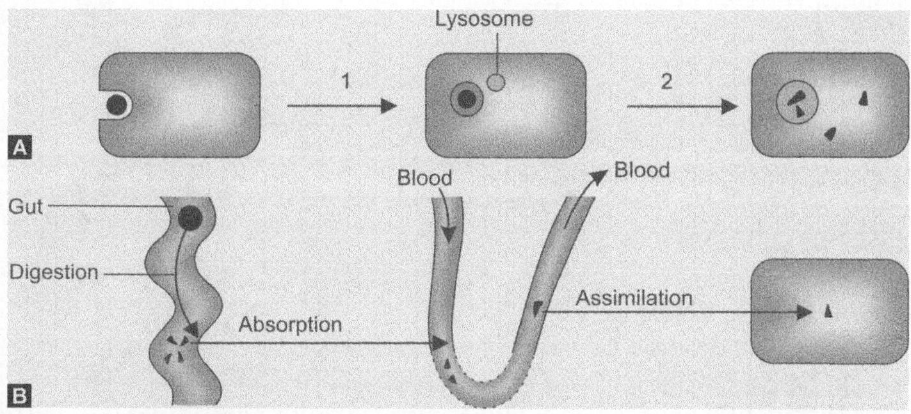

Figs 8.1A and B The process of digestion in unicellular and multicellular organisms. (A) In unicellular organisms, the cell ingests 'food' (1) by phagocytosis. The food is 'digested' (2) with the help of lysosomes. The digested products diffuse into the cell; (B) In multicellular organisms, food enters the gut where it is digested. The digested products are absorbed from the gut into the blood. The blood delivers these products to individual cells depending on the needs

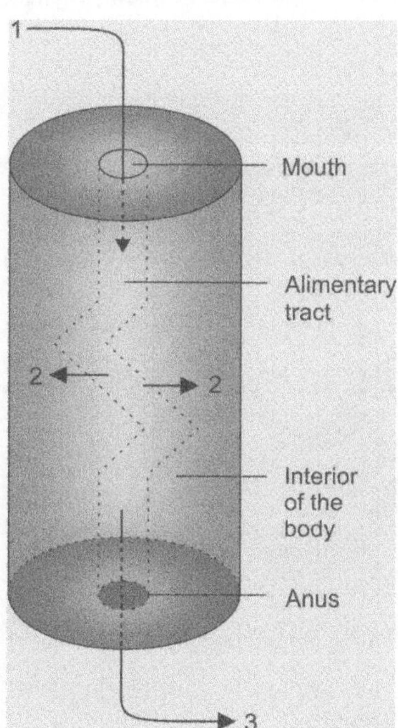

Fig. 8.2 The alimentary canal is essentially a tube passing through the body. The food ingested (1) is not really inside the body unless it is absorbed (2). Whatever is not absorbed is eventually lost in feces (3), and is hence lost to the body (Reproduced from Bijlani RL. Eating Scientifically. New Delhi: Orient Longman, 1974, Fig. 6, p. 22)

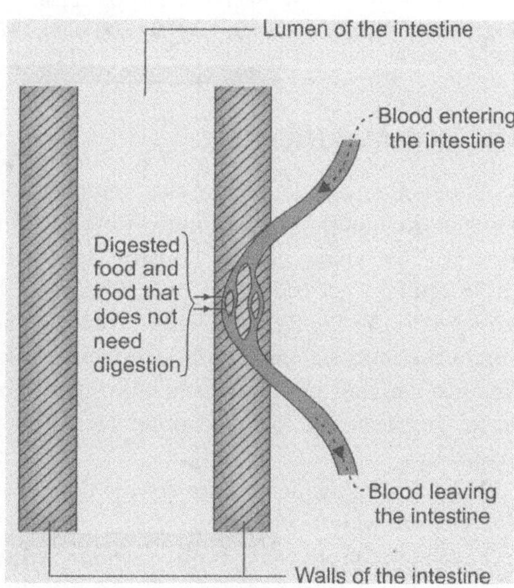

Fig. 8.3 Absorption. During absorption, food enters the blood coming to the intestine and leaves with the blood leaving the intestine. Once absorbed into the bloodstream, food circulates all over the body, and is used as and when required (Reproduced from Bijlani RL. Eating Scientifically. New Delhi: Orient Longman, 1974. Fig. 7. p. 24)

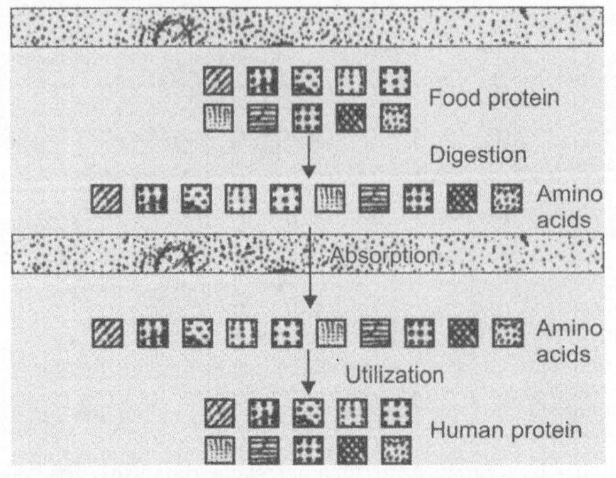

Fig. 8.4 Digestion, absorption and assimilation. Here the three processes have been illustrated diagrammatically using protein as an example. The processes are broadly similar for other nutrients. During digestion, the nutrient molecules are broken down into component molecules. During absorption, the component molecules cross the intestinal mucosa to enter the bloodstream. The absorbed products are assimilated or utilized as building material, as shown here, or as fuel (Reproduced from Bijlani RL. Eating Scientifically, New Delhi: Orient Longman, 1974, Fig. 8. p. 26)

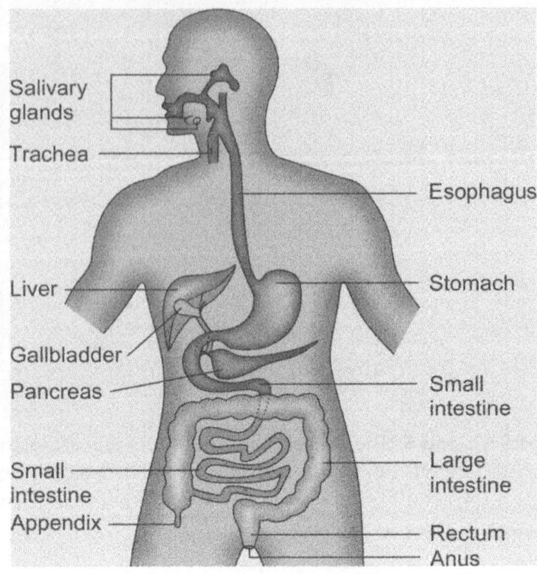

Fig. 8.5 The alimentary tract (Reproduced from Bijlani RL. Eating Scientifically, New Delhi: Orient Longman, 1974, Fig. 5, p. 21)

FUNCTIONAL ANATOMY

The alimentary tract is a long and complex tube starting at the mouth and continuing upto the anus (Fig. 8.5). The typical plan of construction of the gastrointestinal tract (GIT) has been illustrated by a cross section in Figure 8.6. Digestion takes place partly in the mucosal epithelium. Absorption takes place through the mucosal epithelium. The large surface area required for absorption (Fig. 8.7) is provided by:

a. The folds into which the mucosa is thrown, as seen even with the naked eye,
b. Finger-like projections (**villi**; *singular*, **villus**) along the mucosal surface, seen under the light microscope, and
c. Dense and fine folds (**microvilli**) into which the epithelial cell membrane on the lumenal side is thrown, seen only under the electron microscope.

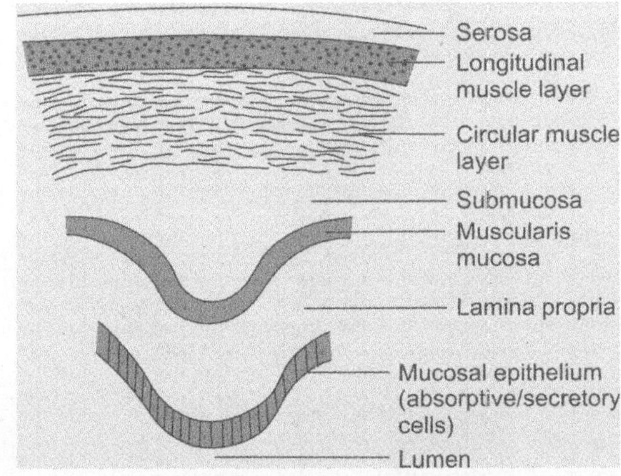

Fig. 8.6 Typical structural plan of the gastrointestinal tract

Blood Supply

The GIT and associated structures receive their blood supply from branches of the aorta: the celiac artery, the superior mesenteric artery and the inferior mesenteric artery. Liver receives blood from the hepatic artery, which is a branch of the celiac

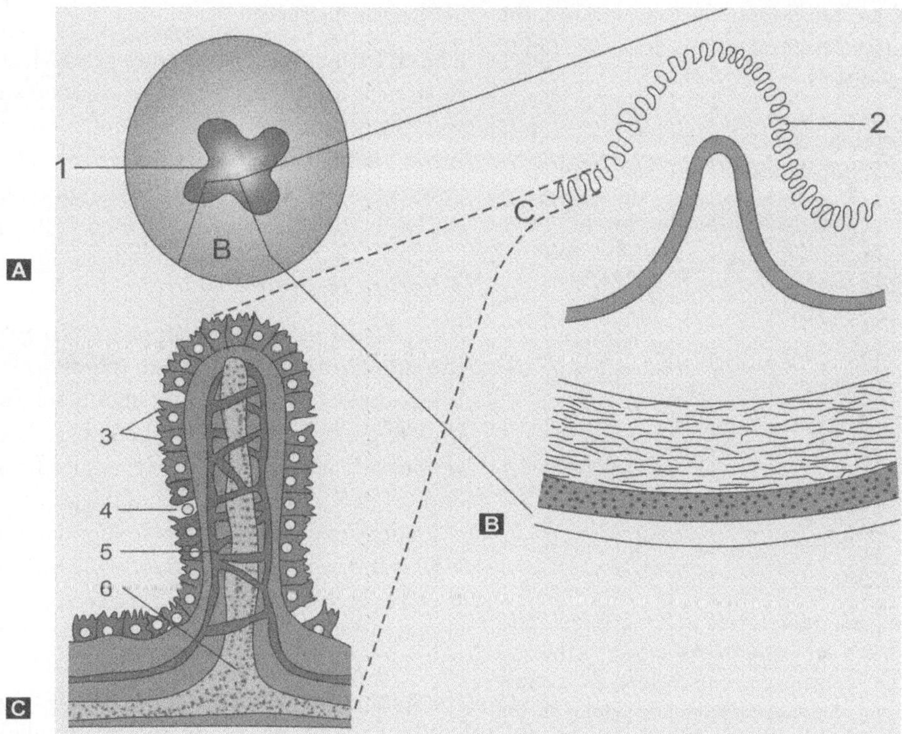

Figs 8.7A to C The surface area of small intestine is enormously increased by repeated folding. Increasing levels of magnification reveal more and more minute folds. (A) Naked eye view; (B) Low power magnification of the sector marked 'B' in (A); (C) High power magnification of the villus marked 'C' in (B). 1, valvulae conniventes; 2, villi; 3, microvilli; 4, goblet cell; 5, blood vessel; 6, lymphatic. The valvulae conniventes, villi and microvilli increase the surface area of the small intestine three -, ten - and twenty-fold respectively, giving a total multiplication of 600-fold. (Reproduced from Bijlani RL, Manchanda SK. The Human Machine: how to prevent breakdowns. New Delhi: National Book Trust, India, Revised edition, 1999, Fig. 23, p. 71)

artery. All the blood that leaves the GIT, pancreas and spleen, is drained by the portal vein, which carries it to the liver. Thus the liver receives blood from two sources: the hepatic artery and the portal vein. The blood leaving the liver leaves it in the hepatic vein. The portal vein gives the liver an opportunity to sample all the material that is absorbed in the GIT.

Nerve Supply

The gastrointestinal tract is lined by smooth muscle. The musculature responds to stretch by contraction. This response does not require nerve supply. But the GIT does have a nerve supply which further improves its motor and secretory activity. The neural elements of the gut may be considered under three headings:

1. Enteric nervous system
2. Afferent nerves
3. Efferent nerves.

Enteric Nervous System

Two important neural networks within the wall of the gut have been known for a long time: Auerbach's plexus and Meissner's plexus. The neuronal organization of these plexuses resembles a reflex arc (Fig. 8.8). The enteric nervous system ensures that the gut responds to mechanical or chemical stimuli present in the lumen. The interconnections between neighboring segments of the gut ensure that the response results in purposeful movement (i.e. either propulsion or mixing). The enteric nervous system makes the gut so self-sufficient that cutting the extrinsic afferent and efferent nerves does not lead to a serious abnormality.

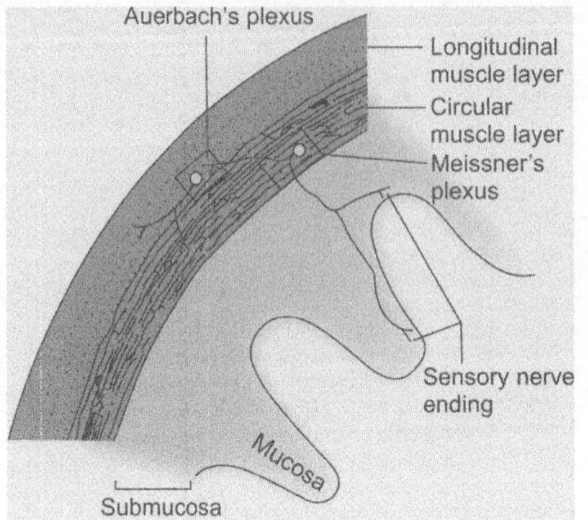

Fig. 8.8 Diagrammatic representation of the neuronal circuitry of Meissner's and Auerbach's plexus. The cell bodies seen in the Meissner's plexus belong to sensory neurons which bring information from the lumen of the gut. The cell bodies seen in the Auerbach's plexus belong to motor neurons which supply smooth muscle of the gut

Afferent Nerves

The GIT has afferent nerve endings which are sensitive to stretch, chemical stimuli and osmotic stimuli. The mesentery, pancreas and capsule of the liver also have nerve endings which are sensitive to painful stimuli. Afferent nerve fibers originating in gut travel either in the vagus nerve or in the dorsal roots of the spinal cord.

Efferent Nerves

The efferent nerve fibers supplying the gut belong to the autonomic nervous system (parasympathetic and sympathetic). These nerves modulate rather than initiate gastrointestinal (GI) activities. The activities modulated are (a) motility, (b) exocrine secretions, and (c) endocrine secretions of the gut.

The parasympathetic nerve supplying most of the GIT is the vagus nerve (Fig. 8.9). The left half of the transverse colon, rectum and anal canal are, however, supplied by the sacral parasympathetic nerves (S2-S4). The sympathetic nerves to the GIT originate in the spinal cord segments T5 - L2.

In general, parasympathetic stimulation increases GI motility and secretion while sympathetic

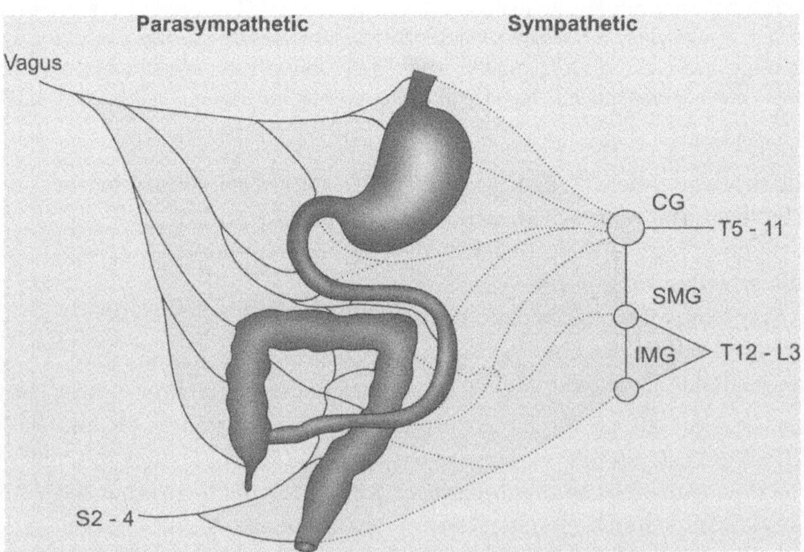

Fig. 8.9 Diagrammatic representation of parasympathetic (continuous lines) and sympathetic (dotted lines) innervation of the gastrointestinal tract. S2–4, second through fourth sacral segments of the spinal cord; T5-11, fifth through eleventh thoracic segments of the spinal cord; T12-L3, twelfth thoracic through third lumbar segments of the spinal cord; CG, celiac ganglion; SMG, superior mesenteric ganglion; IMG, inferior mesenteric ganglion

stimulation decreases them. The responses follow the general pattern that parasympathetic activity dominates under relaxed conditions while sympathetic activity helps the body in emergency situations. Eating and digestion are primarily activities reserved for relaxed conditions and unsuitable in an emergency. Therefore it is appropriate that parasympathetic nerves facilitate GIT activity while sympathetic nerves inhibit it.

Interaction between Enteric Nervous System and Autonomic Nervous System

The enteric nervous system and the autonomic nerves to the GI tract are not entirely independent of each other. The autonomic nerves affect the gut not only indirectly but also by modifying the activity of neurons in the myenteric and submucous plexuses (Fig. 8.10).

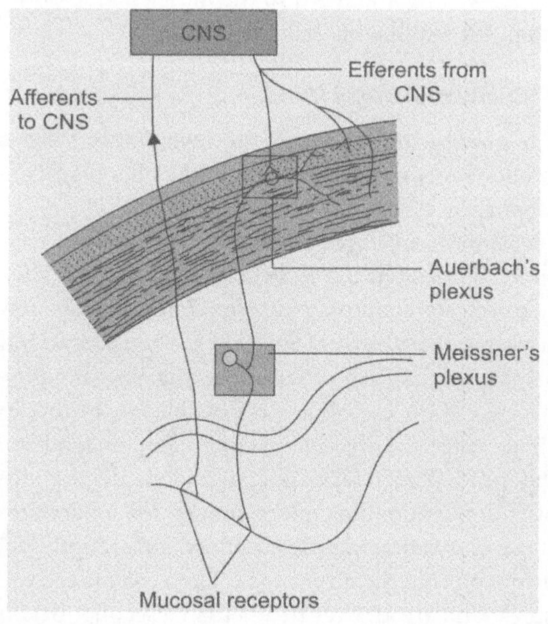

Fig. 8.10 Simplified view of the neural organization in the gut. There is an intrinsic network consisting of the Meissner's and Auerbach's plexuses, on which is superimposed control from the central nervous system (CNS). In addition, central neural reflexes affect gastrointestinal function directly as well

Higher Neural Influences

Many parts of the brain, including the cerebral cortex and limbic system affect the final autonomic output. That is why GI activity is frequently affected by our thoughts and emotions.

To summarize, the primitive intrinsic ability of the GIT to regulate its own activity is assisted by the enteric nervous system. The regulation becomes finer with the help of the autonomic nerves. The autonomic nerves, in turn, are affec-ted by higher regions of the central nervous system. Thus gastrointestinal activity is determined by the integrated output of local and general neural activity.

FOOD IN THE MOUTH

Food starts its journey in the mouth, where we chew it. Chewing, or mastication, is useful, although it may not be essential. Chewing is beneficial in at least four ways:

i. It makes digestion easier.
ii. It prevents damage to the GIT which may possibly arise from some hard food.
iii. It binds the food into a bolus by mixing it with saliva. That makes swallowing easier.
iv. It prevents overeating. Chewing takes time. Besides the quantity of food, it is the time we take to eat that determines when we feel full and stop eating. Thus by prolonging the time taken to eat, chewing makes us eat less than what we may otherwise.

Salivary Secretion

We have three pairs of salivary glands — parotid, submandibular and sublingual. They empty their secretion into the mouth through their ducts. The ducts also play some part in modifying the composition of the salivary secretion, or saliva. The three salivary glands differ in the type of cells that constitute them, and as a result also in the type of secretions they produce. The parotid glands are composed almost entirely of serous cells. Serous secretion is thin and watery. Sublingual cells are made up of mucous cells. Mucous secretion is thick and viscous. Submandibular glands have both serous and mucous cells.

Saliva contains amylase, mucin, electrolytes, antibodies and, of course, a lot of water to dissolve them all. The electrolyte composition is, to some extent, determined by the rate of salivary secretion. This happens because the primary secretion is modified by the ducts. Faster the secretion, less the time available for the modification by the ducts.

Functions of Saliva

Saliva contains the enzyme amylase, which hydrolyses starch into the disachharide maltose. Although not much time is available for the digestion of starch in the mouth, the small amount that is digested improves the taste of food. The food becomes sweet because starch is tasteless while maltose is sweet. The action of salivary amylase stops when food reaches the stomach because the pH of gastric juice is too acidic for amylase activity to continue.

Besides its digestive function, saliva helps bind the food into a bolus, which is more convenient to swallow. Saliva also helps oral hygiene in many ways. First, it washes away food particles and sugar which could otherwise support the growth of bacteria. Secondly, saliva contains thiocyanate, which is bactericidal. Finally, saliva contains the IgA class of antibodies.

In some animals, such as dogs, evaporation of sweat plays an important role in regulation of body temperature.

Regulation of Salivary Secretion

Salivary secretion is regulated primarily by neural mechanisms. Information about the presence of food is conveyed to the brain by olfactory, visual, or taste receptors. Regions of the brain which receive this information are connected to the superior and inferior salivary nuclei which, in turn, control salivary secretion through the activity of sympathetic and parasympathetic nerves. Stimulation of parasympathetic nerves to the salivary glands produces a large volume of watery secretion. Stimulation of sympathetic nerves to the salivary glands produces a small volume of sticky (viscous) secretion.

Swallowing

Swallowing, also called deglutition, starts as a voluntary act but soon becomes involuntary. When we feel that the food has been chewn enough, we collect it into a bolus and push it backwards. Structures in the back of the mouth are particularly sensitive to touch. As soon as the bolus touches these structures, the swallowing reflex is inititated. The swallowing reflex, like all other reflexes, is an involuntary act. That is how the voluntary stage of swallowing passes on to the involuntary stage.

Impulses from the touch receptors located in the mouth and pharynx are conveyed to the swallowing center in the medulla oblongata. The most important nerve responsible for conveying information from the mouth to the swallowing center is the superior laryngeal nerve (a branch of the vagus nerve). After due processing of the information in the swallowing center, efferent impulses are conveyed by cranial nerves V, VII, X and XII to the muscles which bring about the swallowing reflex.

The Swallowing Reflex

The swallowing reflex, or the involuntary stage of swallowing, may be divided into the pharyngeal and esophageal stages.

Pharyngeal stage: The mouth is below the nose, while the esophagus is behind the trachea. These anatomical relations create an unavoidable criss-crossing of pathways (Fig. 8.11). The food and air passages cross each other in the pharyngeal region. Because of the crossing, it is possible for the food or air to enter the wrong passage. Entry of food into the wind pipe (trachea) can lead to death. Most of the events taking place during the pharyngeal stage of swallowing are designed to prevent food from entering the air passage. These events are very quick, and are all over in less than a second. Briefly, the events are:

i. The soft palate rises to block the posterior nares; this prevents food from coming out through the nose.

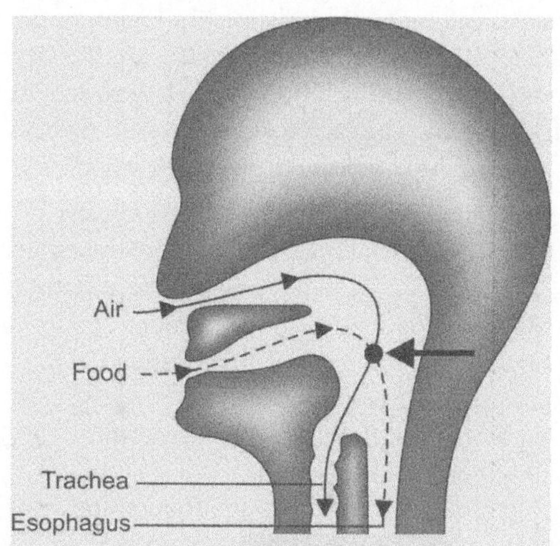

Fig. 8.11 The anatomical relations create an inevitable criss-crossing of food and air pathways

ii. The pharyngeal opening is reduced to a narrow slit, which allows only small quantities of food to pass at a time.
iii. The vocal cords are brought together (adducted), closing the superior opening of the larynx.
iv. The epiglottis swings back to cover the superior opening of the larynx. Therefore the food cannot come in contact with even the adducted vocal cords. The arrangement is comparable to a double door.
v. The larynx is pulled upwards and forwards. This may be verified by placing the tips of two fingers over the thyroid cartilage of the larynx (Adam's apple), and then swallowing a little saliva. Raising the larynx raises also the epiglottis. Thus the food being swallowed does not come in contact even with much of the epiglottis. Instead, most of the food slips along the gutters on either side of the epiglottis rather than go over it.
vi. Breathing stops very briefly (**apnea**) during swallowing. This further ensures that food would not get sucked into the airways during swallowing. The apnea during swallowing is so brief that it is hardly noticed, but it is always there.
vii. The superior constrictor of the pharynx contracts, initiating a peristaltic wave that travels all the way down to the esophagus.
viii. The upper esophageal sphincter (UES) relaxes, letting the bolus enter the esophagus. The UES is a 2-4 cm long high pressure zone (HPZ). The high pressure in the UES region prevents reflux of esophageal con-tents into the pharynx from where they might be aspirated into the respiratory tract. The UES also prevents air from entering the esophagus during inspiration.

Esophageal stage: Once the food has negotiated the UES, it rapidly moves down the esophagus. Three forces may contribute to this movement of the food: pharyngeal contraction, gravity, and esophageal peristalsis. Esophageal peristalsis is a wave of contraction that milks the contents down the esophagus. As in the rest of the gut, it is in the form of a ring of contraction which squeezes the contents. The region next (distal) to the ring relaxes to receive the contents from the squeezed region. When the contents have moved, the region of the gut around the contents contracts to squeeze them, while the region distal to it relaxes to receive them. This goes on till the contents have moved up to the end of the esophagus. To visualize the process, imagine moving a tight ring along a rubber tube.

Once the food reaches the lower end of the esophagus, the lower esophageal sphincter (LES) relaxes and lets the contents pass on to the stomach. LES is a mere thickening of smooth muscle extending over about 3 cm of distal esophagus. The pressure in the LES region (10-40 mm Hg) is higher than the pressure in either the stomach or the rest of the esophagus. Thus, it normally neither allows the contents of the stomach to enter the esophagus, nor does it allow the esophageal contents to enter the stomach. Not only that, if the stomach is distended, or the gastric pressure increases due to any reason, the pressure in the LES increases further. Thus any possibility of gastric contents entering the esophagus is actively resisted. On the other hand, if the lower end of the esophagus is distended, as during swallowing, the LES relaxes briefly, its pressure drops, and the esophageal contents enter the stomach. By responding differently to gastric distension and esophageal distension, the LES prevents gastric contents from entering the esophagus, but allows food to travel from the esophagus to the stomach during swallowing.[1]

FOOD IN THE STOMACH

We have seen above how the food is delivered to the stomach. In the stomach, food is exposed to the gastric juice, which is acidic. Gastric juice initiates the digestion of proteins.

The structural organization of the stomach follows the scheme typical of the alimentary canal (Fig. 8.6). The three types of glands seen in the stomach and their principal cell types are indicated in Figure 8.12. The characteristic glands of the stomach are the oxyntic glands (Fig. 8.13) which occupy the largest area in the gastric mucosa. The secretory products of the various cell types in the stomach are given below:[2]

Peptic (chief) cells: Pepsinogens
Oxyntic (parietal) cells: Hydrochloric acid, Intrinsic factor
Mucous cells: Mucus
Endocrine cells: Gastrin
Several other hormones
Enterochromaffine cells: Serotonin
Enterochromaffine-like cells (ECL): Histamine

	CELL TYPE			
	Peptic (chief)	Oxyntic (Parietal)	Mucous	Endocrine
Cardiac glands			xx	x
Oxyntic glands	xx	xx	x	x
Pyloric glands		x	xx	xx

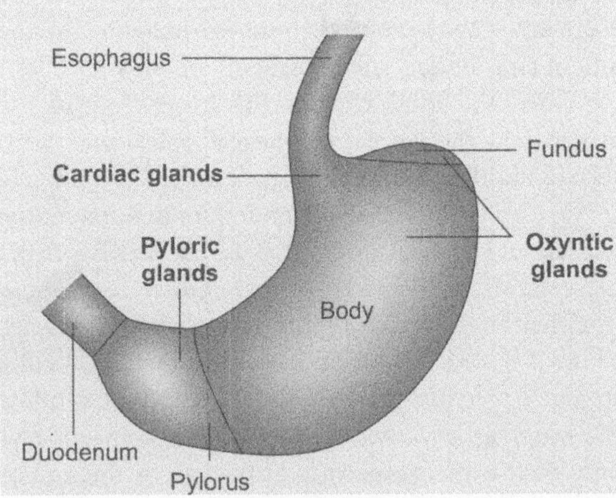

Fig. 8.12 The three types of glands in the stomach and their principal cell types

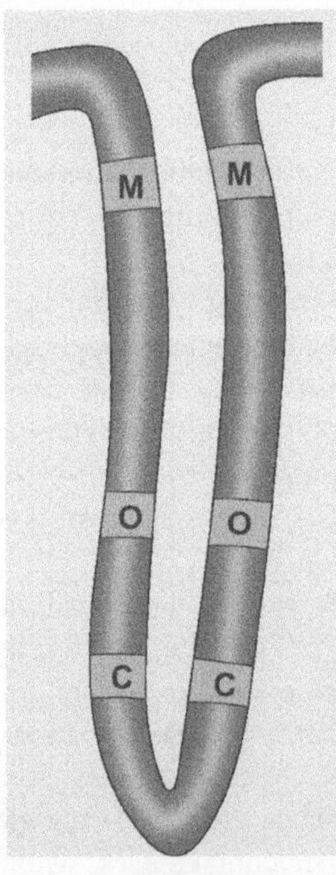

Fig. 8.13 Diagrammatic structure of an oxyntic (fundic) gland and predominant location of different cell types in it. C, chief or peptic cells; O, oxyntic or parietal cells; M, mucous cells

[1]In fact, all sphincters of the gut behave like this. Rather, they are able to function as sphincters because they behave like this.

[2]It is good to be aware of the large number of secretory products of the stomach but the list need not be remembered.

The products of the peptic and oxyntic cells are secreted into the lumen and constitute the gastric juice. Mucus lines the mucosal surface of the stomach. The products of endocrine cells have either an endocrine or paracrine action.

Regulation of Gastric Secretion

Regulation of gastric secretion usually refers to the regulation of acid and pepsin secretion. Fluctuations in acid and pepsin secretion generally parallel each other. Most of our knowledge in this area is based on studies on the regulation of acid secretion.

Gastric secretion is accurately timed to match meal times. The secretion begins when the food is about to enter the stomach, and continues till food leaves the stomach (Fig. 8.14). This coordination between taking food and gastric secretion has at least two advantages. Firstly, it ensures that the stomach works to produce its juice only when it is really required. Secondly, continuing secretion while the stomach is empty would expose the wall of the stomach to its own secretion. In such a situation a part of the wall itself might get digested, leading to a peptic ulcer.

Agents that Stimulate Parietal Cells

1. *Acetylcholine:* Acetylcholine is released in the stomach by the vagus nerve. It stimulates parietal cells directly, and also indirectly by stimulating the release of gastrin and histamine. The action of acetylcholine on the stomach is blocked by atropine.
2. *Gastrin:* Gastrin is a hormone produced by the G cells, which are present largely in the mucosa of the antrum of the stomach. Meals are associated with a rise in serum gastrin level. Several other observations also indicate that gastrin has a physiological role in the regulation of gastric secretion.
   As mentioned above, gastrin release is stimulated by acetylcholine. Hence vagal stimulation releases gastrin. In addition, distension of the gastric antrum and some chemicals present in the stomach (specially acid, peptides and amino acids) also stimulate release of gastrin. Thus several factors preceding and accompanying ingestion of food stimulate gastrin release.
   Gastrin stimulates parietal cells directly, and also indirectly by stimulating the release of histamine.
3. *Histamine:* Histamine is a very potent stimulator of gastric acid secretion. There are at least two sources of histamine in the stomach: mast cells and ECL cells. Mast cells release histamine during the inflammatory response. Physiological meal-related histamine is released by ECL cells. Histamine acts directly on parietal cells via H_2 receptors to stimulate acid secretion.

Interaction between acetylcholine, gastrin and histamine: All these agents stimulate gastric secretion. If more than one of these agents is given simultaneously, the secretory response is greater than that seen with

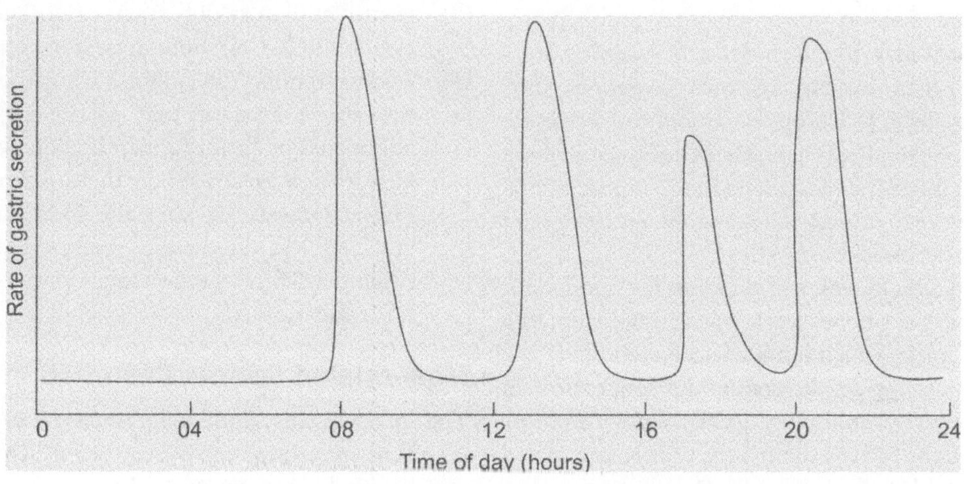

Fig. 8.14 Gastric secretion is synchronous with meals

any of them alone. This phenomenon is known as potentiation. For example, the secretory response to acetylcholine and histamine given together is greater than the combined effect of the same quantity of acetylcholine and histamine given one at a time. This is expressed by saying that histamine potentiates the effect of acetylcholine, or that acetylcholine potentiates the effect of histamine.

Specific antagonists to each of the three major stimulants of gastric secretion are now known. The antagonists block the effects of the stimulating agent. The effect of acetylcholine on the stomach is blocked by atropine, the effect of gastrin is blocked by proglumide, and the effect of histamine is blocked by cimetidine or ranitidine. The effect of an antagonist extends partly to other agents as well. For example, atropine inhibits the secretory response to acetylcholine completely and also the secretory response to gastrin or histamine partly. This happens due to loss of the potentiating effect of acetylcholine, a small quantity of which is constantly available in the background. A small quantity of histamine also seems to be a part of the background.

A tentative model to explain the action of various stimulants of gastric secretion and their interaction has been shown in Figure 8.15.

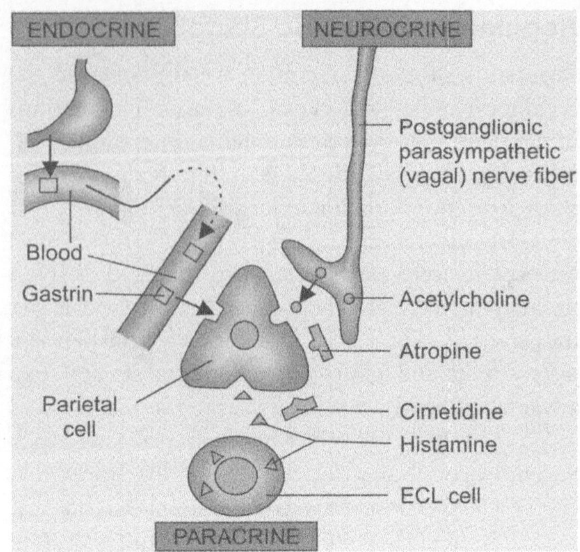

Fig. 8.15 Endocrine, neurocrine and paracrine factors which influence acid secretion by the parietal cell. The figure shows the simplified situation in which the three factors may be assumed to act independently on independent receptors. Atropine and cimetidine molecules have also been shown schematically to illustrate how they might block acetylcholine and histamine (H_2) receptors respectively. ECL cell, Enterochromaffin-like cell

Agents that Inhibit Parietal Cells

Parietal cells may get inhibited by withdrawal or suppression of the stimulants named above. Other factors which may inhibit gastric acid secretion are:

1. *Acid:* Acid inhibits its own secretion, thus exercising a check on the amount of acid secreted. Several mechanisms possibly contribute to the inhibition. First, acid in the stomach inhibits release of gastrin. Secondly, entry of acid into the duodenum reflexly inhibits acid secretion. Finally, entry of acid into the duodenum releases hormones such as secretin from the duodenum, which inhibit acid secretion.
2. *Somatostatin:* Somatostatin inhibits gastric acid secretion by inhibiting gastrin and histamine secretion. Somatostatin secretion is stimulated by acid in the stomach, by the hormones released by entry of acid in the duodenum, as well as by adrenaline.
3. *Food:* Entry of food into the duodenum releases gastric inhibitory polypeptide (GIP) and cholecystokinin (CCK). Both these hormones inhibit acid secretion. You might have gathered from the above account that gastric secretion is stimulated by factors which operate while food is in the stomach. When there is no food, as between meals, or after the food has started entering the duodenum, gastric secretion is inhibited. Thus secretion takes place only when it is really needed.

Meal-related Gastric Secretion

The mechanisms underlying meal-related gastric secretion may now be reconstructed. The process may be divided into three phases.

Cephalic Phase

The mouth starts watering (due to salivary secretion) even before food enters the mouth. Similarly, gastric secretion also begins before food enters the mouth. This is called the cephalic (*kephale,* head) phase of gastric secretion, because it is triggered by the mere thought or awareness of food. Sight, smell or thought of food are enough to initiate the cephalic phase of gastric secretion. The cephalic phase of gastric secretion is mediated by the vagus nerve. The pathway involved is as shown in Figure 8.16. Vagus stimulates gastric secretion not only by directly stimulating the parietal cells but also by releasing gastrin.

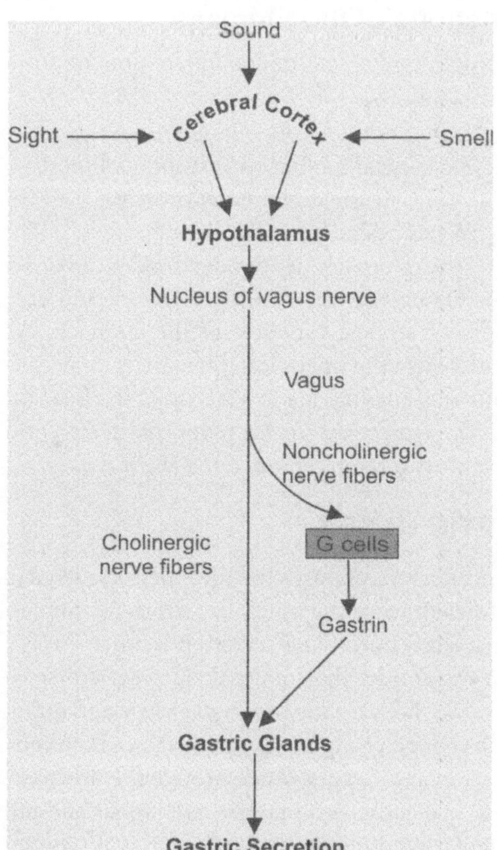

Fig. 8.16 Neural pathway involved in the cephalic phase of gastric secretion

Gastric Phase

When the food reaches the stomach, the rate of gastric secretion increases further. Since this increase is associated with the presence of food in the stomach, it is called the gastric phase of secretion. The mechanism underlying the gastric phase of secretion involves two factors: distension due to the presence of food in the stomach, and chemical stimuli arising from the food present in the stomach.

Distension: Information about distension of the stomach is conveyed to the central nervous system by the vagus nerve. After processing in the central nervous system, nerve impulses travel down the efferent fibers of the vagus nerve to stimulate gastric secretion (Fig. 8.17).

Chemical stimuli: The most potent stimuli for gastric secretion are proteins. Partially digested proteins are even more effective than intact proteins. Products

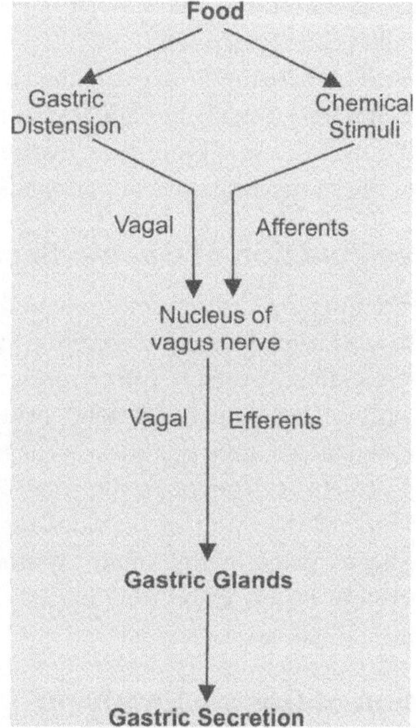

Fig. 8.17 Neural pathway involved in the gastric phase of gastric secretion

of protein digestion (peptides) stimulate release of gastrin, which in turn, stimulates gastric secretion.

Cephalic and gastric phase account for most of the meal-related gastric secretion. But some secretion does take place during the intestinal phase as well.

Intestinal Phase

Presence of food in the small intestine induces both stimulation and inhibition of gastric secretion. But on the whole, there is more inhibition than stimulation. Moreover, the mechanisms which stimulate gastric secretion during the intestinal phase are poorly understood. The mechanisms which *inhibit* gastric secretion during the intestinal phase are both neural and humoral.

Neural mechanisms: Food stimulates intestinal mucosal receptors. As a result, gastric secretion is reflexly inhibited. The reflex is known as entero-gastric reflex.

Hormonal mechanisms: Entry of food into the intestine releases several GI hormones which can inhibit gastric secretion. These hormones may be together called enterogastrone.

As a result of these inhibitory mechanisms gastric secretion becomes gradually less and less as more and more food enters the small intestine. By the time all food leaves the stomach, gastric secretion also stops.

Digestive Function of Gastric Secretion

Gastric secretion plays only a minor role in digestion. The digestive enzyme in gastric secretion is pepsin. Pepsin breaks down proteins into peptides. Pepsin is active only at acidic pH. All food protein may not be broken down into peptides by pepsin. The remaining protein is digested in the small intestine. Secondly, further digestion of peptides into amino acids also takes place in the small intestine. Thus gastric secretion brings about only partial digestion of proteins.

Regulation of Gastric Emptying

The natural tendency of a full stomach to empty is inhibited by several neural and humoral mechanisms. As a result, the stomach empties only slowly, allowing time for digestion in the stomach as well as for neutralization of acid in the duodenum.

Distension of the stomach by food initiates a vago-vagal reflex which slows down gastric emptying.

Food in the stomach releases gastrin from the stomach. Gastrin also inhibits gastric emptying.

Food stimulates the release of cholecystokinin (CCK) and gastric inhibitory polypeptide (GIP) from the duodenum. Both these hormones inhibit gastric emptying.

Acid, which enters the duodenum from the stomach, releases secretin from the duodenum. Secretin also inhibits gastric emptying.

As a result of all these mechanisms, the emptying of a meal from the stomach takes about four hours.

Functions of the Stomach

The functions of the stomach may now be summarized as follows:

1. To provide space for a large meal.
2. Mechanical mixing and crushing of food.
3. To initiate the digestion of proteins.
4. To synthesize intrinsic factor.

If the stomach is removed surgically, symptoms during the early postoperative period are due to loss of storage function of the stomach. A few months after the operation, the patient may develop pernicious anemia due to absence of intrinsic factor. Thus the symptoms are due to loss of the first and the last of the functions enumerated above.

PEPTIC ULCER

Peptic ulcer may be a gastric ulcer or a duodenal ulcer. Both result from the injury caused to the mucosa by gastric secretion. The secretion in such cases may have more acid than normal. However, this is not always so. It seems the health of gastric and duodenal mucosa depends upon a proper balance between acid secretion and factors which protect the mucosa. The major protective mechanisms are *mucus* and *prostaglandins*. In addition, the duodenum is also protected by neutralization of acid by pancreatic and biliary secretions.

It is logical to assume that peptic ulcer may result from excessive acid secretion, or defective protective mechanisms.

Factors which Increase Secretion

Genetic Factors

The tendency to secrete more acid may be inherited.

Food

Some items such as alcohol, cola drinks, tea and coffee increase gastric acid secretion.

Psychosomatic Factors

Anxiety and prolonged mental stress also increase acid secretion.

Factors which Decrease Mucosal Defence

Defective Mucus

In some cases the quality of the mucus may be poor, reducing its efficiency as a protective mechanism.

Drugs

Drugs which impair mucosal defence include aspirin, non-steroidal anti-inflammatory drugs (e.g. phenylbutazone) and corticosteroids.

Alcohol

Alcohol reduces mucus production in the stomach.

Smoking

Smoking reduces mucus production as well as pancreatic secretion.

Helicobacter Pylori

Helicobacter pylori is a bacterium which commonly lives in the stomach and causes gastritis. It is frequently associated with peptic ulcer.

In short, peptic ulcer is a multifactorial disease. Some of the factors may be more important in one patient, while some other factors may be important in another.

PANCREATIC SECRETION

From the stomach, the food moves into the small intestine. In the small intestine, it is acted upon by the pancreatic secretion and bile. We shall first talk about the pancreas and its secretion.

Pancreas has an exocrine and an endocrine part. Here we shall deal with only the exocrine part. The secretion of the exocrine pancreas is called the pancreatic juice. Pancreatic juice has an alkaline pH due to the presence of a high concentration of bicarbonate ions. Pancreatic juice also contains enzymes for the digestion of carbohydrates, proteins, fats and nucleic acids.

Regulation of Pancreatic Secretion

Like the gastric secretion, pancreatic secretion is also switched on when it is needed, and switched off when it is no longer required. This regulation is achieved by a combination of hormonal and neural mechanisms.

Hormonal Mechanisms

When food reaches the duodenum, gastric secretion should be switched off and pancreatic secretion should be switched on. Nature ensures that both these ends are achieved by employing the same hormones for both. In this way the effort required by the body is also reduced to the minimum. The two principal hormones involved in the regulation of pancreatic secretion are secretin and cholecystokinin.

Secretin is secreted by the duodenum. It is released most readily by the entry of acid from the stomach into the duodenum. Its action on the pancreas is to release a large volume of bicarbonate-rich (and hence alkaline) watery secretion.

Cholecystokinin (CCK) is also secreted by the duodenum. It is released most readily by the entry of fats and partially digested proteins into the duodenum. Its action on the pancreas is to release an enzyme-rich secretion.

Observe that acid stimulates secretin secretion, which in turn stimulates alkaline pancreatic secretion which neutralizes the acid. On the other hand, nutrients stimulate CCK secretion, which in turn stimulates secretion of pancreatic enzymes which digest nutrients. Thus the composition of the pancreatic juice is adjusted according to the requirements.

Neural Mechanisms

Pancreatic secretion is affected by parasympathetic as well as sympathetic neural influences. The *parasympathetic* nerve supplying the pancreas is the vagus nerve. Stimulation of the vagus nerve increases pancreatic secretion. The *sympathetic* nerve supplying the pancreas is the splanchnic nerve. Stimulation of the splanchnic nerve decreases pancreatic secretion. The decrease may, however, be secondary to the vasoconstriction brought about by sympathetic stimulation.

BILE

Bile is secreted by the liver and stored in the gallbladder. Besides storing it, the gallbladder also concentrates the bile and adds mucus to it. The major constituents of bile are bile salts, bile pigments, and cholesterol. Chemically, bile salts are sodium glycocholate, sodium taurocholate and related compounds. Their important property which helps in fat digestion is to reduce surface tension. Bile salts are absorbed in the terminal ileum. After absorption, they travel in the portal vein to reach the liver. They are secreted in bile once more to reach the duodenum. Thus most of the bile salts undergo repeated use: the phenomenon is called *enterohepatic circulation*. A small fraction of bile salts which is not absorbed in the terminal ileum reaches the colon. In the colon, bacteria modify bile salts chemically. The bile salts as originally secreted by the liver are called *primary*; after bacterial modification, they are called *secondary bile salts*. Some of the secondary bile salts are also absorbed from the colon and undergo enterohepatic circulation. Recycling of bile salts reduces the need for fresh synthesis of bile salts in the liver.

Regulation of Biliary Secretion

The most important regulators of bile secretion are the bile salts themselves. Bile salts absorbed from the gut stimulate their secretion once again. One of the primary bile salts, chenodeoxycholate (CDC) inhibits fresh synthesis of bile salts. Therefore, if enterohepatic circulation is intact, there is not much of fresh bile salt synthesis.

As in case of pancreatic secretion, secretin stimulates bicarbonate secretion in bile as well. Further, CCK stimulates contraction of the gall bladder which, in turn, delivers bile into the duodenum. Thus the two hormones, secretin and CCK, not only reduce gastric secretion and increase pancreatic secretion but also stimulate bile secretion. All these three events are required simultaneously upon entry of food into the duodenum. Thus employing the same hormones for all the three events combines economy of effort with perfect coordination.

In short, the combined actions of secretin and CCK ensure that:

i. Gastric secretion is smoothly turned off as the food enters the duodenum,
ii. Gastric acid entering the duodenum is promptly neutralized by bicarbonate ions present in pancreatic juice and bile,
iii. Pancreatic juice is secreted rapidly to carry out its digestive functions, and
iv. Bile is secreted and delivered on time to assist the pancreatic juice in fat digestion.

THE SMALL INTESTINE

The small intestine is, in fact quite long. It is about seven meters long in an adult.[3] It has three named divisions: the first 25 cm, **duodenum;** the next three meters, **jejunum;** and the last 4 meters, **ileum.** The small intestine is the site of most of the digestion and absorption. Its mucosal surface is specially adapted for these functions. The mucosal surface is thrown into folds; each fold is thrown into further folds: thus the surface area is enormously increased. The large

[3]It is still called small because its diameter is smaller than that of the large intestine.

surface area is admirably suited for absorption. The folds seen under the microscope are called villi. The villus epithelium is further folded into microvilli on its lumenal surface (see Fig. 8.7). Microvilli can be seen clearly only under the electron microscope. Under the light microscope, microvilli appear like the bristles of a brush, and are therefore together called the brush border. Microvilli not only increase the surface area but also contain enzymes for the final digestion of carbohydrates and proteins: these enzymes are called brush border enzymes.

Carbohydrate Digestion and Absorption

The carbohydrate in our diet is mostly starch. We get starch from cereals and legumes (pulses). The other major carbohydrates in our diet are sucrose (cane sugar) and lactose (the sugar present in milk). In addition, the diet also contains some indigestible carbohydrates **(dietary fiber)**. For all practical purposes, flesh foods contain no carbohydrate.

Starch is first attacked by salivary amylase in the mouth (Fig. 18.18). Amylase breaks down starch into maltose. Starch is tasteless but maltose is sweet. That is why food tastes sweeter after it has mixed with the saliva. But before much starch has been digested, food reaches the stomach. In the stomach, the action of salivary amylase stops because the pH in the stomach is highly acidic. On the other hand the optimum pH for the action of amylase is 6-7. When food reaches the duodenum, it is exposed to the action of pancreatic amylase. Pancreatic amylase also breaks down starch into maltose. Further breakdown of maltose is brought about by the enzyme maltase, which is present in the microvilli (brush border) of the small intestine. Maltase breaks down maltose into glucose. Maltose is a disaccharide: therefore one molecule of maltose gives two molecules of glucose.

Sucrose is also a disaccharide. It is hydrolyzed by sucrase. Sucrase is also present in the brush border. One molecule of sucrose gives one molecule of glucose and one molecule of fructose.

Lactose is also a disaccharide. It is hydrolyzed by lactase. Lactase is also a brush border enzyme. One molecule of lactose gives one molecule of glucose and one molecule of galactose. Maltase, sucrase and lactase are sometimes together called disaccharidases. Some persons, specially the elderly, suffer from lactose intolerance due to lactase deficiency. They cannot digest much lactose. Therefore milk gives them indigestion. Milk may produce in them flatulence, abdominal discomfort and pain, and loose motions. However, they can generally digest satisfactorily small amounts of lactose which are present in tea or curd.

The process of carbohydrate digestion has been summarized in Figure 8.18.

Absorption of Glucose

Glucose is absorbed by active, carrier-mediated, coupled transport (Fig. 8.19). Active means that the transport needs energy, and is therefore possible against the concentration gradient. Carrier-mediated means that there is a specific protein in the cell membrane which binds glucose outside the cell and transfers the glucose towards the inside of the cell. Coupled means that the same carrier also binds to something else so that two substances can be transported simultaneously without using additional energy. Glucose transport is coupled to sodium transport.

Absorption of Fructose and Galactose

Fructose and galactose are the other major monosaccharides generated by digestion of carbohydrates.

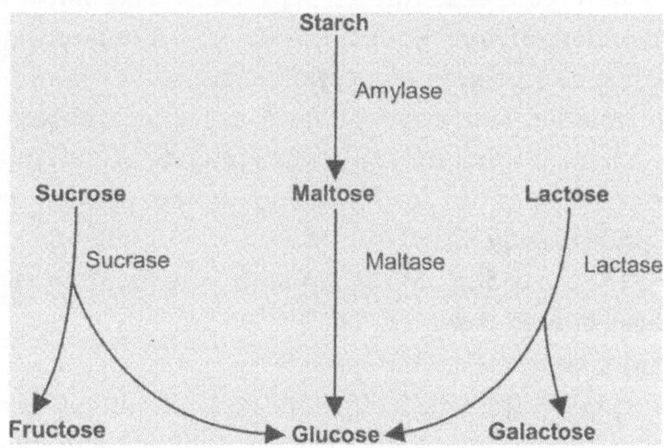

Fig. 8.18 Digestion of carbohydrates

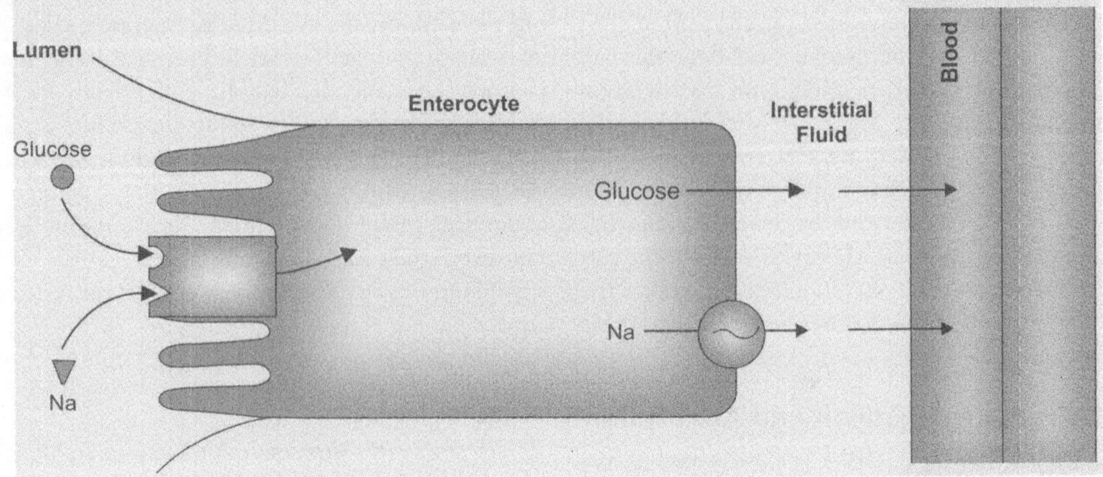

Fig. 8.19 Diagrammatic representation of the mechanism of glucose absorption

Fructose is transported by facilitated diffusion, which means that the process is passive but carrier mediated. Galactose is absorbed by the same mechanism as glucose. The carrier protein for glucose and galactose is also the same.

Protein Digestion and Absorption

The digestion of proteins begins in the stomach with the help of the enzyme pepsin. Pepsin is active in an acidic medium, and is therefore able to hydrolyze proteins in the stomach. Pepsin breaks down proteins into peptides. Further digestion of proteins is brought about by pancreatic enzymes. The principal pancreatic proteolytic enzymes are trypsin, chymotrypsin and carboxypeptidases. Trypsin and chymotrypsin are endopeptidases, which means that they split a protein or peptide chain somewhere in the middle. Carboxypeptidases are exopeptidases, which means that they split one amino acid at a time from the carboxy-terminal end of the protein or peptide (Fig. 8.20).

The final digestion of proteins is assisted by the brush border enzymes. The major proteolytic brush border enzymes are dipeptidase and aminopeptidase. Dipeptidase splits each dipeptide molecule into its two constituent amino acids. Aminopeptidase splits one amino acid at a time from the amino-terminal end of small peptides.Thus finally all protein is converted into amino acids before getting absorbed (Fig. 8.21).

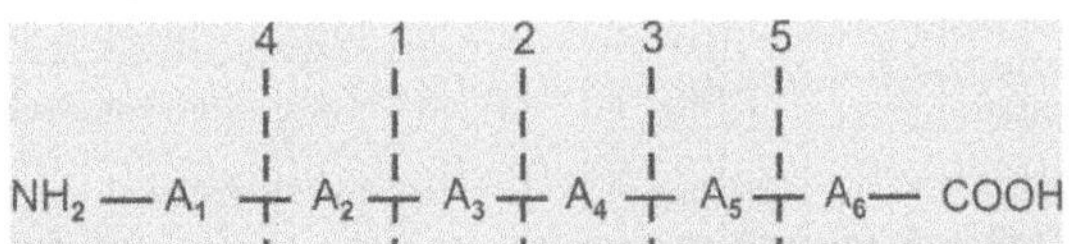

Fig. 8.20 Protein molecule is made up of a large number of amino acids. For simplicity, here a protein has been illustrated by a chain of six amino acids, A_1 through A_6. An endopeptidase may hydrolyze a peptide bond in the middle, i.e. at positions, 1, 2 or 3. An exopeptidase hydrolyzes peptide bonds only at the ends, i.e. at positions 4 or 5. An enzyme which acts at 4 splits the N-terminal amino acid (A_1), and is therefore called an aminopeptidase. An enzyme which acts at 5 splits the C-terminal amino acid (A_6), and is therefore called a carboxypeptidase

Absorption of Amino Acids

The mechanism of amino acid absorption is similar to that for glucose. It is an active, carrier-mediated sodium-coupled process. But the special feature of amino acid absorption is that there are several classes of carrier proteins which are specific for a particular chemical class of amino acids. For example, there are specific carrier proteins for neutral amino acids,

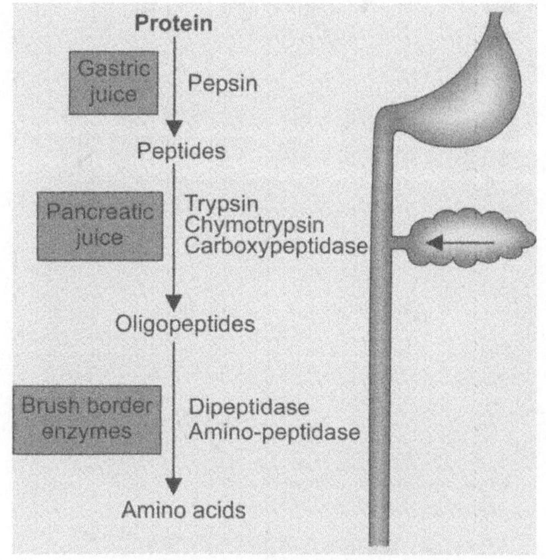

Fig. 8.21 Digestion of proteins

dibasic amino acids, and dicarboxylic amino acids. Several amino acids are transported by more than one of these carriers. The significance of multiple mechanisms for absorption of the same amino acid is that the absorption of every essential amino acid may be adequate even if one of the mechanisms of absorption is defective.

Fat Digestion and Absorption

Most of the dietary fat is in the form of long chain triglycerides. Digestion of triglycerides begins in the duodenum. It needs both bile and pancreatic juice. Bile emulsifies fats while pancreatic juice contains the enzyme, lipase, which hydrolyzes triglycerides.

Bile salt molecules have a fat soluble end and a water soluble end. That is why bile salts break fat globules into small particles which mix well with water (Figs 8.22A and B). The process is called emulsification. Emulsification increases the surface area on which lipase may act. It also makes fat 'dissolve' in the watery contents of the small intestine. However, emulsification also creates a problem. It hides fat molecules so that they are not directly exposed to the action of lipase. Nature has solved this problem

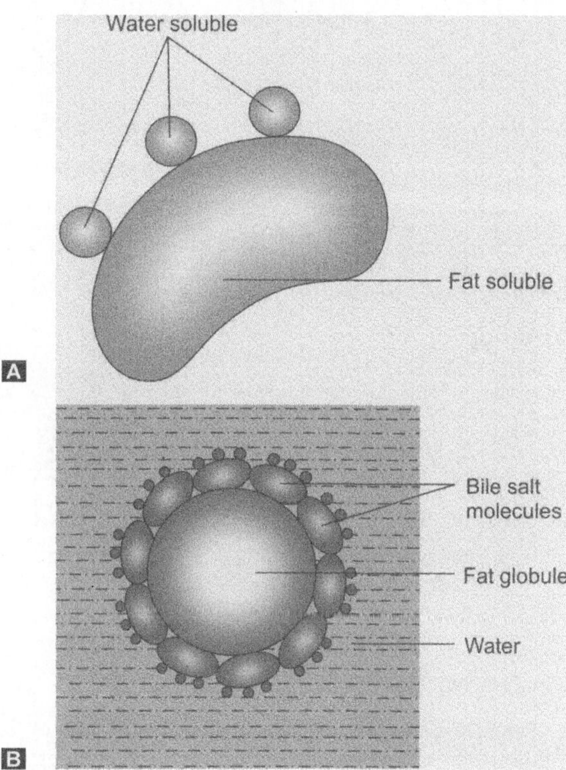

Figs 8.22A and B The role of bile salts in fat digestion. (A) Diagrammatic representation of a bile salt molecule; (B) A fat globule enclosed in bile salt molecules. This is how fat becomes miscible in water with the help of bile salts

by having in the pancreatic juice one more enzyme, called colipase. Colipase alters the shape of bile-fat micelles in such a way as to expose fats to the action of lipase.

Lipase hydrolyzes triglycerides into fatty acids and monoglycerides. Fatty acids and monoglycerides are lipid soluble substances. Therefore they are easily transported across the cell membrane of intestinal epithelium.[4] In the intestinal epithelial cells (enterocytes), fatty acids and monoglycerides again form triglycerides (Fig. 8.23). Triglycerides

[4]Lipid soluble substances can be transported across cell membranes easily because cell membranes also have a lipoid structure.

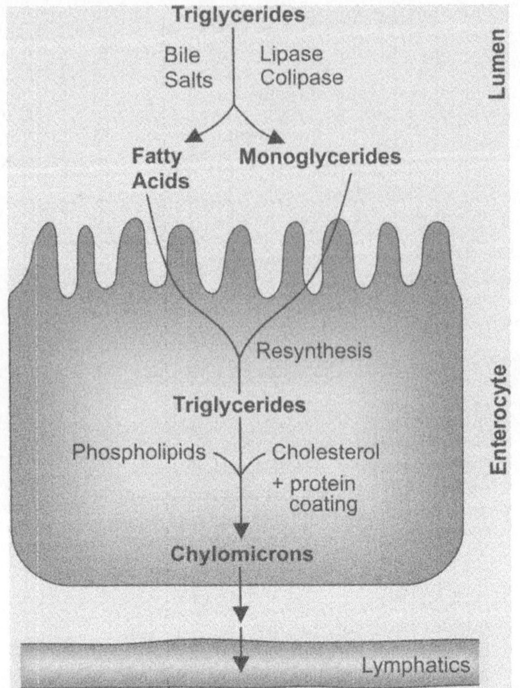

Fig. 8.23 Schematic diagram showing the process of digestion and absorption of long chain triglycerides

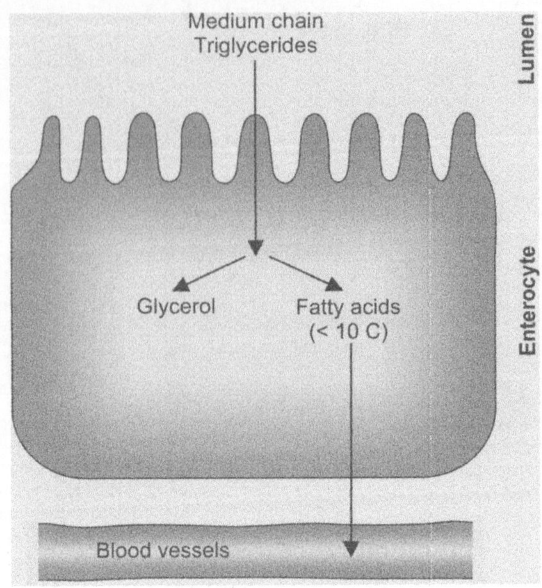

Fig. 8.24 Schematic diagram showing the process of digestion and absorption of medium chain triglycerides

synthesized in the enterocytes join other lipids such as phospholipids and cholesterol, and acquire a protein coating. The protein coating helps in keeping these lipids 'dissolved' in the watery body fluids. Packets of triglycerides, phospholipids, cholesterol and proteins are called **chylomicrons**. Chylomicrons are transported across the enterocyte and enter the lymphatics. Since lymph eventually joins the blood circulation, chylomicrons also finally enter the bloodstream.

The above description applies to digestion and absorption of long chain triglycerides, i.e. triglycerides having fatty acids with a chain length of more than 10 carbon atoms. Fatty acids having a chain length of less than 10 carbon atoms are called medium chain fatty acids. Medium chain triglycerides (MCT) can be transported intact into the enterocytes (Fig. 8.24). Therefore absorption of MCT needs neither bile nor pancreatic enzymes. MCT are hydrolyzed in the enterocytes into fatty acids and glycerol. Further, medium chain fatty acids are absorbed directly into the bloodstream rather than lymphatics. Since the digestion and absorption of MCT is not dependent on pancreatic enzymes, MCT can serve as dietary fat even for patients with pancreatic insufficiency. The only important dietary fat containing significant quantities of MCT is coconut oil.

Water and Electrolyte Absorption

Water and electrolytes need no digestion. They are absorbed as such in the small and large intestine. There is a common misconception that water and electrolytes are absorbed primarily in the large intestine. But, in fact, the small intestine absorbs more water than the large intestine. But the large intestine absorbs most of the water entering it. Therefore the consistency of the intestinal contents changes from liquid to semi-solid as they pass through the large intestine (Table 8.1). There is no active mechanism for absorption of water. Water is absorbed in association with solutes, both electrolyte and non-electrolyte.

Table 8.1 Fluid exchange in the intestine

Region	Fluid entering (L)	Fluid absorbed (L)	% absorbed	Capacity for absorption (L)
Small intestine	8.0	6.5	81.2	12.0
Large intestine	1.5	1.3	86.7	5.0

Absorption of Cyanocobalamin (Vitamin B_{12})

It was in the 1930s that William Castle observed that:

a. Patients of pernicious anemia showed marked improvement if fed meat which had been incubated in normal gastric juice, and
b. Neither meat nor normal gastric juice alone could bring about the improvement.

These observations suggested that normal gastric juice contains some factor essential for absorption of an anti-anemic nutrient present in meat. The factor was named intrinsic factor, and the nutrient was later shown to be vitamin B_{12}. Now we know some more details about the mechanism, which are briefly as follows:

Dietary vitamin B_{12} is generally associated with proteins. Gastric and pancreatic proteases release it from the proteins. Then vitamin B_{12} forms a complex with the intrinsic factor. Intrinsic factor is a glycoprotein secreted by parietal cells of the stomach. The B_{12}-intrinsic factor complex travels essentially unchanged through the stomach and much of the small intestine. The complex attaches itself to receptors which are present only in the distal ileum. Then B_{12} is released from the complex into the enterocytes, from where it is absorbed into the bloodstream.

Absorption of Iron

An adult has about 4 g of iron in the body, which is about the quantity which gives a medium-sized nail. Once iron is in the body, it is kept safely. Adult males lose only about 1 mg/24 h; menstruating women lose about 2 mg/24 h. Iron content of the body is kept constant by regulation of iron absorption.

The mechanism of iron absorption differs somewhat depending upon the source of iron.

Absorption of Heme Iron

Heme iron is the iron present in compounds such as hemoglobin and myoglobin. Heme is released from these proteins by proteolytic enzymes of the gut. Then heme is converted into hemin. Hemin is taken up by intestinal epithelium. Iron is released from hemin intracellularly by the enzyme heme oxygenase. The iron so released is handled in the same way as nonheme iron. Heme iron absorption is not much affected by the presence of other dietary constituents. That is one reason why heme iron absorption is much better than absorption of nonheme iron. Heme iron may be obtained from animal sources.

Absorption of Nonheme Iron

Nonheme iron has to be first converted into ferrous form before it can be absorbed. Therefore gastric acid and ascorbic acid (vitamin C), which help in keeping iron in the ferrous form, facilitate absorption. Animal foods such as meat or fish, but not egg, milk and cheese, also improve nonheme iron absorption. Phytates and oxalates, which are present in several plant foods, form insoluble complexes with iron. That is why phytates and oxalates decrease iron absorption. Calcium facilitates iron absorption by competing with iron for forming complexes with phytates and oxalates. Tea also reduces nonheme iron absorption by forming insoluble iron tannate.

After entering the intestinal epithelium, heme and nonheme iron are treated in the same way. In the epithelial cells (enterocytes), iron may form a complex with a protein, apoferritin. The combination of iron and apoferritin is called ferritin. The iron which *does not* form ferritin may be absorbed into the bloodstream. In the blood, iron is transported in combination with the protein, transferrin.

Regulation of Iron Absorption

Absorption of iron is regulated according to iron requirement of the body. Normally, the amount of iron absorbed is equal to the daily iron loss, i.e.

about 1 mg/day in men and 2 mg/day in women. This quantity is much smaller than the amount of iron consumed in the diet everyday (about 20 mg/day). Thus only 5-10 percent of the dietary iron is absorbed. But when the iron requirements are high, e.g. due to blood loss, up to 25 percent of the dietary iron may be absorbed.

Regulation of iron absorption to match the requirements is achieved by an interesting mechanism. When the iron requirement is high, the amount of apoferritin synthesized in the intestinal epithelium is low. Therefore less of the iron that enters the cell from the intestinal lumen is retained as ferritin, and more is absorbed.[5] Iron in ferritin is lost from the body when intestinal cells containing the ferritin are shed into the lumen. Intestinal cells are continually shed into the lumen and are replaced by new cells. In addition there is some regulation also at the lumenal surface by increased synthesis of receptors for iron on the lumenal surface of the intestinal epithelium when the iron requirements are high. This is the present version of the classical *mucosal block theory* of iron absorption. New research is continuing to throw more light on the mechanism of regulation of iron absorption.

THE LARGE INTESTINE

The large intestine, or colon, receives undigested and indigestible food from the small intestine. Its main functions are absorption, fermentation, storage and defecation.

Absorption

The colon absorbs mainly water and some electrolytes. *Water* is absorbed in the colon by a passive process. It is driven by the osmotic gradient generated by sodium absorption. The colon is presented with about 1500 mL of water everyday, of which more than 90 percent gets absorbed. The maximum capacity of the colon for water absorption is about 6 liters per day. Thus there is a physiological reserve of about 4500 mL which may be useful in diarrhea. *Sodium* is absorbed in the colon by active transport. The colon is presented with about 200 mEq of sodium everyday, more than 95 percent of which is absorbed. The maximum capacity of the colon for sodium absorption is about 800 mEq. *Chloride* absorption in the colon is passive, secondary to sodium absorption. The colon is presented with about 100 mEq of chloride everyday, more than 95 percent of which is absorbed. *Potassium* can be both absorbed as well as secreted by the colon. The overall direction of transport depends on the concentration of potassium in the lumen of the large intestine. If the concentration is above 15 mM, the net result is absorption. If the concentration is below 15 mM, the net result is secretion. Normally, about 10 mEq of potassium is presented to the colon everyday, of which about half is absorbed. The maximum capacity of the colon for potassium absorption is about 40 mEq per day. *Bicarbonate* can also be both absorbed as well as secreted by the colon. But the net result is normally secretion. However, if the concentration of bicarbonate in the lumen is above 25 mM, there is net absorption. The secreted bicarbonate reacts with acids produced by fermentation in the colon to form carbon dioxide, which may be expelled in the gaseous form.

[5]Reason out how the same mechanism will result in less absorption when the iron requirement is low.

Fermentation

Colon is dark, moist, neither very acidic nor alkaline, and has 'food' which stays there a long time. These are ideal conditions for microbial growth. Therefore, the colon has a large population of microorganisms—bacteria, protozoa, and even fungi. Among these, we know relatively more about bacterial activity in the colon. Bacteria not only metabolize food available in the colon, but also affect the person (host) in whose colon they live. Metabolic utilization of food by bacteria is called **fermentation**. Part of the energy released by fermentation is utilized by bacteria, and part by the host.

Carbohydrate Fermentation

Carbohydrates in the colon include undigested starch, indigestible carbohydrates (fiber), and carbohydrate components of intestinal secretions and sloughed (shed) enterocytes. Fermentation of carbohydrates in the colon leads to the formation of volatile fatty acids (VFA), carbon dioxide, hydrogen and methane (Fig. 8.25). The gases are eliminated from the body as flatus or in the expired air, but more than 90 percent of VFA are absorbed.

VFA include acetate, propionate and butyrate. Butyrate is the preferred fuel for colonic epithelial cells. In addition, butyrate and other VFA increase the division of normal cells but suppress the division of cancer cells in the colon. Therefore VFA may have a role in protection against colorectal cancer. Propionate is metabolized in the liver. Acetate is metabolized like acetate from other sources. Besides these specific effects, VFA also make a small contribution to the energy supply of the host. Thus bacteria help us get some energy from that part of our food which would have otherwise been wasted.

Protein Fermentation

Proteins in the colon include a small amount of undigested protein, and the protein components of secretions and sloughed cells. Bacteria can ferment proteins, peptides as well as amino acids. Fermentation of proteins in the colon leads to the formation of VFA, carbon dioxide and ammonia (Fig. 8.26). VFA and carbon dioxide are handled as described above. Part of the ammonia is utilized by bacteria for synthesizing amino acids for their own use. Part of the ammonia is absorbed into the circulation: this part is converted into urea in the liver. Some of this urea may return to the colon through the circulation. Bacteria can metabolize urea into ammonia. Thus there is an enterohepatic circulation of ammonia and urea (Fig. 8.26).

Fermentation of Fats and Related Compounds

Bacteria ferment triglycerides into glycerol and fatty acids. Glycerol is fermented further but fatty acids are degraded only if retained in the colon for at least four days. Degradation of fatty acids yields hydrogen, acetate and, in some cases, carbon dioxide.

Cholesterol, which has not been absorbed in the small intestine, is also fermented in the large intestine to form neutral sterols. About 25 percent of the bile acids delivered to the small intestine also reach the large intestine. Bacteria convert primary bile acids into secondary bile acids by dehydroxylation. Secondary bile acids are partly absorbed by the large intestine,

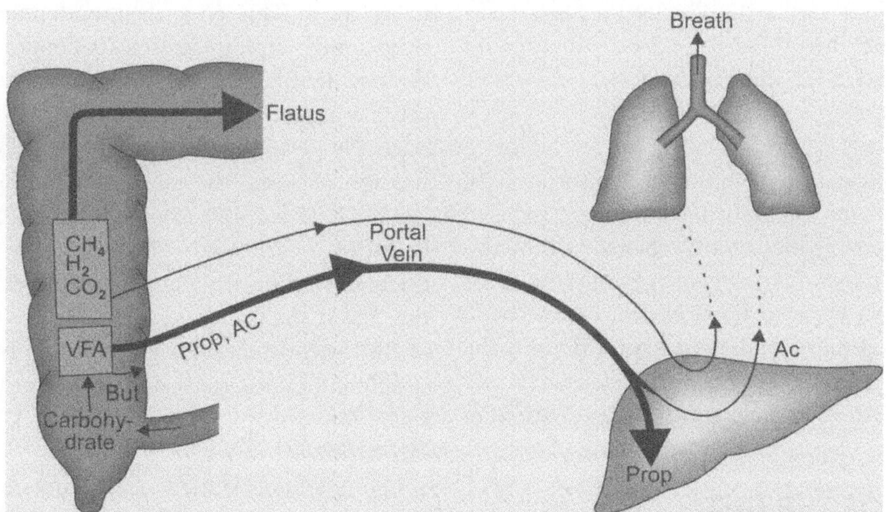

Fig. 8.25 Fermentation of carbohydrates in the colon. VFA, volatile fatty acids; But, butyrate; Prop, propionate; Ac, acetate. Thick arrows represent the major route followed by the products of fermentation

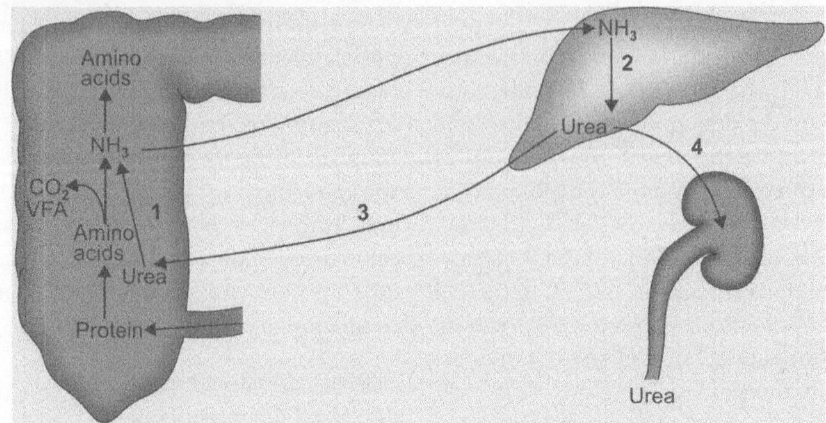

Fig. 8.26 Fermentation of proteins in the colon and enterohepatic circulation of ammonia and urea. Urea may be fermented to form ammonia (1), which travels to the liver. The liver converts ammonia into urea (2). Urea may be excreted by the kidneys (4), or it may return to the colon by circulation (3). In liver disease, formation of ammonia (1) is reduced by using antibiotics which reduce bacterial population in the colon. In renal diseases, it would be helpful to reduce the necessity for renal excretion of urea (4). Details in text

and partly excreted in the feces. The absorbed bile acids undergo enterohepatic circulation.

Beneficial Effects of Intestinal Microflora

Intestinal bacteria have many beneficial effects. They improve the immunological defence mechanisms. They synthesize some vitamins, viz. vitamin K and several members of the vitamin B complex group (cyanocobalamin, folate, pyridoxine, biotin, pantothenate and riboflavin). Finally, they help us in obtaining some energy from the food which could not be absorbed in the small intestine.

Storage

Colon has efficient mechanisms for absorption of water. Therefore the volume of its contents gets reduced remarkably. Secondly, the pattern of colonic motility also favors storage rather than expulsion. Finally, the colon has considerable capacity for distension. As a result, food residue generally spends more than 20 hours in the colon. Expulsion from the colon takes place usually once a day during defecation. Defecation will be discussed in the next section on gastrointestinal motility.

MOTILITY OF THE GUT

We have so far taken for granted that the food moves from one part of the gut to the next to be processed further. But food does not move spontaneously—it moves as a result of movements of the gut. Movements of the gut are of two types: those which move the contents further (**propulsive movements**), and those which mix the contents (**mixing movements**). Often propulsion and mixing may result from the same movement.

Smooth muscle cells of the gut are interconnected by low resistance bridges. Therefore, once excited, excitation spreads from one part of the gut to the next. This type of smooth muscle is called **single unit** smooth muscle (Chapter 13) and the arrangement is called a **functional syncytium**. The cell membrane of gastrointestinal smooth muscle is relatively permeable to ions. Because of continuous leakage of ions, the resting membrane potential (RMP) is about –60 mV. Further, the permeability fluctuates cyclically. Therefore the RMP also fluctuates cyclically. The rhythm of RMP is called the **basal electrical rhythm** (BER). The frequency of BER is constant for a given region of the gut, but is different in different parts of the gut. During these cyclic fluctuations, if the RMP crosses the threshold for excitation, an action potential or a burst of action potentials is fired. Action potentials are associated with contraction (Fig. 8.27). Some special characteristics of movement of different regions of the gut have been discussed below.

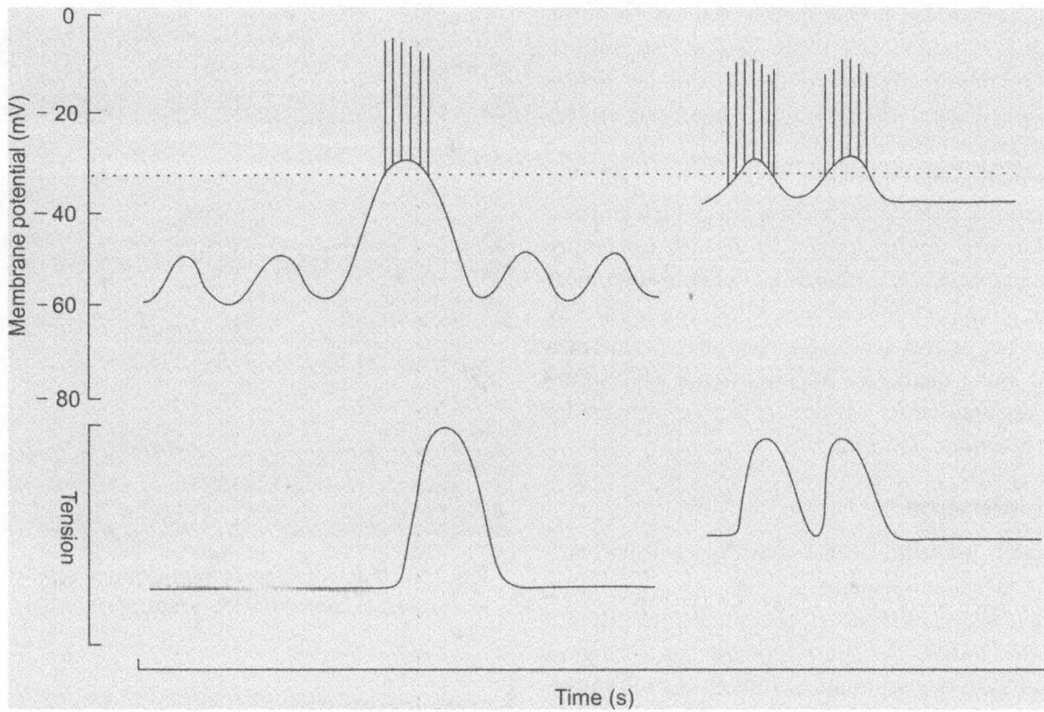

Fig. 8.27 Relationship between electrical activity (upper panel) and mechanical activity (lower panel) in gastrointestinal smooth muscle. When the basal electrical rhythm, crosses a threshold value (dotted line), there is a burst of spikes, which is associated with a wave of contraction

Stomach

The BER of stomach is about 3 per min. Therefore gastric contractions also have a frequency of about 3 per min. Gastric contractions are of four types: mixing contractions, propulsive contractions, hunger contractions and migrating motor complex.

Mixing contractions are seen soon after ingestion. These are gentle waves, the peak pressure being only about 10 mm Hg. These waves serve to mix the food with the gastric juice. As time passes, the waves get stronger. When the pressure reaches about 60 mm Hg, they are called *propulsive contractions*, because now they can propel the food towards the duodenum. But the pyloric sphincter allows only a small fraction of the propelled food to pass into the duodenum; the remaining food is thrown back into the stomach with some force. This results in agitation and consequent mixing of the contents. Thus the so-called propulsive waves result in both propulsion and mixing.

Hunger contractions occur between meals if the interval between meals is long. These are strong contractions, the peak pressure being about 100 mm Hg. Unlike other contractions of the stomach, hunger contractions are perceived consciously, as everyone knows through personal experience.

Besides hunger contractions, one more type of contraction is also seen between meals. It occurs every 60-180 min. It consists of a wave of propulsive contraction starting from the stomach and moving along the entire small intestine. When the wave reaches the terminal ileum, it fades away but a new wave immediately starts from the stomach. This repetetive process goes on for 4 to 7 min. Since the activity migrates from the stomach through the entire small intestine, and since it is associated with a well defined complex of electrical activity, it is called the **migrating motor complex** (MMC). The function of MMC possibly is to empty the stomach *completely*. It may help to remove from the stomach the residue of a meal. It may also remove gastric secretion, swallowed saliva, cellular debris and refluxed duodenal secretion which may collect in the stomach between meals. The quantity of these items which collect between meals is so small that they cannot activate those movements which empty a normal meal from the stomach. But MMC can empty these items. MMC is inhibited by the entry of a meal into the stomach. That is why MMC are seen only between meals and serve to empty the residue of a meal or small quantities of other items which may collect between meals. MMC seems to be initiated by the gut hormone, motilin.

Small Intestine

The small intestine shows both propulsive and mixing types of movements.

Propulsive movements of the small intestine are called **peristalsis**. Peristalsis consists of a ring of contraction in one segment, and receptive relaxation in the immediately distal segment. This results in propulsion of contents from the contracted segment to the relaxed segment. This is promptly followed by contraction of the segment which was earlier relaxed, and relaxation of the segment distal to it. Thus a wave of contraction travels distally, resulting in propulsion of the contents (Fig. 8.28). A mental picture of peristalsis may be formed by encircling a rubber tube tightly with a finger, and moving the finger along the tube. Peristalsis is seen even if the intestine is deprived of its extrinsic nerve supply. Just stretching of a segment of the intestine is enough to initiate peristalsis.

Mixing movements of the small intestine are of two types: segmentation and pendular movements. In **segmentation**, rings of contraction appear at irregular intervals of distance, the average distance being about 1 cm. These contractions seem to divide the intestine into a series of segments. Functionally, segmentation churns the contents, resulting in mixing. **Pendular movements** move the food alternately to one side and then the other. The pattern of movements resembles the motion of a pendulum, and hence the name.

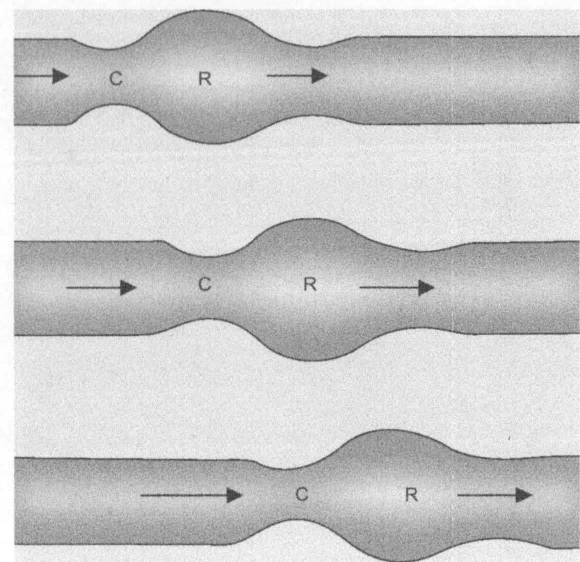

Fig. 8.28 Diagrammatic representation of a peristaltic wave. C, contraction; R, receptive relaxation

Large Intestine

The major mixing movement of the large intestine is *segmentation*. But segmental contractions of the large intestine are stronger than those in the small intestine. Stronger contractions are needed here because the contents are semi-solid whereas in the small intestine the contents are liquid. Strong segmental contractions of the large intestine mix the contents and keep renewing the material in contact with the mucosa. This facilitates absorption of water.

Propulsion of large intestinal contents is quite slow. It becomes somewhat faster after a meal: the phenomenon is called **gastrocolic reflex**. But really significant propulsion takes place only one to three times per day as a result of powerful peristaltic movements. These movements are called **mass peristalsis**.

In the large intestine, the pressure is higher in the anus and rectum than in the proximal parts. That is why normally there is no tendency for the large intestine to empty itself. But during defecation reflex, the pressure becomes temporarily lower in the rectum and anal canal.

Defecation Reflex

Defecation reflex is induced by distension of the rectum. Information about distension of the rectum is conveyed to the spinal cord. After appropriate processing in the central nervous system, the motor response is mediated by parasympathetic fibers originating in sacral segements (S2 - S4) of the spinal cord. Activation of these nerve fibers leads to a wave of propulsive contraction extending from the descending colon to the rectum. Simultaneously there is relaxation of the internal anal sphincter. In addition, during the defecation reflex, the pudendal nerve is also activated, which leads to *contraction* of the external anal sphincter. While contraction of the rectum and relaxation of the internal anal sphincter favor defecation, contraction of the external anal sphincter prevents defecation. This apparently paradoxical response makes it possible to control defecation voluntarily. External anal sphincter is a voluntary muscle. If the conditions under which the defecation reflex has been activated are suitable, reflex contraction of the external anal sphincter is voluntarily inhibited, thereby allowing evacuation. On the other hand, if the conditions are unsuitable, reflex contraction of the external anal sphincter is voluntarily reinforced, thereby achieving postponement of evacuation.

The basic defecation reflex is further controlled by factors which are normally associated with defecation. Toilet training consists in gradually establishing an association of defecation with time of the day, place and posture. Once the association is established, defecation becomes a lifelong conditioned reflex.

GASTROINTESTINAL FUNCTION TESTS

A large variety of chemical and radiological tests, endoscopy and biopsy provide valuable information about gastrointestinal function. But here we shall discuss only some commonly performed tests which have a strong physiological basis.

D-xylose Absorption Test

This is a test for assessment of carbohydrate absorption. D-xylose is a poorly metabolized monosaccharide which is absorbed with the help of the same carrier as glucose. Since it is not metabolized much, after absorption it is excreted in urine. Therefore, poor excretion in urine indicates poor absorption (Fig. 8.29).

The test is performed in the fasting state by giving 25 g d-xylose orally. About half of the dose is absorbed, and of the quantity absorbed, half is excreted in urine and half is metabolized. Thus one can expect about 6 g to appear in the urine. Good urine flow is ensured by administering 3-4 glasses of water during the 5 hours immediately following the administration of d-xylose. Absorption is considered normal if more than 4 g of xylose appear in the urine over the 5-hour period.

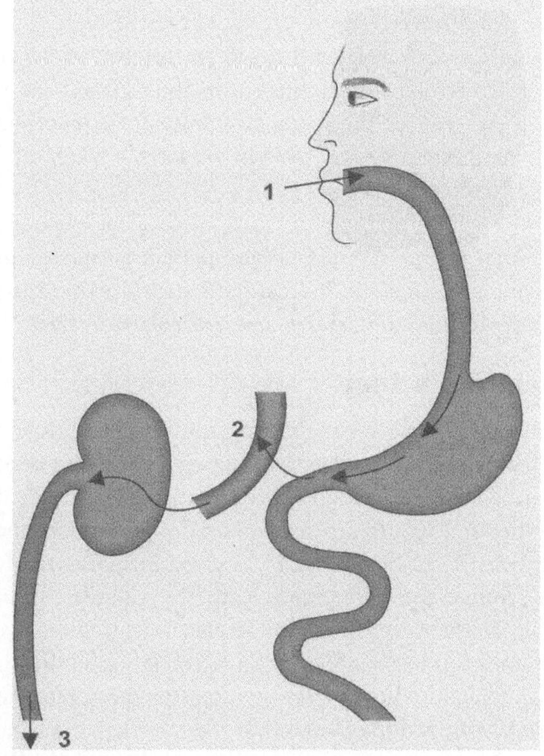

Fig. 8.29 The D-xylose test. The ingested substance (1) is absorbed (2) into the bloodstream. The circulation carries it to the kidneys where it is excreted (3). Urinary excretion depends on gastrointestinal absorption. Therefore the amount excreted (3) in a given time indirectly gives an idea of the amount absorbed (2)

Fecal Fat

This is a test of fat absorption. It is based on the principle that if fat absorption is below normal, fat excreted in the feces will increase. For performing this test, the subject is given an 80-100 g fat diet, and the stool is collected for 3 days. The normal fecal fat excretion on such a diet is 3-5 g. If the amount is more than 6 g per day, it indicates malabsorption.

Fecal fat is a highly valuable test because:

a. Digestion and absorption of fat need pancreatic secretion, biliary secretion as well as enterocyte function. If any of these is defective, fecal fat may be high.
b. Almost the entire length of the small intestine takes part in fat digestion and absorption. Therefore even if only a part of the small intestine is defective, fecal fat may be high.
c. Fat is not degraded much by colonic bacteria. Therefore almost the entire unabsorbed fat is excreted in the feces. In contrast, unabsorbed carbohydrate and protein are largely fermented in the colon.

Because of all the above reasons, fecal fat is usually the first test performed on any patient suspected to have malabsorption. If fecal fat is high, further tests are performed to find the cause of malabsorption.

Schilling's Test

This is a test for assessment of vitamin B_{12} absorption. It is based on the principle that if a person does not need much vitamin B_{12}, the absorbed vitamin will be excreted in the urine to a significant extent. For performing the test, first 1 mg of vitamin B_{12} is given intramuscularly to saturate the body stores with the vitamin. Then 1 microgram of ^{57}Co-cyanocobalamin (radioactive vitamin B_{12}) is given orally. An adequate urine flow is maintained by giving enough water to the subject to drink. Absorption of vitamin B_{12} is considered normal if more than 7 percent of the radioactivity is excreted over a period of 24 h following ingestion.

FUNCTIONS OF THE LIVER

A complete list of functions of the liver would be very long and is quite unnecessary. Most of the functions of the liver are best discussed individually with the relevant organ systems. However a few selected functions have been discussed briefly below.

Secretion of Bile

Secretion of bile involves two types of activities: picking up of appropriate metabolites from the blood, and passing them on to biliary canaliculi as such, or after making some chemical changes. Hepatocytes, accordingly, have asymmetric surfaces. The basolateral or sinusoidal surface picks up substances from the blood, while the apical surface secretes components of bile into the biliary canaliculi. Bile flows from the canaliculi into the biliary duct system. During its stay in the gall bladder, bile gets concentrated. Bile is periodically discharged into the duodenum as and when required.

Two of the components of bile which are extensively metabolized in the liver are bilirubin and bile salts. Bilirubin metabolism has already been discussed in Chapter 4. Hence here we will discuss only the role of liver in bile salt metabolism.

Bile Salt Synthesis

The liver synthesizes bile salts from cholesterol. Firstly it is bile *acids* which are synthesized. The bile acids synthesized are cholic acid and chenodeoxycholic acid. Then bile acids are conjugated with glycine or taurine to form *bile salts.*

Bile Salt Secretion

Bile salts are secreted by the liver cells into biliary canaliculi.

Bacterial Metabolism

Upon reaching the intestines, bile salts are exposed to the action of bacteria residing in the gut. Bacteria deconjugate bile salts and then convert cholic acid into deoxycholic acid, and chenodeoxycholic acid into lithocholic acid. The bile salts formed as a result of bacterial action are called secondary bile salts.

Intestinal Absorption

Most of the bile salts secreted into the intestine are absorbed. The absorbed bile salts travel in the portal vein and thereby reach the liver once again.

Hepatic Uptake and Secretion

Bile salts returning to the liver in the portal vein are taken up from the sinusoids by hepatocytes. The secondary bile salts picked up in this fashion are *not* altered back into the primary form. Uptake is rapidly followed by secretion of bile salts into the canaliculi. When bile is secreted into the duodenum, the bile salts again reach the intestine.

Absorption of bile salts in the intestine, their passage through the liver and secretion back into the intestines is called **enterohepatic circulation**. Because of enterohepatic circulation, there is very little need for fresh bile salt synthesis. However, if enterohepatic circulation is interrupted, there is a marked increase in bile salt synthesis in the liver.

Metabolic Functions

The liver can carry out almost all metabolic reactions. Therefore it is also a regulator of metabolism.

Carbohydrate Metabolism

The liver can utilize glucose as fuel. It can also utilize glucose for synthesis of glycogen, which it stores. The liver can produce glucose by breaking down glycogen. It can also produce glucose from non-carbohydrate sources. Therefore liver is the principal regulator of blood glucose level. When the blood glucose level is high, liver acts as a net glucose consumer. When the blood glucose level is low, liver acts as a net glucose producer. The switch occurs with great accuracy because of the sensitivity of the liver to a wide variety of hormones.

Lipid Metabolism

Liver can carry out lipolysis as well as lipogenesis. In the well-fed state, lipogenesis predominates. During starvation, and in diabetes, lipolysis predominates. Lipolysis generates ketone bodies which can serve as fuel in several parts of the body but not in the liver itself. Liver also manufactures phospholipids and cholesterol. As noted above, liver utilizes cholesterol for the synthesis of bile acids.

Protein Metabolism

Besides routine amino acid transformations, the liver has a few unique and indispensable functions in protein metabolism. First, it is the only organ where albumin is synthesized. Secondly, it is the only organ which transforms ammonia into urea. Finally, it also manufactures most of the globulin fraction of plasma proteins.

Immunological Functions

It is a common observation that globulin levels are raised in liver disease. Most of the rise is in the gamma globulin fraction. It seems that the normal liver receives several antigens in the form of intestinal microorganisms. The microorganims are phagocytosed by the macrophages in the liver (Kupffer cells); the macrophages possibly also degrade the antigens so that they are no longer antigenic. A diseased liver cannot perform these functions properly. Hence the intestinal microorganisms do act as antigens in liver disease, giving rise to excessive production of antibodies (gamma globulins).

Other Functions

Some other functions of the liver have been enumerated below:

1. All the blood that returns from the intestines passes through the liver before entering the general circulation. The liver detects harmful substances in the blood and either eliminates them or converts them into harmless substances (detoxification). The liver detoxifies several drugs, dyes, insecticides and food additives, and also alters the chemical structure of several hormones.
2. The liver stores vitamins A, D and B_{12}, and iron.
3. The liver is the site of hemopoiesis during the first few weeks of life, and in emergencies later on as well throughout life.
4. The liver manufactures fibrinogen, prothrombin and Factors V, VII, IX and X, which are all essential for coagulation of blood.

LIVER FUNCTION TESTS

Liver function is usually assessed by performing a battery of biochemical tests. The common functions have been grouped below in terms of the type of liver function which they test.

Tests of Detoxification and Excretory Function

Serum Bilirubin

Serum bilirubin normally ranges from 5-17 micromol/L (0.3-1.0 mg/100 mL). An increase in serum bilirubin level gives rise to jaundice. Jaundice has been discussed in Chapter 4.

Urinary Bilirubin

Normal urine does not contain any bilirubin. Therefore the presence of bilirubin in the urine indicates disease. Only bilirubin conjugated with glucuronic acid appears in the urine. Hence presence of bilirubin in urine suggests that jaundice has some obstructive element. On the other hand, absence of urinary bilirubin in the presence of jaundice indicates unconjugated hyperbilirubinemia.

Urinary Urobilinogen

The normal urinary urobilinogen excretion is only 0.2-0.3 mg per day. An increased excretion is a sensitive indicator of liver dysfunction. Further absence of urinary urobilinogen indicates total biliary tract obstruction.

Bromsulphalein Excretion

Bromsulphalein (BSP) is a dye which is handled by the liver in the same way as bilirubin. Thus the liver cells take up BSP, conjugate it and excrete it in bile. The test is performed by injecting a standard amount of the dye intravenously. Then venous blood is sampled from the other arm at 5, 25 and 45 min after the commencement of the injection. If the blood level of the dye at 5 min is considered 100 percent, the level at 45 min is generally less than 8 percent and in any case normally less than 14 percent. If more BSP than that is still present in blood at 45 min, it indicates impaired excretion into the bile, and hence impaired liver function.

Rose Bengal Excretion

In this test, ^{131}I-rose bengal is administered intravenously, and its hepatic uptake is assessed by scanning for radioactivity. Its fecal excretion may also be estimated from fecal radioactivity.

Tests of Protein Metabolism

Serum Proteins

Liver is the only source of albumin in the body. Therefore serum albumin level falls in liver disease. On the other hand, as discussed above, serum globulin levels increase in liver disease. Therefore it is useful to do total serum proteins and also to determine separately the albumin and globulin fractions. Absolute albumin and globulin levels are more informative than albumin/globulin ratio because the levels of the two fractions change independently. However, changes in serum proteins are neither seen in early stages of liver disease, nor are they specific for a particular liver disease.

Flocculation Tests

These tests are based on the observation that if serum albumin is low and globulins are high, adding certain reagents to the serum results in flocculation, precipitation or turbidity. Popular tests in this category are *cephalin-cholesterol flocculation test* and *thymol turbidity test*.

Coagulation Tests

Since liver is the site of synthesis of several coagulation factors, *prothrombin time* also reflects protein synthesis in the liver.

Tests of Bile Acid Metabolism

Serum Bile Acids

An increase in serum bile acids is one of the most sensitive tests for detecting minimal liver damage. Even more sensitive may be the bile acid concentration two hours after a meal.

Serum Cholesterol

Hypercholesterolemia is commonly seen in patients having extrahepatic biliary obstruction, which is essentially due to failure of the liver to excrete cholesterol.

Tests of Bile Duct Patency

Obstruction of the biliary tract may be extrahepatic due to a stone or a tumor. It could also be intrahepatic. Some intrahepatic obstruction is a common feature of most liver diseases. Hence the importance of tests for the patency of the biliary passages.

Alkaline Phosphatase

Biliary obstruction leads to an increase in the level of alkaline phosphatase. The various mechanisms which might contribute to this are:

a. Alkaline phosphatase of biliary origin is regurgitated into the bloodstream.
b. There is an increase in the synthesis of alkaline phosphatase at the canalicular membrane. The enzyme is solubilized, probably by the retained bile acids. Then it is regurgitated into the blood stream.
c. Bone alkaline phosphatase in the process of being excreted by the liver may also be regurgitated into the bloodstream.

Measurement of alkaline phosphatase is usually done in International or King-Armstrong Units. The normal range is 35-130 IU/L or 3-13 KA Units.

Other Enzymes

Other enzymes which are also elevated in obstructive liver disease include 5-nucleotidase, leucine aminopeptidase and gamma-glutamyl transpeptidase. Some of these enzymes may be determined in addition to alkaline phosphatase as confirmatory tests.

Bile Pigments

Absence of urinary urobilinogen, absence of fecal bile pigments, and increase in the blood level of conjugated bilirubin provide additional evidence of biliary obstruction.[6]

[6]Reason out why these changes occur in biliary obstruction.

Tests of Hepatocellular Damage

Hepatocellular damage is usually assessed by estimating serum levels of a set of enzymes.

Transaminases

Serum glutamic oxaloacetic transaminase (SGOT), also called aspartate transaminase (AST), and serum glutamic pyruvic transaminase (SGPT), also called alanine transaminase (ALT), are released from liver cells if these cells are damaged by a disease process. Therefore their level rises in hepatocellular damage. Their level rises also in myocardial infarction by a similar mechanism but ALT is relatively more specific for liver disease. Although the normal values of these enzymes vary considerably in different laboratories, AST is usually 5-40 IU/L and ALT 5-35 IU/L.

Lactic Dehydrogenase

Serum lactic dehydrogenase (LDH) level rises in hepatocellular damage as well as liver tumors. But its value is limited because the change is very non-specific.

Conclusion

Besides the above laboratory tests, imaging tests such as ultrasound also make a very useful contribution to assessment of liver function. Further, since only one-fifth of liver is enough to maintain normal function, negative laboratory tests do not necessarily mean that liver is normal. But if some tests are positive, it means that damage is possibly quite significant.

QUESTIONS

1. How much is the esophageal pressure?
2. Why does esophageal pressure reflect the intrathoracic pressure?
3. What are the disorders which may result from LES dysfunction?
4. Why are patients having diarrhea given orally solutions containing both sugar and salt?

5. What is the difference between the route by which glucose is absorbed and that by which fat is absorbed?
6. What are medium chain triglycerides?
7. Why does a person with lactose intolerance have flatulence?
8. How can a person having lactose intolerance tolerate curd?
9. Explain briefly why laxatives should not be used in constipation.
10. How should constipation be treated?
11. What is the difference between a valve and a sphincter?

ANSWERS

1. Esophageal pressure is normally negative (i.e. below the atmospheric pressure) and reflects the intrathoracic pressure.
2. Esophagus is located in the thoracic cage where the pressure is negative. Being a thin-walled toneless structure, esophagus reflects the pressure of its surroundings. That is why the esophagus also shows fluctuations in pressure which are synchronous with respiration.
3. Failure of the esophagus to relax adequately during swallowing is called **achalasia**. Achalasia makes swallowing difficult. Excessive tendency of the LES to relax gives rise to reflux of gastric contents into the esophagus. Since the gastric contents are acidic, the reflux may lead to inflammation of the esophagus, which in turn leads to the experience described as heart burn. The phenomenon is called **reflux esophagitis**.
4. Patients having diarrhea:
   a. Need energy because their food intake is poor and fecal losses heavy, and
   b. Lose water and salts.

   All these deficiencies can be met by solutions containing sugar and salt. Fortunately the combination is also appropriate because glucose and sodium absorption are coupled to each other. Hence giving sugar and salt in the same solution results in more efficient absorption than giving either alone. Giving the solution orally is easier, cheaper and safer than giving glucose saline intravenously. Absorption of the orally administered solution may be incomplete but is considerable even in diarrhea. Therefore, except in very severe cases, oral replenishment of water, electrolytes and energy deficit is preferable.
5. Glucose is absorbed into the bloodstream whereas fats (except medium chain triglycerides) are absorbed into lymphatics.
6. Medium chain triglycerides (MCT) are fats in which the fatty acid chain has less than 10 carbon atoms. These fats do not have to be digested by lipase. They can be directly absorbed into the bloodstream. Therefore MCT are useful for feeding a person with pancreatic enzyme deficiency. Pancreatic enzyme deficiency occurs in pancreatitis. Çoconut oil is an important dietary source of MCT.
7. A person with lactose intolerance has lactase deficiency. Therefore he cannot digest lactose. Undigested lactose reaches the large intestine, where it gets fermented. Fermentation leads to formation of gaseous products, which cause flatulence.
8. A person with lactose intolerance cannot digest milk, but can tolerate curd because some of the lactose in the curd has been fermented by the bacteria which convert milk into curd.
9. Laxatives stimulate intestinal motility so strongly that they empty out more of the large intestine than happens during normal defecation. The result is that the next morning, the colon is still not full enough to create the urge for defecation. It may take three days or more for the fullness in the colon to reach that level. In the meantime, the person feels that she is severely constipated, gets impatient, and takes one more dose of the laxative. Now she needs to wait another three days or more for the natural urge for defecation to occur! That is why laxatives tend to be habit-forming, and should be avoided. However, once a laxative has been taken, one should be patient

and give enough time for the colon to fill up again.

10. Constipation should be treated with high fiber foods, and plenty of water (so that fiber can hold it and achieve adequate fecal bulking as well as softening). Physical exercise and mental relaxation also help. If all that does not work, a spoon or two of ispaghula husk *(Isabgol)* – a rich source of fiber – may be taken with plenty of water. Most of all, the patient needs reassurance. It is not important to pass a motion everyday – we all differ in our bowel habits. What is really important is that the stool, when it is passed, should not be very hard. Soft consistency of the stool can be ensured by taking enough of dietary fiber.
11. A valve is a flap like structure which allows flow only in one direction. A sphincter is a ring of thick musculature to guard a passage. When the muscle contracts, the passage is closed. When the muscle relaxes, the passage is open. A sphincter may only be functional; i.e. it may not have a structural basis. There may be no muscular ring. Instead, there may be only a high pressure zone. When the pressure in this zone drops, the passage is open.

CHAPTER

9 Nutrition and Metabolism

"Fad diets are bad diets."

—STANLEY DAVIDSON

Chapter Outline

- Energy Metabolism
- Carbohydrates
- Fats
- Proteins
- Vitamins
- Minerals
- Recommended Dietary Allowances
- Balanced Diet
- Nutrition during Pregnancy and Lactation
- Nutrition during Infancy and Childhood

Nutrition covers every interaction between man and his food. But in medicine or nursing, nutrition generally refers to the interaction of food with the human body in health and disease. The physiology of nutrition includes digestion, absorption and intermediary metabolism of nutrients in health, and it can help understand the altered nutritional requirements in disease.

The essential chemical constituents of food fall in six major groups. Each of these six is called a **nutrient**. The six nutrients are carbohydrates, proteins, fats, vitamins, minerals and water. Food has two main functions in the body. First, it provides energy; and secondly, it serves to form new living matter (Fig. 9.1). Formation of new living matter is necessary throughout life for replacement of wear and tear. In addition, during childhood, new matter has to be formed also for growth.

Food is measured in terms of its energy value. In nutrition and metabolism, energy has conventionally been measured in kilocalories (kcal), often simply called the Calorie (spelt with a capital C). One kilocalorie is the amount of heat required to raise the temperature of 1 kg of water from 14.5 °C to 15.5 °C. Recently joule has been adopted as the universal unit of energy, including food or metabolic energy. One joule is the energy required to move a mass of 1 kg through one meter by a force of 1 newton acting on it.

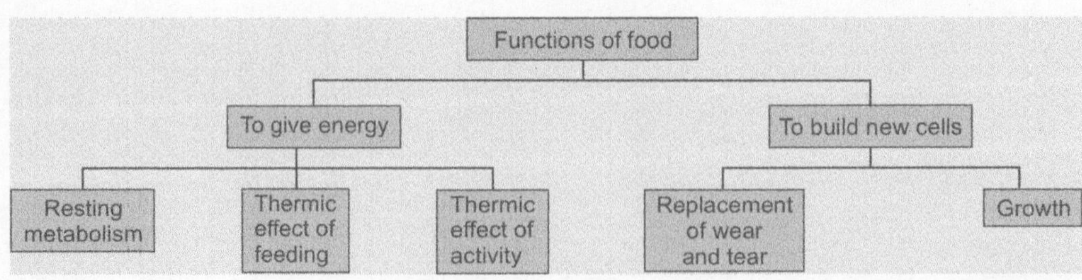

Fig. 9.1 Functions of food

One newton is the force which imparts an acceleration of 1 m per sec per sec to a mass of 1 kg. For metabolism, 1000 joules, or one kilojoule (kJ), is a more suitable unit. Interconversion of units may be performed using the relationship 1 kcal = 4.184 kJ, or 1 kJ = 0.239 kcal.

ENERGY METABOLISM

Staying alive needs constant expenditure of energy. Energy is supplied to the body in the form of food. Over the long run, energy expenditure and energy intake should be equal.

Energy Intake

Of the six nutrients, only three, i.e. carbohydrates, proteins and fats can give energy. Although vitamins, minerals and water do not give energy, they are essential for utilizing the energy-giving nutrients. The energy content of foods or nutrients may be determined in the laboratory by bomb calorimetry. In a bomb calorimeter, the food is completely burnt (oxidized) in the presence of oxygen. The heat released during the process is measured by noting the rise in temperature of a know quantity of water which it can produce. The energy yield of nutrients, by bomb calorimetry, and in the body, is given in Table 9.1. The discrepancy in the case of proteins is because in a bomb calorimeter, protein is oxidized completely whereas in the body protein catabolism leads to excretion of urea which can yield some more energy upon oxidation.

Energy Expenditure

The total energy expenditure of a living organism has three main components : basal metabolic rate (BMR), thermic effect of feeding (TEF), and thermic effect of activity (TEA).

BMR is the minimum rate of energy expenditure which would keep the organism alive. BMR is difficult to measure because basal conditions are difficult to achieve. Therefore usually only the resting metabolic rate (RMR) is measured. RMR is measured at rest in the awake state. RMR accounts for 60-75% of the daily energy expenditure.

TEF is the energy required for digestion, absorption, utilization and storage of nutrients. It accounts for about 10% of the daily energy expenditure.

TEA is the energy expenditure on physical activity. Since physical activity varies a lot from time to time and person to person, its contribution to the daily energy expenditure is highly variable.

Besides BMR, TEF and TEA, some energy may also be spent on various stresses, e.g. cold stress.

The major components of daily energy expenditure have been shown in Figure 9.2.

Table 9.1 Energy content of nutrients

Nutrients	*Energy content (kcal/g)*	
	By bomb calorimetry	*Physiological*
Carbohydrate	4	4
Fat	9	9
Protein	5.4	4*

*Why is the physiological calorific value of proteins less than the bomb calorimetric value? If you do not know it, try to think it out. Then look for the answer in the text.

Basal Metabolism

Basal metabolism is the energy cost of simply staying alive. This energy is used for activities such as beating of the heart, breathing, urine formation, and maintenance of resting membrane potential of excitable cells. Basal metabolism is usually measured by indirect calorimetry.

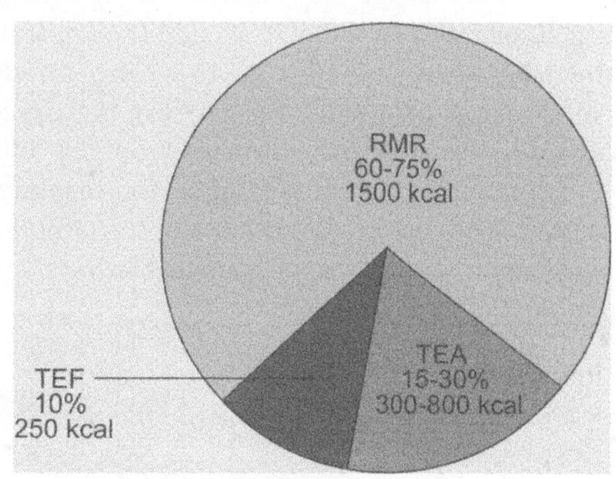

Fig. 9.2 The major components of daily energy expenditure. The values shown are approximate figures for a healthy adult. RMR, resting metabolic rate; TEA, thermic effect of activity; TEF, thermic effect of feeding

Indirect calorimetry: Indirect calorimetry is based on the principle that oxygen consumption is related to energy production in the body. This is so because energy is produced in the body by combustion of nutrients in the presence of oxygen. For an average mixed diet, the body produces 4.825 kcal or 20 kJ of energy for each liter of oxygen consumed.

The subject should be in the basal state, which theoretically means a state of perfect physical, mental and glandular rest. Physical rest is easily ensured by making the subject lie down on a comfortable couch in a relaxed posture. Glandular rest refers to the secretory activity of the alimentary canal. Although absence of secretion cannot be ordinarily achieved, a considerable reduction in activity can be obtained by having the subject report in the post-absorptive state. For that, the subject should have had his last meal 14 h earlier. Since the test is generally conducted in the morning, in practice this requirement means that the subject should report fasting, the last meal being an early dinner or supper the previous evening. Mental rest is the most difficult of the three requirements of the basal state to achieve. A quiet, relaxed, and cheerful atmosphere and a comfortable temperature are conducive to mental relaxation but cannot guarantee it. A man on a railway platform may be much more relaxed than one in a sound-proof air conditioned room.

When the subject reports for the test, he is received warmly, explained the procedure, and then made to lie down on the couch. He is allowed some time for getting accustomed to the persons and the apparatus in the laboratory, and also to breathing through the mouthpiece of a spirometer. Then his oxygen consumption is recorded on the spirometer till a consistent and steady record is obtained for six minutes at a stretch. From the six-minute oxygen consumption, basal metabolic rate may be calculated as follows:

Suppose the 6-min oxygen consumption	=	1200 mL
Then oxygen consumption	=	1200 × 10 mL/h
	=	12000 mL/h
	=	12 L/h
Assuming that the caloric equivalent of oxygen	=	5 kcal/L oxygen,
Basal metabolic rate (BMR)	=	5 × 12 kcal/h
	=	60 kcal/h

If the body weight of the subject is 60 kg,

$$\text{BMR} = \frac{60}{60}\ \text{kcal / kg / h}$$

= 1.0 kcal/kg/h

BMR is commonly expressed in terms of surface area of the body.

Surface area may be calculated by using Du Bois and Du Bois' formula, i.e.

$S = 71.84 \quad W^{0.725} \times L^{0.425}$

where S is surface area in sq cm,

W is body weight in kg, and

L is height in cm.

Alternatively, surface area may be determined by consulting a nomogram (Fig. 9.3). Suppose this subject's height is 160 cm. Then his surface area by Dubois' formula

$= 71.84 \times 60^{0.425} \times 160^{0.725}$

$= 71.84 \times 5.7 \times 39.6$

= 16215.7 sq cm

= 1.6 sq m

Using the nomogram also, his surface area is 1.6 sq m.

Hence BMR = 60/1.6 kcal/sq m/h

= 37.5 kcal/sq m/h

Since basal conditions are difficult to obtain, and even when all efforts are made to achieve the basal state, it cannot be guaranteed, it is preferable to call the metabolic rate measured under resting conditions simply the resting metabolic rate (RMR). Calling the measurement RMR instead of BMR is not merely a matter of semantics but rather a question of intellectual honesty. We should not claim to have measured what we cannot, and should call our measurement what it really is.

The RMR measured on a subject can be interpreted in terms of published tables based on multiple measurements on large number of subjects under carefully controlled conditions. Then the measured RMR is expressed in terms of the percentage deviation from the value predicted for the subject from the tables. A deviation of up to ± 15% is considered within normal limits.

As an approximation, the normal RMR of a healthy adult male is 1 kcal/kg body wt/h. Assuming

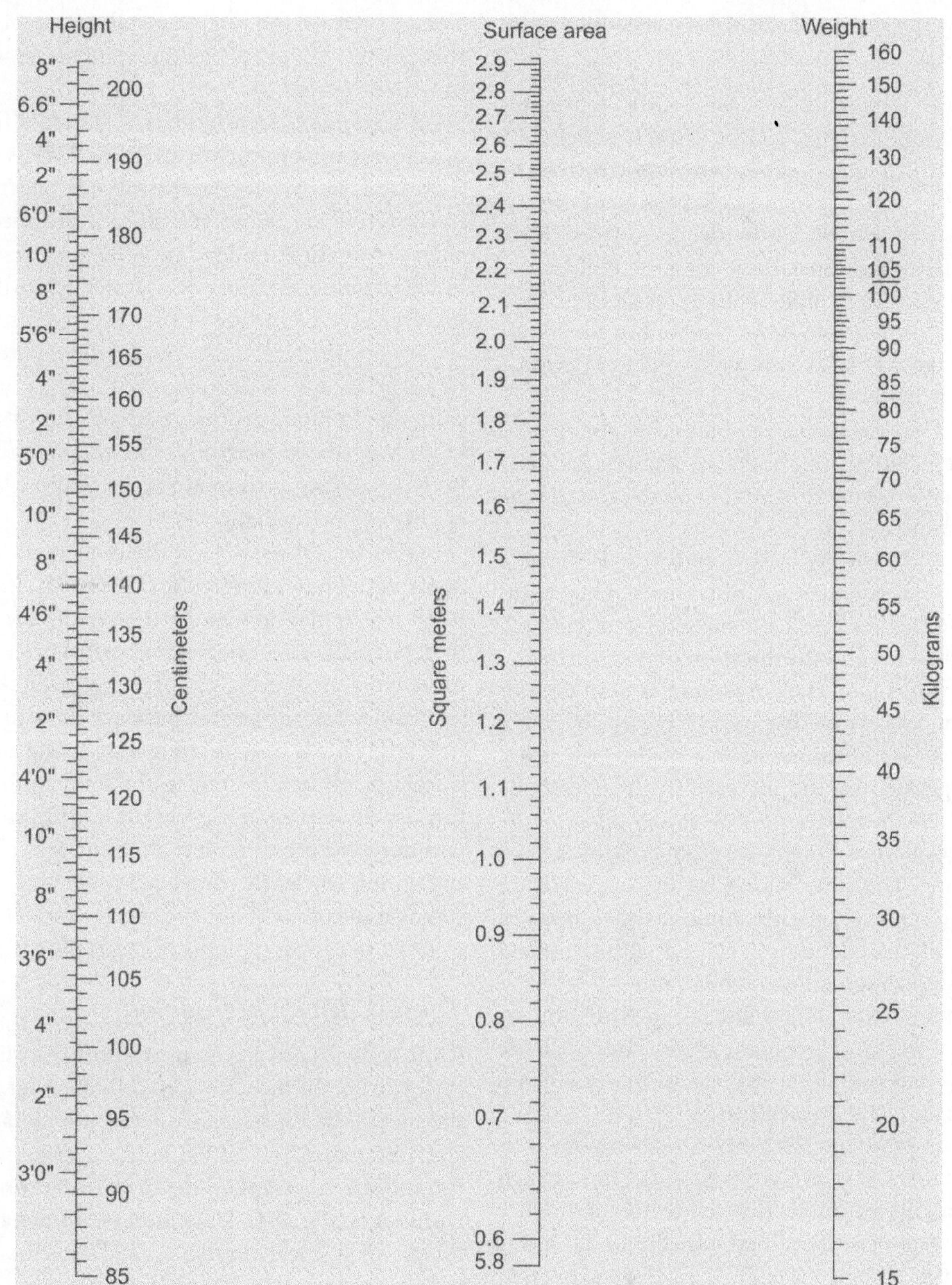

Fig. 9.3 A nomogram for calculation of surface area from height and weight. A ruler which joins the points corresponding to the height and weight of a person will cut the line for surface area at the correct value

the body wt to be 60 kg, the RMR works out to about 1500 kcal/day.

Physiological variations in RMR: RMR represents tissue metabolic activity. Hence RMR is affected by any factor which alters cellular metabolic activity or alters the metabolically active cell mass.

Age: The metabolic rate declines from birth onwards. The high metabolic rate of children is probably due to metabolic activity associated with growth, e.g. protein synthesis. The fall in metabolic rate in old age may be at least partly due to a decrease in lean body mass.

Sleep: The metabolic rate falls by about 10% during sleep. The fall may be due to decreased activity of the sympathetic nervous system, or decreased tone of skeletal muscles.

Exercise: Physically active individuals have a higher RMR than sedentary individuals. Thus regular exercise has an effect on metabolic rate which extends much beyond the duration of the exercise.

Sex: The metabolic rate of women is 6-10% lower than that of men. This effect may be partly due to the difference in sex hormone profile of the two sexes. This is suggested by the increase in the metabolic rate of women during the post ovulatory phase of the menstrual cycle, presumably due to increased level of progesterone. The other reason for the sex variation may be the relatively higher adipose tissue mass of women as discussed later in relation with the effect of body composition on metabolic rate.

Pregnancy: There is a slight fall in RMR during the first 18 weeks of pregnancy. But after that the RMR rises steeply due to increase in maternal lean body mass and fetal metabolism.

Body composition: The body is not homogenous in terms of metabolic rate. Adipose tissue has a much lower metabolic rate than other tissues. Hence higher the percentage of adipose tissue in the body, lower the RMR per kg body weight. If RMR is expressed per kg fat free mass or per kg lean body mass, much of the variation due to age and sex disappears.

Pathological variations in RMR.

Fever: There is an approximately 13% rise in RMR for each degree centigrade rise in body temperature. This is because the rate of metabolic reactions (like that of other chemical reactions) increases with a rise in temperature.

Abnormal activity of thyroid: Thyroid hormones have a profound influence on RMR. RMR is markedly increased in hyperthyroidism, and decreased in hypothyroidism. However, since more specific tests such as protein bound iodine (PBI),and tri-and tetra-iodothyronine levels are now available, RMR has lost its value as a diagnostic test for thyroid disorders.

Undernutrition and overnutrition: There seems to be an adaptive decrease in RMR as a result of prolonged undernutrition, and an adaptive increase in prolonged overnutrition. The adaptation helps the body in adjusting to food supply without an undue change in body weight.

Obesity: Obesity is a heterogenous disorder. Some varieties of obesity are associated with reduced RMR which may, at least partly, explain the tendency to deposit fat. These individuals pay a price for being more efficient at utilizing their energy intake.

Tumors: Some cancer patients show an increase in RMR. This is thought to be due to the addition of metabolically active mass to the body in the form of tumor cells. However, in a recent study in which RMR was done both before and after surgical removal of the tumor, the RMR continued to be high even after removal of tumor. Thus the mechanism of elevation of RMR in cancer patients remains obscure.

Thermic Effect of Feeding

RMR is measured in the postabsorptive state. From this, you might have imagined that eating may alter the metabolic rate. It is true that the metabolic rate starts increasing about 0.5 h after a meal, stays high for about 2 h, and then declines to the resting level within 4 h (Fig. 9.4). This increase in metabolic rate following a meal, earlier called specific dynamic action, is now called the thermic effect of feeding (TEF) or dietary induced thermogenesis (DIT). TEF represents the energy expenditure incurred on utilizing the food, and has therefore been compared to a tax. TEF is partly due to the additional secretory and muscular work that the digestive tract has to

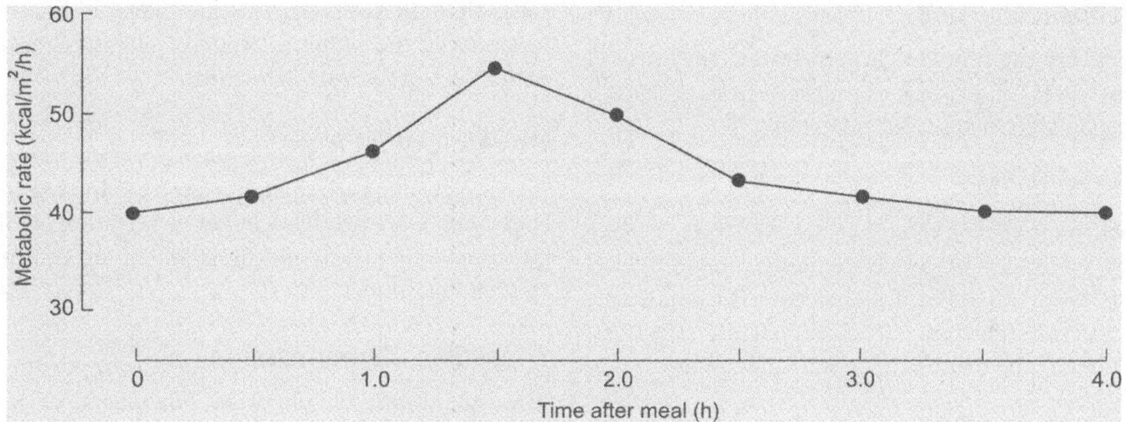

Fig. 9.4 Thermic effect of feeding

undertake to digest and absorb the meal. Part of the TEF is due to the energy spent by the liver and other tissues for breaking down, storing or transforming the nutrients present in the meal. Therefore the magnitude of TEF depends on the nature of the meal. The magnitude of TEF is greater after a protein meal than after a carbohydrate or fat meal. But small variations in nutrient composition of a mixed meal do not affect its TEF much. The TEF of a mixed meal seems to depend mainly on its total energy content and amounts to about 10% of the ingested energy.

TEF is enhanced by sympathetic neural activity. TEF may be one of the regulators of caloric balance. Several studies indicate that some forms of obesity may be at least partly due to reduced TEF. Thus on a comparable caloric intake, some individuals may be able to save more energy for depositing fat by virtue of having a lower TEF.

Thermic Effect of Activity

The energy expenditure during a physical activity may also be measured from the oxygen consumption during the activity by indirect calorimetry. By subtracting the resting metabolic requirements during the activity from the total energy expenditure during the activity, the energy cost of the physical activity may be calculated. TEA is the most flexible and variable part of energy expenditure which can be altered voluntarily. Apart from the energy cost during the activity itself, regular physical activity influences also the RMR. The RMR of physically active individuals is higher than that of sedentary individuals. The effect seems to be due to the higher sympathetic nervous system activity in active individuals.

The energy expenditure on a large variety of everyday activities has been worked out. Knowing the daily activities of an individual and the duration of each activity, the daily energy expenditure may be calculated. In a state of energy balance energy expenditure should equal intake. Knowledge of the total energy required for RMR, TEF and physical activities gives us the most rational estimate of the desirable energy intake of an individual.

CARBOHYDRATES

Carbohydrate is the main constituent of the most commonly eaten foods such as cereals and pulses. In an Indian diet 60-80% of the energy comes from carbohydrates.

Chemistry

Carbohydrates contain carbon, hydrogen and oxygen. Hydrogen and oxygen in carbohydrates are in the same proportion as in water. Cabohydrates are classified into monosaccharides, disaccharides, polysaccharides and complex carbohydrates.

Monosaccharides

These are the simplest carbohydrates. They may be pentoses ($C_5H_{10}O_5$), e.g. ribose, or hexoses ($C_6H_{12}O_6$), e.g. glucose, fructose and galactose.

Disaccharides

Each molecule of disaccharides ($C_{12}H_{22}O_{11}$) yields two molecules of monosaccharides upon hydrolysis. Some disaccharides of nutritional importance are sucrose (glucose + fructose), lactose (glucose + galactose) and maltose (glucose + glucose).

Polysaccharides

Each polysaccharide molecule ($C_6H_{10}O_5$)x yields a large number of monosaccharide molecules upon hydrolysis. Polysaccharides of nutritional importance are starch, cellulose, hemicellulose and pectin. Glycogen is the storage polysaccharide in animals. It is stored in the liver and muscles.

Complex Carbohydrates

These include mucopolysaccharides and glycoproteins. **Mucopolysaccharides** (glycosaminoglycans) contain sugar derivatives such as amino sugars, uronic acids, and sialic acids. Mucopolysaccharides form the ground substance or packing material in bone and connective tissue. **Glycoproteins** are protein molecules contaning some carbohydrate. These are constituents of cell membranes.

Sources

Cereals are the most important dietary source of carbohydrates in the Indian diet. Pulses, potato and banana are other appreciable sources of carbohydrate. All these sources supply carbohydrate in the form of starch. Other important sources of carbohydrate are sugar, which is chemically sucrose, and milk, which supplies lactose.

Cellulose, hemicellulose, pectins and related compounds may be obtained from cereals, pulses, fruits and vegetables. Refined grains have much less of these compounds than unrefined (whole) grains because their concentration is much higher in the husk than in the kernel. Beans have appreciable amounts of the raffinose group of oligosaccharides which are apt to cause flatulence.

Physiological Role

Physiologically, carbohydrates may be divided into those which are readily digested by secretions of the gastrointestinal tract, and those which are resistant to such digestion.

Digestible Carbohydrates

The quantitatively important members of this group are starch, sucrose and lactose. All digestible carbohydrates provide 4 kcal/g. Further, all digestible carbohydrates either yield glucose on digestion, or yield monosaccharides which can be converted into glucose in the body. Glucose can yield some energy anaerobically by glycolysis (Embden-Meyerhoff pathway), and a lot more energy aerobically (Krebs cycle). Alternatively, glucose may be converted into the storage form glycogen, or into triglycerides, or into a limited number of amino acids. In spite of the basic fact that all digestible carbohydrates may be used in one of these ways, all digestible dietary carbohydrates are not alike. Some physiological differences between individual members of this group and their pathophysiological significance have been discussed below.

Glycemic response: After oral ingestion of a carbohydrate food the blood glucose level starts rising, reaching a peak between 0.5 and 1.0 h. The level returns to the fasting level 2-3 h after ingestion. Monitoring the postprandial glycemia after ingestion of a standard dose of glucose forms the basis of the oral glucose tolerance test. It has been observed that the degree and pattern of rise in postprandial glycemia depends not only on the amount of carbohydrate but also on the type of carbohydrate ingested and a variety of other factors. In general, the rise is less steep after ingestion of complex carbohydrates (e.g. starch) than after ingestion of simple carbohydrates (e.g. sucrose or glucose). Other factors which reduce postprandial glycemia include :

a. Inadequate chewing of food
b. Inadequate cooking of starch
c. Presence of indigestible substances (dietary fiber) in food
d. Large particle size of food
e. Presence of enzyme inhibitors in food
f. Presence of protein or fat in association with carbohydrate.

The postprandial glycemia in response to a 50g-carbohydrate portion of the food may be quantified and compared to the response to an equivalent carbohydrate (CHO) load in the form of a reference food. The reference food in current use is white bread. The result is expressed as glycemic index (GI).

$$GI = \frac{\Delta AUC \text{ after 50 g CHO as text food}}{\Delta AUC \text{ after 50 g CHO as white bread}} \times 100$$

where Δ AUC is the incremental area under the 3-h postprandial plasma glucose curve (Fig. 9.5). The GI of a few common foods is given in Table 9.2. Using foods with low GI forms the physiological basis of a rational diet for diabetes mellitus.

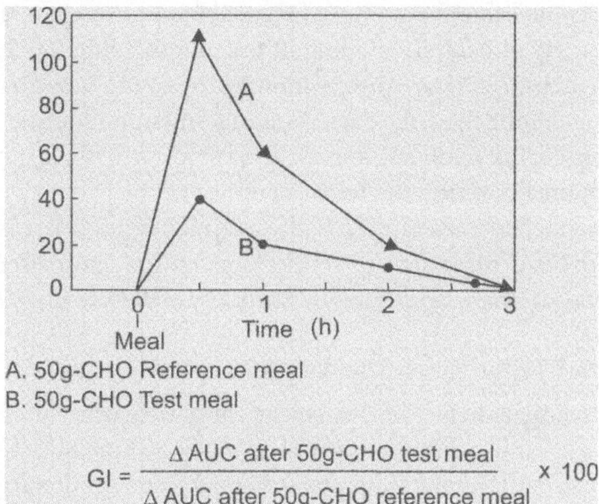

Fig. 9.5 The glycemic index. Note that the plasma glucose levels plotted in the graph are incremental values, i.e. values above the fasting level. Hence the 0 h level (fasting) is 0 mg/dl. Δ AUC, incremental area under the 3-h plasma glucose curve; CHO, carbohydrate (Reproduced from Bijlani RL. Nutrition: A Practical Approach. New Delhi: Jaypee, 1992, Fig. 5.40, p. 136)

Energy intake: Although every carbohydrate provides 4 kcal/g, in practice energy intake is influenced by the source of carbohydrate. The reason is that the amount of carbohydrate required for achieving satiety differs with the food. In general, satiety is achieved at a meal if consuming it takes about 20 min irrespective of its energy content. Sugar adds energy to a food without adding to its volume or the time required to consume it. In fact, by making the food more palatable, sugar may reduce the time taken to consume it. Sugar enters the body so pleasantly, imperceptibly and effortlessly that it adds appreciably to the energy intake quite silently . In contrast starchy foods take time and effort to chew, and are less palatable than sugar. Therefore we are likely to ingest much more carbohydrate if the meal consists of a sugar-containing food than if it consists of a starchy food. As a result, the energy intake is generally higher on sweets than on starchy foods although both sugar and starch provide 4 kcal/g. That is why those who consume more sweets are prone to grow overweight.

Table 9.2 Glycemic index of common foods

Foods	*GI*
Potatoes, cornflakes	80-90
Whole wheat bread, white rice	70-79
Brown rice, bananas	60-69
Buckwheat, frozen peas	50-59
Peas, beans	40-49
Many legumes, milk, ice cream, peanuts	< 40

(From Bijlani RL. *Nutrition: A Practical Approach,* New Delhi: Jaypee, 1992, p. 137)

Nutritional status: One seldom eats pure starch or sugar. Starch generally forms a part of grains which provide, in addition, protein, vitamins and minerals. In contrast, sugar often forms a part of foods which provide little else of value. That is why such foods are called junk foods. They crowd out the appetite but do not provide a balanced mixture of nutrients. Therefore the nutritional status is likely to be better on starchy foods than on sugary foods.

Dental health: Sucrose is a suitable substrate for a variety of bacteria residing in the mouth while starch is not. Therefore, within minutes of eating a sugar-containing food, the bacteria start fermenting sucrose-producing acidic substances. Acid tends to dissolve the enamel covering the teeth. Removal of the protective enamel coat eventually leads to dental caries. That is why it is important to wash the mouth as soon after consuming a sweet food or drink as possible.

Indigestible Carbohydrates: Dietary Fiber

Although dietary fiber includes substances other than indigestible carbohydrates also, this is an appropriate place to discuss the physiological role of dietary fiber. Dietary fiber is obtained from plant foods, and consists of a heterogenous group of chemicals, most of them polysaccharides residing in the cell walls, which share the physiological property of being resistant to digestion by the endogenous enzymes of the human gastrointestinal tract (Fig. 9.6). Each point in this definition merits comment. The fact that dietary fiber is obtained only from plant foods is almost axiomatic. Most of the substances considered part of the fiber complex are polysaccharides but a notable exception is lignin which consists of substituted phenylpropane polymers. Most of the components of dietary fiber reside in the cell wall but pectin is found also intracellularly. Although all constituents of fiber are resistant to hydrolysis by digestive enzymes of the gut, a small but finite part of starch is also resistant to such digestion. This fraction of starch has been named resistant starch, and its proportion in a food may change with the stage of ripening, cooking or

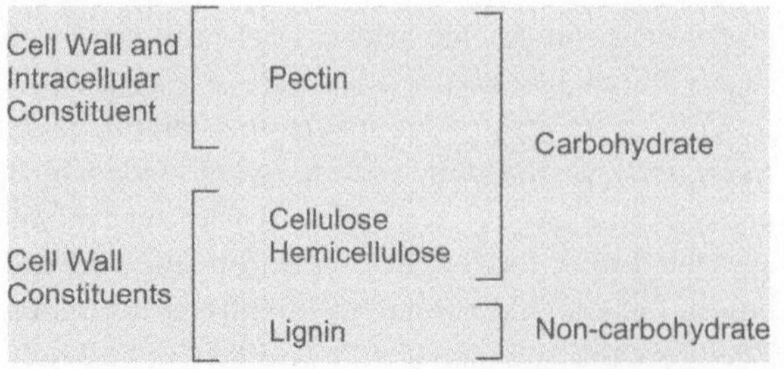

Fig. 9.6 Major constituents of dietary fiber

storage. Physiolgically, resistant starch also behaves like dietary fiber. Further, resistant starch, most of the pectin, and a part of hemicellulose and cellulose are fermented by bacterial flora of the large intestine.

Physiological role of dietary fiber: Although fiber is not digested, it is neither a passive nor redundant part of the diet. Its physiological significance, which is becoming increasingly clear, extends beyond the gut.

Gastrointestinal effects: A high fiber meal is bulky in relation to its caloric content. The bulk increases further in the stomach due to the water-holding properties of dietary fiber. Larger volume of a high fiber meal coupled with its higher viscosity slows down the rate of gastric emptying. In the small intestine too, fiber prolongs the residence time of food by slowing down the motility. But the effects of fiber on large intestinal motility are quite different. Dietary fiber, which starts as a relatively small constituent of the diet, becomes a major constituent of the material delivered to the large intestine. Therefore the volume of the colonic contents depends greatly on the fiber content of diet. Fiber, together with the water that it holds, increases the volume and viscosity of the contents of the large intestine. This stimulates the motility of the large intestine and increases the volume, softness and frequency of evacuation of fecal matter.

Besides motility, fiber also affects the digestive and absorptive functions of the gut. By providing relatively inert space-occupying material, fiber spreads out the digestive function over a longer length of the small intestine. Further, by binding bile salts, and by interposing a mechanical barrier between nutrients and the absorptive surface, fiber reduces the efficacy of absorption. However, because of the great physiological reserve of the intestine, nearly complete absorption is achieved even on high fiber diets by utilizing a longer length of the small intestine.

Effects on glucose metabolism: It has already been mentioned that glycemic response to a carbohydrate meal is reduced if the meal also includes dietary fiber. This is thought to be secondary to the gastrointestinal effects of fiber. Since fiber slows gastric emptying, and spreads absorption over a longer segment of the small intestine, the rate of delivery of digested carbohydrate to the absorptive surface is reduced. Hence the postprandial glycemia is reduced.

Effects on lipoprotein metabolism: Some components of dietary fiber reduce blood cholesterol level. This is thought to be mainly due to the bile salt binding effect of dietary fiber (Fig. 9.7). Bile salt binding by fiber increases the fecal excretion of bile salts and correspondingly reduces the amount available for entero-hepatic circulation. Hence the need for *de novo* synthesis of bile salts in the liver is increased. Increased synthesis of bile salts increases the utilization of cholesterol for this purpose thereby reducing the blood level of cholesterol.

Pathological implications of dietary fiber deficiency: We have become specially aware of the importance of fiber in the diet during the last three decades. The credit for this goes to Surgeon Captain T.L. Cleave, Denis Burkitt and Hugh Trowell, all of them British doctors who spent considerable part of their career in Africa. They were struck by the virtual absence in Africa of several diseases which are very common in Europe and North America. They attributed the difference in the disease pattern to diet. Cleave emphasized the excess of sugar, while Burkitt and Trowell elaborated on the deficiency of fiber in the Western diet. Cleave crystallized his thinking in terms of evolution. He hypothesized that the changes in Western diet were too rapid for evolution to keep pace with. Hence the human species is poorly adapted to a diet high in refined carbohydrates. Therefore such a diet predisposes to several diseases. Burkitt and Trowell proposed the fiber hypothesis and tried to explain the mechanisms whereby fiber deficiency might lead to diseases of the modern civilization. Thus it was the absence of fiber which made us realize the importance of fiber in the diet.

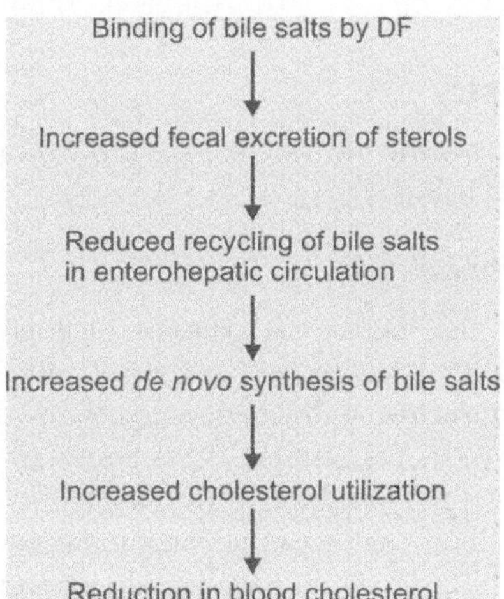

Fig. 9.7 The principal mechanism by which dietary fiber lowers the concentration of cholesterol in blood. DF, dietary fiber

Constipation: The role of fiber in making the fecal matter soft and bulky has been discussed above. That makes fiber important in the prevention and treatment of constipation as well as its sequelae such as piles and varicose veins.

Cancer: Epidemiological as well as experimental studies suggest that dietary fiber protects us from cancer of the large intestine. The mechanisms possibly responsible for the protection include dilution of carcinogens by the water held by fiber; reduction in the duration of contact between carcinogens and colonic mucosa due to stimulation of motility by fiber; and binding of carcinogens to fiber.

Obesity: It was discussed earlier that starchy foods take longer to chew than sugary foods. Among starchy foods, those in which fiber is still intact take more time and effort to chew than those from which fiber has been removed. Further, as mentioned above, fiber slows down gastric emptying. Both these mechanisms promote satiety, and limit energy intake. Finally, fiber limits energy intake by displacing energy-yielding nutrients. Fiber adds to the weight and volume of food but makes only a negligible contribution to energy intake. Thus fiber reduces the energy density of food.

Diabetes mellitus: The reduction in postprandial glycemia brought about by fiber has been discussed earlier. Thus high fiber foods reduce the peak requirement of insulin during the postprandial phase. Further, a high fiber diet has also been shown to improve carbohydrate tolerance possibly by increasing the peripheral sensitivity to insulin. Both these mechanisms make high fiber diets a rational choice for prevention as well as treatment of diabetes mellitus.

Atherosclerosis and coronary artery disease: The possibility that some varieties of dietary fiber lower serum cholesterol has been mentioned earlier. Further, fiber has a beneficial effect on obesity and diabetes. Since hypercholesterolemia, obesity, diabetes and atherosclerosis often form one interrelated complex in the same individual, high fiber diets are thought to be useful for all these metabolic disorders associated with overnutrition. Coronary artery disease is merely a specific instance of atherosclerosis in which the coronary arteries have been affected by the disease process.

Carbohydrate Requirements

There is no strictly scientific reason why carbohydrate is essential in the diet. It is often said that fats burn in the flame of carbohydrates. This concept is based on the fact that only carbohydrates can supply the oxaloacetate required to keep the Krebs cycle running. The minimum amount of carbohydrate required for this purpose can be derived from gluconeogenic amino acids. Thus it is theoretically possible to have a satisfactory diet devoid of carbohydrates. In practice, however, carbohydrates are an abundant and inexpensive nutrient. Any diet devoid of carbohydrates would be highly inconvenient, unpalatable, expensive, and needlessly lop-sided. It was previously believed that at least diabetics should have a low carbohydrate diet. But it was shown in 1935 by Himsworth, and once again in recent studies, that a high carbohydrate diet actually improves carbohydrate tolerance, possibly through up-regulation of insulin receptors. Thus a high carbohydrate diet of the type common in India is a healthy diet. We need no longer be apologetic about the high carbohydrate diet of Indians, and defend it on grounds of poverty or blind tradition. The traditional Indian diet can stand on its scientific merit, and can well serve as a model to shape a healthy diet for normal persons as well as patients of diabetes mellitus.

FATS

Fats are a concentrated source of energy. One gram of fat provides 9 kcal energy, as compared to carbohydrates and proteins which provide only 4 kcal/g each. Because of the great chemical resemblance between dietary fat and body fat, the two are sometimes confused. However, dietary fat undergoes digestion, and after absorption may enter several alternative metabolic pathways, many of which may not lead to its forming body fat. On the other hand, if the energy intake exceeds energy requirements, excess of fat is deposited in the body. This happens even if the excess intake is in the form of carbohydrates and proteins. Thus body fat may be synthesized from non-fat sources.

Besides serving as a concentrated source of energy, *dietary fat* also makes the diet palatable, and helps in the absorption of fat soluble vitamins. Presence of fat also imparts satiety value to the diet by reducing the rate of gastric emptying.

Body fat, in the forms of trigiycerides, serves the function of storing energy which is drawn upon several times a day during the postabsorptive phase, and more heavily during fasting or starvation. Besides that, fat also insulates the body against changes in environmental temperature. Specific fats or their derivatives also help form cell membranes, myelin, steroid hormones and prostaglandins. Fats required for most of these functions can be synthesized in the body even if the diet contains no fat except that a small quantity of essential fatty acids is necessary in the diet.

Chemistry

Dietary fats generally belong to one of the categories described below.

Triglycerides

Most of the dietary fat consists of triglycerides. Chemically, triglycerides are esters of glycerol and fattty acids. Individual triglycerides differ in two respects : the number of carbon atoms in the constituent fatty acids, and the dergee of saturation of the carbon chains of the constituent fatty acids. Dietary triglycerides have predominantly long chain fatty acids. i.e. they have 16 or more atoms in the carbon chain. With respect to saturation, fatty acids may be saturated (no double bond), monounsaturated (one double bond), or polyunsaturated (more than one double bond). Polyunsaturated fatty acids (PUFA) are further classified into n-3 PUFA and n-6 PUFA depending on the position of the first double bond, counting from the methyl end of the fatty acid molecule. Animal fats are generally saturated while vegetable fats are generally unsaturated. Hydrogenation of vegatable fats makes them saturated.

Other Lipids

Besides triglycerides, food also contains small amounts of *cholesterol*. The cholesterol content of a dietary fat is frequently confused with its effect on serum cholesterol level. Vegetable fats contain no cholesterol. Animal fats may contain a small quantity of cholesterol. The only major source of cholestrerol in the Indian diet is egg. On the other hand the impact of dietary triglycerides on serum cholesterol depends on the degree of saturation. In general, saturated fats raise serum cholesterol while polyunsaturated fats lower it.

Another group of fats present in the food in small quantities are the *phospholipids* such as lecithin. Phospholipids are relatively soluble in water, and serve to keep fats emulsified.

Sources

Triglycerides, which are the predominant form of dietary fat, may be obtained from vegetable or animal sources. Although fats from either source yield 9 kcal/g there are important differences between them. Vegetable fats are generally unsaturated while animal fats are generally saturated. Important exceptions are coconut oil, palm oil and hydrogenated vegetable oil, which are saturated; and fish oils, which are unsaturated. Some further details of physiological significance are that vegetable oils obtained from oil seeds and other seeds such as corn or rice provide n-6 PUFA while green leaves and fish oils have n-3 PUFA. Coconut oil has a significant amount of saturated medium chain triglycerides. Palm oil is a reasonably balanced mixture of saturated and monounsaturated fats. The important differences between saturated and unsaturated fats have been given in Table 9.3. The physiological effects of different categories of unsaturated fats have been compared in Table 9.4. In view of the undesirable effects of excess of saturated as well as unsaturated fats, and the absence of complete information about the effects, it is desirable to avoid extremes. A moderate intake of fat providing a mixture of saturated fat, monounsaturated fat, n-3 PUFA and n-6 PUFA seems to be the safest course for a healthy person.

Cholesterol is a compound which belongs only to the animal kingdom. Therefore plant foods do not contain any cholesterol. Among animal foods, egg and brain are specially rich sources of cholesterol. The cholesterol content of a few foods is given in Table 9.5. Egg is the only high cholesterol food consumed commonly on a regular basis in India. Since one egg contains about 250 mg cholesterol, and

Table 9.3 Saturated and unsaturated fats compared

Saturated fats	*Unsaturated fats*
Source	
Animal fats Coconut oil Palm oil*	Most vegetable oils, specially corn oil, sesame oil and sunflower oil
Hydrogenated oils	Fish oils
Physical state	
Solid at room temperature	Liquid at room temperature
Stability	
More stable, longer shelf life	More prone to rancidity due to oxidation
Associated nutrients	
Fat soluble vitamins	Vitamin E
Effect on serum cholesterol	
Tend to raise serum cholesterol; hence increase the risk of atherosclerosis	Tend to lower serum total and LDL cholesterol; hence decrease the risk of atherosclerosis
Undesirable effects of excess	
Rise in serum cholesterol	Increase in vitamin E requirement

*Palm oil has monounsaturated fatty acids also

experts recommend that the daily cholesterol intake should be less than 300 mg, we can have one egg per day and still stay within the permissible limit.

Essential Fatty Acids

Essential fatty acids (EFA) are those fatty acids which serve important functions but cannot be synthesized in the body, and must therefore be supplied in the diet. Three unsaturated fatty acids, viz, linoleic acid (an n-6 PUFA with 2 double bonds), linolenic acid (an n-3 PUFA with 3 double bonds) and arachidonic acid (an n-6 PUFA with 4 double bonds) have traditionally been considered EFA. But arachidonic acid can be derived from linoleic acid. Hence only linoleic acid and linolenic acid are truly EFA.

Functions of EFA

The important functions of EFA fall in two categories: as suppliers of lipid components of cell membranes and as precursors of regulatory molecules.

Cell membranes: Linoleic acid, linolenic acid, and their derivatives form components of membranes which bind cells and organelles. There is a certain degree of flexibility in the exact molecules used as membrane constituents. The fatty acid composition of membranes is influenced by the type of fatty acids present in the diet. However, the physicochemical properties of membranes with different composition may not be the same. In case of brain and retina, an n-3 PUFA, docosahexaenoic acid (DHA) is a

Table 9.4 Different categories of unsaturated fats compared

	Monounsaturates (e.g. oleic acid)	*n-3 PUFA (e.g. linolenic acid)*	*n-6 PUFA (e.g. linoleic acid)*
Sources	Olive oil Palm oil Mustard oil	Mustard oil, rapeseed oil, soyabean oil, beans, green leafy vegetables, fish and fish oils	Most vegetable oils, e.g. corn oil, sesame oil, sunflower oil, groundnut oil, soyabean oil, rice bran oil
Essentiality	Not essential	Essential	Essential
Effects on serum cholesterol	No direct effect. Reduce total and LDL cholesterol if used as replacement for saturated fat. No effect on HDL cholesterol	Reduce total and LDL cholesterol. No consistent effect on HDL cholesterol	Reduce total, LDL and HDL cholesterol
Important metabolic products	Nil	Prostaglandins (3-series) Thromboxane (TXA_3) Leukotrienes (5-series) Docosahexenoic acid (DHA)	Prostaglandins (2-series) Thromboxane (TXA_2) Leukotrienes (4-series)
Physiological effects of metabolic products		PGI_3 inhibits platelet aggregation. TXA_3 is a weak platelet aggregator. Leukotriene B_5 is a weak inducer of inflammation. DHA is an important constituent of brain and retina.	PGI_2 inhibits platelet aggregation. TXA_2 is a strong platelet aggregator. Leukotriene B_4 is a strong inducer of inflammation. Hence excess may promote atherogenesis in spite of lowering serum cholesterol.
Dietary recommendation	A good replacement for a substantial part of saturated fat	A good replacement for a substantial part of saturated fat. A basic minimum intake essential	A good replacement for a substantial part of saturated fat. A basic minimum intake essential. Cannot replace –3 PUFA

Table 9.5 Cholesterol content of foods

Food	*Cholesterol content (approximately)*
Meat, chicken, fish	100 mg/100 g
Liver, kidney	300 mg/100 g
Brain	> 2000 mg/100 g
Egg, one	250 mg
Egg yolk, one	250 mg
Egg white, one	0 mg
Milk, whole	40 mg/glass
Ice cream	50 mg/small cup
Butter	35 mg/tablespoonful
Fish oils	500 mg/100 g
Vegetable oils	0 mg/100 g
Nuts and oil seeds	0 mg/100 g

(From Bijlani RL. *Nutrition: A Practical Approach*. New Delhi: Jaypee, 1992: 147)

membrane component which has been studied extensively. DHA can be derived from linolenic acid, or obtained from breast milk or fish oils. If DHA supply is deficient, brain and retina incorporate an n-6 PUFA closely resembling DHA. But incorporating the substitute instead of DHA impaires retinal function and makes the brain more susceptible to damage by environmental toxins and alcohol.

Regulatory molecules: EFA are the precursors of regulatory molecules such as prostaglandins, thromboxanes and leukotrienes. But the exact type of molecules derived from linolenic acid are different from those derived from linoleic acid (Table 9.4). On balance, it appears preferable to have the type of molecules derived from linolenic acid (an n-3 PUFA).

Thus from the point of view of membrane structure as well as regulatory molecules, it appears preferable to use linolenic acid instead of lenoleic acid. In any case, it is better to tip the balance in favor of linolenic acid when a mixture is being consumed. This point has become important now because in traditional diets, the ratio of n-6 to n-3 PUFA was around 1:1. But with the popularization of vegetable oils during the last few decades, a ratio of 25:1 is not uncommon. Since no human population has tried such lopsided diets long enough, it is considered prudent to restore the balance.

Deficiency

Deficiency of EFA on any reasonably normal diet is virtually unknown. EFA deficiency may be induced in experimental animals with the help of a specially formulated diet. Clinically, EFA deficiency may occur in infants fed on a fat-free formula, or in patients on total parenteral nutrition if EFA are omitted from their nutrition. EFA deficiency does not occur even if all visible fat is omitted from the diet. The small quantity of fat present in cereals, pulses and leafy vegetables (invisible fat) is sufficient to supply the minimum requirement of EFA.

Requirements

The minimum EFA requirement has been estimated to be 7.5 g for adults and 0.5-1% of the energy intake for infants. Canada has recommended for its population separate allowances for n-3 and n-6 PUFA with an n-3 to n-6 ratio of 1:6.

The Lipid-coronary Connection

Atherosclerosis is a fairly common disease of the elderly. It is an arterial disease with a multifactorial etiology, and is characterized by deposits of fatty material in the intimal layer. Although atherosclerosis is a generalized disorder, its impact is felt maximally in organs which (a) have end arteries (i.e. no anastomoses), and (b) are vital for survival. Coronary arteries are essentially end arteries, and heart is a vital organ. Hence the impact of atherosclerosis is felt acutely in the heart. The fact that atherosclerotic deposits are lipid suggested that excess of lipids in the diet might lead to these deposits. There does seem to be a connection, but in spite of decades of intensive research, the connection is still far from clear.

Although the impact of atherosclerosis is felt relatively late in life, the precursor of the lesion are fatty streaks in arteries which appear in childhood in genetically susceptible individuals. Therefore it has been suggested that for maximum benefit sound nutrition should be started early, and followed life-long.

Biochemistry of Atherosclerosis

Since cholesterol esters are a major component of atherosclerotic deposits, it was natural to examine the blood cholesterol levels of susceptible individuals. Extensive population studies have established that blood cholesterol levels are a rough index of susceptibility to atherosclerosis and ischemic heart disease. The predictive value is further increased if instead of total cholesterol level we consider the levels of low density lipoprotein cholesterol (LDL-C) and high density lipoprotein cholesterol (HDL-C). High LDL-C levels and low HDL-C levels indicate a high degree of susceptibility to ischemic heart disease (Table 9.6). It is considered desirable to have a total plasma cholesterol level below 230 mg/dL and the LDL-C level below 130 mg/dL.

The basis of these biochemical indices can be understood if atherosclerosis is considered to be a disorder of cholesterol balance. Cholesterol is a normal constituent of the body with vital functions. It is a constituent of cell membranes, and the precursor of steroid hormones and bile salts. The body has mechanisms for synthesizing cholesterol from acetate. The liver can synthesize as much as 2 g cholesterol per day, which is many times the amount ordinarily present in the diet. The synthesis of cholesterol is regulated by requirements, the key enzyme being hydroxymethylglutaryl coenzyme A reductase (HMG CoA reductase). Higher the intake of dietary cholesterol, lower the synthesis in the body. However, the mechanism can be overwhelmed by very high levels of dietary cholesterol. Hence very high cholesterol intakes do raise blood levels of cholesterol, thereby suggesting that limiting cholesterol intake may help prevent atherosclerosis. Besides dietary cholesterol itself, the other dietary variable affecting serum cholesterol is the degree of saturation of dietary fat as discussed already.

Table 9.6 Normal limits of blood cholesterol

	Normal limit	
	mmol/L	mg/dL
Plasma cholesterol	< 7.8	< 300
Serum VLDL-C	< 0.65	< 25
Serum LDL-C	< 4.4	< 170
Serum HDL-C	> 0.9	> 35

(Based on Weatherall DJ, Ledingham JGG, Warrell DA, Eds. Oxford Textbook of Medicine, Oxford: Oxford University Press, 2nd Edition, 1987: 29.7.)

The next important question is regarding the biochemical link between blood levels of cholesterol, LDL-C and HDL-C, and atherosclerosis. To understand this link, atherosclerosis may again be considered a disorder of cholesssterol balance at cellular level. In atherosclerosis, the amount of cholesterol entering the cells in the arterial wall exceeds that metabolized or expelled by them.

There are at least three ways in which circulating lipoproteins can enter the arterial wall: ultrafiltration, LDL receptor pathway, and uptake of modified LDL by 'scavenger receptors'. Ultrafiltration is not a significant mechanism in this case. The LDL receptor pathway discovered by Brown and Goldstein, for which they also received the Nobel Prize, has attracted considerable attention. In this scheme, LDL binds to receptors on the cell surface, is internalized and decomposed. The LDL-derived cholesterol inhibits de novo cholesterol synthesis and also reduces LDL receptor synthesis, thereby maintaining a check on cholesterol accumulation in the cell. It was believed that a disturbance of these regulatory mechanisms may be responsible for accumulation of cholesterol in arterial cells. But now we know that LDL receptor pathway is a major mechanism in the liver but not in the arterial wall. A reduced number of LDL receptors may be responsible for some varieties of familiar hyperlipoproteinemia but may not explain the pathogenesis of atherosclerosis. The mechanism currently thought to be responsible for the link between LDL and atherosclerosis is the uptake of modified LDL by 'scavenger receptors'. LDL can be oxidatively modified by arterial endothelial cells, smooth muscle cells as well as macrophages. The modification has two aspects. Firstly, there is peroxidation of the polyunsaturated fatty acid components in the lipid moiety of LDL, leading to generation of free radicals which are potentially cytotoxic. Secondly, there is a change in the protein moiety of LDL leading to recognition by 'scavenger receptors' but loss of recognition by Brown and Goldstein's LDL receptors. The modified LDL binds to scavenger receptors present on the surface of macrophages. The free radicals associated with modification of LDL may be responsible for damaging the macrophages leading to the formation of foam cells. In adddition, modified LDL also acts as a chemo-attractant for monocytes. This might be responsible for adhesion of monocytes to endothelial cells. Thus the chemotactic effect of modified LDL may be a fundamental event in the genesis of fatty streaks. In short, a basic step in pathogenesis of atherosclerosis seems to be the uptake of oxidatively modified LDL by arterial macrophages leading to cholesterol accumulation and free radical damage (Fig. 9.8)

Dietary Recommendations for Coronary Heart Disease

Since lipoprotein profile is an objective, easily measurable variable, a diet suitable for coronary heart disease and other forms of atherosclerotic disease is one which improves the lipopprotein profile. Current dietary recommendations for prevention and treatment of coronary heart disease are as follows:

1. The total dietary fat should be reduced so that it provides less than 30 percent of the energy intake.
2. Saturated fats should provide less than 10 percent of the energy intake and so should polyunsaturated fats. The intake of mono-unsaturated fats should be increased. In the Indian context it means restricting ghee, butter and hydrogenated oils, and replacing these by vegetable oils.
3. Cholesterol intake should be less than 300 mg per day. Since one egg contains about 250 mg per day, and the Indian diet has no other significant source of cholesterol, taking one egg per day still leaves cholesterol intake in the permissible range.
4. Sodium intake should be less than 3 g per day.
5. Alcohol intake should be less than 60 mL ethanol per day.
6. It is considered generally desirable to replace refined foods by high-fiber unrefined foods.
7. Energy intake should be reduced, if necessary, to maintain normal body weight.

The above recommendations would benefit not only atherosclerosis but also diabetes, which are both disorders associated with overeating. However, both atherosclerosis and diabetes are multifactorial diseases, and diet is only one of the factors which can contribute to their causation or prevention.

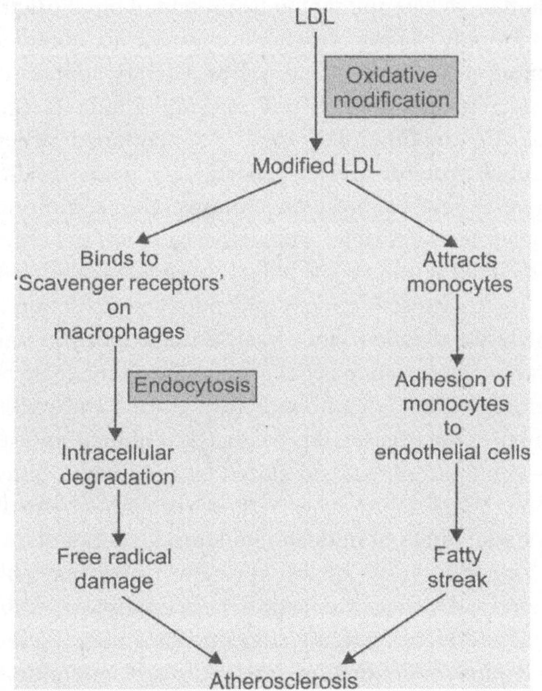

Fig. 9.8 The oxidative modification of LDL as a mechanism for the LDL-atherosclerosis linkage

PROTEINS

Proteins are one of the three macronutrients which yield energy in the body. Although proteins can yield 4 kcal/g, they are preferentially utilized for other more specific purposes which cannot be served by any other nutrient. This gives proteins a somewhat special status among nutrients; hence the name protein (*proteios*, first). Proteins are specially important for building up new living matter. Therefore their requirement is relatively higher in growing children, during pregnancy and lactation, and during convalescence. However, obsession with protein has been responsible for many faulty concepts and loop-sided nutrition interventions. Here we shall try to arrive at a balanced approach to the place of proteins in diet.

Chemistry

Proteins are large molecules, their basic units being alpha-amino acids. The amino acids are joined to each other through—CONH—linkages. There are 20 different amino acids present in animal proteins. Each protein molecule may have thousands of amino acid molecules. If just 26 letters of the alphabet can make thousands of words, it is easy to imagine that the variety of proteins possible is truly astronomical. The large variety makes it possible for proteins to play highly specific roles as enzymes, antigens, antibodies, hormones and receptors. The proteins of each individual of a species are somewhat different; the proteins of individuals belonging to different species are more different; the proteins of plants and animals are still more different from each other in their amino acid make up. It is not an exaggeration to say that the way a cell looks, and the way it behaves depends on the proteins it synthesizes.

Essential Amino Acids

Of the 20 amino acids, 11 can be synthesized in the body from non-protein sources if necessary. But 9 amino acids cannot be synthesized by the human body. These nine amino acids are called essential amino acids. Essential amino acids must be supplied by the diet in quantities commensurate with their requirements for satisfactory nutrition. This is necessary because the structure of each protein is coded with great precision in the genetic material of the organism. While this precision guarantees precise construction of protein molecules, it also means that all the amino acids required for a particular protein should be available in adequate quantity. If even a single amino acids is deficient, the amino acid chain on the ribosomes will be constructed only till the point where the deficient amino acid is required. The chain cannot continue further till the deficient amino acid is provided. Therefore all of the twenty amino acids should be available in approximately the same proportion in which they are required for protein synthesis. While the deficit of nonessential amino acids can be made up by endogenous synthesis, essential amino acids must be available from dietary protein.

Protein Quality

From the above discussion it is clear that dietary protein should provide essential amino acids in the proportion in which they are required for protein synthesis. A protein which does so is called a good quality protein. Naturally, the more a dietary protein resembles human proteins in its amino acid profile, the better will be its quality. Since human proteins are more similar to animal proteins than to plant proteins, animal proteins have a better quality than plant proteins.

Sources

Protein, in the quantity required, is readily available in plant as well as animal foods. Protein of plant origin, commonly called vegetable protein, is obtained mainly from cereals and pulses. Dietary sources of animal protein include milk and milk products, egg, and fish and other flesh foods. As mentioned earlier, animal proteins are, in general, of a better quality than vegetable proteins. Among the commonly consumed vegetable proteins, cereals are generally deficient in lysine while pulses are generally deficient in methionine. If cereals and pulses are combined, the lysine deficiency of cereals is made up by pulses, and the methionine deficincy of pulses is made up by cereals. Hence a combination of cereals and pulses can provide a reasonably balanced combination of all essential amino acids required by the human body. That is the reason why even those vegetarians who do not take much of milk and milk products can obtain reasonably good quality protein from vegetable sources. This fact seems to have been discovered by trial and error by many ancient civilizations. Cereal and pulse combinations are the staple diet almost throughout India. Rice and soyabean are the staple diet in China, while corn and beans are the staple diet in Latin American countries. This fact has been rediscovered through the experimental method by present day scientists. Studies performed at the National Institute of Nutrition have clearly shown that the growth rates of animals brought up on a combination of cereals and pulses are comparable to those of animals brought up on animal proteins.

Protein Requirements

Protein is a unique nutrient in that its quantitative requirement depends partly on the quality of dietary protein. As quality deteriorates, the quantity required to meet nutritional needs increases. The reasons for the importance of protein quality reside in the uses to which proteins are put in the body, and the structure of the protein molecule. In the body, proteins form structural elements such as cell membranes and collagen fibers, or function as enzymes, hormones and antibodies. These are all specific functions which only a specific protein can perform. They are unlike the function of providing energy which can be performed by a wide variety of carbohydrates, fats or proteins almost equally well. Hence for proteins to be useful, specific proteins must be synthesized in the body. Specific proteins have a rigidly prescribed amino acid sequence, which can be satisfied by a relatively small quanity of good quality proteins. If the quality is poor, a large intake is necessary to provide the essential amino acids in the required quantity and ratio. The large intake may also leave behind a large amount of redundant amino acids which may be used as fuel. Taking the day to day variations in dietary protein quality into account, and providing a reasonable margin of safety, it has been recommended that adults should take about 1 g/kg body weight protein per day. This protein may come from a judicious mixture of vegetable proteins, or from animal proteins, or a mixture of vegetable and animal proteins. The recommended intake of 1 g/kg body weight means that a 60 kg person should take 60 g protein per day. 60 g protein has an energy value of 240 kcal, which is about 10% of the daily energy intake. Cereals have about 10% protein, and pulses have about 20% protein. Hence a mixture of cereals and pulses is not only satisfactory in quality, it can also meet the quantitative protein requirement. Children need more protein per unit body weight, but they need also more energy per unit body weight. Therefore a cereal-pulse mixture can meet the protein requirement of children as well. Fortunately cereals and pulses are readily available and widely acceptable items of the diet. These common foods can meet the protein requirement of children as well as adults, and there is no need for any exotic supplements.

VITAMINS

Vitamins and minerals are needed in very small amounts, and are therefore called micronutrients. But the small requirement does not mean they are unimportant. They have extensive involvement in metabolic reactions as cofactors and coenzymes. Most of the vitamins cannot be synthesized in the body, and must therefore be provided in the diet. Vitamins are classified into fat soluble (Vitamins A, D, E and K), and water soluble (Vitamin B complex and vitamin C).

Vitamin A

Vitamin A comprises a group of compounds closely related to retinol, collectively called retinoids. In food, vitamin A may be present as retinoid compounds or as the precursors of vitamim A, the carotenoid pigments. Carotenoids are all closely related to beta-carotene. Beta-carotene is transported intact into the enterocytes. In enterocytes, some of it is split : each molecule of beta-carotene yields two molecules of vitamin A. The remaining part of beta-carotene is absorbed intact into the bloodstream. It is quite possible that beta carotene may have some functions independent of retinol. Retinol can be stored in the body in the liver, and carotene in the adipose tissue. The stores can be mobilized in times of need.

Sources

The important sources of vitamin A are liver, egg yolk, butter, and fortified hydrogenated oils or margarine. Carotenoid precursors of vitamin A are found in green and yellow vegetables. Carrots are an exceptionally rich source of carotene; in fact that is the basis of the name carotene (carota, carrot).

Functions

The best understood function of vitamin A is its role in vision. In the eye, it forms a component of the rod pigment, rhodopsin. Rhodopsin functions by getting decomposed into retinaldehyde and opsin by light. The reaction is reversed in darkness. Repeated decomposition and synthesis results in loss of some vitamin A which has to be replaced from the bloodstream. Vitamin A is a component of the cone pigments also.

Other functions of vitamin A include maintenance of the integrity of epithelial tissues, growth, bone remodeling and reproduction.

The role of vitamin A in differentiation of epithelial cells has drawn considerable attention. In vitamin A deficiency, many mucus-secreting cells are replaced by keratinized cells. In vitamin A deficient cells in cultures, keratinizing cells can be converted into mucus-producing cells by addition of vitamin A to the culture medium. Vitamin A also induces the transformation of some malignant cells in culture into epithelial cells. The mechanism by which vitamin A influences differentiation is not certain but considerable experimental evidence exists for two hypotheses, which are not mutually exclusive. According to one hypothesis, vitamin A affects the transcription of certain cellular proteins. According to the other hypothesis, vitamin A alters the cell surface glycoproteins in a wide variety of cells.

Requirements

The ICMR recommended dietary allowance of Vitamin A for adults is 600 micrograms of retinol per day. If a part of the intake is in the form of beta-carotene, the intake has to be correspondingly increased because the bioavailability of beta-carotene is only about 25 percent. About 100 g of carrots or any of a large variety of green leafy vegetables can meet the daily requirement of vitamin A. It is not essential to meet the daily requirement on a daily basis because the liver can store about 50 days' supply of vitamin A. If excess of vitamin A is consumed during the season when carrots and green vegetables are readily available, it can be stored in the liver and used when the supply is deficient. Therefore, it is really a pity that vitamin A deficiency is one of the commonest nutritional deficiencies in India.

Deficiency

One of the earliest manifestations of vitamin A deficiency is prolongation of the time taken by the eye for dark adaptation. Aggravation of this handicap leads to the symptom of night blindness. In more serious and prolonged deficiency there are visible lesions in the eyes, such as Bitot spots, xerophthalamia, keratinization of the cornea, and sometimes corneal ulceration. The ulcer may heal with fibrosis leading to corneal opacity which may result in partial or total loss of vision. Vitamin A deficiency is a common preventable cause of blindness in India.

Derangement of epithelial tissues in vitamin A deficiency may lead to frequent respiratory tract infections and diarrhea, and dry skin lesions.

Vitamin D

Vitamin D is a collective term for a group of related substances, two of which are particularly important. One of them is ercalciol (ergocalciferol, vitamin D_2), which we get from vegetable sources. The other is calciol (cholecalciferol, vitamin D_3), which we get from animal sources. 7-dehydrocholesterol in the skin, when irradiated with short ultraviolet rays of the sun, yields calciol. 7-dehyrocholesterol is a normal constituent of the skin. That is why even persons who do not take enough vitamin D in diet do not get deficient in the vitamin if they receive some exposure to sunlight regularly.

Sources

In the diet, vitamin D may be obtained from liver, eggs, milk, butter, fish liver oils, and fortified hydrogenated oils. But in tropical countries like ours there is one more easy way to get vitamin D: through irradiation of 7-dehydrocholesterol in the skin by sunlight. In fair-skinned individuals it has been estimated that a 15-minute exposure of hands and face to the summer sun can yield enough vitamin D to satisfy one day's requirement of the vitamin. Ultraviolet rays cannot penetrate clouds, window glass, clothing or skin pigment. In spite of these barriers, even dark-skinned persons can manufacture substantial amounts of vitamin D if a reasonable part of the body is exposed to sunlight for a few hours every day. That is why vitamin D is also known as sunshine vitamin.

Functions

After intestinal absorption, cholecalciferol is converted into 25-hydroxycholecalciferol in the liver. The cholecalciferol that is synthesized in the skin by irradiation is also transported to the liver for the conversion. 25-hydroxycholecalciferol is transported in the bloodrsteam to the kidneys where it is further converted into 1, 25-dihydroxy cholecalciferol [1,25-$(OH)_2D_3$]. 1,25-$(OH)_2D_3$ is the active form of vitamin D. The active form of vitamin D has a profound influence on calcium and phosphorus metabolism. The influence is mediated mainly through actions on the intestine, bone, and kidneys.

In the *intestine*, vitamin D stimulates the synthesis of calcium and phosphorus binding proteins. These two proteins enhance the intestinal absorption of calcium and phosphorus respectively.

In the *kidneys*, vitamin D stimulates the reabsorption of calcium and phosphorus, thereby reducing their urinary loss and increasing their blood level.

In the *bone*, vitamin D promotes deposition of calcium. Bone mineralization is achieved by elevating the plasma calcium level. While on one hand vitamin D promotes deposition of calcium in bones, it also stimulates mobilization of calcium from bone fluids. This may be a mechanism for regulating plasma calcium level, or to allow modeling and remodeling of bones. Bone modeling and remodeling are important to shape the bones in accordance with the stress imposed on them.

The overall result of the actions of vitamin D is to prevent hypocalcemia, and to achieve adequate calcium and phosphorus deposition in the bones while at the same time allowing their modeling and remodeling.

Requirements

A person needs about 400 International Units (IU) of vitamin D per day irrespective of age. One IU is equal to 0.025 micrograms of cholecalciferol.

Deficiency

Vitamin D deficiency manifests as rickets in children. The bones are poorly calcified. Therefore the bones are too weak to bear the weight of the body. Hence the child develops bowing of legs. The ribs are also deformed. Characteristically, there is a swelling at costochondral junctions. These regularly spaced swellings on the chest look like beads of a *mala* (or rosary); the appearance has been described as rachitic rosary.

In adults vitamin D deficiency is rarer than in children. When it does occur, it manifests as poorly calcified bones which fracture with even mild trauma. The condition is known as osteomalacia (osteon, bone; malakia, softness).

Vitamin E

Vitamin E is a group of substances known as tocopherols. The most biologically active member of the group is d-alpha-tocopherol.

Sources

The major natural source of vitamin E are the vegetable oils. The vitamin E content of vegetable oils varies a lot from one oil to another. In general, the vitamin E content of an oil is directly related to its polyunsaturated fatty acid (PUFA) content. This is remarkable because our requirement of vitamin E also increases with our dietary intake of PUFA.

Functions

The main role of vitamin E in the body is as an antixodant. Free radicals which can be quenched (neutralized) by antioxidants are formed during metabolic reactions and also enter the body from the environment (e.g. ozone and nitrogen dioxide). Gradual accumulation of free radical damage is thought to be one of the contributors to the process of aging. Besides quenching free radicals, antioxidants are also required for preventing the oxidation of PUFA in cell membranes. The composition of cellular and subcellular membranes seems to be somewhat flexible. Higher the PUFA content of the diet, more is the amount of PUFA incorporated in the membranes. Therefore our vitamin E requirement varies with our PUFA intake. Antioxidants such as vitamin E protect these membranes against oxidation damage. The membranes most susceptible to oxidation damage are those of the red blood cells. Damage to red cell membranes by oxidation results in hemolysis.

The antioxidant role of vitamin E overlaps at least partly with the similar role of other antioxidants in the body such as glutathione peroxidase.

The presence of vitamin E in vegetable oils also protects the PUFA in these oils against atmospheric oxidation. Oxidation of PUFA in the oils is responsible for their rancidity.

Requirement

It is considered advisable to take about 10 mg vitamin E per day. This allowance is based on a moderate PUFA intake. However, if the PUFA intake increases, the vitamin E intake also increases simultaneously because the content of the two is related in vegetable oils. Therefore a conscious intake of about 10 mg vitamin E per day takes care of our needs irrespective of the PUFA intake.

Deficiency

In experimental animals, vitamin E deficient diets lead to sterility in males, resorption of the fetus, and muscular dystrophy. In human beings, vitamin E deficiency is extremely rare. That is why it was once thought that human beings may not need vitamin E. But now it is generally agreed that human beings also need vitamin E. Rarity of deficiency is because the vitamin is readily available in the quantities required through any ordinary diet. In human beings, deficiency may be seen in premature infants and in adults having intestinal malabsorption. The major manifestation of vitamin E deficiency in human beings is hemolytic anemia.

Vitamin K

Vitamin K is a group of chemicals collectively called quinones. The most important members of the group are phylloquinone, found in plants, and menaquinone, synthesized by bacteria and found in animal tissues.

Sources

Most of us get our supply of vitamin K from green leafy vegetables and from bacterial synthesis in the large intestine. Since absorption from the large intestine is poor, we are able to use only a part of the vitamin K that is synthesized. But still the diet and bacterial synthesis are ordinarily quite sufficient for our vitamin K requirements. Vitamin K deficiency occurs only if a person has malabsorption, or is on antibiotics (why?), or is taking a vitamin K antagonist such as dicumarol.

Functions

Vitamin K is required for the synthesis of prothrombin and coagulation factors VII, IX and X in the liver. In case of prothrombin, vitamin K catalyzes the conversion of a glutamic acid residue in the prothrombin precursor into gamma-carboxy-glutamic acid.

Requirements

Human vitamin K requirement has been estimated to be 0.4 microgram/kg body weight/day. However, half of this requirement can perhaps be met by intestinal bacterial synthesis, and only half needs to be supplied in the diet. An intake of 30 micrograms/day would prevent deficiency in all healthy adults.

Deficiency

Vitamin K deficiency is rarely due to poor intake. It is generally due to malabsorption, vitamin K antagonists or antibiotics. Liver disease may give rise to a similar picture. The manifestations are bleeding tendency, prolonged prothrombin time, and low serum prothrombin level.

Thiamine

Thiamine is popularly known as vitamin B_1. As the name suggests, it is a sulphur (*thio*) and nitrogen (*amine*) containing compound.

Sources

The most important sources of thiamine in the Indian diet are cereals and pulses. More than 90% of the thiamine in grains resides in the husk and germ, which are both removed during milling. That is why the poor man's diet consisting almost exclusively of polished rice has been associated with thiamine deficiency. Repeated washing of rice, soaking of legumes for a long time in water which is discarded, and use of baking soda to hasten the cooking of legumes, are all practices which enhance the loss of thiamine from the diet. Besides whole grains, other sources of thiamine in the diet include vegetables, milk and milk products, and various flesh foods, specially pork.

Functions

The active forms of thiamine are thiamine pyrophosphate (TPP) and thiamine diphosphate (TDP) which are both coenzymes in carbohydrate metabolism. TPP is too large a molecule to pass through the enterocyte membrane intact. It is split in the intestine, and then resynthesized by body cells as and when required.

Requirements

Since the main role of thiamine is in carbohydrate metabolism, the requirement depends on the energy intake, which in turn should be guided by the energy requirements. An intake of 0.5 mg thiamine per 1000 kcal energy intake is ordinarily quite satisfactory. While in alcoholics the intake of thiamine may be poor due to malnutrition, the requirement is actually increased because thiamine is involved in the metabolism of acetaldehyde, an intermediate compound in alcohol metabolism. Thiamine requirement may also be increased in heavy tea drinkers because of the presence of a heat-stable thiaminase in tea.

Deficiency

Mild deficiency may give rise to vague symptoms such as anorexia, depression, mental confusion and instability of mood. Severe deficiency gives rise to *beriberi*, which may take two forms. In wet beriberi, damage to the heart muscle leads to edema and eventually heart failure and death. In dry beriberi, there is loss of body tissue resulting in emaciation. In both wet and dry beriberi, there is numbness of limbs due to peripheral polyneuritis, and mental confusion or irritability, probably due to the involvement of the central nervous system.

Riboflavin

Riboflavin is popularly known as vitamin B_2. It is a compound with an intensely yellow color.

Sources

Whole cereals are a good source of riboflavin. However, refining of cereals results in loss of up to 60% of their riboflavin content. Milk and milk products, and flesh foods are also good sources of riboflavin.

Functions

Riboflavin is a component of the two coenzymes, flavin mononucleotide (FMN) and flavin adenine dinucleotide (FAD). FMN and FAD occur in cells in combination with proteins known as flavoproteins. FMN and FAD act as hydrogen or proton acceptors in biological oxidation reactions in mitochondria. Riboflavin is also involved in the conversion of tryptophan into another B vitamin, niacin (see below). Riboflavin is also required for conversion of another B vitamin, folic acid (see below) into its coenzyme form. Thus riboflavin plays an indirect role also in the functions attributed to niacin and folic acid.

Requirements

Because of its involvement in energy metabolism, riboflavin requirement is also related to energy intake. An allowance of 0.6 mg/1000 kcal meets the requirements of all age groups satisfactorily.

Deficiency

Clinical manifestations of riboflavin deficiency are centered around the mouth. There may be cracks at the corners of the mouth *(angular stomatitis)*, lips may be inflamed *(cheilosis)* (*cheilos*, lip), and tongue may become smooth and purplish red *(glossitis)*. These symptoms appear only after the deficiency has been present for many months, and disappear promptly on administration of riboflavin.

Niacin

Niacin is a group of compounds including nicotinic acid and nicotinamide, which all have similar biological activity. The names derive from the fact that the vitamin was first obtained by oxidation of nicotine, and this form was called nicotinic acid.

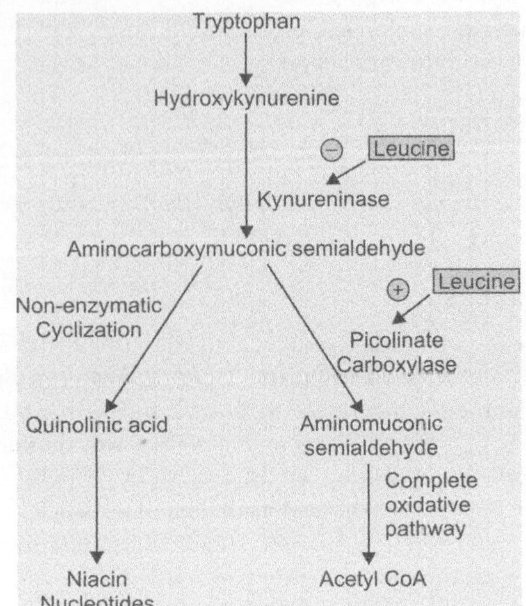

Fig. 9.9 Some of the metabolic pathways of tryptophan. The pathway on the left shows the conversion to niacin. That is why tryptophan deficiency may lead to niacin deficiency. Leucine inhibits kynureninase and activates picolinate carboxylase. That is why excess of leucine reduces the synthesis of niacin from tryptophan.

Sources

Niacin is present in cereals but more than 90% of the vitamin resides in the husk. Niacin may also be obtained from legumes and flesh foods. Besides using preformed niacin, the body can also synthesize niacin from the amino acid tryptophan (Fig. 9.9). Maize protein is very poor in tryptophan. That is why niacin deficiency is common among populations subsisting almost exclusively on maize (*makki*). Maize protein is very poor in tryptophan.

It has been observed in India that populations subsisting almost exclusively on jowar (*Sorghum vulgare*) also develop niacin deficiency. But jowar protein is not deficient in tryptophan. It was first pointed out by Gopalan and Srikantia from the National Institute of Nutrition, Hyderabad, in 1960 that jowar protein has a particularly high leucine content which may be the factor responsible for the pellagragenic effect of jowar. It was also observed that isoleucine could correct the pellagragenic effect of leucine. It has been subsequently observed that leucine inhibits kynureninase competitively, and also increases the diversion of aminocarboxymuconic semialdehyde into the total oxidative pathway (Fig. 9.9). Both these actions of leucine reduce the conversion of tryptophan into niacin, and thereby predispose to pellagra. The leucine hypothesis is one of the most brilliant pieces of nutrition research to have originated from India. But the hypothesis is still highly controversial because not all subsequent studies done elsewhere support it. One possible reason is that high dietary leucine has to be accompanied by a marked dietary deficiency of both tryptophan and niacin to precipitate pellagra. Many investigators have not ensured this in their experiments and have therefore failed to reproduce the Indian findings. In human populations subsisting on jowar, the combination of high leucine intake and low intake of tryptophan and niacin does exist, and is possibly responsible for the high incidence of pellagra.

It would also be observed in Figure 9.9 that conversion of tryptophan into niacin needs at least three other vitamins—thiamine, riboflavin and pyridoxine. Hence a deficiency of any of these vitamins might also lead to niacin deficiency. That is one reason why it is so difficult to separate clearly the manifestations of deficiency of individual members of the vitamin B complex. The other reason is that the sources of different vitamins also overlap. Hence a diet deficient in one vitamin is generally deficient also in other vitamins. Therefore in practice we generally come across multiple nutritional deficiency in the same person rather than an isolated deficiency of a single substance. Syndromes due to deficiency of a single vitamin can be produced only by using specially designed diets, as is done in studies conducted for academic reasons.

Functions

Niacin is a component of the coenzymes nicotinamide adenine dinucleotide (NAD) and nicotinamide adenine dinucleotide phosphate (NADP). NAD and NADP participate in redox reactions by accepting and transferring hydrogen. Thus, like thiamin and riboflavin, niacin also plays a vital role in utilization of carbohydrates, proteins and fats in all cells of the body.

Requirements

Since niacin is involved in energy metabolism, its requirements are also related to energy intake. A niacin intake of about 7 mg/1000 kcal is generally satisfactory. However, the entire quantity need not be preformed niacin. Part of the requirement can be met by conversion of tryptophan into niacin. Quantitatively, the yield is 1 mg of niacin from about 60 mg of tryptophan.

Deficiency

Clinically, niacin deficiency manifests as pellagra. Pellagra affects the function of gastrointestinal tract, skin and nervous system giving rise to the symptom complex of the three Ds, diarrhea, dermatitis and dementia. The dermatitis of pellagra affects clearly demarcated areas on parts of the body exposed to sunlight. The neural involvement may initially produce headache and irritability. But severe deficiency eventually leads to psychiatric symptoms such as hallucinations, delusions and depression.

Pantothenic Acid

Pantothenic acid is a compound incorporating an alanine moiety and a pantoic acid moiety.

Sources

Pantothenic acid is widely distributed in plant as well as animal foods. Refining of cereals and heat processing result in appreciable loss of pantothenic acid as well as several other vitamins.

Functions

The body uses pantothenic acid to synthesize coenzyme A (CoA). Coenzyme A further activates acetate to form acetyl CoA. Acetyl CoA is a vital reactant in the Krebs cycle. Thus pantothenic acid is essential for obtaining energy from carbohydrates, fats or proteins. Acetyl CoA is also a precursor of triglycerides, cholesterol, hemoglobin and acetylcholine synthesized in the body.

Requirements

Based on the intake data of healthy individuals, the pantothenic acid requirement of adults has been estimated to be 4 to 7 mg/day.

Deficiency

Because of its ubiquitous nature, clear pantothenic acid deficiency is rare in human beings. Mild deficiency may, however, give rise to nonspecific symptoms such as poor resistance to stresses like infection.

Biotin

Biotin is a group of closely related compounds. The naturally occurring d-biotin is cis-tetrahydro-2-oxothieno (3,4-d)-imidazoline-4-valeric acid.

Sources

Biotin is a ubiquitous vitamin present in appreciable amounts in almost all foods. Particularly rich sources include liver, kidney, yeast and legumes. Biotin synthesized by bacterial flora of the gut also makes a small contribution to our biotin intake.

Functions

Biotin is a coenzyme for a large number of carboxylation reactions. These reactions occur during oxidation of carbohydrates and fats, and synthesis of fatty acids. Biotin is also required for some deamination reactions, protein synthesis, and conversion of tryptophan into niacin. Thus biotin has vital roles in carbohydrate, fat as well as protein metabolism.

Requirements

The biotin requirement of adults has been estimated to be 100-200 micrograms/day. Intestinal bacteria also seem to make a substantial contribution to biotin supply of the body.

Deficiency

Under ordinary circumstances biotin deficiency is unknown. It may be induced experimentally by combining a low biotin diet with raw egg white. Raw egg white contains a protein, avidin, which binds biotin. The complex cannot be absorbed by the intestines, thereby inducing biotin deficiency. Heat denatures avidin, and therefore cooked egg white does not induce biotin deficiency. Although this fact is widely talked about, it is not of much practical importance. It has been found that a person has to take the whites of about 25 raw eggs a day to get biotin deficiency !

Pyridoxine

Pyridoxine, also called vitamin B_6, comprises of a group of at least three related compounds, pyridoxol, pyridoxal and pyridoxamine, all with similar biological activity.

Sources

The richest sources of pyridoxine are high protein foods such as meat, egg and liver. Considerable quantities are also present in grains, specially in the husk. Fruits, vegetables and milk are poor as sources of pyridoxine.

Functions

The biologically active form of pyridoxine is pyridoxal phosphate (PLP). PLP is a coenzyme in several reactions in protein metabolism such as transamination, deamination, and decarboxylation of amino acids. Decarboxylation is involved in the synthesis of serotonin, histamine and norepinphrine from amino acids. Pyridoxine is also required for conversion of tryptophan into niacin.

Requirements

Since pyridoxine is required for protein metabolism, its requirements depend on protein intake, and are thought to be about 0.02 mg/g dietary protein.

Deficiency

Pyridoxine deficiency is rather uncommon. But when it does occur, it may result in poor growth, anemia, and neurological symptoms such as nervousness, irritability, insomnia and convulsions.

The common antitubercular drug, isoniazid (INH) is a pyridoxine antagonist. Since pyridoxine is involved in conversion of tryptophan into niacin, INH may also precipitate niacin deficiency. That is why patients on INH are also given vitamin B complex, specially pyridoxine and niacin.

Folic Acid

Folic acid, or folacin, is pteroylglutamic acid. Its molecule is a combination of pterin, para-aminobenzoic acid, and glutamic acid. The vitamin, as present in food, may have one to seven glutamic acid residues per molecule. The extra glutamic acid residues are removed in the gastrointestinal tract.

Sources

As its name suggests, folic acid (*folium*, leaf) is abundant in green leafy vegetables. It may also be obtained from fruits, wheat germ, liver, kidney and yeast.

Functions

Folic acid, in the form of tetrahydrofolic acid (THFA), is required as a coenzyme for all single carbon transfer reactions in the body. It is also involved in the synthesis of purines and pyrimidines, which form a part of DNA and RNA molecules. Hence folic acid is particularly important for the integrity of rapidly dividing cells such as blood cells. Its other role in physiology of blood is in the synthesis of the porphyrin moiety of the hemoglobin molecule.

Requirements

The ICMR recommends 100 micrograms of folate intake per day for adult males and nonpregnant females, and 300 micrograms per day for pregnant females. These levels of intake not only prevent deficiency but also maintain normal blood levels of folate.

Deficiency

Folate deficiency is fairly widespread thoughout the world. The deficiency is specially common during pregnancy. Its best studied and most prominent manifestation is a variety of megaloblastic anemia. A similar anemia may sometimes be due to the deficiency of vitamin B_{12} and it is important to distinguish between the two as discussed later in the chapter.

Cobalamin

Cobalamin, or vitamin B_{12}, is a complex molecule containing cobalt and resembles hemoglobin in its structure. It exists in many forms : as cyanocobalamin, which is synthesized by bacteria; and as hydroxycobalamin and methylcobalamin, which are found in dairy products.

Sources

Vitamin B_{12} is unique in that it is available only in animal foods. It is synthesized by bacteria residing in the rumen of animals, absorbed, and stored in tissues. Bacteria residing in the human colon also synthesize vitamin B_{12} but it cannot be absorbed from there. Therefore human beings must have their supply of vitamin B_{12} from animal foods, viz. milk and milk products, liver, kidney and other flesh foods.

Functions

The active form of vitamin B_{12} is the cobamide coenzyme, which can be synthesized from the dietary vitamin B_{12} with the help of riboflavin, niacin and manganese.

Vitamin B_{12} supplies methyl groups for the synthesis of DNA. Therefore the vitamin is important for cell division, and its deficiency specially affects rapidly dividing cells such as blood cells.

Vitamin B_{12} also has a unique role in neural function, the precise nature of which is not understood. Some plausible suggestions are that the role may be related to the participation of vitamin B_{12} in carbohydrate metabolism in neurons or in lipid metabolism in the myelin sheath.

Requirements

Vitamin B_{12} is required in very small amounts; quantities even less than 1 microgram per day seem sufficient. It has been recommended by ICMR that about 1 microgram per day be consumed as a safe allowance. However, this allowance need not necessarily be supplied on a daily basis because in a well nourished individual, the liver stores about 1 mg vitamin B_{12} which can last 1000 days in case of lack of dietary vitamin B_{12}.

Deficiency

Vitamin B_{12} deficiency is rare in India. When it does occur, it is generally due to special circumstances. It may be either due to poor absorption due to deficiency of the gastric intrinsic factor, or due to a strictly vegetarian diet from which even milk and milk products are completely excluded.

The deficiency manifests as a variety of megaloblastic anemia known as pernicious anemia. It is called pernicious because, if not treated in time, it progresses to a serious form in which the central nervous system is involved. The typical neural lesion of pernicious anemia is subacute combined degeneration of the spinal cord, which involves defective myelination of peripheral nerves as well as of the posterior and lateral columns of the spinal cord.

It is important to distinguish between vitamin B_{12} and folic acid deficiency because if folic acid is given in vitamin B_{12} deficiency, the megaloblastic anemia does respond but the neurological lesions continue to progress silently. Thus the improvement in anemia is deceptive and may lead to an unjustified complacency. It has been hypothesized that neurological damage in vitamin B_{12} deficiency is due to the requirement of B_{12} for conversion of propionate into methylmalonate. The hypothesis is probably incorrect because available evidence points against it, but it has been mentioned here because no better explanation has been proposed so far.

Folate-B_{12} Interaction

The facts that deficiency of either folate or vitamin B_{12} gives rise to similar type of anemia, and that not only folate deficiency anemia but also vitamin B_{12} deficiency anemia responds to folate therapy, have a metabolic basis. The conversion of deoxyuridylate into thymidylate is made possible by donation of a one-carbon unit by 5,10-methylene tetrahydrofolic acid (THFA). Regeneration of 5,10-methylene THFA requires that 5-methyl THFA donate its methyl group to B_{12} which acts as an intermediary in conversion of homocystine into methionine. Hence in vitamin B_{12} deficiency, 5-methyl THFA accumulates, giving rise to a deficiency of 5, 10-methylene THFA required for thymidylate synthesis. The phenomenon has been called methylfolate trap. The trap can be properly corrected by giving vitamin B_{12} . But it can also be temporarily circumvented by giving excess of folic acid which can generate 5,10-methylene THFA.

Ascorbic Acid

Ascorbic acid is popularly known as vitamin C.

Sources

In contrast with vitamin B_{12}, vitamin C is found only in plant foods. It is well known that the richest sources of vitamin C are amla (*Emblica officinalis*), lime, lemons and oranges. But substantial amounts are also present in potato and fresh green vegetables. However the high vulnerability of vitamin C to heat and oxidation reduces the intake to levels far below those predicted from food composition tables.

Functions

Vitamin C is essential for hydroxylation of proline and lysine residues in connective tissue during the synthesis of collagen. Vitamin C is also involved in the formation of dentin in the teeth, and the neurotransmitters norepinephrine and serotonin in the central nervous systmem. Vitamin C also functions as an antioxidant in the body.

Requirements

Although the requirements are controversial, the recommended intake of 40 mg per day is sufficient to prevent any obvious manifestations of deficiency. Larger intakes may be required after major injuries or surgery to facilitate formation of connective tissue during healing. Whether large doses of vitamin C improve the resistance of the body to common cold and other infections is still not settled. Vitamin C, in a dose of about 1 g per day, may reduce the severity of symptoms of common cold. However, such large doses should not be taken beyond a few days at a time because of the possible adverse effects. First, high doses increase the requirement, and thus induce dependence on large intakes. Second, since vitamin C is excreted as oxalic acid, high doses may increase the formation of renal stones.

Deficiency

Severe form of vitamin C deficiency is called scurvy. It affects particularly tissues where connective tissue is functionally more important, such as blood vessels, leading to abnormal petechial hemorrhages under the skin. Bleeding of the gums is a common symptom. Bleeding in joints may lead to joint pains. In addition, there is generalized weakness, and flaccidity of muscles which may give rise to the frog posture in infants.

Vitamin Pills: Yes or No

Vitamins are a unique class of nutrients to which even some highly acclaimed specialists have ascribed almost magical effects. No wonder, different doctors often give contradictory advice to healthy persons on whether to take a vitamin supplement regularly. On one hand, taking a pill is far less expensive and far more convenient than ensuring an equivalent intake of vitamins through the diet. This is so because of the high susceptibility of vitamins to losses during storage, cooking, processing, etc. In view of this uncertainty, many doctors feel justified in advocating the regular use of a supplement as a sort of insurance against vitamin deficiencies. The practice is generally harmless. On the other hand, the complacency generated by the vitamin supplement may lead to neglect of nutrition in other respects. Vitamins are not a substitute for a balanced diet. Further, taking an excess of some vitamins may make the body accustomed to high intakes. If due to any reason the supplement is then discontinued, the person finds it difficult to manage on a normal vitamin intake. The result is that in spite of a normal intake, the person shows signs of vitamin deficiency. There is no absolute deficiency, but there is a relative deficiency because the requirements have become abnormally high due to prolonged high intakes of the vitamin. This phenomenon has been shown in case of vitamin C. Although even moderately high intakes of most vitamins are quite safe, toxicity has been observed following large doses of vitamins A, D, E and K, and niacin and pyridoxine. The beneficial effects of large doses of antioxidant vitamins such as vitamin E, vitamin C, or beta-carotene, which are in vogue these days are also controversial. The arguments for and against regular use of vitamin supplements have been given in Table 9.7.

In view of the above discussion it is clearly not possible to give a definite verdict on the question of regular vitamin supplements. If there is the slightest doubt about the diet being deficient in vitamins, a supplement should be taken. If a person is under physical or mental stress, a supplement should be taken because stress increases vitamin requirements.

Table 9.7 Pros and cons of regular vitamin supplementation

Pros	*Cons*
Inexpensive	Neglect of balanced diet
Convenient	Getting accustomed to high intake
Insurance against deficiency	High doses are not absolutely safe
Harmless	Not enough evidence that excess is useful

If a person feels more comfortable having the insurance cover of a daily vitamin pill, even then the supplement may be taken. But under all these circumstances, the supplement taken should be one which supplies vitamins in doses which are fairly close to the recommended daily allowances (RDA). Supplements containing a much larger dose than the RDA of any vitamin should not be taken except for short periods on medical advice. Finally, in our age of excessive dependence on science and technology it is well to remember that the human race has survived and thrived through much of its past without vitamin supplements. If it has been possible for thousands of years, it is possible even now.

MINERALS

Like vitamins, minerals are also nutrients which are required only in small quantities but perform vital functions in the body. When a food is burnt, for instance in a bomb calorimeter, a small quantity of ash is left behind. Minerals are present in the ash. More than twenty minerals are now considered essential nutrients. Nutrient minerals are classified into macronutrients and micronutrients depending on their relative tissue content. Micronutrients are also called trace elements. In general, animal foods are a better source of minerals than plant foods. In cereals and legumes, the minerals are concentrated in the outermost layers, i.e. the husk. Therefore refining of food grains results in considerable mineral (and vitamin) loss.

Here we shall discuss only a few selected minerals (calcium, phosphorus, iron, iodine, zinc and selenium) and related substances called electrolytes (sodium, potassium, and fluorine). The selection is based on considerations such as the quantity in the body, relative importance as a nutrient, prevalence of deficiency, and the level of our knowledge about the nutrient.

Calcium

The body of an adult has about 1 kg calcium, of which about 99 percent is in bones and teeth.

Sources

The best sources of calcium in the diet are milk and milk products. Grains not only have less calcium, their calcium is less efficiently absorbed. In areas where water has a high mineral content, drinking water may provide upto a quarter of the daily calcium requirements.

Functions

Quantitatively, the most important functions of calcium reside in bones and teeth. In bone, calcium salts are deposited on the collagen matrix, thereby imparting rigidity to the bones. In teeth, calcium salts are deposited in dentin and enamel.

Although quantitatively less significant, calcium has several other very important functions in the body. Calcium ions are essential for the generation of thromboplastin during the process of clotting. A normal calcium ion concentration is essential for normal neuromuscular excitability. Calcium ions are also involved in the activation of several enzymes in the body.

Requirements

Calcium requirements have been difficult to establish for various reasons. The absorption of calcium is affected by a very large number of factors such as vitamin D, lactose, and phosphorus content of the diet, and also the body's need for calcium. Dietary fiber, oxalates and phytates may reduce the absorption of calcium. High protein diets may increase urinary calcium excretion. However, in India the recommended dietary allowance in healthy adults is 400 mg per day under ordinary circumstances, and 1000 mg per day during pregnancy and lactation.

Deficiency

There is no clear calcium deficiency syndrome. This may be because of the remarkable adaptation to low intakes by improvement in absorption and reduction in calcium excretion. However, calcium metabolism shows abnormalities in vitamin D deficiency, hypo- and hyperparathyroidism, and senile osteoporosis.

Phosphorus

The body of an adult has about 600 g phosphorus, of which about 90 percent is in bones and teeth.

Sources

Phosphorus is widely distributed in foods. The concentration of phosphorus is particularly high in protein rich foods. Aerated soft drinks and processed foods contain considerable amounts of phosphorus. Excessive consumption of these foods may unduly lower the calcium/phosphorus ratio of the diet.

Functions

Phosphorus is required for a wide range of body functions. The key molecules involved in energy transactions of the body, ATP, ADP and AMP, contain phosphorus. Phosphorylation of enzymes is a key step in mediating the action of various hormones, neurotransmitters and neuroactive peptides. Phosphate groups form a part of DNA and RNA molecules. Although these are all vital and generalized functions of phosphorus, quantitatively the most significant contribution of phosphorus is in the form of calcium salts in bones and teeth.

Requirements

It is desirable that the phosphorus intake should be less than twice the calcium intake. The ICMR recommendation is that phosphorus intake should be equal to calcium intake, i.e. 400 mg per day under ordinary circumstances, and 1000 mg per day during pregnancy and lactation.

Deficiency

Phosphorus deficiency is unknown in human beings under ordinary circumstances. Special circumstances in which it may occur include renal dialysis, and excessive use of antacids containing aluminium hydroxide, which reduces phosphorus absorption.

Iron

The body of an adult has about 4 g iron, roughly the same as the amount in a medium-sized nail. About two-thirds of the body iron exists in the form of hemoglobin. The remaining iron is in the form of myoglobin, cytochromes, transferrin, ferritin, and storage iron (hemosiderin).

Sources

The important sources of iron in the food are green leafy vegetables, potatoes, legumes, fruits and flesh foods, specially liver. In grains, iron is concentrated in the husk. Milk is a poor source of iron. It is thought that in olden days when cooking in iron utensils was common, the utensils contributed significant amounts of iron to the diet.

Food iron is often divided into heme iron and nonheme iron. The intestinal absorption of heme iron is much better (upto 30 percent may be absorbed) than that of nonheme iron. The factors affecting absorption of iron have been discussed in Chapter 8.

Functions

The most significant function of iron is in oxidation-reduction reactions. It contributes to this function in the form of hemoglobin and myoglobin by carrying oxygen, and in the form of cytochromes as an electron carrier. Thus iron is essential for generation of energy through metabolic reactions.

The other functions of iron include antibody production and synthesis of purines, which are a component of DNA and RNA.

Requirements

Iron is a highly protected mineral. The body loses very little iron through the usual routes of excretion. An adult man loses only about 1 mg iron per day, and a woman upto 2 mg per day due to menstrual losses. However, because of poor intestinal absorption from mixed cereal diets prevalent in India, the food should contain about thirty times as much iron as the quantity lost every day. The ICMR recommendation is that an adult man should take 28 mg iron per day, an adult nonpregnant woman 30 mg per day, and a pregnant woman 38 mg per day. Supplying this quantity of iron through the diet on a regular basis can be very difficult because the consumption of green vegetables is extremely poor in India. The problem is compounded by chronic intestinal blood loss due to hookworm infestation, which increases the iron requirement considerably. Therefore supplying iron through fortification of common salt has been given serious consideration. Salt is a suitable vehicle for fortification because it is consumed regularly in predictable amounts by all sections of the society. A long series of studies done at the National Institute of Nutrition, Hyderabad, has shown that fortifying salt with a mixture of ferric orthophosphate (3500 mg/kg) and sodium hydrogen sulphate (5000 mg/kg) gives a combination which provides 1 mg iron/g of salt. The bioavailability of iron from the combination is equivalent to that from ferrous sulphate. The color of the combination is not different from that of common salt, and its color or chemistry do not alter appreciably on storage.

Deficiency

Iron deficiency leads to a microcytic hypochromic anemia, which has been discussed in Chapter 4.

Iodine

Iodine metabolism in the body is intimately linked to thyroid function (Chapter 11).

Sources

The iodine content of water and foods, both plant and animal, varies from one region to another, and depends on the iodine content of the soil in the region. In general, areas far removed from the sea coast, such as hilly areas, have an iodine-deficient soil. In order to make up for this deficiency salt is iodized in these areas by adding potassium iodate at a level which achieves an iodine concentration of at least 30 ppm at the manufacturers' level. This makes it reasonably sure that an iodine content of at least 15 ppm is present at the consumers' level. Assuming a daily salt intake of 10 g, iodized salt containing 15 ppm iodine supplies 150 micrograms of iodine everyday.

Functions

Iodine functions in the body in the form of thyroid hormones.

Requirements

The requirement of iodine is a meagre 1 microgram/kg body weight.

Deficiency

Iodine deficiency has long been known to be endemic in the sub-himalayan belt in India. Now it has been discovered that less frequent but still endemic levels of iodine deficiency exist not only in hilly areas but also in coastal areas and the plains in other parts of the country. Iodine deficiency may be direct due to deficient intake, or indirect due to consumption of foods containing antithyroid substances (or goitrogens). Goitrogens are present in many plants of the genus Brassica such as cabbage, turnip, radish, etc. Although not much data is available on goitrogen consumption in India, there are pockets with endemic goiter where the frequency of goiter cannot be accounted for by the urinary iodine excretion levels, which are quite high. These observations suggest that the high prevalence of goiter may be due to consumption of goitrogens. The compounding effect of goitrogens on iodine deficiency exists in its worst form in Central Africa where goitrogen consumption is high due to the staple being cassava. Iodine deficiency leads to various forms and degrees of thyroid disorders as discussed in Chapter 11.

Zinc

Zinc is a mineral which has been added to the list of essential nutrients relatively recently. The body of an adult contains about 2 g zinc, about 75 percent of which is in bones. Other tissues with relatively high concentration of zinc are skin, hair and testes. Circulating zinc is concentrated in red blood cells. Serum zinc is largely bound to proteins. Use of oral contraceptive pills leads to a fall in serum zinc levels.

Sources

Cereals and legumes contain significant amounts of zinc but the absorption of zinc from these sources is limited by phytic acid. Flesh foods, particularly sea foods, are very good sources of zinc, but are not a part of the regular diet for a large majority of mankind. Because of these difficulties, it seems that at least a marginal deficiency of zinc may be quite widespread throughout the world.

Functions

Zinc is a part of several enzymes known as metalloenzymes. These enzymes include carbonic anhydrase, carboxypeptidase, alkaline phosphatase, DNA polymerase and RNA polymerase. It is also a cofactor in the activation of zinc-dependent enzymatic reactions, e.g. the synthesis of collagen.

At a functional level, zinc seems to be essential for normal growth, reproductive function, wound healing, and normal acuity of the sense of taste and smell. Current state of our knowledge still does not allow correlating the enzymatic functions with gross functions.

Requirements

Based on data from zinc balance studies and the reasonable assumption that only 25 percent of dietary zinc is absorbed, it has been recommended that an adult should take 15 mg zinc per day. The requirements are slightly higher during the growth spurt, pregnancy and lactation.

Deficiency

Zinc deficiency was first discovered in Iran in 1961 as the cause of a prevalent syndrome characterized by poor growth and slow sexual development. It was found that the deficiency was due to a diet consisting almost exclusively of unleavened whole wheat bread. Because of the high fiber and phytate content of diet, the absorption of zinc from such a diet is very poor. Zinc deficiency is also prevalent in Egypt where the problem is compounded by loss of zinc through blood loss due to hookworm infestation. Now it is generally felt that milder forms of zinc deficiency are extremely common in many other countries, including the developed countries.

Besides poor physical and reproductive growth, poor wound healing, loss of appetite, diminished acuity of taste and smell, and several skin disorders have been attributed to zinc deficiency.

Zinc deficiency may also be precipitated by iron supplements. Iron and zinc possibly share some intestinal transport mechanisms. Therefore large doses of iron reduce the absorption of zinc, thereby precipitating zinc deficiency.

Selenium

Selenium is an essential nutrient required in very small amounts. The selenium content of diet depends on the selenium content of soil. Since the selenium content of soil varies considerably from one region to another, both selenium deficiency and toxicity of dietary origin are known.

Source

If the soil of the region where the food has originated has adequate selenium, food will have adequate selenium. Selenium is present in both plant and animal foods and its content is higher in foods with higher protein content. Refining of grains, and boiling of vegetables results in considerable loss of selenium.

Functions

Selenium is a part of the antioxidant system of the body. It is incorporated in glutathione peroxidse, an enzyme which prevents peroxidation of fats present in cellular and subcellular membranes. Thus the functions of selenium overlap with those of vitamin E. Hence the role of selenium, like that of other antioxidants, may be to retard the aging process and to prevent cancer.

Requirements

The recommended intake for selenium is 1 microgram per kg body weight.

Deficiency and Toxicity

It has been claimed that the incidence of cancer in a region is inversely related to the selenium content of the soil. While this statement may not be strictly true, selenium deficiency possibly does predispose to some cancers.

Keshan disease, characterized by degeneration of cardiac muscle, is prevalent in some parts of China. Selenium has been shown to have a beneficial effect in the disease.

Taking selenium in high doses for a long time has been reported to cause loss of hair.

Sodium

Sodium is the principal cation of the extracellular fluids. It suggests that the most primitive forms of life probably originated in sea water. The concentration of sodium in the intracellular fluids is kept low by a pump in the cell membrane which continually pumps sodium ions out of the cell.

Sources

Considerable amount of sodium is present naturally in food. But consuming some additional sodium as sodium chloride to improve the taste of food is an almost universal practice.

Functions

As the principal cation of extracellular fluids, sodium is the major contributor to the osmotic pressure of these fluids. In this way sodium helps regulate the total fluid volume of the body as well as the balance between extracellular and intracellular fluids.

Sodium, as sodium bicarbonate, forms a part of the bicarbonate-carbonic acid buffer system of the body. In this way sodium helps regulate the pH of body fluids.

Hence by regulating osmolarity and pH of extracellular fluids, sodium makes important contributions to maintenance of constancy of the internal environment. It provides the cells an optimal and relatively constant environment in which they can function normally.

Requirements

There are certain minimum urinary, fecal and cutaneous losses of sodium which have to be replaced. In addition, considerable amounts can be lost in sweat in hot environment. All these losses can be replaced by an intake of about 150 mg sodium. But a diet containing only 150 mg sodium has a very poor taste. Therefore most of us voluntarily consume much more sodium than the minimum requirement. In tropical climates, additional sodium losses in the sweat enhance the requirements. From the viewpoint of prevention of heart disease, experts currently recommend a sodium intake of less than 3 g/day, which corresponds to a sodium chloride intake of less than 7.5 g/day. This quantity would usually be more than enough to meet the requirements even in tropical climates.

Deficiency and Excess

Sodium requirement is so little in relation to its liberal supply in foods that sodium deficiency is essentially unknown. However, consuming much more sodium than we need is thought to be responsible for a tendency towards high blood pressure. Therefore those with hypertension, or at risk of atherosclerosis, are advised to restrict sodium in the diet. Sodium restriction is also advised when there is accumulation of excess extracellular fluid (edema). Sodium restriction may be achieved by avoiding the use of table salt, and eliminating from the diet preserved foods and pickles, chutneys, snacks, processed and preserved foods, and salted butter.

Potassium

Potassium is the principal cation of the intracellular fluid. Since the concentration of potassium in intracellular fluid is normally constant, measurement of body potassium is one of the methods for determining intracellular fluid volume as well as cell mass of the body. The cell mass derived from total body potassium is close to the lean body mass because adipose tissue has very little intracellular fluid and hence very little potassium.

Sources

Potassium is an almost universal constituent of food, specially of fruits and vegetables. It may be lost in cooking water. On the other hand, additional potassium may be present in the form of additives in processed foods.

Functions

Potassium is an essential contituent of cells. Hence potassium is required when cell mass has to grow, as during body growth. Potassium is one of the two major ionic participants in maintenance of resting membrane potential and genesis of action potential, the other participant being sodium. Potassium ions form one of the minor mechanisms for maintenance of acid base balance of the body. In acidosis, potassium ions start leaving the cells to enter extracellular fluids in order to regulate the extracellular pH.

Requirements

The minimum potassium requirement of an adult is about 2 g per day. Many persons take as much as three times the minimum requirement, which seems to be harmless.

Deficiency

Potassium deficiency may occur due to excessive loss, as in diarrhea, vomiting, heavy sweating, use of digitalis (a drug for some heart diseases), or use of diuretics (drugs which increase urinary volume). Heavy potassium loss from the body may cause weakness and muscle cramps. Potassium deficiency is best corrected through natural foods, e.g. oranges, lemons or lime.

Fluorine

Fluorine is an element of which both deficiency and excess are harmful and are known to occur in different parts of the world.

Sources

The principal source of fluorine is drinking water which contains fluorine in the form of fluorides.

Functions

Fluorine is deposited in bones and teeth in the form of fluorapatite crystals. In the bones, these crystals reduce mineral resorption and thereby prevent osteoporosis. In the teeth, presence of fluorapatite crystals in enamel confers resistance to acids, thereby preventing dental cavities.

Requirements

The fluoride requirement of the body seems to be about 2 mg per day. This requirement is optimally met when drinking water has 1 ppm fluoride.

Deficiency and Excess

The main ill effect of fluoride deficiency is dental caries. This is often quantified in terms of the DMF index, which includes the decaying, missing and filled teeth. In areas where fluoride deficiency is prevalent, fluoridation of water is one way to supply adequate fluoride to the population. Other methods include the use of sodium fluoride tablets. Some benefit is also obtained by topical application, as by using a fluoride containing toothpaste.

The ill effects of excess fluoride intake (fluorosis) also manifest in teeth and bones. If fluoride intake is excessive during development of teeth, the dental enamel shows mottling. The degree of mottling can vary from slight discoloration to extensive chalkiness of the surface. The teeth may show pitting and chipping due to erosion of the mottled areas. But even severley mottled teeth are resistant to dental caries. In fluorosis, bones show excessive deposition of calcium. Even the ligaments may show calcification. As a result there is pain in the joints, and the vertebral column may become stiff. Skeletal fluorosis is a much more serious problem than dental fluorosis.

At molecular level, studies by Dr AK Susheela and her colleagues have shown that in fluorosis collagen synthesis is reduced, and the colla-gen that is synthesized is inadequately cross-linked.

In India fluorosis is endemic in Andhra Pradesh, Haryana, Punjab, Tamil Nadu and Uttar Pradesh. Newer belts of endemic fluorosis have been identified recently so that now about twelve states are known to be seriously affected by the problem. Since the major problem in our country is fluorosis rather than fluorine deficiency, there is no justification for fluoride toothpastes in India.

Mineral Supplements

Fortunately fads about minerals are not as widespread as those about vitamins. Even so, the arguements for and against regular supplementation apply as much to minerals as to vitamins (see Table 9.7). One should particularly avoid supplements containing many times the normal requirement of iron, zinc or any other mineral because of their potentially harmful effects.

RECOMMENDED DIETARY ALLOWANCES

Nutrition experts have prepared for ready reference a list of essential nutrients and the quantity of each which, in their opinion, will meet the needs of nearly every member of a healthy population. The quantities recommended are called recommended dietary allowances (RDAs). In spite of the limitations and pitfalls of RDAs, they have some value, specially when dealing with a population. Application of RDAs to guide or evaluate the intake of an individual needs caution and may lead to erroneous conclusions.

A summary of the RDAs of a few selected nutrients is presented in Table 9.8. Glance through the Table to get a feel of it; you need not remember it. The purpose of including it in the book is for you to know that such Tables exist for you to consult as and when necessary.

BALANCED DIET

A balanced diet is a satisfactory diet from the scientific point of view. It provides adequate quantities of all essential nutrients.

Table 9.8 Recommended dietary allowances for Indians (Indian Council of Medical Research, 1990)

Group	Particulars	Body weight (kg)	Recommended dietary allowance							
			Energy (kcal/d)*	Protein (g/d)*	Calcium (mg/d)	Iron (mg/d)	Vitamin A** (μg/d)	Vitamin C (mg/d)	Folic Acid (μg/d)	Vitamin B_{12} (μg/d)
Man	Moderate work	60	2875	60	400	28	600	40	100	1
Woman	Moderate work	50	2225	50	400	30	600	40	100	1
	Pregnant***		+300	+15	1000	38	600	40	400	1
	Lactation									
	0-6 mo		+ 550	+ 25	1000	30	950	80	150	1.5
	6-12 mo		+ 400	+ 18	1000	30	950	80	150	1.5
Infant	0-6 mo	5.4	108 kcal/kg	2.05 g/kg	500		350	25	25	0.2
	6-12 mo	8.6	98 kcal/kg	1.65 g/kg	500		350	25	25	0.2
Children	1-3 y	12.2	1240	22	400	12	400	40	30	1
	4-6 y	19.0	1690	30	400	18	400	40	40	1
	7-9 y	26.9	1950	41	400	26	600	40	60	1
Boys	10-12 y	35.4	2190	54	600	19	600	40	70	1
Girls	10-12 y	31.5	1970	57	600	34	600	40	70	1
Boys	13-15 y	47.8	2450	70	600	28	600	40	100	1
Girls	13-15 y	46.7	2060	65	600	41	600	40	100	1
Boys	16-18 y	57.1	2640	78	500	30	600	40	100	1
Girls	16-18 y	49.9	2060	63	500	50	600	40	100	1

*Unless specified otherwise.
**As retinol. For beta-carotene, the allowance is four times as much.
***2nd or 3rd trimester.

Framing a Balanced Diet

Framing a balanced diet for an individual incorporates two basic steps : to determine the scientific specifications of the diet, and to translate the specifications into a diet which the individual is likely to accept.

Scientific Specifications

These depend mainly on the age, sex, body weight and habitual physical activity of the individual. After examining these factors, we determine the energy intake which would be adequate for the individual. For this purpose, we make use of the RDAs. The next step is to determine the desirable minimum protein intake on the basis of RDA. For example, for a 50 kg moderately active woman, the diet should provide 2225 kcal and at least 50 g protein everyday. 50 g protein would provide 200 kcal. The remaining 2025 kcal can be obtained from a rather flexible mixture of carbohydrates and fats. The diet should also provide at least the RDA of vitamins and minerals.

Translating the Specifications into a Diet

The leap from chemistry to kitchen involves four basic steps:

1. Know the patient well. Find out her usual dietary pattern, likes and dislikes.
2. Keeping the patient's preferences and scientific specifications in mind, frame a provisional diet.
3. Using food composition data from published tables, calculate the composition and energy content of the provisional diet. Examine how far the scientific features of the provisional diet deviate from the predetermined specifications.
4. Make adjustments in the provisional diet so that the diet finally prescribed to the patient meets the scientific specifications exactly.

In short, framing a balanced diet for an individual needs three types of information:

1. Recommended dietary allowances, to determine the specifications of the diet to be framed.
2. Patient's dietary preferences, to guide the foods to be included in the diet.
3. Food composition data, to ensure that the quantities of different foods included are just right for meeting the specifications.

In the Indian context, these aims can be generally achieved quite simply by including in the diet:

1. A mixture of cereals and pulses as the major source of energy. This automatically ensures adequate quantity and satisfactory quality of dietary protein. If the grains are not highly refined, it also ensures adequate fiber intake.
2. Vegetables, preferably green and at least partly raw. This ensures adequate vitamin and mineral intake.
3. Some milk and milk products, and some visible fat, to introduce variety in the diet and to improve its palatability.

Thus it is quite easy to frame a balanced diet using locally available, generally acceptable and relatively inexpensive foods, provided priority is given to scientific specifications of the diet rather than taste, fads and customs associated with food.

NUTRITION DURING PREGNANCY AND LACTATION

Nutrition during pregnancy and lactation needs special consideration because these are both periods of extremely rapid growth. During pregnancy, the fetus which weighs only 15 g at 12 wk grows to 3000 g by 40 wk of pregnancy. This amounts to a 200-fold growth in 28 wk, which is unparalleled during any other phase of life. The maternal tissues, specially uterus, breasts and placenta also show significant growth during pregnancy. During lactation, the rate of growth is much less rapid but the absolute growth is still considerable. A 3 kg newborn grows by 3 kg during the first 6 months of life, often entirely on breast milk. The nutritional implications of rapid growth are two-fold. First, the energy intake has to be appropriately increased. Second, the nutrients required for tissue growth such as proteins, vitamins and minerals should form a relatively larger fraction of the diet. It has been shown through several studies, on both human beings and animals, that malnutrition during pregnancy affects both the mother and the child adversely. The mother may get emaciated and develop anemia, osteoporosis or osteomalacia. The baby may be born prematurely, and may have a low birth weight in relation to the duration of gestation (small for date).

Nutritional Requirements during Pregnancy

Let us consider briefly the special nutritional considerations required during pregnancy in terms of individual nutrients.

Energy

A woman gains about 10 kg in body weight during pregnancy. Most of this gain in weight takes place during the second and third trimester. Hence the energy intake also needs to be increased only during this phase. The ICMR recommends an additional intake of 300 kcal during the second and third trimester of pregnancy.

Nutrients

The protein intake also needs to be increased during pregnancy. This can be achieved easily if most of the additional energy intake is in the form of a cereal-pulse mixture.

Not much additional calcium intake is necessary during pregnancy if the intake before pregnancy was satisfactory. This is so because gastrointestinal absorption improves during pregnancy in response to enhanced needs. However, it is desirable to achieve a calcium intake of about 1 g/day during pregnancy.

An iron supplement is often necessary during pregnancy to meet the recommended intake of 38 mg per day. However, one should take care not to raise the hemoglobin level above 11g/100 mL blood. There is some physiological hmodilution during pregnancy. Hence 11 g/100 mL is the physiological upper limit of hemoglobin concentration. Higher levels than that raise the viscosity of blood, thereby reducing placental blood flow which may prove harmful.

Deficiency of folic acid is fairly common in India due to inadequate consumption of green leafy vegetables. The deficiency is aggravated during pregnancy due to enhanced demands. Therefore it has been recommended that a pregnant woman should take 400 micrograms folic acid per day instead of the 100 micrograms required when not pregnant. It is difficult to supply 400 micrograms of folic acid from the diet. Therefore supplements are essential, but there is no justification for giving amounts as large as 15 mg provided by some supplements.

Other Considerations

Besides energy and nutrients, some other special considerations are necesary during pregnancy because of frequent attacks of nausea and vomiting, limited capacity to eat at one meal, constipation, and some peculiar cravings. These problems can be helped by small frequent meals, a high fiber diet, and due attention to reasonable and harmless cravings.

Nutritional Requirements during Lactation

Although a woman should continue to eat for two during lactation, she may not be as conscious of it during lactation as during pregnancy. In fact, the absolute growth of the baby is greater during lactation than during pregnancy. Hence, the nutritional requirements during lactation are even greater than during pregnancy.

Energy

A lactating woman secretes about 800 mL of milk everyday during early pregnancy, which provides about 550 kcal to the infant. The mother converts food energy into milk energy with an efficiency of about 80 percent. But she deposits some additional fat during pregnancy which she should lose during lactation. Therefore the ICMR recommends an additional intake of 550 kcal/day during the first 6 months of lactation. If lactation continues longer, the milk output is often reduced. Therefore the additional allowance for the next 6 months of lactation is 400 kcal/day.

Nutrients

The requirement for protein, iron, calcium and vitamins continues to be high during lactation. Therefore the general principles applicable during pregnancy also apply during lactation. The additional needs for nutrients can be met more easily if the additional energy intake is in the form of a well balanced diet.

Other Considerations

Condiments and spices should be avoided during lactation because their odor may enter the milk thereby making it unpleasant for the baby. Frequent meals make it easier to achieve the desired energy intake.

NUTRITION DURING INFANCY AND CHILDHOOD

Besides the hackneyed importance of looking after children well for the sake of the future of the world, there are also important physiological reasons why the nutrition of children deserves special attention. Childhood is a period of rapid growth. Therefore children need more energy in relation to their body weight, and also need more of body building ingredients. Hence the quantity as well as quality of a child's diet assume importance. Further, much of the postnatal brain growth takes place during the first two years of life. Any retardation in mental development due to poor neurogenesis is essentially irreversible. And the impact of suboptimal mental faculties on the quality of life is more serious than that of poor growth. Finally, the capacity of a child's stomach, and consequently meal size, is limited. Therefore in order to meet their enormous nutritional requirements, children have to eat more frequently, and find an increase in the caloric density of their meals beneficial.

Nutrition from Birth Onwards

The recommended dietary allowances for different age groups from birth onwards are given in Table 9.8. Up to the age of 6 months, all nutritional requirements can be, and ideally should be, met by breast milk. Breast feeding may be continued longer, but after the age of 6 months, breast milk, or any milk that the child is taking, should be supplemented with semisolid foods. After the age of one year, the quantity of supplements should steadily increase, and their consistency should become more solid. Finally, by the age of about two, the child should be able to eat almost everything which the adults in the family eat. With this brief outline as a background, we shall now discuss some important points of interest in child nutrition.

Advantages of Breastfeeding

One may ask why a newborn must be breastfed. Is there no other way of providing adequate nutrients to an infant ? Don't we have the example of a whole generation of highly successful bottlefed individuals in western Europe and north America? If they have achieved good physical and mental growth, and a long life span, in spite of being bottlefed, why can't we ? First, the West is also turning to the breast; and secondly, the brief 20th century Western experiment cannot be duplicated simply anywhere and at any time due to important socioeconomic reasons. Hygiene is the first casualty in bottlefed babies in developing tropical countries like India. In order to provide a clean bottle, nipple and milk, thorough boiling and refrigeration are essential. The parents often cannot afford even the fuel required for boiling, leave aside the refrigerator. The cost of formula feeds is also so high that the parents often dilute the feed excessively to stretch the supply. The result is that the child gets inadequate quantities of unhygienic feed. If a child could be given adequate quantity of formula feeds in a hygienic manner, satisfactory feeding can be achieved, as the Western experience has shown. But even this satisfactory bottle feeding is not as good as breast feeding because of some special features of breast milk, which have been summarized below:

1. Breast milk is sterile.
2. Breast milk is convenient to give and is generally readily available.
3. Breast milk is delivered to the baby at the right temperature.
4. Breast milk is neither too concentrated nor too dilute.
5. Breast milk is inexpensive. Ordinary foods such as cereals, legumes and vegetables are converted into milk with more than 80% efficiency, so that breast milk costs about the same as the simple food which the mother eats.
6. There is rarely a chance of allergy to breast milk.
7. Breast milk is easily digestible.
8. There is no danger of overfeeding a breast fed baby.
9. Breastfeeding brings the mother and the child physically and psychologically closer to each other.
10. Suckling stimulates oxytocin release, which besides ejecting milk from the breast, also contracts the uterus. Contraction of the uterus after delivery helps in speedier and more complete involution of the uterus.
11. Breastfeeding inhibits ovulation and normal menstrual cycles, thereby inducing a contraceptive effect which helps in spacing out children and limiting the size of the family.
12. Women who breastfeed are less likely to get breast cancer.
13. The composition of breast milk changes with the age of the child. From delivery until 5 days postpartum, the milk, known as colostrum, has a lower energy content but much higher lactoferrin and antibody content than mature milk. The concentration of these

proteins continues to be high in transitional milk which is secreted from the 6th to the 15th day postpartum. High concentration of these proteins is likely to protect the newborn against infections. Mature milk is secreted from the 15th day postpartum. Slow changes in the composition of mature milk continue throughout lactation but the significance of these changes is not understood.

14. It has been observed that in mothers who deliver prematurely, the concentration of antibodies continues to be high longer than in mothers who deliver full-term babies. This may provide welcome additional protection to the vulnerable premature infant. There are other differences also in the composition of preterm milk as compared to term milk, the significance of which is not understood. It is tempting to believe that changes in the composition of breast milk with the age and maturity of the infant are related to the changing nutritional reuirements of the infant. Such tailor-made milk would be difficult to provide from any other source.
15. The composition of breast milk differs from one species to another. The well known differences between cow's milk and human milk have been shown in Table 9.9. However, today we know that this comparison is superficial and incomplete. There are finer differences between human and cow's milk in terms of the nature of proteins, their amino acid profile, the fatty acid profile of fats, and micronutrient composition. The awareness of innumerable biochemical differences between animal milk and human milk has made scientists realise that any attempt to manipulate the composition of animal milk to make it mimic human milk is doomed for failure. A few unique biochemical features of human milk, the significance of which is known, are given below.

Anti-infective Properties

Human milk has a high count of lymphocytes, neutrophils and macrophages which confer non-specific as well as specific immunity. The high concentration of antibodies, specially in colostrum, transitional milk and preterm milk has already been mentioned. Lactoferrin is an iron binding protein which competes with iron-demanding bacteria for iron available in the gastrointestinal tract thereby reducing the growth of these bacteria. The lactoferrin concentration of human milk is much higher than that of animal milk. The concentration of lysozyme, an anti-bacterial enzyme, is 3000 times higher in human milk than in cow's milk. All these features make the anti-infective properties of human milk superior to those of any other milk.

Digestive Properties

Casein present in human milk is more easily digested than that in cow's milk. The higher concentration of lactoferrin in human milk possibly prevents iron overload during the first few months of iron adequacy. The presence of folate and cobalamin binding proteins in human milk suggests that these proteins assist the absorption of the corresponding vitamins. The higher concentration of lactose in human milk promotes calcium absorption. There are several lipases also present in breast milk, the most important of which is the bile salt stimulated lipase (BSSL). Milk lipases assist the endogenous lipase in lipid digestion, which is an important function because lipid digestion is poor in the newborn, specially the preterm newborn.

Growth Factors

The human milk has been found to have several growth promoting factors such as epidermal growth factor (EGF), insulin and somato-medin-C.

In summary, now it is considered well established that breast milk is the best for the baby, and human breast milk is superior to animal milk for the human infant. No substitute can come close to breast milk even under the best circumstances. And, under the circumstances prevailing in tropical developing countries like India, breast milk substitutes are simply disastrous.

Supplements

As regards semisolid and solid supplements for children above 6 months of age, simple supplements are the best. These include *khichri*, chapati and *dal*, chapati made from mixed *atta* (e.g. wheat and soyabean or wheat and Bengal gram), banana, mashed boiled potato with curd, toast, biscuits, boiled vegetables, and fruits.

The Protein Myth

There is a widespread notion that since children need more protein, they should have special high-protein foods. Let us examine this concept critically (Table 9.10). If we compare the needs of an adult with those of a one-year old child, we find that the child needs only 6 percent of its caloric intake in the form of protein while an adult needs 8 percent. Since a mixture of cereals and pulses provides at least 10 percent of the calories in the form of proteins, the mixture can serve as a staple for both children and adults. This is so because although children need more protein per kg body weight, they also need more energy per kg body weight. That is why children do not need any special high protein foods. The main concern in both child and adult nutrition is to provide adequate quantity of food in the form of ordinary foods such as cereals and pulses. If the quantity of food (energy content) is enough, quality (protein content) takes care of itself (Table 9.10).

Table 9.9 Comparison of the composition of human milk and cow's milk

	Per 100 g milk	
	Human milk	*Cow's milk*
Water (g)	87	87
Energy (kcal)	70	70
Carbohydrate (g)	7	4.8
Fat (g)	3.8	3.7
Protein (g)	1.2	3.3

Tips for Feeding Children

Although the same foods can meet the nutritional requirements of children and adults, children need some special consideration because children are not simply small adults. First, children have a small stomach and therefore their capacity to eat is limited. Therefore their heavy nutritional needs can be met only by increasing the meal frequency and by increasing the caloric density of food. The caloric density may be increased by adding butter or oil to foods whenever feasible. Some other tips for feeding children are given below :

1. New foods should be introduced one at a time. This facilitates discovery of the child's preferences and also identification of any food to which the child may be allergic.
2. The child should be served a varied menu with love and tact.
3. There should be no rigidity about forcing on the child a food which the child dislikes.
4. Junk foods such as cold drinks and candy should be minimized. These foods may crowd out the appetite leaving little room for better foods. The disadvantage of junk foods is that they may provide energy but not the proteins, vitamins and minerals which are coupled with calories in better foods.

Table 9.10 Protein requirements of an adult compared with those of a child

		Recommended allowance		*Protein-energy*	
Age	*Body weight (kg)*	*Energy (kcal)*	*Protein (g)*	*Protein calories*	*Protein calories/ total energy (%)*
Adult*	60	2875	60	240	8.3%
1 year	9	909	13.5**	54	5.9%

* Moderately active male

** On the basis of 1.5 g/kg body weight

(From Bijlani RL. *Nutrition: A Practical Approach*, New Delhi: Jaypee Brothers, 1992; 78).

With these general principles in mind, a child can be provided a satisfactory diet without much hassle or expense.

QUESTIONS

1. Do animal foods provide carbohydrate?
2. How does saturation of dietary fat affect lipoprotein metabolism?
3. Can vitamin D be considered a hormone?
4. Why is rickets uncommon in children having protein energy malnutrition?
5. How can vitamin K antagonists or antibiotics induce vitamin K deficiency?
6. Why is the urine yellow a few hours after taking a tablet of vitamin B Complex?
7. Why is vitamin B complex customarily given to patients on antibiotics?
8. What are food-based dietary guidelines?
9. For each of the following statements, indicate whether it is true or false:
   A. Mustard oil is a healthy cooking medium
   B. No plant food contains cholesterol
   C. Animal proteins are essential for a balanced diet
   D. Cereals provide us carbohydrate whereas pulses provide us proteins
   E. Adults should take about 500 g of vegetables and fruits per day.

ANSWERS

1. Animal foods do not supply much carbohydrate. Milk contains lactose, the concentration being 4.4 g/100 mL in cow's milk. Muscle and liver contain a small amount of glycogen. But much of muscle glycogen is lost during rigor mortis.
2. As a general rule, saturated fats raise serum cholesterol, monounsaturated fats have no effect on serum cholesterol, and polyunsaturated fats lower serum cholesterol.

   Saturated fats raise primarily LDL cholesterol by reducing LDL receptor mediated uptake. Thus the fractional clearance of LDL cholesterol is reduced, raising its serum level.

   Although monounsaturated fats have no known direct effect on serum cholesterol, if monounsaturated fats replace part of the saturated fat in the diet, the LDL cholesterol raising effect of saturated fats is reduced, and thereby LDL cholesterol is lowered.

   Polyunsaturated fats lower total and serum LDL cholesterol through mechanisms which are not completely understood. Some of the possible mechanisms are:

   i. Suppression of hepatic fatty acid and triglyceride synthesis, thereby reducing VLDL secretion by the liver. Since LDL is derived from VLDL, lower VLDL secretion may reduce also LDL levels.
   ii. Inhibition of apoliopoprotein B synthesis. Apolipoprotein B is a part of the LDL molecule. Reduction in its synthesis may reduce LDL levels.

      In terms of their effect on serum cholesterol fractions, and their other effects which can affect atherogenesis, n-3 PUFA differ from n-6 PUFA (Table 9.4).
3. A suggestion has been made that since vitamin D has to be modified in the body before it is biologically active, it should be considered a hormone. Comparison with the thyroid hormones would illustrate the point.

	Vitamin D	*Thyroid hormones*
Precursor present	Yes, vitamin D_2 or vitamin D_3	Yes, iodine in diet
Organ(s) where precursor transformed	Liver and kidney	Thyroid gland
Product	1,25-dihydroxy cholecalciferol	Tetra-and tri-iodothyronine
Target organs	Intestine, bones and kidneys	All parts of the body
Mode of transport to target organs	Bloodstream	Bloodstream

Further, the active form of vitamin D has a structure resembling steroid hormones, and acts, like the steroid hormones, by influencing protein synthesis in target cells.

However, in spite of all these similarities, vitamin D is conventionally not considered a hormone. Besides convention, the only justification for this practice probably is that the dietary and biologically active forms of vitamin D are not markedly different in chemical structure.

4. Children with protein energy malnutrition show poor growth. Since vitamin D is required for bone growth, vitamin D deficiency is unlikely to manifest itself if the bones are not growing.
5. Vitamin K antagonists compete with vitamin K in the liver and thereby inhibit prothrombin synthesis.

   Antibiotics may eliminate the gastrointestinal bacteria which synthesize vitamin K, and thereby reduce supply of the vitamin to the host.
6. Tablets of vitamin B complex often have much larger quantities of vitamins than the body can use immediately. Since vitamin B complex is not stored in the body, the excess ingested is exerted in the urine. Riboflavin is intensely yellow in color and imparts its color to the urine.
7. This is because antibiotics may eliminate or at least reduce the bacterial population of the intestine, thereby curtailing the supply of vitamins synthesized by these bacteria. However, not all antibiotics reach the large intestine in amounts sufficient to alter the bacterial population significantly, and there is no vitamin for which the bacterial source is generally critical (except perhaps vitamin B_{12} in strict vegetarians). But the practice of medicine can be quite different from theory. If there is the slightest justification for giving relatively harmless substances such as vitamins, most physicians would like to give them. An additional justification is that vitamin requirement may be increased in these patients due to stress of the infection for which antibiotics are being given.
8. Food-based dietary guidelines (FBDGs) differ from RDAs in being based on foods rather than nutrients. For example, 'Prefer whole grains to refined grains', or 'Take 400 g of vegetables and 100 g of fruits everyday' are FBDGs. Since we take foods rather than nutrients, FBDGs are easier to use in practice than RDAs. FBDGs may be qualitative rather than quantitative, and take into account the sociocultural context and habitual dietary pattern of the population. Hence RDAs all over the world are very similar but FBDGs are region-specific.
9. A. True. Mustard oil is one of the very few vegetable oils with a significant n-3 PUFA content.

   B. True.

   C. False. A mixture of cereals and pulses gives protein of good quality, and if the mixture is the staple diet, it also gives the required quantity of protein.

   D. False. In addition to carbohydrate, cereals also provide protein. In addition to protein, pulses also provide carbohydrate. The composition of a typical cereal is: carbohydrate 70%, protein 10%, water 20%. The composition of a typical pulse is: carbohydrate 60%, protein 20%, water 20%. Further, since the quantity of cereals consumed is generally much more, they may provide us more protein than pulses. The significance of pulses lies in complementing the cereal protein in terms of the limiting amino acids. That is why the mixture of cereal and pulse protein is much better in quality than either alone.

   E. True. We need that much vegetables and fruits to meet our requirements of vitamins, minerals, antioxidants and water-soluble dietary fiber. This may be achieved in practice by taking five helpings of vegetables/fruits per day: two at lunch, two at dinner, and one at some other meal.

CHAPTER

10 Excretory System

"Sips of water is all it takes, To keep the kidneys shipshape"

—RAMESH BIJLANI

Chapter Outline

- Functional Anatomy
- Mechanism of Urine Formation
- Role of Kidneys in Acid-base Balance
- Physiology of Micturition

Metabolic reactions in the body are associated with formation of waste products. These waste products would be harmful to the body if allowed to accumulate. They have to be removed from the body in order to keep the internal environment of the body suitable for cellular activity. The waste products include carbon dioxide (which is removed by the lungs) and urea, which is removed by the kidneys. Kidneys also remove other water-soluble waste products, metabolites and drugs from the body. In addition, kidneys adjust the rate of hydrogen ion excretion to maintain the acid-base balance of the body. Further, kidneys adjust the rate of urine formation to maintain water and electrolyte balance of the body. Thus kidneys make several important contributions to homeostasis.

FUNCTIONAL ANATOMY

We have two kidneys each, which are bean-shaped organs. Urine formed by the kidneys is conveyed to the urinary bladder by ureters. The urinary bladder empties its contents through the urethra (Fig. 10.1). A longitudinal section of the kidney shows that the outer layer (cortex) is granular while the inner layer (medulla) is striated, and that a set of about six calyces open into the renal pelvis, which in turn narrows to form the ureter.

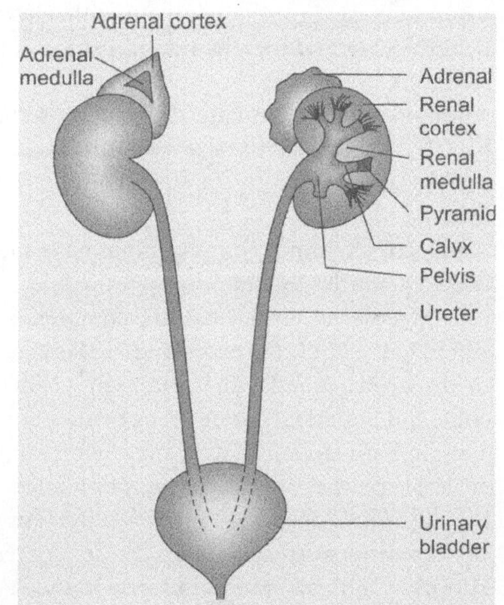

Fig. 10.1 The urinary system and adrenal glands. The right adrenal and left kidneys have been shown in longitudinal section

The structural and functional unit of kidney is called a nephron (Fig. 10.2). Each kidney contains about one million nephrons. Thus both kidneys together have about two million nephrons. Each nephron consists of a cup-shaped structure called the Bowman's capsule, which continues into a long tubule having a characteristic shape and several named

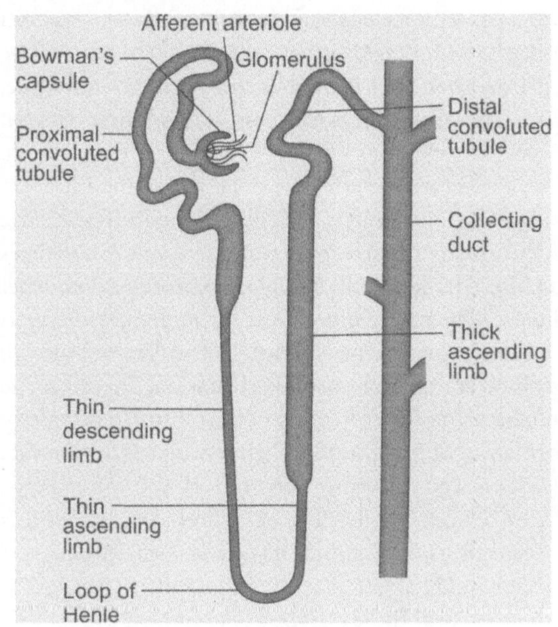

Fig. 10.2 Schematic representation of a nephron

segments with different structural and functional features. We shall learn something about different portions of the nephron in the next few pages.

MECHANISM OF URINE FORMATION

The first step in formation of urine is filtration. As blood passes through the glomerular capillaries, it gets filtered into the Bowman's capsule. The filtrate has a composition similar to plasma except that it does not contain any protein. The filtrate is modified in the remaining parts of the nephron in two ways. First, most of water and electrolytes are removed from the filtrate and returned to the blood. All glucose, amino acids and other useful substances are also returned to the blood. This process is called reabsorption. Second, some substances are removed from the blood and added to the filtrate. This process is called secretion.

The fluid remaining at the end of the nephrons leaves the kidneys as urine. Urine contains mainly those substance which it is essential for the body to lose. These unwanted substances are dissolved in a rather small amount of water (Fig. 10.3).

The overall process of urine formation resembles the method we often use for cleaning a dirty, overcrowded desk. First we remove everything from the desk (as in filtration). Then we replace on the desk things which we want to keep (as in reabsorption). We throw the unwanted things in the dustbin. On second thought, we may remove some more articles from the desk and put them in the dustbin (as in secretion). When we are sure that the dustbin has only those things which we do not want, we empty it into the main dustbin (comparable to urinary bladder).

Now we shall study the processes in individual segments of the nephron one by one.

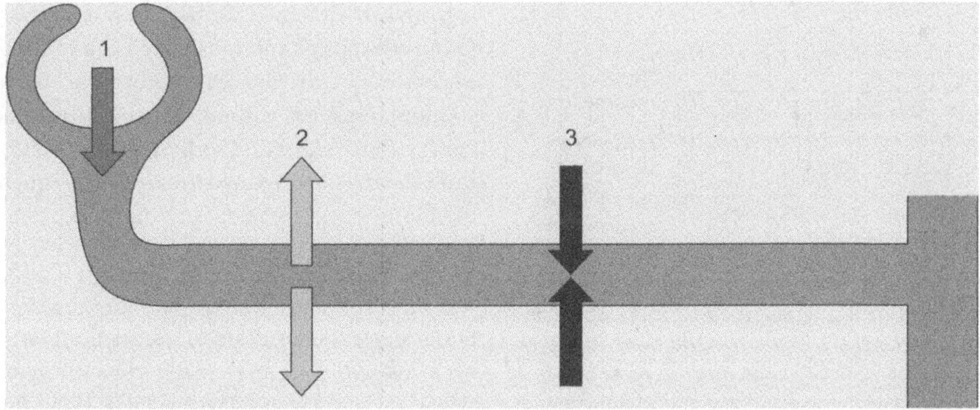

Fig. 10.3 The three basic processes involved in formation of urine. 1, Filtration; 2, Reabsorption; 3, Secretion (Reproduced from Bijlani RL, Manchanda SK. The Human Machine. New Delhi: National Book Trust, India, 1990, Fig. 29, p. 77)

Glomerular Filtration

Glomerulus is a ball of capillaries which fits closely in the cup-shaped Bowman's capsule. Blood flows into the glomerular capillaries through the afferent arteriole. Blood leaves the glomerulus through the efferent arteriole.

The blood passes through the glomerular capillaries at a pressure of about 60 mm Hg, which is higher than the pressure in capillaries anywhere else in the body. The high pressure facilitates filtration. For filtration, the filtered fluid has to pass through three layers: the capillary endothelium, the basement membrane, and the epithelium of Bowman's capsule (Figs 10.4A and B, Plates 4A and 4B). The endothelial layer has openings about 100 nm in diameter. The basement membrane has a glycoprotein network which allows only molecules smaller than 10 nm in diameter to pass through. The epithelial cells of the Bowman's capsule show foot processes. The foot processes of neighboring cells fit each other. The gaps between foot processes are about 23 nm wide. Thus the filtration surface is like a three-layered sieve. The openings of the three layers are not in one line. Therefore the effective pore size of the filtration surface is only about 6 nm (Plate 4A and B). Because of this small pore size, only water and small molecules get filtered. Blood cells and plasma proteins do not get filtered. The rate of blood flow through the kidneys in an adult human being is about 1100 mL/min. 1100 mL of blood contains about 600 mL plasma. Therefore the renal plasma flow (RPF) is 600 mL/min. The rate of formation of the filtrate, i.e. glomerular filtration rate (GFR) is 120 mL/min. Thus out of 600 mL plasma, 120 mL fluid, or one-fifth, gets filtered. If the GFR is 120 mL/min, how much filtrate is formed per day? What would happen if all the filtrate were to be lost as urine? Answer these questions before you go further.[1]

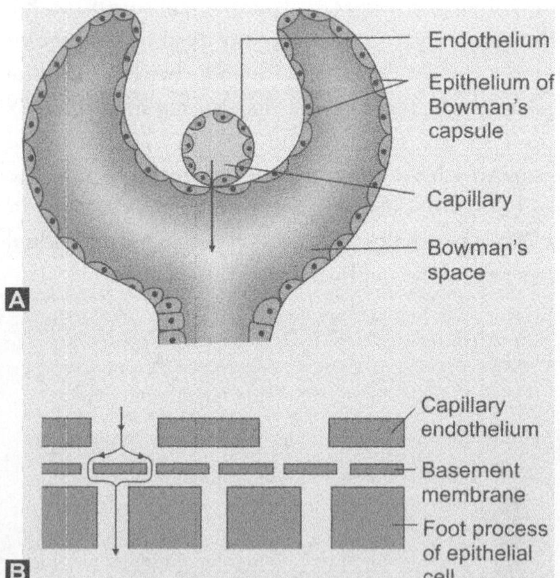

Figs 10.4A and B Diagrammatic representation of structural features of the filtration surface. (A) Bowman's capsule with one capillary. The arrow indicates the layers through which the capillary fluid has to pass before it appears as ultrafiltrate in the Bowman's space; (B) The three principal layers of the filtration surface. The arrows indicate the path traversed by the ultrafiltrate

Proximal Tubule

The proximal tubule is lined with cuboidal epithelial cells. These cells have a brush border or microvilli, on the lumenal surface. They also have several mitochondria. The microvilli increase the surface area for reabsorption. The mitochondria generate energy for the reabsorptive mechanisms.

The proximal tubule reabsorbs an enormous amount of fluid. It reabsorbs about two-thirds of the glomerular filtrate. The mechanism of reabsorption is primarily designed for active transport of sodium. Other substances are transported as a result of sharing a common carrier with sodium, or secondary to sodium transport without expenditure of additional energy. Since water and sodium are both absorbed, the fluid leaving the proximal tubule is very much reduced in volume but it remains isotonic with plasma.

[1]Filtrate formed per day = 120 × 60 × 24 mL = 172800 mL = 172.8 L. This volume would fill about ten medium-sized buckets. We cannot afford to lose so much water because we cannot drink so much water. Reabsorption of water reduces the rate of urine formation to about 1.5 L/day, or 1 mL/min, i.e. less than 1% of the rate of filtration. Thus the kidneys reabsorb more than 99% of the filtrate.

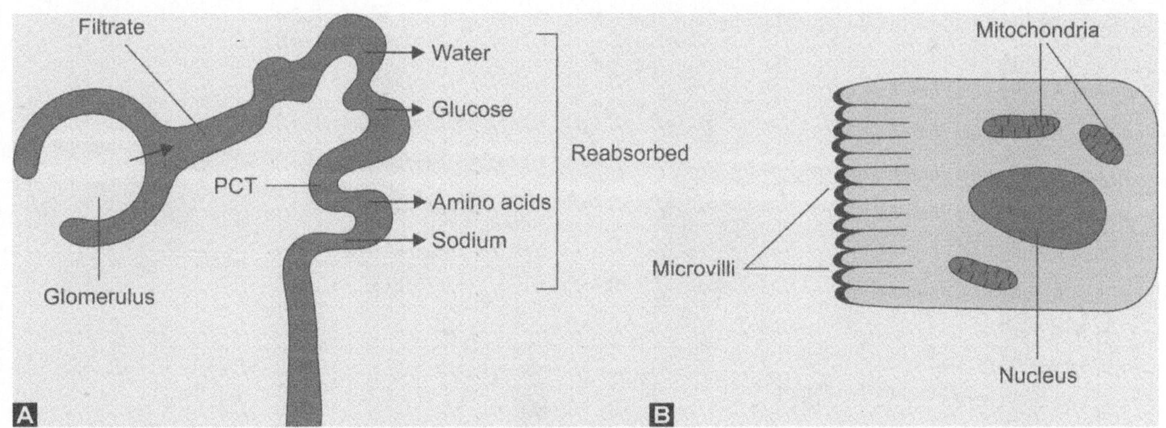

Figs 10.5A and B Reabsorption in the proximal convoluted tubule (PCT). (A) About two-thirds of water and sodium, and all the glucose and amino acids filtered by the glomerulus are reabsorbed in the PCT; (B) An epithelial cell lining the PCT. Microvilli increase the surface area of the lumen

Besides reabsorption of water, sodium and other electrolytes, proximal tubule also reabsorbs glucose and amino acids. These substances are useful for the body and are reabsorbed completely. Therefore these substances normally do not appear in the urine. However, there is a limit to the amount that can be reabsorbed. In case of glucose, the limit is crossed when the plasma glucose level is above 180 mg/dL (10 mmoles/L). The plasma glucose level of 180 mg/dL is called the renal threshold for glucose.

In short, what leaves the proximal tubule is fluid which has been reduced to one third in volume, and which does not contain any glucose or amino acids (Figs 10.5A and B).

Loop of Henle

The proximal tubule continues as a thin straight tube which goes 'down' towards the renal medulla. Therefore it is called the thin descending limb. The descending limb is thin because its epithelial cells are flat. These cells have no brush border and very few mitochondria. As these structural features suggest, the reabsorption in this limb is less than in the proximal tubule and is passive. The most striking feature of the descending limb is its high permeability to water and absence of any permeability to sodium. Reabsorption of water in the descending limb increases the concentration of electrolytes. Therefore as the fluid moves towards the loop, its osmolarity increases. In some nephrons which have long loops, by the time fluid reaches the bend of the loop, the osmolarity is four times the osmolarity of plasma, i.e. 1200 mOsmL[2]. The movement of water out of the descending limb is due to osmosis because the osmolarity of the peritubular fluid also increases from cortex towards the medulla (Figs 10.6A and B).

The descending limb takes a U-turn at the bend of the loop of Henle (like a hair-pin) and moves 'up' towards the renal cortex. Therefore this limb of the loop of Henle is called the ascending limb. In long-looped nephrons, the ascending limb is first thin, and then thick. In other nephrons (the majority), the ascending limb has only a thick regment. It is thick because its epithelial cells are cubodial. The peculiarity of the ascending limb is *absence of any permeability to water.* But it has mechanisms for *reabsorption of sodium.* Reabsorption of sodium reduces the osmolarity of tubular fluid. Hence, by the time the fluid reaches the distal tubule, its osmolarity is only about 100 mOsm/L, i.e. it is hypotonic (Figs 10.7A and B).

You might have noticed that in the loop of Henle, both water and sodium are reabsorbed from

[2]Obviously, the osmolarity of plasma is 300 mOsm/L.

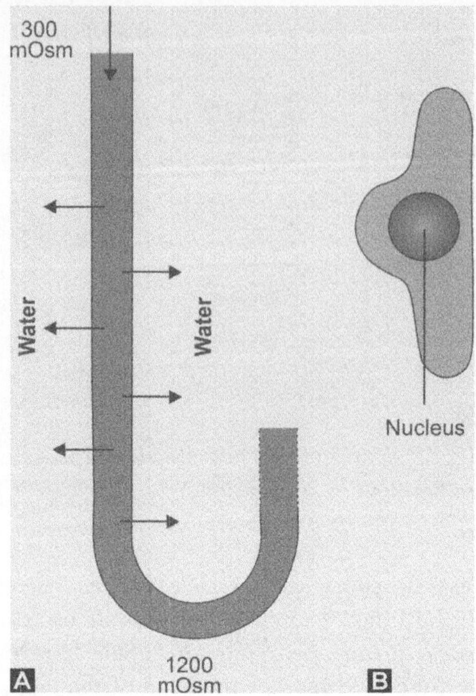

Figs 10.6A and B Reabsorption in the descending limb. (A) The thin descending limb is primarily a site of water reabsorption. As a result, osmolarity of the tubular fluid may rise up to 1200 mOsm at the tip of the loop of Henle; (B) An epithelial cell lining the thin descending limb

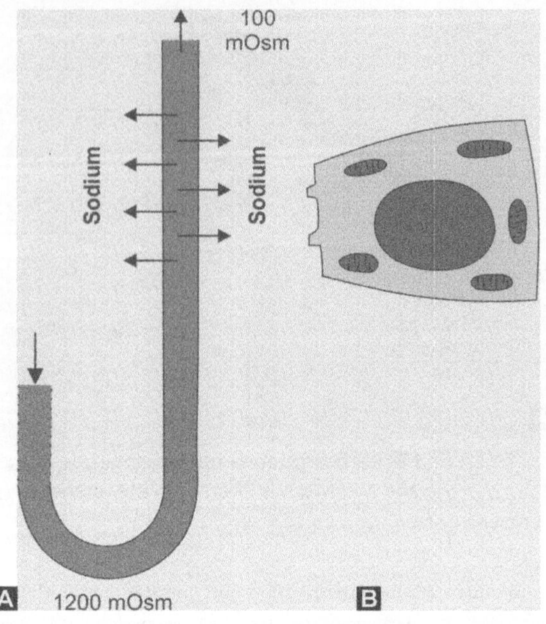

Figs 10.7A and B Reabsorption in the ascending limb. (A) The ascending limb is primarily a site of sodium reabsorption. As a result, osmolarity of the tubular fluid may fall to 100 mOsm at the end of the ascending limb; (B) An epithelial cell lining the ascending limb

the tubular fluid. But the reabsorption is broken into two instalments. First, water is reabsorbed in the descending limb. Then, sodium is reabsorbed in the ascending limb (Fig. 10.8). The advantages of this arrangement are:

a. There is minimal expenditure of energy. Water is transported entirely passively (by osmosis). Part of the sodium is also transported passively (by diffusion).[3]
b. A high concentration gradient is achieved. Starting with a tubular fluid of 300 mOsm/L, a concentration of 1200 mOsm/L is achieved. This is made possible although tubular epithelial cells cannot individually achieve a gradient of more than 200 mOsm/L.
   This occurs because fluid in the two limbs of the loop of Henle moves in opposite directions. Therefore the process is said to incorporate a countercurrent multiplier system.
c. The distal tubule is delivered a hypotonic fluid. Now the distal tubule and collecting duct have the choice of leaving the urine hypotonic, making it isotonic, or making it hypertonic up to the extent of 1200 mOsm/L. This 'decision' is taken according to the requirements of the fluid balance of the body.

The Distal Tubule and Collecting Duct

The distal tubule and collecting duct are essentially one functional unit. These segments of the nephron are lined largely with cuboidal cells which grow progressively taller in the distal portions

[3]As the highly concentrated fluid from the bend moves up in the ascending limb, it is exposed to peritubular fluid with lower sodium concentration. Therefore sodium diffuses out of the ascending limb along the concentration gradient.

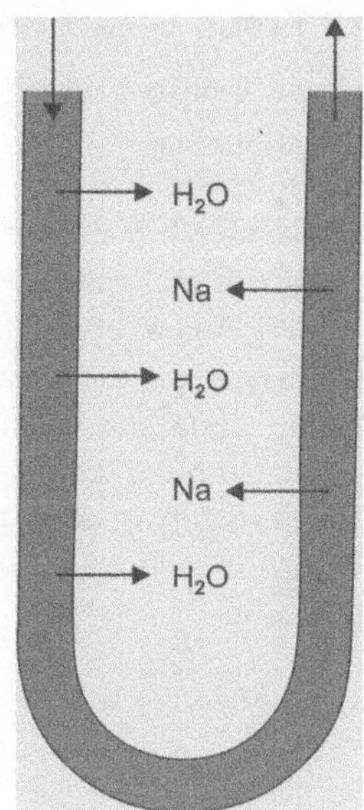

Fig. 10.8 The overall result of reabsorption in both the limbs of the loop of Henle is reabsorption of both water and sodium

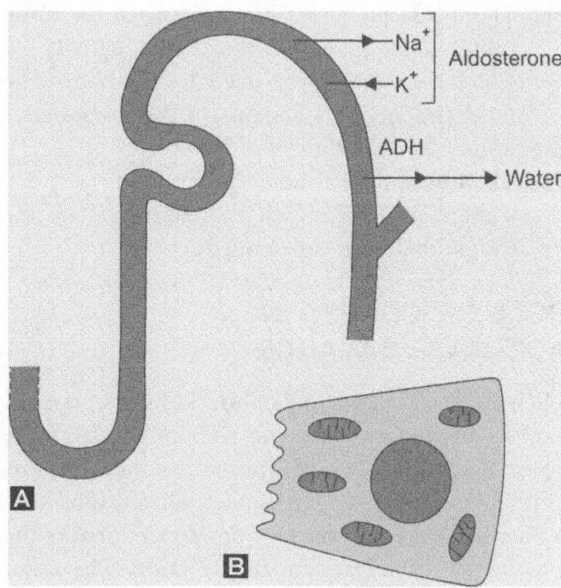

Figs 10.9A and B (A) Reabsorption in the distal nephron is regulated by aldosterone and ADH; (B) An epithelial cell lining the distal nephron

of the collecting duct till they become columnar. Most of these segments are sensitive to the action of aldosterone. Under the influence of aldosterone, sodium is reabsorbed and potassium is secreted. The most remarkable feature of the distal tubule and collecting duct is that they are ordinarily impermeable to water but become permeable under the influence of antidiuretic hormone (ADH). Permeability makes possible reabsorption of water (Figs 10.9A and B). Reabsorption of water makes the urine concentrated and reduces the urinary loss of water from the body. Thus this region of the nephron helps regulate the fluid balance of the body (Fig. 10.10).

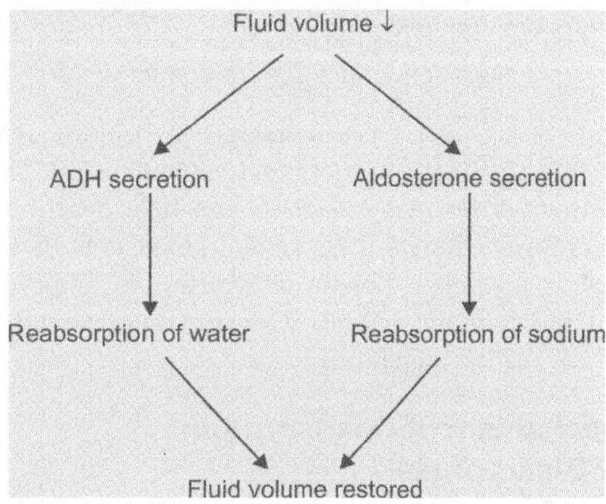

Fig. 10.10 Hormonal regulation of fluid balance by the kidneys

Functional Segments of the Nephron

From the above discussion, it is clear that the nephron has four functional segments:

a. The *filtering segment* consisting of the Bowman's capsule, into which glomerular capillaries filter plasma.
b. The *conserving segment* consisting of the proximal tubule, which conserves water, electrolytes, glucose and amino acids by reabsorption on a massive scale.
c. The *concentrating segment* consisting of the loop of Henle, which reabsorbs water and sodium step by step, further conserving these essential constituents of the body.

d. The *regulating segment* consisting of the distal tubule and collecting duct, the activity of which depends on the needs of the body. The fluid and electrolyte status of the body determines the secretion of aldosterone and ADH. The hormones, in turn, determine how much sodium and water will be reabsorbed by the distal tubule and collecting duct.

ROLE OF KIDNEYS IN ACID BASE BALANCE

We have so far talked only of how kidneys can regulate the amount of water and sodium lost from the body. The filtrate has many more substances, the loss of which is regulated. One such important substance is bicarbonate. Bicarbonate is one component of the bicarbonate buffer system of the body. The other component of the buffer is carbonic acid (H_2CO_3), which is nothing but dissolved carbon dioxide. As you know, bicarbonate component of the buffer prevents acids from lowering the pH of body fluids much. For example,

$$NaHCO_3 + HCl = NaCl + H_2CO_3$$

Thus bicarbonate has converted hydrochloric acid (a strong acid) into carbonic acid (a weak acid). The body produces many acids in metabolic reactions. Bicarbonate buffers these acids immediately. If we lose too much bicarbonate in the urine, the body will not be able to buffer acids. The kidneys prevent this loss by reabsorbing bicarbonate.

Mechanism of Reabsorption of Bicarbonate

A long section of the nephron (proximal tubule, thick segment of ascending limb, distal tubule and collecting duct) can reabsorb bicarbonate. The mechanism is as shown in Figure 10.11. Note that the reabsorption is indirect. The bicarbonate that is reabsorbed is not the same as the bicarbonate in the tubular fluid. Carbon dioxide, which diffuses easily across cell membranes, acts as a vehicle for carrying bicarbonate into the epithelial cell.

Generation of Fresh Bicarbonate

The kidneys not only reabsorb bicarbonate but also generate fresh bicarbonate which is added to the body fluids. This also happens in the same regions of the nephron in which bicarbonate is reabsorbed. The mechanism is as shown in Figure 10.12. Note that the mechanism is very similar except that the source of carbon dioxide here is not the filtrate but the cell itself.[4] Also note that simultaneously hydrogen ions are secreted into the tubular lumen. That is why urine is normally acidic (pH about 6). However, urine is not as acidic as it could be because tubular fluid also has buffers.

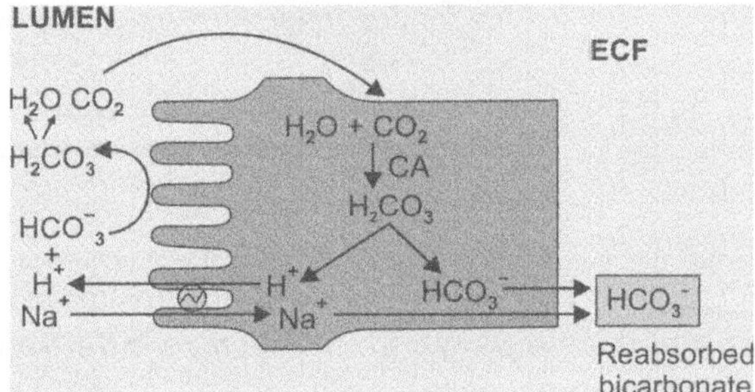

Fig. 10.11 Mechanism of reabsorption of bicarbonate. CA, carbonic anhydrase

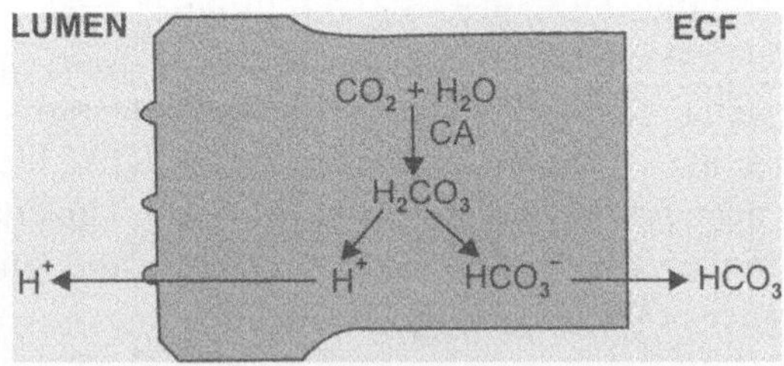

Fig. 10.12 Mechanism of generation of new bicarbonate ions and secretion of hydrogen ions in the distal nephron. CA, carbonic anhydrase

[4]The carbon dioxide is produced in the cell by metabolic reactions. Some carbon dioxide may also be taken from the blood.

Buffers in Tubular Fluid

The kidneys use two main buffers to buffer the tubular fluid: ammonia and phosphates.

Ammonia Buffer

Ammonia is produced in tubular epithelial cells from amino acids such as glutamine. Ammonia diffuses into the tubular fluid. In the tubular fluid, ammonia combines with hydrogen ions to form ammonium ions (Fig. 10.13). Thus hydrogen ions get excreted as ammonium salts, which are much less acidic than hydrogen ions.

Phosphate Buffer

Phosphates are present in tubular fluids in high concentration. Hydrogen ions are buffered by phosphates as shown in Figure 10.14.

Regulation of Acid-base Balance

The amount of bicarbonate reabsorbed by the kidneys, or the amount of fresh bicarbonate generated by the kidneys is not fixed. It gets altered in response to the requirements of acid-base balance of the body. Thus the kidneys help in regulating acid-base balance of the body by altering the concentration of bicarbonate in body fluids.

An integrated picture of regulation of acid-base balance is given in Chapter 19.

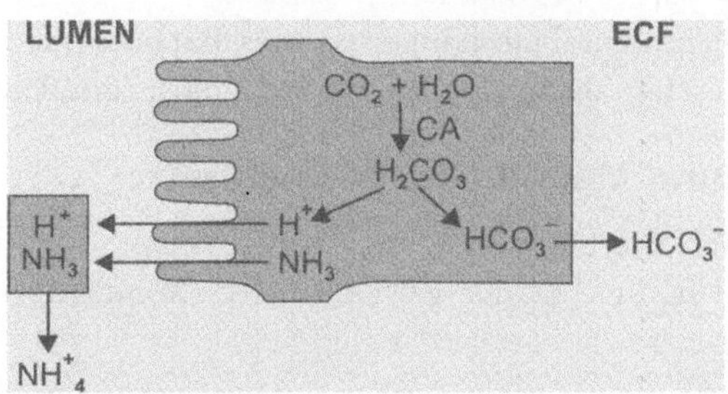

Fig. 10.13 Buffering action of ammonia in the renal tubules. CA, carbonic anhydrase

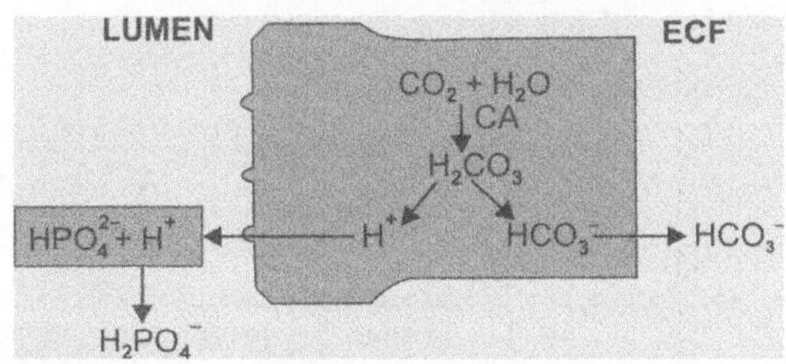

Fig. 10.14 Buffering action of the phosphate buffer in the renal tubules. The phosphate buffer is much more important in the distal nephron than in the proximal nephron

PHYSIOLOGY OF MICTURITION

Urine is formed by the kidneys continuously. It is carried to the urinary bladder drop by drop. It is stored in the bladder till the bladder is full. A full bladder creates a feeling which makes us go to the toilet, where we can pass the urine voluntarily. The act of passing urine is called micturition. Voluntary control (i.e control of will power) includes:

a. The ability to initiate (start) micturition whenever we like, even when the bladder is not full,
b. The ability to terminate (stop) micturition whenever we like, even in the middle of the act, and
c. The ability to postpone (delay) micturition for a considerable period after the bladder is full, if the conditions are not appropriate for the act.

Functional Anatomy

Urinary bladder is lined by transitional epithelium. Transitional epithelium can stretch quite a lot without tearing. The bladder has a thick coat of smooth muscle. At the neck of the bladder is a sphincteric mechanism, called the internal sphincter. The internal sphincter has smooth muscle. There is also an external sphincter around the urethra. The external sphincter is made up of skeletal muscle.

At the upper end of the bladder are the openings of the ureters. Ureters enter the bladder obliquely (Figs 10.15A and B). As a result, when the bladder contracts, the tense bladder wall presses hard against the ureteric openings and closes them shut. That is why during micturition, or while holding urine in a full bladder, urine does not flow back from the bladder into the ureters. Ureters are also furnished with smooth muscle in their walls which aids the flow of urine.

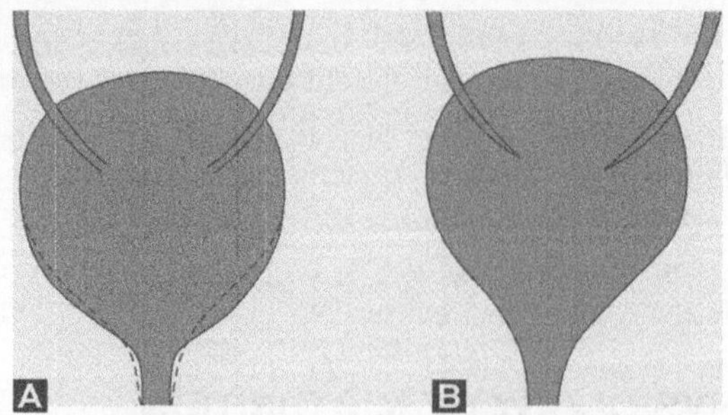

Figs 10.15A and B Distended urinary bladder in a relaxed (A) and contracted (B) state. The dotted lines in A indicate how contraction widens up the opening between the bladder and the urethra

Innervation

The bladder has both sensory and motor nerve supply. Sensory nerves convey information about distension or discomfort. Sensory nerve fibers originating in the bladder travel in pelvic and hypogastric nerves. Motor nerves make the bladder contract or relax.

The sympathetic nerve fibers to the bladder originate in the first two lumbar segments of the spinal cord. The parasympathetic nerve fibers to the bladder originate in the second, third and fourth sacral segments of the spinal cord.

Keeping in mind the general principle that sympathetic activity leads to functions which are useful in an emergency, and parasympathetic activity leads to functions required when one is relaxed, you can predict the effect of these nerves on the bladder. Micturition should be performed when one is relaxed. Accordingly, parasympathetic activity leads to contraction of the bladder. However, whether sympathetic activity relaxes the bladder is not so certain.

It is possible that sympathetic fibers supply only the blood vessels of the bladder.

The external urethral sphincter is a skeletal muscle, and is accordingly supplied by a somatic nerve (pudendal nerve) which originates in the third and fourth sacral segments of the spinal cord.

Mechanics of Micturition

Urine keeps collecting in the bladder till the bladder is full. Then the bladder is emptied almost completely, and the process of refilling starts all over again. Accordingly, there are two aspects of the process: filling and emptying.

Filling of the Bladder

The bladder has a characteristic pressure-volume relationship. When the bladder is empty, the pressure is almost zero. Addition of a small amount of urine to the bladder raises the pressure to about 5 mmHg. But further additions of fluid do not raise the pressure further due to extreme distensibility of the urinary bladder. The bladder pressure remains low till the bladder contains about 200 mL of urine. Thus the bladder can accommodate about 200 mL of urine without much rise in pressure (Fig 10.16).

Emptying of the Bladder

If the bladder is distended beyond the threshold of about 200 mL the pressure rises steeply. Rise in the pressure stretches the smooth muscle of bladder. Stretch leads to contraction. Contraction may empty the bladder. But this simple mechanism would empty only part of the bladder.

The neural mechanism ensures that once micturition starts, the bladder is emptied almost completely.

Neural Mechanism of Micturition

When the bladder is full, stretch receptors in the wall of the bladder get stimulated. Stimulation of

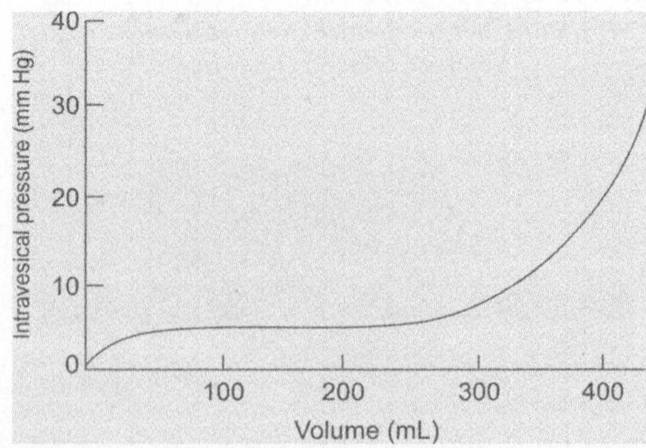

Fig. 10.16 Pressure-volume relationship in the urinary bladder

WHAT IS CLEARANCE

Clearance is a simple concept but is commonly confused. When the kidneys excrete a substance in the urine, they 'clear' the plasma. Therefore clearance is measured in terms of plasma from which the substance is removed in one minute. In other words, clearance is the volume of plasma which is cleared of the substance in one minute.

Suppose the concentration of a substance in urine = U mg/mL
Suppose the rate of urine formation = V mL/min
Then the excretion of the substance = U x V mg/min
Suppose the plasma concentration of the substance = P mg/mL
If P mg of the substance are present in 1 mL plasma,

Then UxV mg of the substance must have come from $= \frac{U \times V}{P}$ mL plasma

Hence clearance of the substance $= \frac{U \times V}{P}$ mL / min

If a substance is freely filtered by the glomeruli but is neither reabsorbed nor secreted in the tubules, the amount excreted will be equal to the amount filtered. In other words, all the plasma that is filtered is cleared of the substance. Hence clearance of such a substance will be equal to the glomerular filtration rate. One such substance is inulin.

Now let us consider a substance which is freely filtered by the glomeruli and is also secreted by the tubules in such large amounts that the plasma leaving the kidneys does not contain the substance at all. In other words, all the plasma that flows to the kidneys is cleared of the substance. Hence clearance of such a substance will be equal to the renal plasma flow. One such substance is para-aminohippuric acid (PAH).

these receptors is conveyed by sensory nerves to a central integrating center in the sacral spinal cord. The output of integration is conveyed by motor nerves to the bladder, which results in contraction of the bladder and relaxation of the internal urethral sphincter. However, this primitive reflex is normally under the influence of impulses from the brain, principally the anterior pons and cerebral cortex. As a result of this influence from the brain, micturition is under voluntary control. We initiate it only when an appropriate opportunity for evacuation is available.

Voluntary micturition involves more than contraction of the bladder. The process is initiated by contraction of the diaphragm and abdominal muscles, and relaxation of muscles of the pelvic floor. That results in a further increase in the intravesical pressure. That leads to removal of the higher inhibitory influences on the micturition reflex. Then the external urethral sphincter is relaxed voluntarily. Then the basic micturition reflex takes over, and the urinary bladder contracts strongly, emptying itself almost completely. When the bladder is empty, flow of urine stops, the bladder relaxes and the external urethral sphincter is closed. The bladder is now ready to fill up again, thus starting the cycle all over again.

QUESTIONS

1. Explain briefly why normal urine does not contain (a) protein, and (b) glucose.
2. How much is the renal clearance of glucose?
3. Why is it good for health to drink plenty of water?

ANSWERS

1. a. Normal urine does not contain protein because plasma protein molecules are too big to get filtered through the glomerular capillaries.
   b. Normal urine does not contain glucose because glucose in the filtrate is completely reabsorbed in the proximal convoluted tubule.

2. The renal clearance of glucose in a healthy person is 0 mL/min. Since glucose is completely reabsorbed in the renal tubules, all the glucose that is filtered is returned to the blood. Therefore no volume of blood is cleared of (i.e. emptied of) glucose. 'No volume' is the same as 0 mL.
3. For several reasons. Plenty of water takes care of sweating losses. It also helps prevent constipation by making available water for dietary fiber to hold. Further, excess water does not normally accumulate in the body–it is excreted in the urine. Hence taking plenty of water makes the urine dilute. Dilute urine is a safe urine from the point of view of two common diseases of the urinary tract: calculi (stones) and urinary tract infection. Calculi are more likely to crystallize in concentrated urine. Concentrated urine is also a good medium for bacterial growth. Therefore urinary tract infections are also more likely if the urine is concentrated (Now the chapter opening quotation will make more sense to you!).

CHAPTER

11 Endocrine System

"One dreamed and saw a gland write Hamlet, drink, At the Mermaid, capture immortality; A committee of hormones on the Aegean's brink, Composed the Iliad and the Odyssey"

—SRI AUROBINDO

Chapter Outline

- Classification of Hormones
- Mechanism of Action of Hormones with Intracellular Receptors
- Mechanism of Action of Hormones with Cell Membrane Receptors
- Hypothalamic and Pituitary Hormones
- Thyroid Gland
- Parathyroid Gland
- Other Hormones Affecting Calcium Metabolism
- Adrenal Cortex
- Adrenal Medulla
- Pancreas
- Gastrointestinal Hormones

In the previous chapters, we have discussed those systems of the body which make a direct contribution to homeostasis by adding nutrients or oxygen to the internal environment, or by removing waste products or carbon dioxide from it. Now we shall turn our attention to systems, which make indirect but important contributions to homeostasis. For example, there are systems, which coordinate the activity of all other systems of the body. One of the systems having the role of a coordinator is the endocrine system.[1]

The endocrine system consists of a set of endocrine glands and endocrine cells. Endocrines (endon, within; krinein, to separate) act by secreting chemical substances called hormones (hormaein, to excite). Endocrine glands have no ducts. Therefore they are also called ductless glands. But there must be a way of carrying the secretions of endocrine glands to their destination. Endocrine glands pour their secretions (hormones) directly into the bloodstream. Since blood travels to all parts of the body, hormones travel to all parts of the body. But not all hormones influence the activity of all cells of the body. In fact, most hormones act in only a few organs (called target organs). If hormones go to all organs, how do they manage to act only in target organs? The answer to this question is that a hormone acts only in those organs which have receptors for the hormone. A receptor is a molecular assembly, which recognizes a specific hormone. The hormone and its receptor form a complex comparable to a lock and key. After the complex has been formed, the action on the target cell begins.

CLASSIFICATION OF HORMONES

Although the hormones may be classified in many ways, here we shall classify them in terms of the localization of the receptor and the nature of the hormone-receptor interaction. Chemically, most hormones belong to one out of two categories. One category is that of steroid hormones. The second is that of peptides and amino acid derivatives. In general, the receptors for steroid hormones are located within the cell whereas the receptors for peptide and related hormones are located on the cell membrane.

[1]The other such system is the nervous system.

An exception is thyroxin, which is an amino acid derivative but has an intracellular receptor. Further, the intracellular receptor may be in the cytoplasm or in the nucleus. And in case of cell membrane receptors, the molecule mediating the effect of the hormones (called second messenger) could be one out of several known. Keeping these criteria in view, a classification of hormones has been presented in Table 11.1.

Table 11.1 Classification of hormones

I. Hormones having intracellular receptors
   1. Thyroid hormones
   2. Glucocorticoids
   3. Mineralocorticoids
   4. Sex hormones

II. Hormones having cell membrane receptors
   a. Second messenger: cAMP
      1. Corticotropin releasing hormone (CRH)
      2. Adrenocorticotropic hormone (ACTH)
      3. Thyroid stimulating hormone (TSH)
      4. Follicle stimulating hormone (FSH)
      5. Luteinizing hormone (LH)
      6. Melanocyte stimulating hormone (MSH)
      7. Antidiuretic hormone (ADH)
      8. Calcitonin
      9. Parathyroid hormone (PTH)
      10. Catecholamines (most actions)
      11. Glucagon
      12. Human chorionic gonadotropin (hCG)
   b. Second messenger: cGMP
      1. Atrial natriuretic factor (ANF)
      2. Nitric oxide (NO)
   c. Second messenger: calcium or phosphatidylinositol (or both)
      1. Thyrotropin releasing hormone (TRH)
      2. Gonadotropin releasing hormone (GnRH)
      3. Antidiuretic hormone (vasopressor action)
      4. Oxytocin
      5. Catecholamines (some actions)
      6. Cholecystokinin (CCK)
      7. Gastrin
   d. Second messenger: a kinase or phosphatase cascade
      1. Growth hormone (GH)
      2. Prolactin
      3. Insulin

Adapted from Granner DK. Hormone action. In Harper's *Biochemistry*. 24th edition, 1996.

MECHANISM OF ACTION OF HORMONES WITH INTRACELLULAR RECEPTORS

The hormone enters the target cell and binds to its receptor. The receptor may be in the cytoplasm or in the nucleus. But even if the receptor is in the cytoplasm, the hormone-receptor complex enters the nucleus. The hormone receptor complex affects the expression of a gene. The effect is mediated through that part of DNA which regulates the expression of the gene. The regulatory region of DNA has a part called the hormone response element (HRE). The hormone-receptor complex binds to the HRE. The binding influences the frequency with which transcription of the gene takes place. The frequency of transcription determines the amount of mRNA formed. The amount of mRNA formed determines the amount of protein coded by the gene that will be synthesized. If the protein is an enzyme, its amount will affect the rate of some chemical reactions in the cell. In this way the hormone may affect some important activities of the target cell (Fig. 11.1).

MECHANISM OF ACTION OF HORMONES WITH CELL MEMBRANE RECEPTORS

Peptide and amino acid-derived hormones (except thyroid hormones) have receptors located on the cell membranes of target cells. The hormone-receptor complex stimulates an enzymatic reaction in the cell membrane. As a result, a substance (called second messenger) is produced. The second messenger enters the cell and influences the function of the cell in a specific way (Fig. 11.2).

The hormone (which may be considered the first messenger) does not enter the target cell. Instead, it sends another molecule to transmit the message: therefore the molecule which enters the cell is called the second messenger. The commonest second messenger is cyclic AMP (cAMP). We shall study its generation in the cell membrane in some detail.

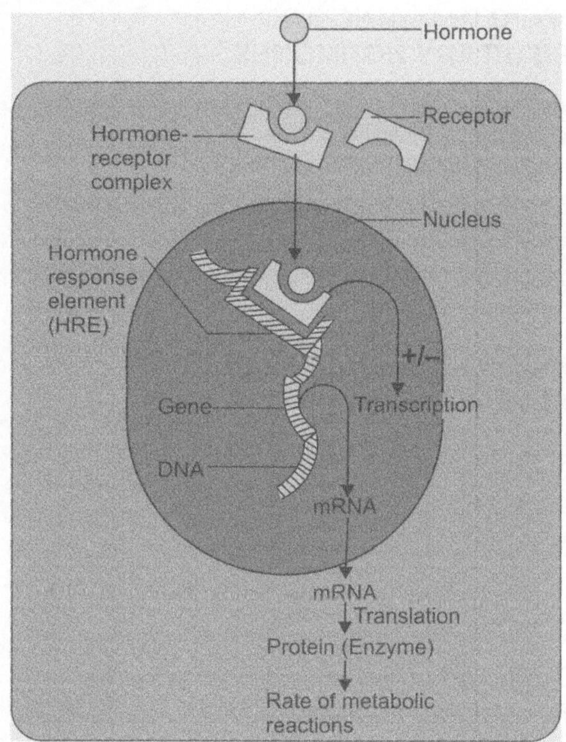

Fig. 11.1 Diagrammatic representation of the mechanisms of action of hormones with intracellular receptors (steroid hormones and thyroid hormones). By affecting the frequency of transcription of a gene (+, stimulation; –, inhibition), the hormone can eventually affect the rate of metabolic reactions in the cell

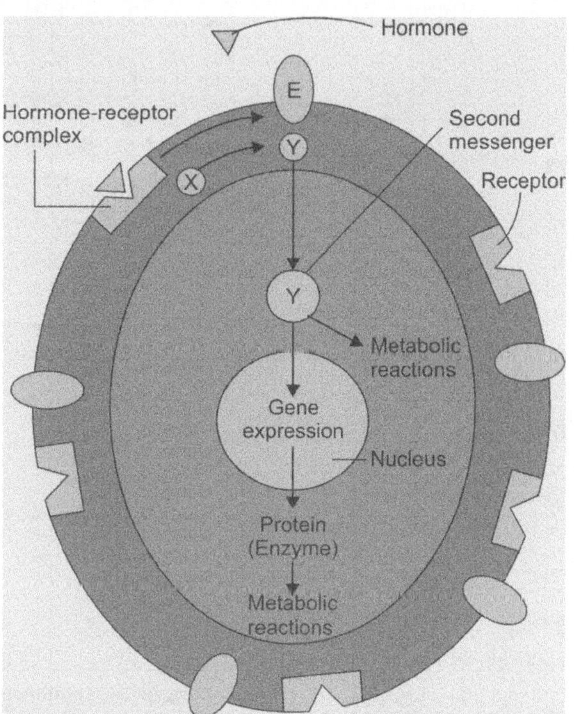

Fig. 11.2 Diagrammatic representation of the mechanisms of action of hormones with cell membrane receptors (peptide and amino acid-derived hormones, except thyroid hormones). The hormone-receptor complex stimulates an enzymatic system (E) which catalyzes the conversion of X to Y. As a result, the rate of formation of Y is increased, and larger amounts of Y enter the cytoplasm. Y (the second messenger) may affect metabolic reactions in the cytoplasm directly, or by influencing gene expression like the steroid hormones (see Fig. 11.1)

Hormone-induced Activation of Adenylyl Cyclase

The hormone-receptor complex triggers the dissociation of the subunits of a membrane protein, called G protein (Figs 11.3A to C). G protein has three subunits: alpha, beta and gamma. Interaction with the hormone-receptor complex triggers the dissociation of the alpha subunit. The alpha subunit, along with the GTP bound to it, then goes and binds to the enzyme adenylyl cyclase, which is also present in the membrane. The alpha subunit-GTP complex activates adenylyl cyclase, which in turn converts ATP into cAMP. While activation of adenylyl cyclase is going on, there is another parallel activity also in progress. The alpha subunit has GTPase activity. Due to this activity, GTP breaks down to GDP. The alpha subunit bound to GDP does not remain bound to the enzyme. It returns to join the beta and gamma subunits. Thus the activation of adenylyl cyclase is a brief reversible event.

Other Second Messengers

Some hormones with cell membrane receptors employ second messengers other than cAMP. One of these messengers is cGMP. Still other hormones either increase the membrane permeability to calcium

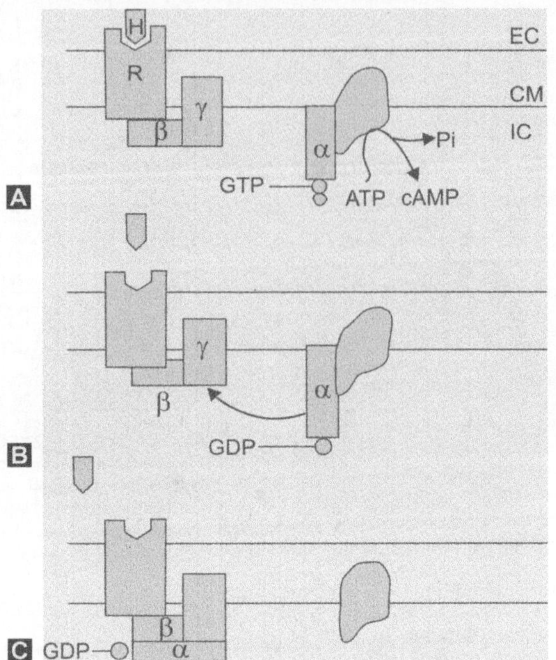

Figs 11.3A to C The role of G-proteins in signal transduction. Diagrammatic representation of the sequence of events involved in the action of a hormone (H) which acts via a G-protein coupled receptor (R). (A) The alpha subunit dissociates from the beta and gamma subunits and interacts with the effector enzyme (adenylyl cyclase). The enzyme is activated and catalyzes the formation of cAMP; (B) The hormone dissociates from its receptor. GTP bound to the alpha subunit is reconverted into GDP; (C) The alpha subunit once again associates with the beta and gamma subunits. Thus, the situation prevailing in (1) is restored. EC, extracellular; CM, cell membrane; IC, intracellular

ions, or release calcium ions from intracellular stores, or both. Calcium combines with the protein, calmodulin. The calcium-calmodulin complex can affect the activity of a large number of enzymes. Some other hormones activate tyrosine kinase and subsequently a cascade of other kinases, finally affecting the process of gene expression. Although the details of action vary with different hormones, the general principles are well illustrated by the mechanism of action of steroid hormones and of the hormones which employ cAMP as the second messenger.

HYPOTHALAMIC AND PITUITARY HORMONES

Hypothalamus is a part of the brain whereas pituitary is an endocrine gland. But one of the functions of the hypothalamus is to produce hormones which are closely related to pituitary function. Pituitary has two main lobes: anterior and posterior. The relationship of the hypothalamus to the two lobes of pituitary is somewhat different.

Hypothalamic Control of Anterior Pituitary

Most of the anterior pituitary hormones are controlled by hypothalamic hormones. The hypothalamic hormones control the release, and in some cases also the production, of the anterior pituitary hormones. The hypothalamic hormones are called releasing hormones.

Transport of Releasing Hormones to the Anterior Pituitary

The releasing hormones are transported to the anterior pituitary in the bloodstream.[2] They diffuse into the hypothalamic capillaries, which join to form the hypothalamo-hypophyseal portal venous system. The portal veins carry the releasing hormones towards the anterior pituitary. In the anterior pituitary they break into another set of capillaries.[3] The releasing hormones diffuse out of these capillaries into the anterior pituitary and influence the release of its hormones (Fig. 11.4).

Action of Releasing Hormones

Most of the releasing hormones increase the release of a specific hormone of the anterior pituitary. The anterior pituitary hormone, in turn, stimulates a target endocrine gland to increase the release or production of its hormone. The action may be

[2]That is why they are called hormones.

[3]Portal venous system is, by definition, the venous system interposed between two sets of capillaries.

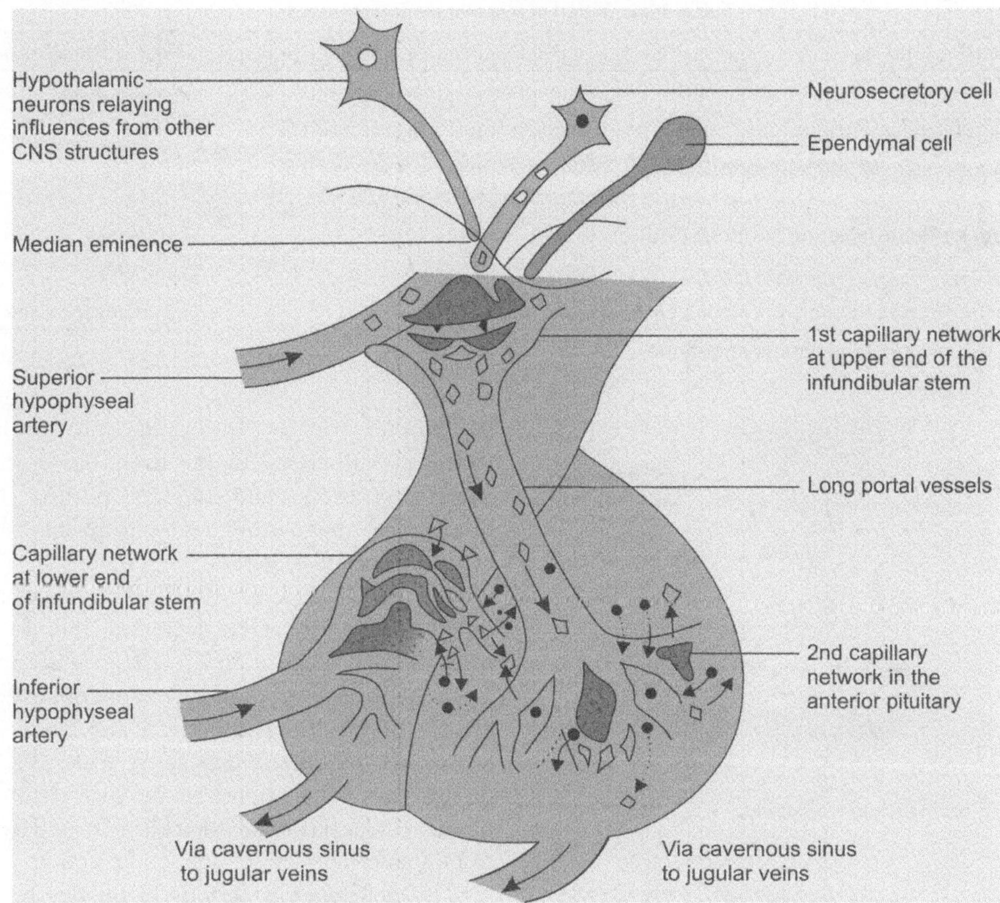

Fig. 11.4 Vascular arrangement linking the hypothalamus and anterior pituitary

illustrated by the hypothalamo-hypophyseal-adrenal axis. The hypothalamus produces the corticotropin releasing hormone (CRH). CRH stimulates the anterior pituitary to release adrenocorticotropic hormone (ACTH). ACTH stimulates the adrenal cortex to release glucocorticoids.

The action of all established releasing hormones is given along these lines in Table 11.2.

Regulatory Role of Hypothalamic and Anterior Pituitary Hormones

Why is the chain of hypothalamus-pituitary-target gland necessary? The chain helps in regulating the level of the hormone of the target gland by a feedback mechanism. An increase in the level of the target hormone inhibits the secretion of the corresponding pituitary or hypothalamic hormone, or both. Similarly, the anterior pituitary hormone inhibits the release of the hypothalamic hormone. In this way the level of the target hormone is brought down. If it falls below normal, the same mechanism works in the opposite direction to bring up the level of the hormone. This is a classical negative feedback mechanism (Fig. 11.5).

Anterior Pituitary Hormones

Anterior pituitary secretes a large number of polypeptide hormones, of which growth hormone

Table 11.2 Action of hypothalamic hormones

Hypothalamic hormones	Target pituitary hormone	Target of pituitary hormone
1. Corticotropin releasing hormone (CRH)	Adrenocortico-tropic hormone (ACTH)	Adrenal cortex
2. Thyrotropin releasing hormone (TRH)	Thyroid stimulating hormone (TSH)	Thyroid
3. Gonadotropin releasing hormone (GnRH)	Follicle stimulating hormone (FSH) Luteinizing hormone (LH)	Gonads
4. Growth hormone releasing hormone (GHRH)	Growth hormone (GH)	Generalized
5. Somatostatin*	GH	Generalized
6. Prolactin release inhibitory hormone (PRIH)*	Prolactin	Not strictly localized

* Inhibits the release of the pituitary hormone

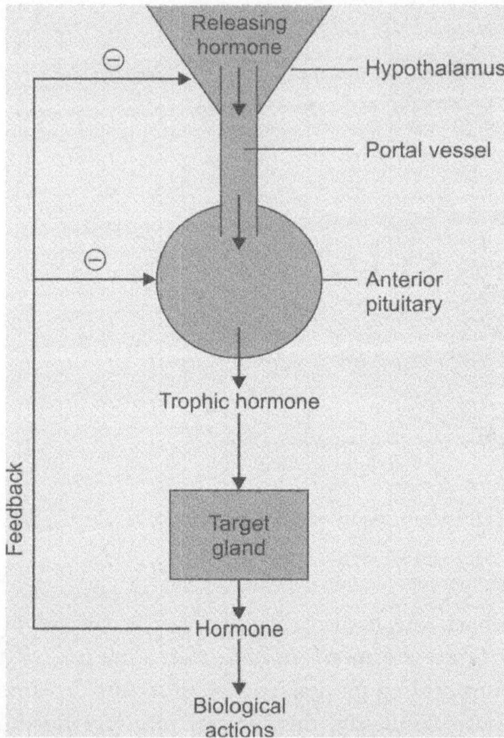

Fig. 11.5 General scheme of regulation of hormone secretion by the hypothalamo-hypophyseal axis

and prolactin have independent actions while others stimulate specific target glands.

Growth Hormone

As its name indicates, growth hormone (GH), is essential for normal growth. The growth is mediated by another peptide, insulin-like growth factor-1 (IGF-1), synthesized in the liver. IGF-1 increases protein synthesis and induces positive balance of calcium, magnesium and phosphate. All these actions promote growth.

GH itself has direct effect on carbohydrate and lipid metabolism. GH decreases the peripheral utilization of glucose and increases gluconeogenesis in the liver. Both these effects are opposite to the actions of insulin, and increase the blood glucose level. GH mobilizes free fatty acids (FFA) and glycerol from the adipose tissue. As a result of this, blood FFA level rises and there is increased oxidation of FFA as fuel.

GH deficiency is serious in infancy because it leads to poor growth. GH deficiency in early life is a significant cause of dwarfism (small height).

GH excess in early life leads to gigantism (tall height). GH excess in an adult does not increase the height further. But it leads to a protrusion of the jaws and enlargement of nose, hands, feet, skull and viscera (acromegaly).

Prolactin

Prolactin (PRL) is structurally similar to GH and can exert similar effects also. But, as its name indicates, PRL is physiologically involved in lactation. In a breast which has been exposed to the action of female hormones (i.e. primed), PRL induces and maintains lactation by stimulating synthesis of milk.

PRL has no known function in males. But its excess in men may lead to gynecomastia and impotence.

Follicle Stimulating Hormone

The name, follicle stimulating hormone (FSH), is based on the action of the hormone in females. But the hormone has a role also in males.

In females, FSH stimulates the follicular cells in the ovary. Thus it promotes the development of ovarian follicle and subsequent secretion of estrogen.

In males, FSH stimulates the Sertoli Cells of the testis and thereby promotes spermatogenesis.

Luteinizing Hormone

The name, luteinizing hormone (LH), is also based on the action of the hormone in females. But the hormone has a role also in males.

In females, LH stimulates the development of corpus luteum and the secretion of progesterone by it.

In males, LH stimulates the Leydig cells (interstitial cells) to secrete testosterone. That is why LH is also called interstitial cell stimulating hormone (ICSH).

Thyroid Stimulating Hormone

As the name indicates, thyroid stimulating hormone (TSH) stimulates the thyroid gland. The stimulation is both short-term and long-term. The short-term effect of TSH is to stimulate the synthesis of thyroid hormones. The long-term effect of TSH is to stimulate the growth of the thyroid gland.

Adrenocorticotropic Hormone

Adrenocorticotropic hormone (ACTH) is also called corticotropin. As its name indicates, ACTH stimulates the adrenal cortex. Short term ACTH stimulation increases the synthesis and release of glucocorticoids from the adrenal cortex. The effect on secretion of mineralocorticoids and adrenal androgens is minimal. Long-term stimulation by ACTH increases the size of the adrenal cortex.

Melanocyte Stimulating Hormone

Melanocyte stimulating hormone (MSH) activity is significant only in animals having a well developed intermediate lobe of the pituitary. In human beings, MSH is essentially absent after birth. MSH disperses the melanin granules in melanocytes of the epidermis. That leads to darkening of the skin.

Posterior Pituitary Hormones

The so-called posterior pituitary hormones are actually synthesized in the hypothalamus. They are transported to the posterior pituitary in the axons of the neurons which synthesize them. They are released by the posterior pituitary into the bloodstream, as and when required, under the influence of an appropriate stimulus.

Antidiuretic Hormone

Antidiuretic hormone (ADH), as the name suggests, reduces the rate of urine formation. ADH is synthesized predominantly in the supraoptic nucleus of the hypothalamus.

The most important stimulus for the secretion of ADH is an increase in the osmolarity of plasma. The increase in osmolarity is sensed by osmoreceptors located in the hypothalalmus. The response to stimulation of the osmoreceptors is an increase in the synthesis and release of ADH.

ADH acts on the distal convoluted tubules and collecting ducts of the kidney. In these parts of the nephron, ADH increases the permeability of the lining epithelium to water. As a result, more water is reabsorbed from the nephron. Hence the urine formed is concentrated, and small in volume. Therefore the rate of urine formation is decreased. Since more water is retained in the body, the osmolarity of body fluids falls. Thus the disturbance which had initiated ADH secretion tends to get corrected. Hence ADH plays an important role in regulation of water balance.

A disease affecting the hypothalamo-hypophyseal tract may reduce ADH secretion. That leads to an abnormal increase in the rate of urine formation. The disease is called diabetes insipidus. A patient of diabetes insipidus has polyuria (high urinary flow) but does not have glucose in the urine. A patient of diabetes mellitus (which is due to insulin deficiency) has polyuria, and the urine has glucose.

ADH is also called vasopressin. This name refers to the capacity of the hormone to bring about vasconstriction and thereby raise the arterial blood pressure. But the vasoconstrictor effect is seen only with pharmacological doses of ADH, not at physiological concentrations.

Oxytocin

Oxytocin is synthesized predominantly in the paraventricular nucleus of the hypothalamus. Oxytocin has two important actions, one which may contribute to parturition (delivery of the baby), and another which is required after parturition.

i. Oxytocin brings about contraction of the uterus. First, distension of the uterus and vagina stimulates secretion of oxytocin. Secondly, the uterus is more sensitive to the action of oxytocin at full term than at other times. The combined result of these two factors is that during partutition, oxytocin brings about uterine contraction, which in turn aids delivery. However, experimental animals whose capacity to secrete oxytocin has been impaired by a lesion of the hypothalamo-hypophyseal tract deliver quite normally. This observation suggests that oxytocin may not be absolutely essential for normal delivery.
ii. Oxytocin brings about contraction of myo-epithelial cells of the mammary gland ducts. This action leads to ejection of milk from the breasts. First, the sensivitity of the myoepithelial cells of the breast to oxytocin is also increased near parturition. Secondly, stimulation of nipples by the suckling baby leads to a reflex release of oxytocin. Both these factors ensure the milk ejection reflex at the right time. Oxytocin is essential for the normal milk ejection reflex.

THYROID GLAND

Thyroid gland is situated in the neck, anterior to the trachea. It consists of two lobes joined by an isthmus (Fig. 11.6). A section of the thyroid shows, under the microscope, clusters of follicles lined by epithelium. The follicles are filled with 'colloid', the secretions of the epithelial cells. An active thyroid has cuboidal or columnar epithelial cells, but very little colloid in the follicles because the secretions are released promptly into the blood stream. On the other hand, an inactive ('resting' or 'lazy') thyroid has follicles lined with flat squamous epithelial cells and full of colloid because whatever secretions are there are stored rather than released. Thus, paradoxical though it may seem, a thyroid having follicles full of colloid is actually inactive (Figs 11.7A to C).

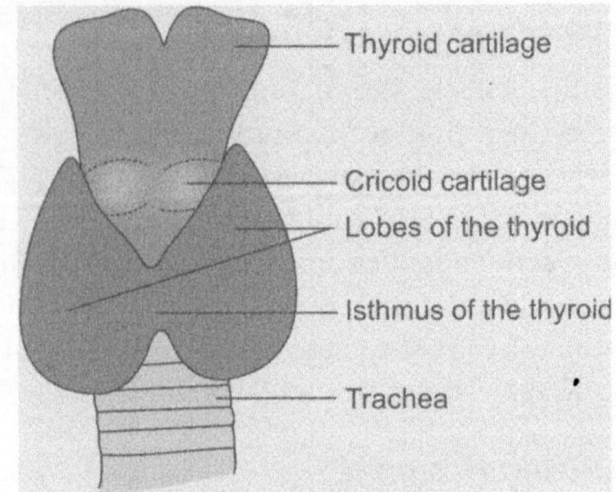

Fig. 11.6 The thyroid gland

Scattered in the connective tissue between the follicles are cells called parafollicular cells. Parafollicular cells contain numerous secretory granules.

Hormones of the Thyroid Gland

The epithelium of thyroid follicles produces two hormones: triiodothyronine (T_3) and tetraiodothyronine (T_4). The parafollicular cells secrete the hormone calcitonin. Because of their functional relationship, calcitonin will be discussed later with parathyroid hormone. Here we shall discuss only T_3 and T_4.

Synthesis of Thyroid Hormones

Synthesis of thyroid hormones, T_3 and T_4 requires iodination of the amino acid, tyrosine. The reaction occurs while tyrosine is still part of a protein molecule: the protein called thyroglobulin. Thyroglobulin is a tyrosine-rich protein. Each thyroglobulin molecule has 5000 amino acid residues, out of which 115 are those of tyrosine. Thyroglobulin is synthesized in the follicular epithelium of the thyroid. Besides

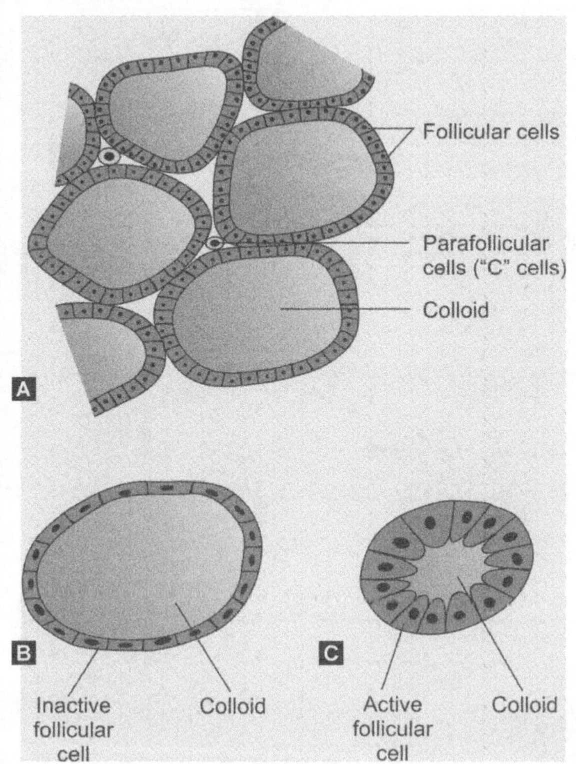

Figs 11.7A to C (A) Histological structure of a moderately active thyroid gland. Note that the follicular cells are cuboidal; (B) Follicle of an inactive thyroid gland. The cells are flat because they are inactive. The follicle is large because it contains a large amount of stored colloid; (C) Follicle of an active thyroid gland. The cells are tall and columnar because they are active. The follicle is small because the thyroid is secreting the hormones rather than storing them as colloid

thyroglobulin, the second requirement for synthesis of thyroid hormones is iodine.

Circulating iodide is captured by the follicular epithelium. Iodide uptake is an energy-dependent process, utilizing a sodium/potassium ATPase. The trapped iodine and the thyroglobulin are both transported to the apical surface of the cell (i.e. the surface facing the follicular lumen). The enzymes for synthesis of hormones are located on the apical surface of the cell. The steps involved in synthesis are:

a. Oxidation of iodide to iodine,
b. Iodination of tyrosyl residues in thyroglobulin to form monoiodotyrosine (MIT) and diiodotyrosine (DIT), and
c. Coupling of some of the iodinated residues to form T_3 and T_4 (Fig. 11.8).

T_3 and T_4 are still a part of the thyroglobulin molecule. They are transported in this form to the lumen of the follicle for storage. Histologically, this stored hormone appears as colloid.

When T_3 and T_4 are required for circulation, the stored hormone, 'attached' to thyroglobulin, is transported back into the follicular cell. The transport is accomplished by phagocytosis. The phagocytosed thyroglobulin-containing vacuole fuses with lysosomes. Lysosomes contain enzymes for hydrolysis of thyroglobulin. Besides a large variety of amino acids, the hydrolysis releases T_3 and T_4, which are secreted into extracellular space. They diffuse from the extracellular space into capillaries, and thus enter the general circulation (Fig. 11.8).

Transport of Thyroid Hormones

On entering the bloodstream, most of the T_3 and T_4 get bound to a plasma protein called thyroxine binding globulin (TBG).[4] The small amount that is free is the one which is responsible for activity of the hormones. Most of the free T_4 is converted by tissues into T_3. Further, T_3 has ten times as much affinity for thyroid hormone receptors as T_4. Therefore T_3 is considered the principal thyroid hormone which finally mediates the metabolic effects.

Functions of Thyroid Hormones

Thyroid hormones have two general effects: stimulation of gene transcription and stimulation of metabolism. These two effects may be interrelated, and can explain most of the other effects.

Calorigenic Effect

Thyroid hormones enhance oxygen consumption, and hence the basal metabolic rate (BMR). This may

[4]Binding prevents renal excretion of the hormones. T_3 and T_4 are small molecules which can be easily filtered and excreted by the kidneys. But TBG, like other plasma proteins, does not get filtered by the kidneys.

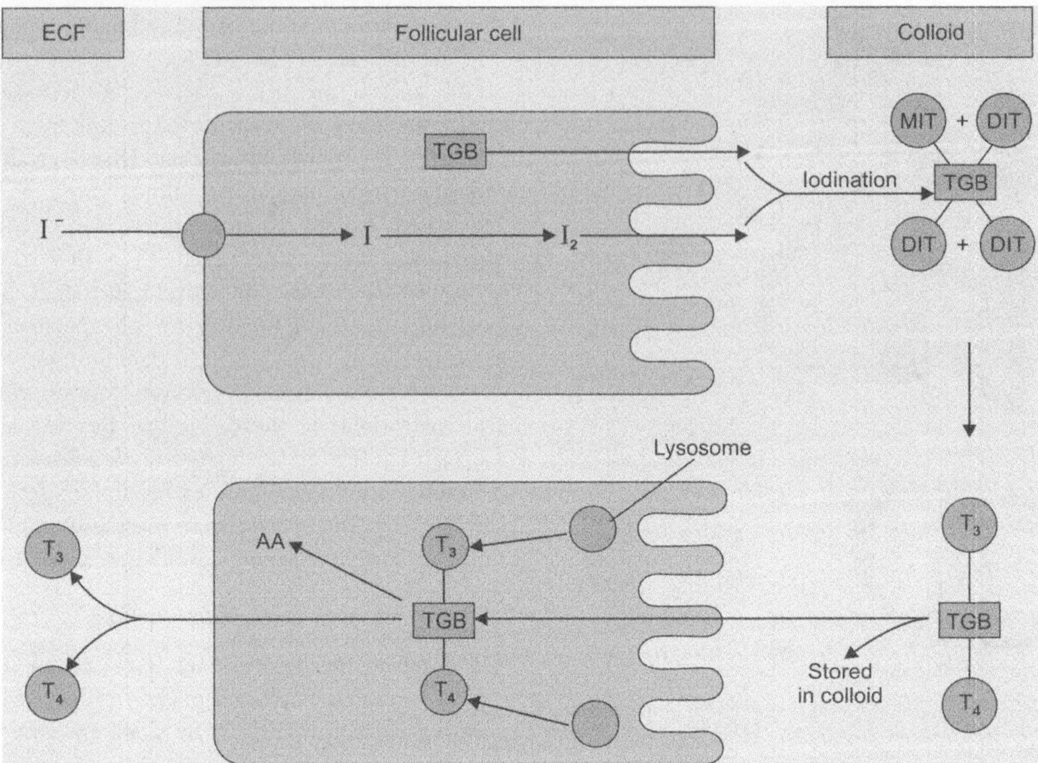

Fig. 11.8 Synthesis and release of thyroid hormones. Iodide is trapped by the follicular cells by means of an iodide pump. The follicular cells also synthesize a protein called thyroglobulin (TGB). Oxidized iodide (i.e. iodine) iodinates the tyrosine residues in TGB to form monoiodotyrosine (MIT) and diiodotyrosine (DIT). Appropriate coupling of MIT and DIT produces triiodothyronine (T_3) or tetraiodothyronine (T_4). Iodination and coupling reactions take place in the extracellular environment, but not necessarily in the lumen of the follicle. T_3 and T_4 may be stored in the colloid in association with TGB. Alternatively, the complex may be internalized and hydrolyzed by lysosomes. In that case, T_3 and T_4 are released into the extracellular fluid (ECF) and thence into the bloodstream. AA, amino acids

be at least partly due to increase in the activity of membrane Na/K ATPase. Thyroid hormones also increase the number and activity of mitochondria, which may be the cause or the effect of increase in oxygen consumption. At very high concentrations, thyroid hormones uncouple oxidation and phosphorylation in mitochondria.

By increasing the metabolic rate, thyroid hormones raise the body temperature, lead to loss of body weight, and increase urinary nitrogen loss.

Growth and Development

Thyroid hormones are essential for normal growth and development. The classical example to illustrate this function is that of tadpoles, which do not change into frogs unless thyroid hormones are available. In human beings also, thyroid hormone deficiency impairs growth and development. The effect is partly because thyroid hormones potentiate the effect of growth hormone.

Effects on Substrate Metabolism

Thyroid hormones increase the rate of absorption from the gastrointestinal tract. They also stimulate glycolysis, gluconeogenesis as well as insulin secretion. They mobilize fats from adipose tissue, leading to an increase in the plasma concentration of free fatty acids. All these effects help in making available substrates for the enhanced metabolic rate.

Systemic Effects

a. *Nervous system:* Thyroid hormones are essential for normal formation of synapses and myelination in the developing brain. That is why if hypothyroidism occurs during intrauterine life, the child is mentally retarded. In later life also, thyroid hormones improve mental alertness.
b. *Cardiovascular system:* Thyroid hormones increase the heart rate, and cardiac output, and consequently also the systolic blood pressure. But the diastolic pressure may fall due to vasodilation in several vascular beds induced by the increased metabolism. The cardiovascular effects of thyroid hormones are partly mediated by their increasing the sensitivity of tissues to catecholamines.
c. *Respiratory system:* Thyroid hormones increase the rate and depth of respiration
d. *Gastrointestinal system:* Thyroid hormones increase gastrointestinal secretion and motility, and as mentioned above, also increase the rate of absorption.

Mechanism of Action of Thyroid Hormones

Thyroid hormones have intracellular receptors. The receptors are located in the nucleus. The hormone-receptor interaction leads to increased transcription, and thereby an increase in protein synthesis. In the anterior pituitary, T_3 enhances transcription of the GH gene. That explains the positive effect of thyroid hormones on growth. In the same way, T_3 possibly influences regulation of specific genes in several other tissues which would explain its other effects such as brain development.

Regulation of Thyroid Secretion

Thyroid secretion is regulated by a classical negative feedback mechanism. An increase in thyroid hormone level suppresses TSH and TRH secretion. On the other hand, a decrease in thyroid hormone level stimulates TSH and TRH secretion (Fig. 11.5). Thus the level is maintained within normal limits.

Disorders of the Thyroid Gland

Hypothyroidism

As the name indicates, hypothyroidism means a decrease in thyroid activity. Its predominant cause is iodine deficiency. Iodine deficiency may occur while the fetus is growing in the mother's womb. Such a child is born a cretin. A cretin is mentally retarded, grows slowly, is constipated and has a hoarse cry. Since the brain continues to grow for only a few years after birth, treatment of cretinism should be started as soon as possible to minimize the degree of mental retardation.

If hypothyroidism occurs in an adult, it gives rise to myxedema. In myxedema, the person has a puffy face, constipation, sleepiness, slow heart rate and slow reactions. He also feels colder than normal persons due to a reduction in basal metabolic rate (BMR). He may also have obesity, anemia, hypercholesterolemia and a swelling in the neck (goiter).

Hyperthyroidism

Hyperthyroidism means an increase in thyroid activity. Hyperthyroidism leads to an increase in BMR, and hence an increased tolerance to cold, excessive sweating, and loss of weight. Other features are an increase in heart rate, insomnia, tremors, nervousness and hyperirritability. In one form of hyperthyroidism (Grave's disease), eyes are very prominent because the eyeballs are pushed outwards (**exophthalmos**).

Goiter

Goiter is a swelling in the neck due to enlargement of the thyroid gland. In case of iodine deficiency, the production of thyroid hormones is decreased. That stimulates the anterior pituitary to produce more TSH. TSH stimulates the thyroid gland, leading to its enlargement. The enlarged thyroid may be able to trap enough iodine from even a deficient supply to achieve normal thyroid hormone production. Or, the thyroid hormone production may improve but still be deficient in spite of enlargement of the thyroid gland. In either case, the goiter will reduce in size if the dietary iodine intake is increased. This may be achieved by taking iodized salt. Since very large areas of India are deficient in iodine, iodization of all salt sold in the market has been adopted as a target, which is likely to be met in the very near future.

In some cases an enlarged thyroid gland (goiter) produces more hormones than a normal thyroid gland. In that case, the patient has hyperthyroidism.

Thus a goiter may be associated with normal thyroid function (euthyroidism), hypothyroidism or hyperthyroidism.

PARATHYROID GLANDS

Parathyroids are four small glands situated behind the thyroid gland, one each at the upper and lower poles of the two lobes (right and left) of the thyroid.

Parathyroid hormone (PTH) is a polypeptide hormone. PTH is the principal regulator of calcium metabolism in the body. PTH has three main actions:

1. PTH brings about dissolution of bone and thereby mobilizes calcium from bones. Thus PTH raises plasma calcium level.
2. PTH reduces renal calcium excretion. This action of PTH also raises plasma calcium level.
3. PTH stimulates the conversion of 25-hydroxy-cholecalciferol (25-OH-D_3) into 1, 25 $(OH)_2$-D_3 by the kidney. 1, 25 $(OH)_2$-D_3 is the biologically active form of vitamin D. 1, 25 (OH)2-D3 stimulates the synthesis of calcium binding protein (CBP) by the intestine. CBP increases calcium absorption by the intestine. Through this action, PTH indirectly increases the calcium content of the body.

Thus all the three actions of PTH improve calcium availability. The action on the bone is an emergency measure to prevent plasma calcium level from falling below the normal level. But this is achieved at the expense of bone demineralization, which weakens the bone. The action on the kidney tries to save calcium by reducing its urinary loss. But this action can have only a limited impact on calcium balance. The third action improves calcium supply of the body. That is the best way to maintain plasma calcium while keeping the bones also well provided with calcium. But being a long-term measure, it needs more time to be effective and also needs adequate supply of calcium and vitamin D in the diet.

Regulation of Parathyroid Hormone Secretion

PTH secretion is regulated mainly by the plasma calcium level. Plasma calcium level is sensed by appropriate receptors in parathyroid cells. Parathyroid cells respond to this information by altering the rate of PTH secretion. As you might expect, low plasma calcium level leads to increased PTH secretion. Conversely, high plasma calcium level leads to a decrease in PTH secretion.

OTHER HORMONES AFFECTING CALCIUM METABOLISM

The body of an adult contains about 1 kg of calcium, 99% of which is in bone. While calcium is important for the strength of bones, the small amount of calcium in circulation is also important. The normal plasma calcium level is about 5 mmol/L (20 mg/dL), of which nearly half is bound to proteins and the other half is ionized. The ionized calcium level needs to be maintained constant for normal neuromuscular excitability. A decrease in ionized calcium level makes nerve and muscle cells hyperexcitable and may lead to tetanic convulsions. An increase in ionic calcium level may lead to coma and death due to paralysis of respiratory muscles.

Besides neuromuscular excitability, calcium ions regulate several other functions. The functions regulated by calcium ions have been enumerated below:

1. Maintenance of neuromuscular excitability.
2. Participation in coagulaltion of blood.

3. Regulation of the activity of several enzymes, e.g. myosin ATPase.
4. Release of neurotransmitters, hormones and several other secretory products.
5. Mineralization.

That is the reason why it is so important to maintain plasma calcium at a normal level. This is achieved mainly by PTH. Other hormones which regulate plasma calcium level are calcitriol and calcitonin.

Calcitriol

Calcitriol is the name now given to 1, 25-dihydroxycholecalciferol, abbreviated as 1, 25 $(OH)_2$-D_3, to indicate that it is a dihydroxylation product of vitamin D_3. Vitamin D_3 may be synthesized from its precursor in the skin under the effect of sunlight, or may be taken in the diet. D_3 is hydroxylated at position 25 in the liver and then at position 1 in the kidney. The final product 1, 25 $(OH)_2$-D_3, has been synthesized in the body, and is released into the circulation. It travels in the bloodstream to its target organ (intestine) where it acts like a steroid hormone to stimulate the synthesis of calcium binding protein (CBP). Thus 1, 25 $(OH)_2$-D_3 (calcitriol) has all the characteristics of a hormone. The 'secretion' of calcitriol is regulated by PTH as discussed earlier.

Calcitonin

Calcitonin, a polypeptide hormone, is secreted by parafollicular cells of the thyroid gland. Its actions are somewhat opposite those of PTH. Calcitonin reduces bone resorption and promotes deposition of calcium in bones. Hence it reduces the plasma calcium level. The significance of calcitonin in adults is uncertain. But in children it may have a role in the remodeling of bones. Calcitonin secretion is regulated by the plasma calcium level. A high calcium level stimulates calcitonin secretion while a low calcium level inhibits it.

ADRENAL CORTEX

Adrenals are a pair of glands situated, as the name indicates, next to the kidneys. In fact, they are placed on top of each kidney. Each adrenal consists of an outer layer called the cortex, and an inner core called the medulla. Functionally, the cortex and medulla are two separate glands.

A section of the adrenal cortex shows three layers under the microscope: zona glomerulosa, zone fasciculata and zona reticularis. The three zones secrete, respectively, three different classes of steroid hormones, viz. mineralocorticoids, glucocorticoids and androgens, with some overlap between the functions of the layers. Zona glomerulosa secretes mineralocorticoids, while both zona fasciculata and zone reticularis secrete both glucocorticoids and androgens.

Mechanism of Action

Steroid hormones have intracellular receptors. The hormone-receptor binding may take place either in the cytoplasm or in the nucleus. The hormone-receptor complex affects the expression of a specific gene in the nucleus. Alteration in the rate of synthesis of the protein expressed by the gene mediates the biological actions of the hormone.

Glucocorticoids

The main glucocorticoid secreted by the human adrenal cortex is cortisol.

Actions of Cortisol

Cortisol has specific effects on carbohydrate, protein and fat metabolism, which can be understood in light of its general effects on immune mechanisms, inflammation and, broadly, the response of the body to stress. The actions have been enumerated below.

1. *Carbohydrate metabolism:* Glucocorticoids stimulate production of glucose from amino acids (gluconeogenesis) and glycogen synthesis in the liver. They reduce the peripheral utilization of glucose in most tissues except brain and heart. When cortisol is present, glucagon and adrenaline are more effective in producing glycogenolysis in muscle. The combined result of these actions is an increase in the level of blood glucose. The improved glucose supply to the brain and heart is useful in stress.

2. *Protein metabolism:* At physiological levels, cortisol promotes protein synthesis. High levels of cortisol, seen in states of stress, promote protein breakdown everywhere in the body except in the liver. The amino acids mobilized by protein breakdown are converted into glucose in the liver and utilized to meet the requirements of stress.
3. *Fat metabolism:* Cortisol promotes lipolysis directly, and also indirectly by facilitating the action of adrenaline and growth hormone. The free fatty acids mobilized by lipolysis are also useful as fuel in states of stress.
4. *Cardiovascular effects:* Glucocorticoids increase contractility of the heart, and thereby increase cardiac output and blood pressure. These are useful actions in states of stress.
5. *Muscle contraction:* Glucocorticoids increase the force of skeletal muscle contraction. This action is also useful in stress.
6. *Role in stress:* Both physical and mental stress stimulate release of ACTH and consequently increased secretion of glucocorticoids. Glucocorticoids help the body in coping up with stress through the actions discussed above.
7. *Anti-inflammatory effect:* In pharmacological doses, glucocorticoids suppress inflammation. Used with adequate precautions, the anti-inflammatory effect of glucocorticoids can be useful in some diseases. Synthetic analogs of glucocorticoids are most commonly used locally to suppress inflammation of the skin in various forms of dermatitis.
8. *Immunosuppressive effect:* In pharmacological doses, glucocorticoids suppress also the immune response. Immune response is a normal and generally desirable response. But sometimes it may need to be suppressed, as in autoimmune diseases and hypersensitivity reactions.

Regulation of Glucocorticoid Secretion

Glucocorticoid secretion is stimulated by adrenocorticotropic hormone (ACTH), which is secreted by the anterior pituitary. ACTH secretion is stimulated by corticotropin releasing hormone (CRH), which is secreted by the hypothalamus, and is delivered to the anterior pituitary by the hypothalamo-hypophyseal portal vessels. The chain is called hypothalamus-pituitary-adrenal axis. The secretion of ACTH and CRH is subject to negative feedback inhibition (Fig. 11.5). The feedback effect keeps glucocorticoid secretion within normal limits. Stress can stimulate the hypothalamus to release more CRH. That in turn increases ACTH secretion. Consequently glucorticoid secretion is elevated in stress.

Excess Glucocorticoid Secretion: Cushing's Syndrome

Excess of glucocorticoids leads to a fat round face and fat deposition in the abdomen but the limbs remain thin. Hair growth at all vulnerable areas of the body is stimulated, e.g. females may develop hairiness over the beard area of the face. The muscles are wasted and bones develop osteoporosis due to protein catabolism. Blood sugar may be raised primarily due to gluconeogenesis. Resistance to infections is impaired due to immunosuppression. The blood pressure is raised. Sodium and water retention occurs due to the weak mineralocorticoid activity of glucocorticoids, which becomes significant when the secretion is excessive.

Deficient Glucocorticoid Secretion: Addison's Disease

Deficiency of glucocorticoids leads to loss of appetite, loss of weight, anemia and weakness. It impairs the capacity of the body to cope up with stress. The blood pressure may be low. Body fluids may be depleted of sodium and water. Blood tests show lymphopenia and eosinopenia. If the deficiency is due to a defect in the adrenal cortex itself, negative feedback leads to elevated ACTH levels. Elevated ACTH levels lead to pigmentation of the skin and mucous membranes.

Mineralocorticoids

The main mineralocorticoid secreted by the human adrenal cortex is aldosterone.

Actions of Aldosterone

Aldosterone acts primarily in the kidney. It increases sodium reabsorption in the distal convoluted tubules and collecting ducts. As the result of this, the body retains sodium. Secondary to sodium retention, water is also retained. Thus aldosterone promotes sodium and water retention. In contrast, aldosterone increases the renal loss of potassium.

Regulation of Aldosterone Secretion

Aldosterone secretion is regulated primarily by two factors: plasma potassium level and renin-angiotensin system

1. *Plasma potassium:* When the plasma potassium level is high, aldosterone secretion is increased. This is understandable because aldosterone increases urinary potassium loss. Thus plasma potassium level itself can regulate aldosterone secretion so that plasma potassium stays within normal limits.
2. *Renin-angiotensin system:* Renin is a hormone released by the kidneys. It is synthesized in the juxtaglomerular cells of the kidney. Some of the important stimulators of renin release are renal ischemia and salt depletion. These changes are also detected by the juxtaglomerular cells. Renal ischemia may be due to a fall in blood pressure, which in turn, may be due to salt and water depletion. Thus the two factors are interrelated.

Renin acts on a plasma protein, angiotensinogen, to form angiotensin I. Angiotensin I is converted by an enzyme, angiotensin converting enzyme (ACE) into angiotensin II. Besides being a potent vasoconstrictor, angiotensin II also releases aldosterone from the adrenal cortex. In addition, angiotensin II also inhibits renin release from the kidney, thereby forming a negative feedback loop.

Excess Aldosterone Secretion: Conn's Syndrome

Excess aldosterone secretion leads to sodium retention and excess potassium loss. Sodium retention leads to water retention. Sodium and water retention may lead to hypertension. Along with excess renal potassium excretion, aldosterone also increases renal hydrogen ion excretion. That leads to alkalosis.

Deficient Aldosterone Secretion

Deficiency of aldosterone has features opposite those of aldosterone excess. Excess sodium and water loss may lead to hypotension. Reduced potassium excretion leads to hyperkalemia. Reduced hydrogen ion excretion leads to acidosis.

Androgens

Adrenals are a significant source of androgens in females, although in males they only supplement, in a small way, the testicular androgen secretion. In females, androgens possibly have an important anabolic function contributing to bone integrity and muscle mass. Androgens of adrenal origin can be converted into estrogens by adipose tissue. These estrogens are the major source of estrogen in males and in postmenopausal females.

Abnormal Secretion: Adrenogenital Syndrome

In some cases of congenital deficiency of enzymes involved in glucocorticoid synthesis, the intermediate compounds accumulate in excess (Fig. 11.9). These compounds can be converted into androgens. Further, deficiency of glucocorticoids leads to increased secretion of ACTH by negative feedback. High levels of ACTH lead to adreno-cortical hyperplasia. The enlarged hyperplastic adrenals cannot still manufacture enough glucocorticoids due to enzyme deficiency but end up making still more androgens. The large amounts of androgens lead to precocious (early) puberty in males, and to appearance of male secondary sexual characteristics in females.

ADRENAL MEDULLA

Adrenal medulla is, functionally, a part of the sympathetic division of the autonomic nervous system (ANS). It is supplied by fibers of the

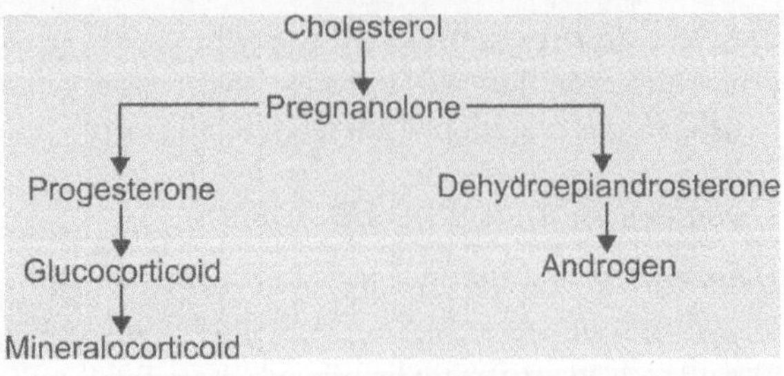

Fig. 11.9 Skeleton of biochemical pathways in adrenal cortex. Deficiency of enzymes for glucocorticoid synthesis leads to increased conversion of pregnanolone into androgen

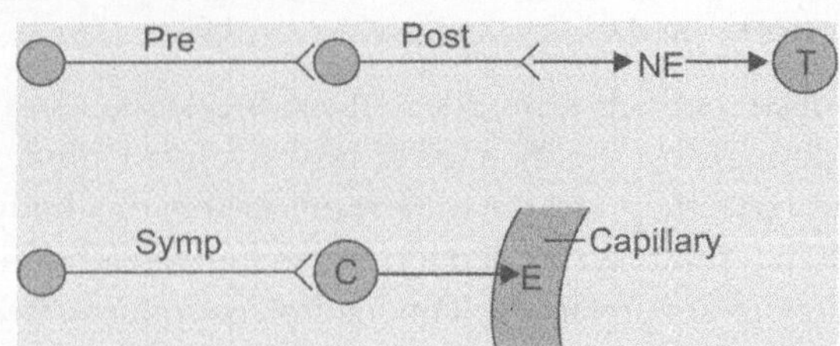

Figs 11.10A and B Adrenal medulla is comparable to postganglionic neurons of the sympathetic nervous system. A. Schematic representation of sympathetic nervous system. Pre, preganglionic neuron; Post, postganglionic neuron; NE, norepinephrine; T, target organ. B. Schematic representation of adrenal medulla and its innervation. Symp, sympathetic nerve fibers supplying the adrenal medulla; C. chromaffin cells of the adrenal medulla; E, epinephrine

splanchnic nerve. These fibers, which are equivalent to preganglionic fibers, terminate on the chromaffin cells of the adrenal medulla. Chromaffin cells synthesize catecholamines–mostly epinephrine, but also some norepinephrine. Thus chromaffin cells are equivalent to postganglionic neurons. But they lack axons. Instead, chromaffin cells of the adrenal medulla release epinephrine directly into the bloodstream. That is why adrenal medulla is an endocrine gland (Figs 11.10A and B). Adrenal medulla is activated whenever sympathetic nervous system is activated. Sympathetic nerves release norepinephrine locally in the organs supplied by them. Adrenal medulla releases epinephrine and norepinephrine into the general circulation so that it can also reach organs outside the reach of sympathetic nerves (e.g. skeletal muscles).

Mechanism of Action

Catecholamines are derived from the amino acid, tyrosine. Like peptide hormones, catecholamines also have cell membrane receptors. Catecholamine receptors are broadly of two types - alpha and beta. Further, each of these has two subtypes, viz. alpha1 and alpha 2, beta1 and beta 2. All these receptors are G-protein coupled receptors. Both the subtypes of beta receptors, when combined with the hormone, lead to an increase in cAMP in the cell which, in turn, mediates the action of the hormone. Alpha 2 type of receptors, in contrast, act by decreasing the level of cAMP in the cell. The action of Alpha 1 receptors is mediated by a change in intracellular concentration of calcium ions.

Besides the difference in second messengers, the classification of receptors also takes into account differences in biological action, and the variation in antagonists which can block individual actions.

Epinephrine acts via both alpha and beta receptors. Norepinephrine acts primarily via only alpha receptors.

Actions of Catecholamines

Like the sympathetic nervous system, catcholamines also help the body cope up with stress. Bodily responses to catecholamines can be generally predicted correctly by thinking what would be helpful to the body in stress. The actions have been summarized in Table 11.3. As seen, the cardiovascular system and respiratory system are made ready for muscular action, and fuel is mobilized for additional effort.

Regulation of Catecholamine Secretion

Regulation of catecholamine secretion is linked up with regulation of autonomic activity. It is controlled by the brain stem reticular formation via the hypothalamus. This aspect, and some other aspects of adrenal medullary function will become clearer after studying ANS (Chapter 17).

Table 11.3 Actions of catecholamines

Alpha receptor actions	*Beta receptor actions*
Vasoconstriction	Increase in rate and force of contraction of heart
Contraction of gastro-intestinal and genitourinary sphincters	Bronchodilation
Relaxation of gastrointestinal tract	Dilatation of blood vessels in skeletal muscles
Glycogenolysis	Glycogenolysis Gluconeogenesis Lipolysis

Excess Catecholamine Secretion

Excess catecholamine secretion may be the result of a tumor of the adrenal medulla called pheochromocytoma. The cardinal feature of pheochromocytoma is hypertension.

PANCREAS

Pancreas is a stucture which may be considered two organs in one. Its exocrine part, which secretes digestive enzymes, has already been considered (Chapter 8). The endocrine part, which secretes hormones, will be discussed here. The endocrine part forms about 1 percent of the weight of the pancreas. Histologically, the endocrine pancreas forms about 1 million clusters (islands) of cells scattered at random throughout the pancreas. These islands are called the islets of Langerhans. The islets have four types of cells which secrete four different hormones. A cells, which form about 25 percent of the islet cells, secrete glucagon. B Cells, which form about 70 percent of the islet cells, secrete insulin. D cells, which form about 5 percent of the islet cells, secrete somatostatin. The F cells, very few in number, secrete pancreatic polypeptide. Somatostatin affects the secretion of insulin and glucagon locally. Pancreatic polypeptide plays a role in the regulation of some gastrointestinal secretions. Here we shall discuss only the major hormones of the pancreas, viz. insulin and glucagon.

Insulin

As mentioned above, insulin is secreted by the B cells of the islets of Langerhans of pancreas. Its deficiency–absolute or effective – is the basic defect in the common disease, diabetes mellitus.

Actions of Insulin

Insulin affects the metabolism of carbohydrates, lipids and proteins, and also stimulates cell division.

1. *Effects on carbohydrate metabolism:* Insulin increases the utilization of glucose and decreases its production by its following actions.
   a. Insulin stimulates oxidation of glucose by glycolysis, specially in the liver and skeletal muscle. Thus insulin favors utilization of glucose as fuel. Thereby, it spares amino acids for protein synthesis and fatty acids for lipogenesis.
   b. Insulin stimulates glycogenesis. In other words, it favors conversion of glucose into its storage form, glycogen. This action is seen in both liver and muscle.
   c. Insulin inhibits synthesis of glucose from non-carbohydrate sources (gluconeogenesis).

   The overall effect of the above actions is a decrease in the blood glucose level.
2. *Effects on lipid metabolism:* Insulin stimulates synthesis of lipids (lipogenesis) and inhibits their breakdown (lipolysis).
3. *Effects on protein metabolism:* Insulin stimulates protein synthesis (anabolism) and inhibits protein breakdown (catabolism).
4. *Effects on cell division:* Insulin enhances the effect of many other growth factors in cell cultures. This suggests that insulin may have a role in stimulating cell division during growth and repair.

Food has two basic functions: to provide energy and to provide material for growth and repair. Insulin helps in utilization of carbohydrate as fuel to obtain energy. Insulin also conserves protein for growth, and stimulates cell division, which is necessary for growth. In addition, insulin also serves to store carbohydrate as glycogen and fats as triglycerides. These reserves are useful when carbohydrate supply is reduced, as between meals and during fasting. Thus insulin helps in making best use of all the major nutrients in our diet.

Mechanism of Action

Although insulin has so many actions, so far we know of only one type of insulin receptor. Insulin is a peptide hormone. Accordingly, insulin receptors are cell membrane receptors. The multiple actions of insulin are the result of the insulin-receptor complex leading to generation of a wide variety of second messengers or intracellular signals. For example, one mechanism by which glucose utilization is enhanced is by translocating glucose transporters to the cell membrane. In this way the transport of glucose into the cells is increased. Another mechanism by which intermediary metabolism is affected is by activation or inhibition of various enzymes involved in metabolic reactions. Protein synthesis is stimulated non-specifically by enhanced transport of amino acids into cells. In addition, mRNA synthesis is also increased. Stimulation of specific types of mRNA increases the synthesis of specific proteins, including some enzymes. The expression of some specific genes may even be inhibited. For example, insulin inhibits the expression of the gene for a key enzyme required for gluconeogenesis. That is how insulin inhibits glucose production by gluconeogenesis. Finally, insulin also stimulates DNA synthesis under some circumstances. This may explain the effect of insulin on cell division.

Regulation of Insulin Secretion

The most important regulator of insulin secretion is the concentration of glucose in the plasma. When the plasma glucose level is above the fasting level (80-100 mg/dL), insulin secretion is turned on. As the plasma glucose level increases further, insulin secretion also increases. Maximum secretion of insulin occurs at a plasma glucose level between 300 and 500 mg/dL. This arrangement is logical and works very well because:

a. Insulin reduces plasma glucose level. Thus the regulatory mechanism has the features of a negative feedback control system.
b. Plasma glucose level rises after a meal. Insulin helps in making best use of the various components of the meal, viz. carbohydrates, proteins and fats.

In fact, the pancreas is activated in anticipation of the rise in plasma glucose by gut hormones, specially GIP. GIP is secreted in response to the presence of glucose in the small intestine. Thus even before glucose has been absorbed, GIP reaches the pancreas through the bloodstream and stimulates insulin secretion. This is called **enteroinsular axis**.

Regulation of Plasma Glucose

Regulation of plasma glucose is closely linked to the regulation of insulin secretion. As the above discussion indicates, insulin secretion would prevent the plasma glucose from rising much above the fasting level. That is why even after a heavy meal, plasma glucose generally stays below 200 mg/dL in healthy persons.

But it is equally important to ensure that plasma glucose does not fall very low. Some organs such as the brain do not function normally at low plasma glucose levels. Fortunately there are several hormones which raise plasma glucose level. One of them is built into the islets itself, viz. glucagon (see below). Epinephrine and cortisol are stimulated by stress, including that of hypoglycemia, and bring the plasma glucose back to normal. In addition, growth hormone also increases plasma glucose level. Thus there are several hormones which raise plasma glucose, and only one (insulin) which lowers plasma glucose. But the physiological mechanisms regulate the secretion of all these hormones in such a way that plasma glucose always stays within the normal range.

Pathophysiology of Diabetes Mellitus

Diabetes mellitus, commonly called simply diabetes, is due to an effective deficiency of insulin. There may be an actual decrease in insulin secretion (absolute deficiency), or the body may be resistant to the action of insulin (relative deficiency). Insulin resistance may be due to insulin antibodies in circulation, a decrease in insulin receptors, or antibodies to insulin receptors.

The features of diabetes mellitus can be easily understood in light of the actions of insulin. Insulin promotes glucose utilization. Therefore in insulin deficiency, glucose is poorly utilized. Hence the plasma glucose level becomes high (hyperglycemia). The renal threshold for glucose reabsorption is plasma glucose level of about 180 mg/dL. If the hyperglycemia of diabetes exceeds this level, glucose appears in the urine (glucosuria). The presence of glucose in renal tubules exerts an osmotic effect, thereby reducing reabsorption of water. Therefore the volume of urine formed increases (polyuria). Excessive urinary loss of water activates the mechanisms of thirst. Therefore the patient drinks too much water (polydipsia). Since his glucose utilization is poor, the body behaves as if the person is not eating enough. Hence the food intake mechanisms are also activated, and the patient eats more (polyphagia). But since the food fuels are not utilized efficiently due to insulin deficiency, the person loses weight. That is why diabetes is sometimes called the disease of starvation in the midst of plenty. Excessive breakdown of protein adds to the wasting and makes the person further emaciated.

Since insulin inhibits lipolysis, in insulin deficiency lipolysis is increased. Therefore the plasma free fatty acid level is raised. Consequently, free fatty acid oxidation is also increased, which tends to compensate for the decreased glycolysis. However, due to reduced glycolysis, there is a reduction in the amount of fatty acids that can be oxidized to carbon dioxide. Therefore some of the fatty acids are only partially oxidized, forming ketone bodies (ketosis). Excessive loss of water in the urine may lead to some dehydration and disorders of electrolyte and acid-base balance.

Together with ketosis, these disturbances may lead to ketoacidosis and even coma in severe uncontrolled diabetes.

Glucagon

Glucagon is secreted by the A cells of the isets of Langerhans of pancreas.

Actions

The actions of glucagon are somewhat opposite those of insulin.

1. Glucagon stimulates glycogenolysis in the liver but not in muscle. Breakdown of glycogen yields glucose.
2. Glucagon stimulates production of glucose from amino acids (gluconeogenesis). Both glycogenolysis and gluconeogenesis tend to raise plasma glucose level.
3. Glucagon stimulates lipolysis. Breakdown of lipids yields free fatty acids, which may be oxidized completely to carbon dioxide, or incompletely to form ketone bodies.

Regulation of Glucagon Secretion

Glucose inhibits glucagon secretion and so does insulin. The action of glucose may be direct, or may be indirectly mediated by insulin.

Glucagon Excess

Glucagon levels are generally high in diabetes mellitus. This may be the result of reduced inhibition by insulin, which is deficient in diabetes.

GASTROINTESTINAL HORMONES

Although the first hormone to be discovered was a gut hormone (secretin), today more is known about hormones secreted elsewhere. One reason possibly is that gut hormones are secreted by specialized cells scattered in the gut rather than by a discrete gland. Secondly, many of the gut hormones have only a paracrine or neurocrine action. In any case, the functions of the major gut hormones are closely related to gastrointestinal function, and have therefore been already discussed at appropriate points in Chapter 8. Here the actions of gut hormones have been summarized in Table 11.4.

Table 11.4 Gastrointestinal hormones

Hormone	*Stimulus for secretion*	*Site of secretion*	*Action*
Gastrin	Presence of food, especially protein, in the stomach. Vagal stimulation	Gastric antrum	Stimulation of gastric secretion.
Cholecystokinin (CCK) or pancreozymin (PZ)	Presence of food, especially fats, in the duodenum	Duodenum	Stimulation of enzyme-rich pancreatic secretion.
Secretin	Presence of acid in the duodenum	Duodenum	Stimulation of bicarbonate-rich pancreatic secretion.
Gastric inhibitory polypeptide (GIP)	Presence of glucose in the small intestine	Small intestine	Inhibition of gastric secretion. Stimulation of insulin secretion. Inhibition of gastric secretion

QUESTIONS

1. How is the hypothalamus related to (a) the anterior pituitary, and (b) the posterior pituitary?
2. Explain briefly why:
   A. A person having hypothyroidism has low thyroxine level but high TSH level
   B. Glucocorticoids (steroids) should be used for treatment of disease with great caution
   C. Adrenal medulla is considered to be structurally and functionally a part of the sympathetic nervous system
   D. A person having diabetes might have glucose in his urine
3. The gland that has both endocrine and exocrine functions is:
   A. Pancreas
   B. Thyroid
   C. Adrenal cortex
   D. Parotid
4. For each of the following statements, indicate whether it is true or false:
   A. In general, the receptors for steroid hormones are located on the cell membrane.
   B. The most common second messenger employed by hormones with intracellular receptors is cyclic AMP.
   C. ADH is also called vasopressin.
   D. Osteoporosis results from calcium deficiency and lack of physical activity.

ANSWERS

1. A. The hypothalamus delivers releasing hormones to the anterior pituitary via the portal circulation. Thus the relationship is vascular.
   B. The hypothalamus delivers ADH and oxytocin to the posterior pituitary via nerve endings. The neurons which manufacture these hormones have their cell bodies in the hypothalamus, and their axon terminals in the posterior pituitary. The hormones are released at the axon terminals. Thus the relationship is neural (Fig. 11.11).
2. A. Hypothyroidism → Low thyroxine → Feedback to the anterior pituitary →Excessive release of TSH → High TSH level
   B. Because:
   - Steroids do not cure any disease. They only suppress inflammation and create a false sense of well being
   - After stopping the steroids, there is rebound exacerbation of disease
   - Steroids have serious side effects such as osteoporosis, gastric ulcer, immunosuppression, diabetes, moon-shaped face, hirsutism (hairiness), etc.
   - If stopped suddenly, endogenous adrenal cortical secretion is dangerously low

C. Sympathetic preganglionic neurons supply cells of the adrenal medulla. Adrenal medullary cells release adrenaline. Therefore adrenal medullary cells are equivalent to postganglionic neurons. The only difference compared to the rest of the sympathetic nervous system is that the secretion of the 'postganglionic neuron' is released into the blood, not in an organ. (For details, see Chapter 17)

D. Because the blood glucose level might exceed the renal threshold for reabsorption (180 mg/dL).

3. A
4. A. False
   B. False
   C. True
   D. True

CHAPTER

12 Reproductive System

"Life is creation."

—CLAUDE BERNARD

Chapter Outline

- Sex Determination
- General Scheme of Reproductive Function
- Puberty
- Male Reproductive System
- Female Reproductive System
- Pregnancy
- Lactation
- Contraception

Reproductive system is different from all other systems of the body in that it makes almost no contribution to homeostasis. Therefore an individual can survive without the reproductive system. But without the reproductive system, there can be no next generation. Without the next generation, the species cannot survive. Unless the species survives, there can be no individual. Thus, indirectly, reproductive system is as essential for survival as any other system of the body.

SEX DETERMINATION

In higher animals like man, the key factor in reproduction is the differentiation of individuals into two types: male and female. These two types called sexes, perform complementary roles in reproduction. Sexual differentiation begins before birth, and continues after birth, assuming high visibility during puberty. Sex is determined by genes. Genes are located on chromosomes. Each cell of a human being has 46 chromosomes. Out of these, only one pair of chromosomes determines the sex of an individual. If both members of the pair are of the type called X, the individual is a female. If only one of the members is X, and the other is of the type called Y, the individual is a male. Sex is determined at conception. If the first cell with which life begins (called zygote) has the sex chromosome combination XX, all cells arising from its division also have the combination XX, and the embryo differentiates into a female. If the zygote has the combination XY, the embryo differentiates into a male. How the zygote may acquire the XX or XY combination will be explained later when we discuss pregnancy (See Table 12.2).

Sex Chromatin

Cells of a female have two X chromosomes while the cells of a male have only one. The extra X chromosome in females gives rise to a characteristic appearance in some cells of the body. In epidermal cells or cells scraped from the oral mucosa, the extra X chromosome (sex chromatin) may be seen as a bit of condensed chromatin near the nuclear membrane. The condensed chromatin is called **Barr body.** In some neutrophils (1-15%) sex chromatin appears as a "drumstick" attached to the nucleus (Fig. 12.1). The Barr body and the drumstick are thought to represent one of the X chromosomes which has turned inactive.

Examination of cells for sex chromatin is useful in cases of doubtful sexual differentiation. In individuals with more than one X chromosome, only one chromosome is active. All the extra chromosomes appear as sex chromatin. Thus the abnormality consisting of

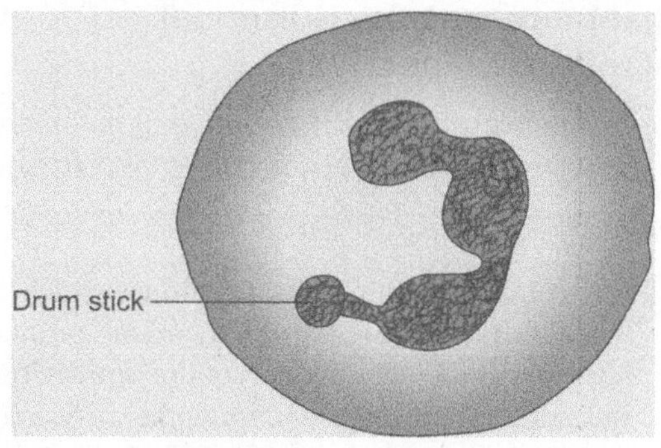

Fig. 12.1 Sex chromatin in a neutrophil, sometimes called drum stick because of its appearance

the chromosomal combination XXX ("superfemale") is charactertized by the presence of two Barr bodies or drumsticks in each cell. "Superfemales" may be detected only if examined for sex chromatin because they do not show any other obvious abnormality.

GENERAL SCHEME OF REPRODUCTIVE FUNCTION

The general scheme of reproductive function is the same in both sexes (Fig. 12.2). The basic reproductive organ in both sexes is the gonad. Gonads have two primary functions: to produce gametes, and to secrete sex hormones. These two functions of gonads are regulated directly by two separate hormones (gonadotropins) of the anterior pituitary. Anterior pituitary gonadotropins are regulated by the gonadotropin releasing hormone (GnRH) secreted by a part of the brain, the hypothalamus. Hypothalamic GnRH secretion is influenced by those parts of the brain which are concerned with emotions (limbic system) and thoughts (cerebral cortex). That is why thoughts and emotions can affect reproductive function. Conversely, several parts of the brain are influenced by sex hormones. That is why thoughts and emotions undergo a dramatic upheaval during puberty when sex hormone secretion increases.

Sex hormones have various target organs. First among them are the gonads. Thus sex hormones, secreted by the gonads, affect gametogenesis by the gonads. The other target organs are responsible for

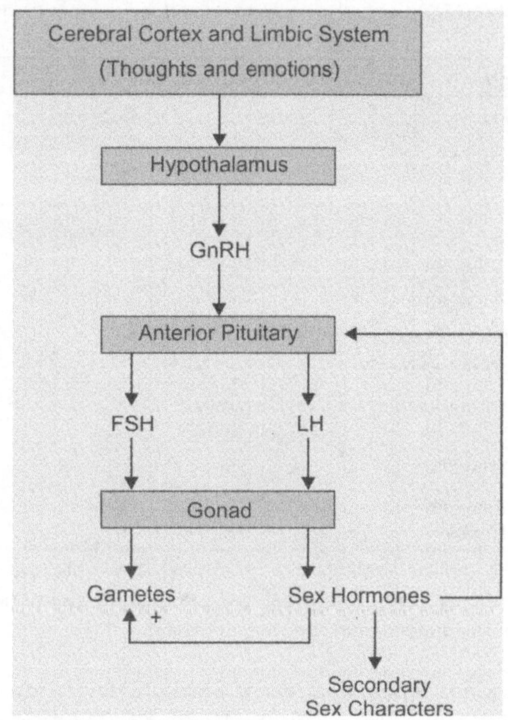

Fig. 12.2 Basic functional organization of the reproductive system

the sex hormones leading to secondary sex characters and the metabolic effects of sex hormones.

Secretion of sex hormones is subject to feedback regulation. In general, sex hormones exert a negative feedback on anterior pituitary gonadotropin secretion.

The general scheme of reproductive function, as expressed in the two sexes, has been depicted in Table 12.1.

PUBERTY

It is common knowledge that children do not show much sexual activity during infancy and childhood. The onset of sexual activity, rather suddenly at the age of about ten, is called puberty. Till puberty, sex hormone secretion, anterior pituitary gonadotropin secretion, and hypothalamic GnRH secretion are low. At puberty, secretion of all these hormones increases. The mechanism of puberty may be resolved into two

Table 12.1 General scheme of reproductive function as expressed in males and females

Organ/function	*In males*	*In females*
Gonads	Testes	Ovary
Gametes	Sperm	Ovum
Hormones	Testosterone	Estrogens Progesterone
Anterior pituitary gonadotropins		
For stimulating gametogenesis	FSH	FSH
For stimulating sex hormone secretion	LH (also called ICSH in males)	LH
Hypothalamic hormone	GnRH	GnRH

FSH, follicle stimulating hormone; LH, luteinizing hormone; ICSH, interstitial cell stimulating hormone; GnRH, gonadotropin releasing hormone.

questions. First, what keeps hormone levels low in childhood; and second, what leads to a sudden increase in hormone secretion at puberty.

Why is Hormonal Secretion Low in Childhood?

The mechanism may be explored step by step.

1. In childhood, gonads are small and secrete only small amounts of sex hormones. But if a child's gonads are stimulated by gonadotropins, they quickly grow and function like adult gonads. Hence low secretion of sex hormones is not due to immaturity of gonads.
2. In childhood, anterior pituitary secretes only small amounts of gonadotropins. But if a child's anterior pituitary is stimulated by GnRH, it is capable of secreting gonadotropins as in the adult. Hence low secretion of gonadotropins is not due to immaturity of anterior pituitary.
3. In childhood, the hypothalamus secretes only small amounts of GnRH. But the hypothalamic content of GnRH is not low during childhood. Hence low secretion of GnRH is probably not due to immaturity of the hypothalamus.

What Increases the Hormonal Secretion at Puberty

1. It was once believed that in childhood, the anterior pituitary gonadotropin secretion is extremely sensitive to the negative feedback effect of sex hormones. Therefore, it was thought, even the low concentrations of sex hormones which are present in childhood are able to inhibit pituitary gonadotropins. But at puberty the sensitivity of the anterior pituitary was thought to decrease dramatically. As the result of this change, gonadotropin secretion increases, leading to stimulation of gonads and a consequent increase in secretion of sex hormones.
   But it has been found that if the gonads are removed during childhood, so that even low levels of sex hormones are not available for inhibiting the anterior pituitary, gonadotropin secretion still does not increase. Thus the low secretion of gonadotropins during childhood is not due to high sensitivity to the negative feedback effect of sex hormones. Hence the increase in secretion at puberty cannot be due to a change in the sensitivity of anterior pituitary.
2. The above discussion indicates that we do not know the mechanism underlying the onset of puberty. There is some evidence indicating that puberty has to wait for the maturation of some part of the brain (probably in the limbic system) which normally influences the hypothalamus. When this part of the limbic system is mature, it stimulates the hypothalamus to secrete more GnRH. GnRH stimulates the anterior pituitary to secrete more gonadotropins. Gonadotropins stimulate the gonads to secrete more sex hormones. That is how puberty sets in.

MALE REPRODUCTIVE SYSTEM

Functional Anatomy

The male reproductive system consists of the testes, the accessory glands, viz. prostate and seminal vesicles, and a system of tubes which carries the products of all these structures outside the body (Fig. 12.3). The testes are made up of long, thin coiled tubes called seminiferous tubules. The male gametes (spermatozoa) are formed in these tubules: the process is called spermatogenesis. Between the seminiferous tubules are interstitial cells or Leydig cells (Fig. 12.4). Interstitial cells secrete testosterone. Seminiferous tubules are open at both ends. Both ends of each seminiferous tubule open into the epididymis, also a long coiled tube. The epididymis opens into the vas deferens. At the distal end, the vas deferens dilates to form the ampulla and also receives the secretions of the seminal vesicles, and continues as the ejaculatory duct. The ejaculatory duct joins the prostatic urethra. The subsequent path of the products of the genital tract is the same as that of the urine. The prostate and urethral glands also contribute to the semen.

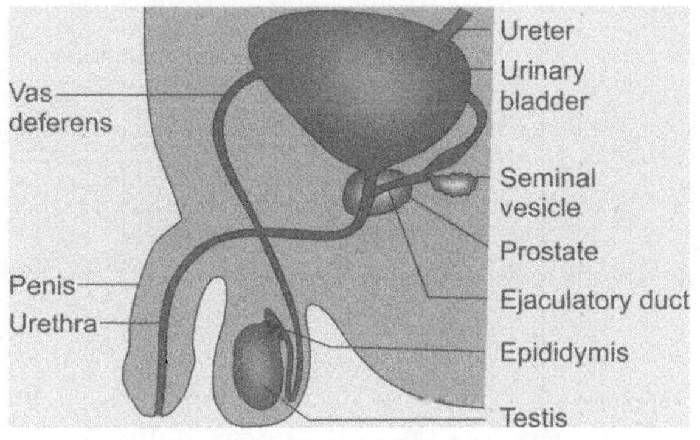

Fig. 12.3 The male reproductive system

Spermatogenesis

Spermatogenesis means the formation of male gametes, called spermatozoa, or simply sperms. Formation of mature sperms capable of fertilizing an ovum is a long process which is completed only in the female genital tract. But the essential steps of spermatogenesis are completed in the testes.

The precursors of sperms are the cells called spermatogonia, which line the outer border of seminiferous tubules. Spermatogonia have a high capacity for cell division. They divide repeatedly, and

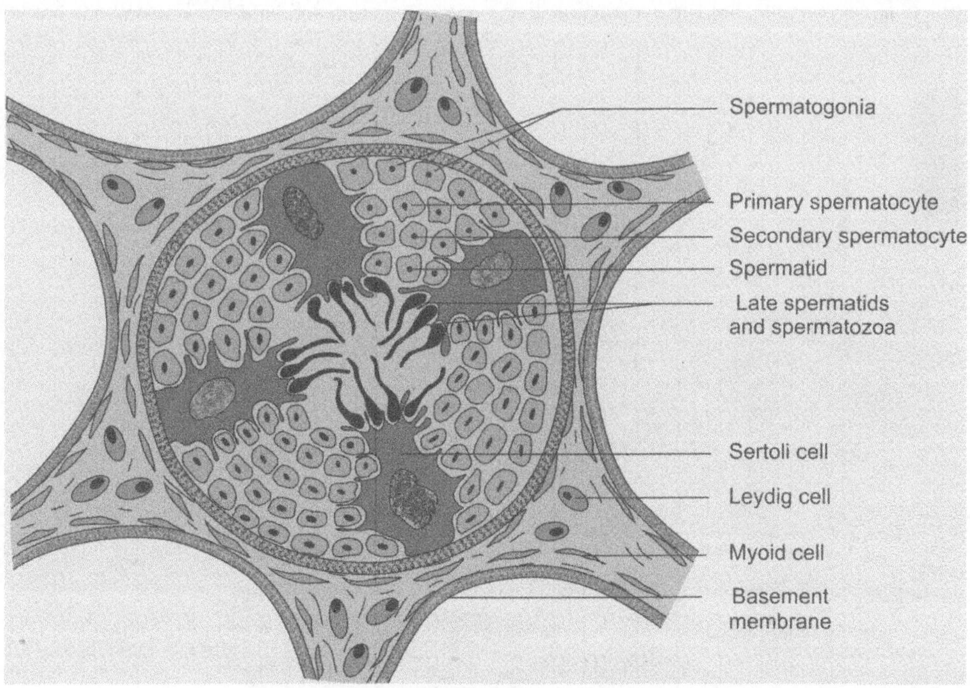

Fig. 12.4 Histology of the testis

some of the daughter cells are slightly differentiated, and migrate centrally in the seminiferous tubule. These cells cross the barrier formed by junctions between adjacent Sertoli cells, and rest in the pockets formed by cytoplasmic processes of Sertoli cells. Here the spermatogonia differentiate into primary spermatocytes. Primary spermatocytes undergo meiosis. The first meiotic division gives rise to secondary spermatocytes. The second meiotic division gives rise to spermatids. Meiotic division reduces the number of chromosomes to half. Hence each spermatid has only 23 chromosomes. Spermatids migrate to occupy pockets between cytoplasmic processes of Sertoli cells towards the lumen of the seminiferous tubules (Fig. 12.5). Here the spermatids undergo further maturation to form spermatozoa.

A sperm consists of a head and a tail (Fig. 12.6). The head consists essentially of the nucleus and the acrosome. The acrosome contains proteolytic enzymes and hyaluronidase. These enzymes help the sperm clear its way towards the ovum while travelling in the female genital tract. The tail resembles cilia in its structure and function. It is responsible for the swimming-like movement of the sperm in the female genital tract. The energy for movement comes from ATP. ATP is generated by the sperm in a proximal segment of the tail.

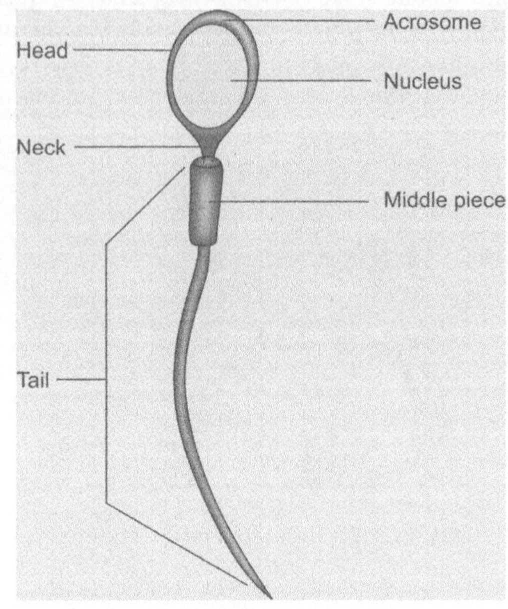

Fig. 12.6 Simplified structure of a sperm

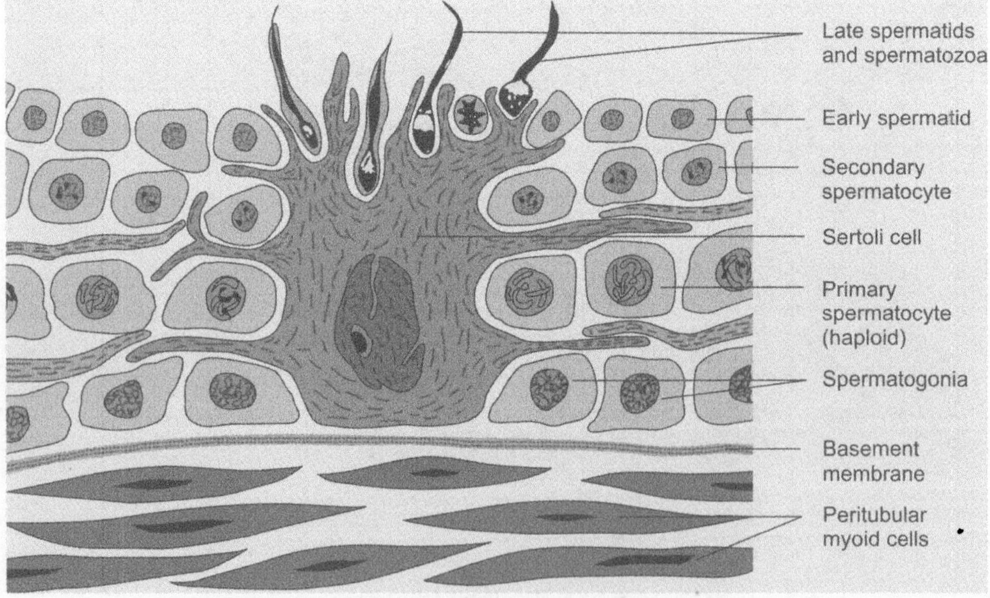

Fig. 12.5 Diagrammatic representation of spermatogenesis

Sertoli Cells

As described above, Sertoli cells nest the developing sperms. But their function is much more than providing mechanical support. Junction between adjacent Sertoli cells forms a barrier (**blood-testis barrier**) which does not allow harmful substances to enter the area where spermatogenesis is going on (Fig. 12.7). Further, since blood vessels do not enter the seminiferous tubules, nutrition to the developing sperms is also conducted by Sertoli cells. Sertoli cells also synthesize inhibin and androgen binding protein (ABP) which have a role in regulation of spermatogenesis.

Hormonal Regulation of Spermatogenesis

The principal hormone directly affecting spermatogenesis is testosterone. Testosterone is synthesized by Leydig cells. It does not have to reach seminiferous tubules by the bloodstream. First, it diffuses into the seminiferous tubules where it affects spermatogenesis. Secondly, Sertoli cells secrete ABP which binds testosterone and helps in increasing its concentration in the seminiferous tubules. As a result of the geographical closeness of seminiferous tubules to the site of synthesis of testosterone and trapping of testosterone by ABP, the concentration of testosterone achieved in the seminiferous tubules is much higher than in the bloodstream. Testosterone stimulates spermatogenesis.

Testosterone secretion is itself subject to feedback regulation by pituitary and hypothalamic hormones. The more important feedback effect of testosterone is on the hypothalamus. Testosterone inhibits the secretion of GnRH from the hypothalamus. Reduced secretion of GnRH reduces FSH and LH secretion from the pituitary. Testosterone also has a direct weak inhibitory effect on LH secretion from the pituitary. Reduced LH secretion reduces testoterone secretion by Leydig cells and thereby depresses spermatogenesis. Reduced FSH secretion inhibits ABP secretion by Sertoli cells. That reduces the ability of seminiferous tubules to trap testosterone. Reduced concentration of testosterone in the seminiferous tubule also depresses spermatogenesis.

Another hormonal mechanism for regulation of spermatogenesis involves **inhibin,** a hormone secreted by Sertoli cells. Increased spermatogenesis leads to secretion of inhibin by Sertoli cells. Inhibin inhibits FSH secretion from the anterior pituitary. Reduced FSH secretion reduces ABP secretion by Sertoli cells and eventually depresses spermatogenesis as discussed above.

The above discussion may give an impression as if regulatory mechanisms have been designed to depress spermatogenesis. But one should remember that reduced testosterone secretion or reduced spermatogenesis act by the same mechanisms to increase spermatogenesis. Thus the mechanisms can work in both directions and are designed to regulate the level of spermatogenesis. The mechanisms involved in hormonal regulation of spermatogenesis have been summarized in Figure 12.8.

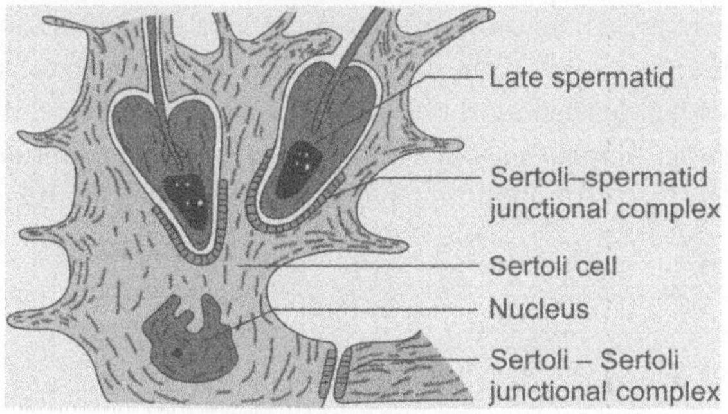

Fig. 12.7 Blood-testis barrier

Semen

Semen is the fluid deposited by the male in the female genital tract. It is the vehicle for carrying sperms to the female genital tract so that one of them can unite with an ovum, if it is available. But the semen is much more than a vehicle: it has several components which are indispensable for the union of the sperm and ovum.

When sperms are shed into the seminiferous tubules, they are still not capable of movement. To these freshly formed sperms is added a fluid secreted by Sertoli cells. Further, as the sperms move into the epididymis, fluid secreted by the epididymis is also added. These fluids contain nutrients for the sperms and also substances for maturation of

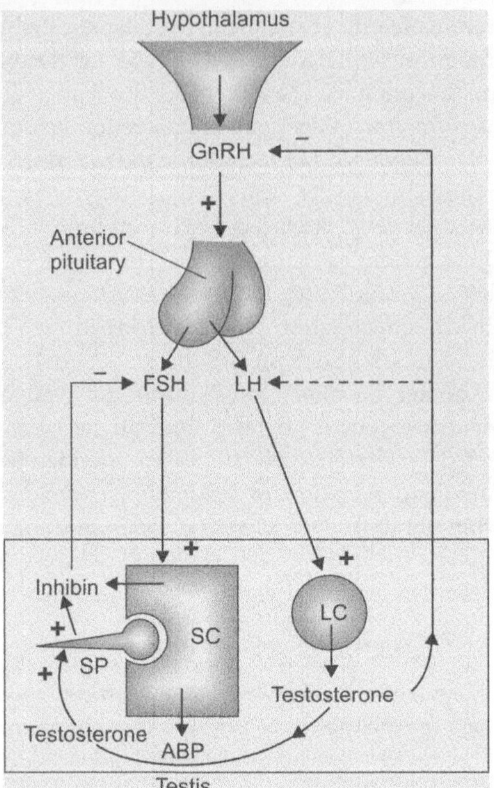

Fig. 12.8 Regulation of spermatogenesis. GnRH, gonadotropin releasing hormone; FSH, follicle stimulating hormone; LH, luteinizing hormone; ABP, androgen binding protein; SP, precursors of spermatozoa; SC, Sertoli cell; LC, Leydig cell

sperms. After staying in the epididymis for about one day, the sperms acquire the capacity to move.[1] From the epididymis, the sperms move into the vas deferens. Vas deferens is the principal site for storage of spermatozoa. The sperms remain viable for at least one month in the male genital tract.

The spermatozoa, along with the fluid in which they are suspended in the vas deferens, form only about 10% of the volume of the ejaculated semen. The other contributions come mainly from the seminal vesicles and the prostate gland.

[1]They acquire the capacity for movement but do not actually move. Several substances present in the male genital tract inhibit sperm motility. The motility is exhibited only after the semen has been ejaculated.

Functions of Seminal Vesicles

Seminal vesicles secrete a fluid which forms about 60 percent of the volume of semen. Besides contributing to volume, the seminal vesicle fluid contains several substances of great functional importance. It contains fructose, vitamin C and several other nutrients for use by the sperms. It contains fibrinogen which helps the coagulation of the semen after ejaculation. It contains prostaglandins which act on the female genital tract in such a way as to facilitate movement of sperms towards the ovum. When the semen is ejaculated, seminal fluid is ejaculated last which helps wash out sperms from the vas deferens and urethra. The mucoid nature of the seminal vesicle fluid is responsible for the stickiness of semen.

Functions of the Prostate Gland

Besides forming about 25 percent of the volume of the semen, the secretions of the prostate gland also have substances of great functional importance. The prostatic fluid contains enzymes for coagulation and also for dissolving the clot. Being alkaline in nature, it neutralizes the acidity of the rest of the semen and also the acidity of the fluids in the female genital tract. This neutralization is one of the factors which makes it possible for sperms to exhibit their motility in the female genital tract. The secretion of the prostate is responsible for the milky color of the semen.

Characteristics of Semen

Semen ejaculated at a time is about 3 mL in volume and contains about 100 million sperms/mL. These sperms represent the product of about 2 days of testicular activity. Therefore, excessive frequency of ejaculation leads to a fall in the sperm count. Normally, sperms with abnormal morphology are less than 20 percent. A larger number of abnormal forms, or a sperm count of less than 40 million/mL, may render the semen infertile.

Deposition of Semen in the Female Genital Tract

Semen is deposited in the female genital tract during sexual intercourse. Psychic sexual stimuli or physical stimulation of male genitalia (generally a combination of both) leads to sexual arousal of the male. The first and most prominent sign of the arousal is erection of the penis. Erection is mediated by parasympathetic nerves arising from segments S2–S4 of the spinal cord. Activation of these nerve fibers leads to nitric oxide mediated dilatation of blood vessels in the erectile tissue of the penis. Dilatation of these blood vessels leads to erection of the penis. Introduction of the erect penis into the vagina provides further tactile stimulation of the glans penis, the most sensitive part of the penis. Stimulation of the glans penis leads to a sympathetic reflex involving segments L1–L2 of the spinal cord and consisting of two components which follow each other in quick succession. The first component is emission. **Emission** consists of contraction of the vas deferens, and then contraction of the musculature of the prostate gland, and then finally contraction of the seminal vesicles. Secretions from all these regions mix in the internal urethra and form the semen. The second component is ejaculation. **Ejaculation** consists of expulsion of semen from the urethra. Since the penis is in the vagina during the sexual intercourse, ejaculation deposits the semen in the vagina.

Fate of Semen in the Female Genital Tract

Soon after the semen enters the vagina, the clotting enzymes of the prostatic fluid and fibrinogen of the seminal vesicle fluid react to form a weak clot. While the sperms are trapped in the clot, they get exposed to vaginal secretions. Vaginal secretions improve the mobility and fertilizing ability of sperms. The clot dissolves after 15-30 minutes. Further exposure to secretions of the female genital tract further improves the mobility and fertilizing ability of the sperms. The beneficial effects of stay in the female genital tract are collectively called **capacitation.** It is so important that without capacitation, fertilization is impossible. Capacitation needs at least one hour but may take much longer. Sperms which have undergone capacitation release some hydrolytic enzymes from the acrosome. As a result, these sperms are able to clear their path and swim easily towards the ovum. First the sperms have to pass through the granulosa cells surrounding the ovum. Then they have to pass through the zona pellucida, the thick membranous covering of the ovum. Then the sperm membrane fuses with the cell membrane of the ovum, and genetic material from the sperm enters the ovum. This final fusion of sperm and ovum is called **fertilization**. Only one sperm participates in fertilization although several approach the ovum and 20-30 sperms may even reach the zona pellucida.

Functions of Testosterone

As mentioned earlier, testosterone is the principal male sex hormone, or androgen. It is secreted mainly by the testes but small quantities are also produced by the adrenal cortex. The role of testosterone in spermatogenesis has already been discussed in detail. Here all the functions of testosterone have been summarized.

Role before Birth

Testosterone is produced from the seventh week of embryonic life onwards. During fetal life it is responsible for the development of male external genitalia, seminal vesicles and prostate. Testosterone also has a role in descent of the testes into the scrotum. Testosterone continues to be produced in significant amounts till about 10 weeks after birth. After that, the production declines to negligible levels till puberty.

Secondary Sex Characteristics

At puberty there is a sudden increase in testosterone secretion which leads to the development of male secondary sex characteristics in boys. These include behavioral changes such as increased interest in girls and aggressiveness, a change in voice, and structural changes such as increased hairiness, specially in the beard and moustache area, pubis and chest, recession of hairline on the scalp, muscular growth, gain in height and increase in secretion of sebaceous glands of the skin leading to acne.

Role in Spermatogenesis

Testosterone stimulates spermatogenesis. In the absence of testosterone, spermatogenesis cannot proceed beyond the spermatid stage. Details of the hormonal regulation of spermatogenesis have been already discussed.

Anabolic Effect

Testosterone stimulates protein synthesis. This effect is responsible for the increase in growth. However, while stimulating bone growth, testosterone also accelerates the fusion of epiphyses of long bones. Therefore after a brief growth spurt, further increase in height becomes impossible.

Mechanism of Action of Testosterone

Like other steroid hormones, testosterone has an intracellular receptor. The cytoplasmic receptor binds to the hormone, and the hormone-receptor complex enters the nucleus where it increases the rate of gene transcription. Increased transcription eventually increases protein synthesis.

Some of the actions of testosterone are mediated by testosterone itself while others are mediated by its derivative, dihydrotesosterone (DHT). For actions mediated by DHT, testosterone is much less potent than DHT.

FEMALE REPRODUCTIVE SYSTEM

Functional Anatomy

The female gonads are a pair of ovaries in the abdominal cavity (Fig. 12.9). The gamete (ovum) discharged from an ovary is generally captured by a funnel shaped structure, the fimbriated end of the Fallopian tube. The ovum is transported in the Fallopian tube towards the uterus. The uterus is the child-bearing organ. The uterus opens into the vagina, which in turn opens towards the exterior.

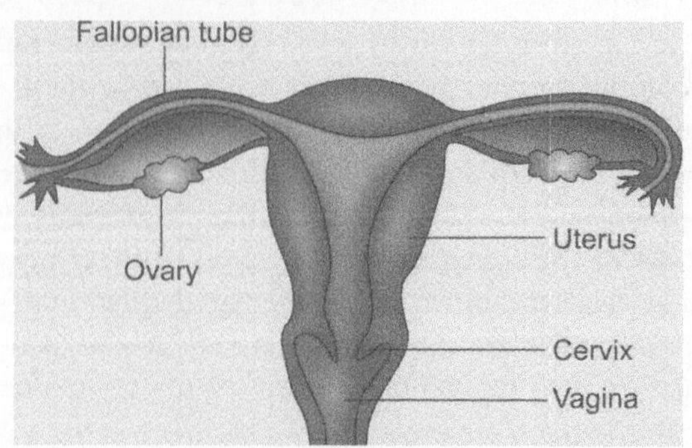

Fig. 12.9 The female reproductive system

The ovary is covered by a single layer of somewhat flattened cuboidal epithelium. In the stroma of the ovary are embedded a large number of immature ova (primary oocytes). Each primary oocyte is surrounded by several stromal cells, called granulosa cells. The primary oocyte together with the granulosa cells forms a primordial follicle. At birth, each ovary of a girl has about one million primordial follicles. Most of these fail to mature and are lost through atresia. A woman produces only one ovum every month during her reproductive period (approximately 15-50 years of age), which comes to about 400 ova in a life-time. No ovum is produced during pregnancy because the monthly ovarian cycle is suspended during pregnancy. The monthly cycle is commonly called the menstrual cycle because it is accompanied by bleeding from the uterus (menstruation) for about 4 days in a month.

The Menstrual Cycle

The menstrual cycle is due to the cyclic secretion of pituitary gonadotropins, which in turn imparts cyclicity to estrogen and progesterone secretion from the ovary. The cycle is accompained by ovarian as well as uterine changes. The cycle begins with puberty (at about age 10 years) but the first menstruation (menarche) is generally a few years later (age 12-14 years).

The average duration of the cycle is 28 days but the normal range is quite wide (20-45 days). The days are numbered in terms of menstrual bleeding, day 1 of the cycle being the first day of menstrual bleeding. Ovulation takes place at about day 14 of the cycle. If the cycle length is shorter or longer than 28 days, the variation is generally in the period before ovulation. That is, the interval between ovulation and end of the cycle is essentially constant at 14 days irrespective of cycle length.

The biological rationale of the cycle is apparently based on the assumption that ovulation may be soon followed by fertilization. The cycle ensures that the fertilized ovum will be received by a well-prepared uterus. If, however, fertilization does not take place, the preparations of the uterus are undone. In the process, the uterine wall breaks down and bleeds, resulting in menstruation. That is why menstrual bleeding has been considered 'uterine tears' shed to mourn the failure of the ovum to get fertilized.

Ovarian Cycle

The first half, i.e. 14 days, of the cycle are occupied by development of the follicles. That is why this phase is also called the **follicular phase**. During the first week of the follicular phase, a few primordial follicles start developing. But by the end of one week, only one follicle continues to develop further, while the remaining follicles become smaller and disappear, i.e. undergo atresia. The follicle that continues to develop finally has a cavity filled with follicular fluid. On one side is the ovum surrounded by granulosa cells. The granulosa cells are further surrounded by two layers of theca cells: theca interna and theca externa (Fig. 12.10). On day 14 of the cycle, the follicle ruptures, the ovum together with a few surrounding granulosa cells is shed into the abdominal cavity, and the remaining follicle forms the corpus hemorrhagicum in the ovary. The process of the ovum being discharged from the follicle is called **ovulation.**

The early growth of follicles is due to the action of FSH secreted by the anterior pituitary. After that, the granulosa cells and theca cells of the follicle start secreting estrogen. Estrogen increases the number of FSH receptors on granulosa cells, which in turn leads to release of more estrogen, resulting in a positive feedback loop. Further, the combined action of FSH and estrogen leads to the expression of LH receptors on granulosa and theca cells. Availability of LH receptors leads to progesterone secretion towards the end of the follicular phase. Further, a finely programmed positive feedback mechanism leads to a sharp increase in LH secretion about 6 hours before ovulation. The LH surge seems to be essential for ovulation. There is also a smaller surge in FSH secretion at the same time as the LH surge.

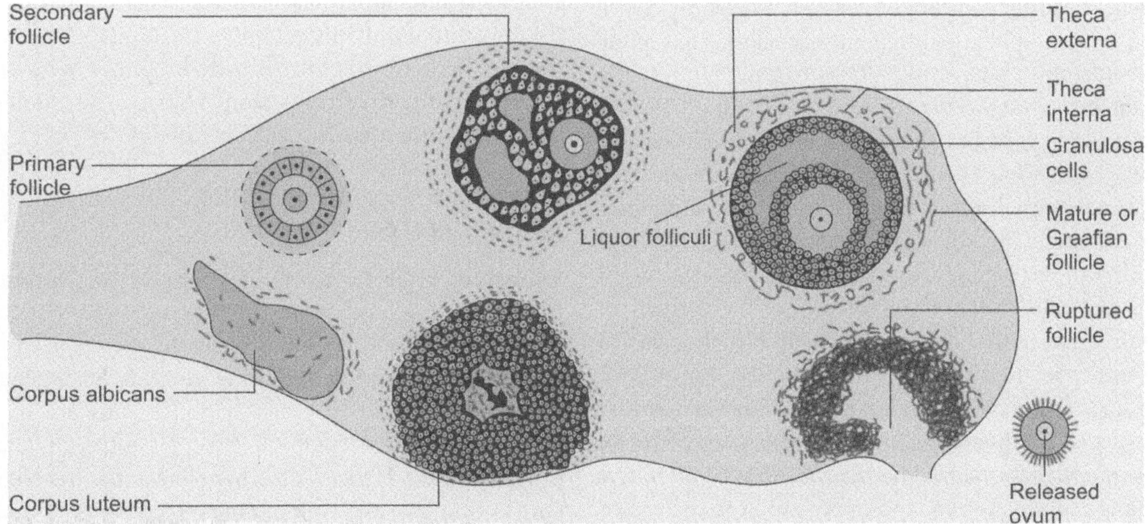

Fig. 12.10 Stages in the life of a Graafian follicle

The second half of the ovarian cycle is called the **luteal phase** because it is associated with the development of the corpus luteum. Corpus luteum develops from the granulosa cells and theca cells still remaining in corpus hemorrhagicum under the influence of the luteinizing hormone (LH). Luteal cells synthesize both estrogen and progesterone. If the ovum is fertilized, the corpus luteum persists for about 3 months. If the ovum is not fertilized, the corpus luteum starts degenerating around day 24 of the cycle. After degeneration, what remains of the corpus luteum is called corpus albicans. Degeneration of the corpus luteum is due to the declining level of LH and increase in the secretion of inhibin by the luteal cells themselves. Inhibin reduces pituitary gonadotropin secretion, specially the secretion of FSH, but also that of LH.

Uterine Cycle

As seen above, towards the end of the menstrual cycle, the corpus luteum degenerates to form the corpus albicans. The degenerated corpus luteum cannot synthesize much estrogen and progesterone. Withdrawal of these hormones leads to breakdown of the uterine wall and bleeding, resulting in menstruation. Conventionally, the onset of bleeding is considered to be the beginning of the menstrual cycle. Bleeding continues for about 4 days. By day 5, the ovarian follicle is sufficiently developed to secrete considerable quantities of estrogen. Under the influence of estrogen, the uterine wall not only starts getting repaired but the endometrial thickness also starts increasing. During menstruation, all superficial uterine epithelium is shed. Under the influence of estrogen, the surface epithelium is restored. In addition, estrogen also leads to proliferation of stromal cells of the endometrium and enlargement of the endometrial glands. The result is that by day 14 of the cycle, the endometrium is about 3-4 mm thick and has well developed glands and blood vessels and an intact epithelium. Since the follicular phase of the menstrual cycle is characterized by proliferative changes in the uterine endometrium, it is also called the **proliferative phase.**

After ovulation (around day 14 of the cycle), the ovarian follicle is transformed into the corpus luteum. Corpus luteum secretes both estrogen and progesterone. While the action of estrogen on the endometrium continues, progesterone accelerates further development of the endometrium. The stromal cells acquire lipid and glycogen deposits. The glands and blood vessels enlarge further and become tortuous. The glands start secreting. The endometrium grows thicker, reaching its maximum (about 6 mm) around day 21 of the cycle. All these changes are designed to welcome the fertilized ovum. The secretions of the uterus provide nutrition to the embryo till it implants. After implantation nutrition is provided by the lipid and glycogen deposits in stromal cells. The enlarged blood vessels bring more blood to the uterus to meet its enhanced metabolic needs. Their tortuosity ensures that they can stretch as the uterine wall thickens further during pregnancy. But if the pregnancy does not take place, the corpus luteum involutes and estrogen and progesterone are withdrawn.

Withdrawal of hormones takes away the support which led to the increase in thickness and growth of glands and blood vessels in the endometrium. As a result, the endometrium becomes thinner. The blood vessels constrict, reducing blood flow to the endometrium. Superficial layers of the endometrium die for want of nutritional support leading to desquamation. Breakdown of tissue includes injury to blood vessels, leading to extravasation of blood. The cellular debris and blood are lost as menstrual flow.

Hormonal Regulation of the Menstrual Cycle

Menstrual cycle involves the interplay of ovarian, pituitary and hypothalamic hormones.

At the beginning of the cycle, the estrogen level is very low and progesterone level is negligible. Therefore, the pituitary and hypothalamus are free from the negative feedback effect of estrogen and progesterone. Hence the hypothalamus secretes GnRH and the anterior pituitary secretes FSH and some LH. FSH stimulates follicular development.

Ovarian follicles secrete estrogen. Estrogen tends to suppress FSH secretion, but progressive follicular development ensures a rise in estrogen level. Around day 11 of the cycle, the estrogen level crosses a certain threshold. Above this threshold level, estrogen has a positive feedback effect on LH secretion, and to some extent also on FSH secretion. This leads to LH and FSH surge. The LH surge is essential for ovulation. After ovulation has taken place on day 14, the corpus luteum starts developing under the influence of LH. Corpus luteum secretes estrogen, progesterone and inhibin. The combined effect of these hormones is to suppress the secretion of FSH and LH by negative feedback effect on the anterior pituitary, and to a lesser extent also on the hypothalamic GnRH secretion. Absence of support from FSH and LH leads to regression of the corpus luteum. Regression of the corpus luteum leads to a sharp decline in estrogen and progesterone levels. Withdrawal of support from estrogen and progesterone leads to menstrual bleeding. Thus one cycle ends and the next cycle begins (Fig. 12.11).

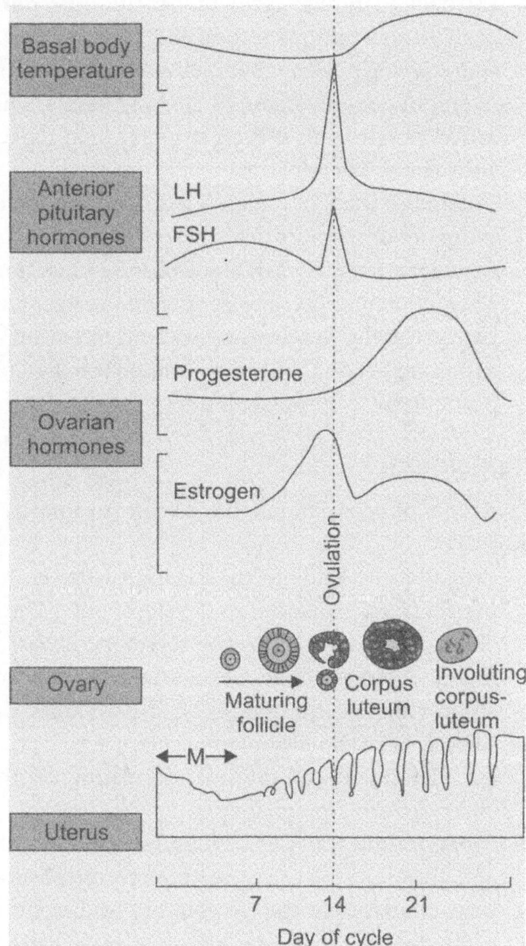

Fig. 12.11 The menstrual cycle. M, menstruation

Ovarian Hormones

The principal ovarian hormones are estrogen and progesterone, and their action on the uterus has been discussed above in relation to the menstrual cycle. During pregnancy, these hormones are also secreted by the placenta and have other functions. In addition, they have other actions as well in the non-pregnant as well as pregnant female, some of which have been summarized below.

Estrogen

The most important estrogen in the human female is beta-estradiol. Its actions have been summarized below:

1. Estrogen is responsible for secondary sex characters of the female which appear after puberty. These include enlargement of the breasts; deposition of fat, specially in the buttocks and thighs; and growth of pubic hair with flattened top pattern.
2. Estrogens increase the size of the uterus by increasing the stromal cells, glands and muscle. These changes form a part of the proliferative phase of the menstrual cycle. They also increase blood flow through the uterus and increase the contractility of the uterus.
3. Estrogens increase the size of the vagina and external genitalia. In the vagina, they also change the epithelium from cuboidal to stratified squamous, which is more resistant to trauma and infection.
4. Estrogens induce the growth of stromal tissue and ducts in the breast, and also lead to deposition of fat in the breast. Thus the breasts become larger and more mature, but estrogens cannot induce secretion of milk.

5. Estrogens induce growth, including bone growth, and are thus responsible for the growth spurt during puberty. But they also hasten union of epiphyses with shafts of the long bones. This action of estrogens is even stronger than that of androgens. Therefore growth is arrested earlier in females than in males. That is why females are generally shorter than males.
6. Estrogens have a weak aldosterone-like action. This action may become significant during pregnancy, leading to water and sodium retention.
7. Estrogens act on the brain to influence behavior, particularly to stimulate libido.

Progesterone

The actions of progesterone have been summarized below:

1. Progesterone leads to thickening of the endometrium and glandular development. These changes form a part of the secretory phase of the menstrual cycle. Progesterone reduces contractility of the uterus. It also reduces the sensitivity of the uterine musculature to oxytocin. These effects prevent expulsion of the embryo during pregnancy.
2. Progesterone leads to development of lobules and alveoli in the breast. Although some secretory changes in the alveoli are induced by progesterone, actual secretion of milk cannot occur without further action of prolactin.

Relaxin

Relaxin is also an ovarian hormone secreted by the corpus luteum. It relaxes the pubic symphysis and other pelvic joints. It also softens and dilates the cervix. These actions facilitate delivery of the fetus.

Menopause

Menopause is the decline in sexual function of women as a result of aging. After the age of about 45, menstruation becomes irregular, and then stops completely by the age of 55 years. There may also be other manifestations, some of which can be quite unpleasant. There may be flashes of warmth radiating from the trunk towards the face. There may be psychological symptoms such as anxiety, tiredness, mood swings and irritability. Reduced bone density is almost universal and may become severe enough to make minor trauma lead to fractures.

Mechanism

Menopause is due to a decrease in the number of primordial follicles in the ovary. After the age of about 45, there are very few follicles left which respond to pituitary gonadotropins. Hence the secretion of estrogen and progesterone falls, and finally stops altogether. The main source of estrogens then is adipose tissue where some adrenal androgens are converted into estrogens. In the absence of ovarian hormones, the negative feedback on the pituitary is removed. Therefore FSH and LH rise to high levels.

Treatment

If the symptoms are troublesome, estrogens may be given. The dose of estrogens may be reduced gradually to achieve a slow withdrawal. The woman should be reassured and family members counselled so that she does not feel unloved or unwanted. Fractures may be prevented by giving adequate dietary calcium and vitamin D.

PREGNANCY

Pregnancy is the process whereby the life of a baby begins in the mother's womb and progresses up to the stage when it is safe to expose the baby to the outside world. The process takes a little more than nine months, and needs coordinated activity of all parts of the baby and the mother for its success. A few major events of pregnancy will be described here with special attention to endocrine changes.

Fertilization

Fertilization is the union of the ovum and the sperm. After the ovum is shed from the ovary (ovulation), the ovum moves towards the Fallopian tube. In spite of the several places where the ovum could possibly wander in the abdominal cavity, almost all ova actually enter the Fallopian tube. The ciliary motion on the inner surface of the fimbriated ends of Fallopian tubes possibly aids this outcome. If sperms are introduced into the vagina around the same time as ovulation, fertilization may take place. Out of the millions of spermatozoa present in one ejaculate, only about a hundred reach the ovum in the Fallopian tube. Even that is a miracle considering how long the journey is for the tiny sperm. The movement of sperms towards the ovum is facilitated by a chemoattractant substance secreted by the ovum, and also hormonal factors (oxytocin and prostaglandins) which set up propulsive waves of contraction in the uterus and Fallopian tubes. When a sperm comes in contact with the surroundings of the ovum (zona pellucida), it releases hydrolytic enzymes from the acrosome (acrosomal reaction). The enzymes aid the penetration of the sperm into the ovum. Once a sperm has entered an ovum, there are mechanisms, not fully understood, which prevent the entry of any other sperm. Then the nucleus of the ovum and the nucleus of the sperm fuse to form a single nucleus. After the fusion, the ovum becomes the zygote. Zygote is the beginning of the baby. In human beings, the nucleus of the ovum has 23 chromosomes and the nucleus of the sperm also has 23 chromosomes. Thus the zygote has 23 pairs of chromosomes. The sex of the baby which the zygote will form is also determined at this stage (Table 12.2). The zygote undergoes repeated cell division. After cell division, it is called the embryo.

Implantation

Implantation is the process by which the embryo sticks to the uterus. The embryo takes about 3 days to travel through the Fallopian tube to reach the uterus.

Table 12.2 Sex of the zygote

Chromosome composition of			
Ovum	*Sperm*	*Zygote*	*Sex*
22 + X	22 + X	44 + XX	Female
22 + X	22 + Y	44 + XY	Male

It takes another 3 days to get implanted, usually in the dorsal wall of the uterus. Thus the embryo is about 1 week old when it gets implanted.

Let us see how implantation takes place. When the embryo comes close to the wall of the uterus, the embryonic cells in contact with the uterus, called trophoblastic cells, proliferate and release enzymes which digest the endometrial (decidual) cells.[2] As a result, the embryo sinks a little in the wall of the uterus, and gets attached (implanted) there.

The trophoblastic cells which are nearest the embryo and are still well organized are called the cytotrophoblast. The cytotrophoblastic cells which 'float' along with decidual cells in a 'soup' of digested cells are called the syncytiotrophoblast.

The Pregnant vs Non-pregnant Uterus

It was mentioned while discussing the menstrual cycle that after ovulation, the corpus luteum secretes progesterone and estrogen, which prepare the uterus for pregnancy. However, if pregnancy does not occur, the corpus luteum regresses about one week after ovulation. But if pregnancy takes place, about one week after ovulation, the embryo gets implanted. At this stage, the syncytiotrophoblastic cells start releasing a hormone, human chorionic gonadotropin (hCG). hCG has properties similar to LH and mediates its effects via the LH receptors. Thus hCG stimulates the corpus luteum, and does not let it regress. The stimulated corpus luteum continues to secrete estrogen and progesterone. Estrogen and progesterone stimulate endometrial growth, vascularity, secretions and nutrient storage, thereby making the uterus a comfortable home for the embryo. After the 10th week of pregnancy, the corpus luteum starts becoming smaller, but continues to function throughout pregnancy. However, by the 6th week, i.e. before the corpus luteum function declines, the placenta starts producing hCG as well as estrogen and progesterone. Thus there are mechanisms for keeping uterus hospitable for the baby throughout pregnancy.

[2]The endometrial cells of pregnancy are called decidual cells.

From the above account, the changing sources of nourishment of the embryo from conception onwards can also be understood. The embryo receives its nutrition successively from:

a. The nutrients stored in the ovum
b. Secretions of the Fallopian tube
c. Secretions of the uterine endometrium
d. Digested decidual cells

The decidual cells continue to supply nutrition to the embryo upto the age of 8 weeks but the placenta also starts supplying some nutrition after the age of 16 days.

The Placenta

As discussed above, the embryo, ovary and uterus together keep making some makeshift arrangement to maintain the uterus in a hospitable state and to continue the supply of nutrients to the embryo. But as the embryo grows up to become the fetus[3], these makeshift arrangements are no longer adequate. In anticipation of this inadequacy, the embryo and uterus together start making the placenta so that it may take over these functions. Although the placenta starts functioning at the age of 16 days, it takes over all nutritional and endocrine functions only at the age of about 8 weeks.

Placenta is a structure in which fetal blood vessels come in close contact with blood sinuses containing maternal blood. The surface area of contact is increased by the fetal vessels growing into folded structures called villi (Fig. 12.12).

Functions of the Placenta

The functions of the placenta may be described briefly as follows:

1. *Supply of oxygen to the fetus:* Oxygen diffuses from the maternal blood to the fetal blood due to a pressure gradient of about 20 mm Hg. Although the gradient is small, it is able to supply the fetal requirements because the oxyhemoglobin dissociation curve of fetal hemoglobin (HbF) is shifted to the left as compared to that of adult

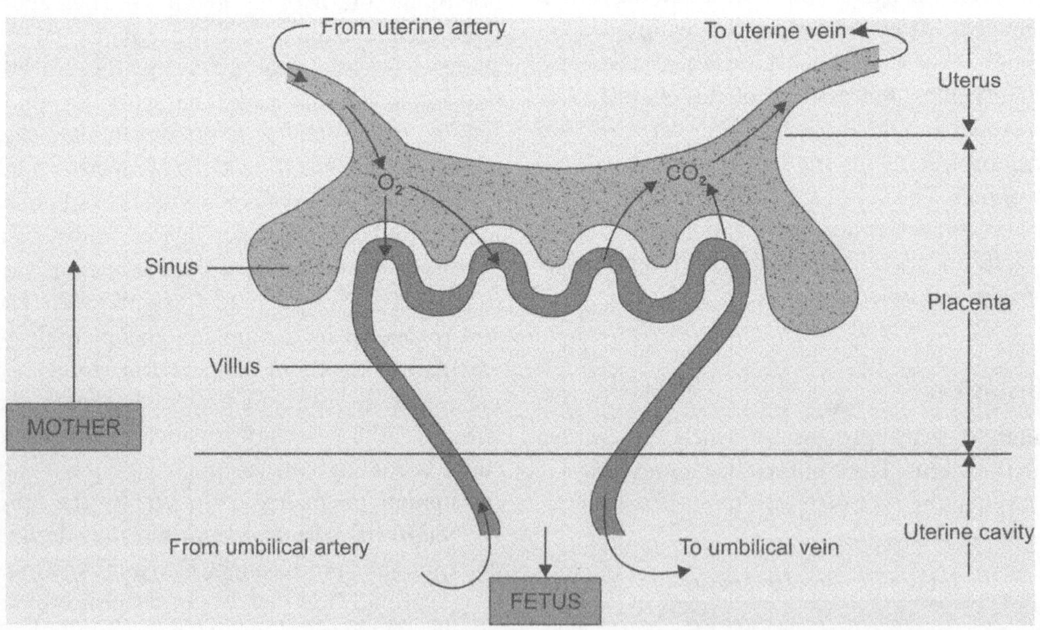

Fig. 12.12 Diagrammatic representation of the placenta

[3]The embryo, even after repeated cell division, remains essentially a round structure till about 9 weeks of age (8 weeks after implantation). At that age, it acquires a shape: a distinct head and trunk, and the outline of major structures is ready. When that happens, it is called the fetus.

hemoglobin (Fig. 12.13). As a result, HbF can carry more oxygen even at a low PO_2. Secondly, the PCO_2 in the fetal blood is high. As carbon dioxide diffuses from the fetal to maternal blood, it raises the PCO_2 of maternal blood and the PCO_2 of fetal blood falls. Rise in PCO_2 of maternal blood facilitates giving up of oxygen by the maternal blood (Bohr effect).[4] On the other hand, fall in PCO_2 of fetal blood facilitates picking up more oxygen by the fetal blood (also Bohr effect). That is why this phenomenon is called double Bohr effect. Thus the placenta supplies oxygen to the fetus.

2. *Removal of carbon dioxide from the fetus:* Carbon dioxide diffuses from the fetal blood to the maternal blood due to a pressure gradient of about 3 mmHg. This small gradient is able to remove carbon dioxide satisfactorily because it is much more soluble than oxygen.
3. *Supply of nutrients to the fetus:* Glucose and other nutrients diffuse from the maternal blood to the fetal blood due to a concentration gradient. For glucose, the diffusion is carrier mediated (facilitated diffusion). This is valuable because glucose is required in much larger amounts than other nutrients.
4. *Removal of waste products from the fetus:* Waste products such as urea, uric acid and creatinine diffuse from the fetal blood to the maternal blood due to a concentration gradient. Then they are removed, along with similar waste products of the mother, by the mother's kidneys.
5. *Secretion of hormones:* Placenta secretes hCG, estrogens, progesterone, human chorionic somatomammotropin (hCS) and relaxin.

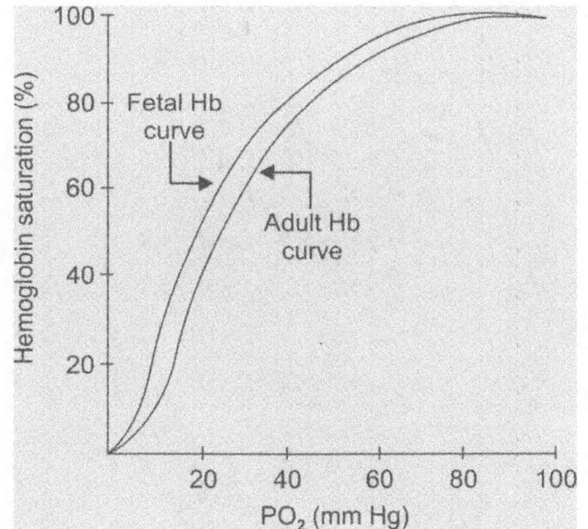

Fig. 12.13 Oxygen dissociation curves for adult and fetal hemoglobin compared

As discussed above, hCG stimulates the corpus luteum to produce estrogens and progesterone.

Estrogens are responsible for the enlargement of the uterus and breasts during pregnancy. Estrogens also relax the ligaments of the pubic symphysis so that the passage becomes easier for the fetus during delivery.

Progesterone inhibits uterine contraction, thereby allowing pregnancy to continue. In addition, it has a trophic effect on the uterus right from the beginning of pregnancy, as discussed already. Further, progesterone also participates in preparing the breasts for lactation.

HCS has a structure and actions resembling prolactin and growth hormone. Like prolactin, it promotes breast development for synthesis of milk. Because of this function, the hormone was previously called human placental lactogen (hPL). In addition, hCS also decreases glucose utilization in the mother, thereby increasing the maternal blood glucose level. This increases the amount of glucose that may diffuse to the fetal blood.

Relaxin, as the name suggests, relaxes—it relaxes two tissues—it relaxes the uterus (like progesterone) and also the pelvic ligaments (like estrogen).

To summarize, the placenta performs for the fetus the functions which are performed after birth by the lungs, gastrointestinal tract and kidneys. In addition, the placenta is also an endocrine organ.

Fetoplacental Unit

The placenta and fetus work together for the synthesis of some steroid hormones. Progesterone synthesized in the placenta is used by the fetal adrenal

[4]If you have forgotten what Bohr effect is, see Chapter 6.

cortex to synthesize the glucocorticoids, cortisol and corticosterone. But the fetus also does something for the placenta. Pregnenolone, an intermediate in the synthesis of steroid hormones, is synthesized by the placenta and passed on to the fetus. Fetal adrenals convert pregnenolone into the androgens, dehydroepiandrosterone (DHEA) and 16-hydroxy DHEA. DHEA and 16-hydroxy DHEA are sent back to the placenta where they are converted into estradiol and estriol respectively. Thus the fetus contributes an important step in the synthesis of placental estrogens. This collaborative activity is referred to as fetoplacental unit (Fig. 12.14).

Parturition

The fetus grows, differentiates and matures in the uterus under the mother's care. About 39 weeks after fertilization, it reaches a stage when it can begin its extrauterine life. The process of delivery of the fetus is called parturition. What precipitates parturition is not fully understood, but two types of factors seem to be involved: mechanical and hormonal.

The mechanical factors arise from the increase in the size of the fetus, increasing progressively the stretch on the uterus. Stretch of smooth muscle is itself a stimulus for contraction.

The hormonal factors in pregnancy are two-fold. First, near term the progesterone level falls. Since progesterone inhibits uterine contraction, a fall in its level increases the excitability of the uterus. Secondly, as term approaches, the number of oxytocin receptors in the uterus increases steeply. Hence the same level of oxytocin becomes more and more effective in inducing uterine contraction.

The onset of labor is generally announced by a sudden increase in uterine contractions, which are somewhat painful. The frequency and strength of contractions and the pain associated with them increase as labor progresses. Simultaneously the cervix becomes softer and dilates progressively. Descent of the fetal head stretches the cervix. Now a positive feedback mechanism leads to delivery of the fetus (Fig. 12.15). Stretch of the cervix leads to contraction of the uterus. Contraction of the uterus pushes the head further down, stretching the cervix further. Hormonal factors add to this mechanical phenomenon. Stretching of the cervix releases oxytocin, which also induces uterine contraction. Voluntary contraction of the abdominal muscles by the mother also contributes to delivery of the fetus.

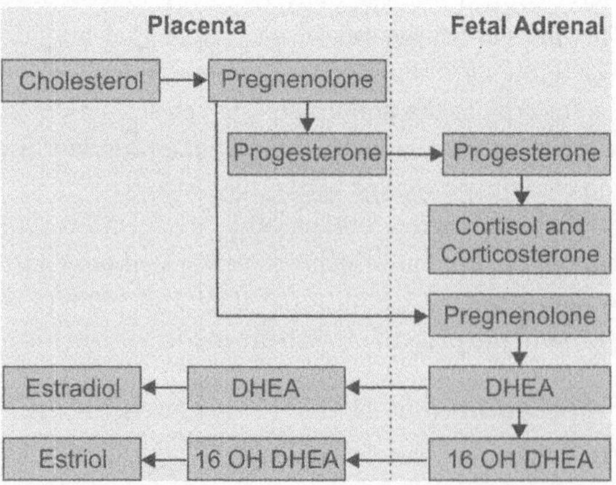

Fig. 12.14 The fetoplacental unit

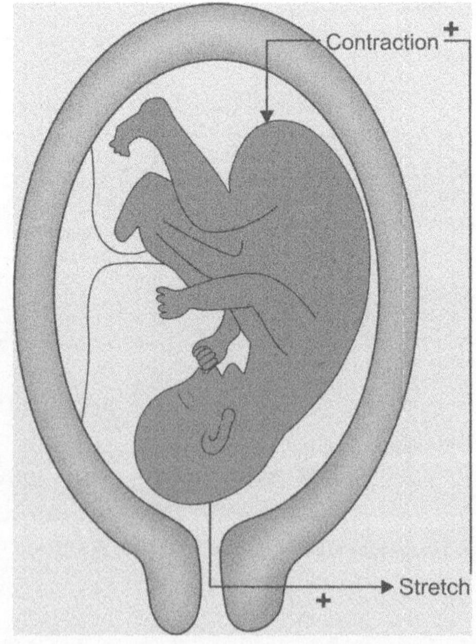

Fig. 12.15 The positive feedback mechanism involved in parturition

After the delivery of the fetus, high oxytocin levels ensure contraction of the uterus to a fairly small size. This produces stress on the attachment of placenta to the uterine wall, leading to separation and eventual delivery of the placenta about 30 min after delivery of the baby.

Further decrease in the size of the uterus (involution) continues for 4-5 weeks after parturition. This is aided by breastfeeding because every feed involves release of oxytocin, which in turn leads to uterine contraction.

LACTATION

Lactation is the process of secretion of milk. The mother's milk can look after the nutritional needs of the baby completely for about 4 months, and partially for a year or more even after that.

The preparation for lactation begins long before it is required. Some development of the breast takes place at puberty. Further development occurs during pregnancy. The development involves the following components:

a. *Proliferation of mammary ducts*: This requires primarily estrogen, but also glucocorticoids (to mobilize amino acids), growth hormone (to mobilize glucose), insulin (to promote protein synthesis) and prolactin. During pregnancy, prolactin is further supplemented by hCS, which has actions similar to prolactin.
b. *Development of lobules and secretory alveoli*: This requires primarily progesterone, but also the other hormones named earlier. The other hormones are required primarily because rapid growth anywhere would need an extra supply of nutrients and enhanced protein synthesis.
c. *Secretion of milk*: This requires primarily prolactin. Secretion of milk is inhibited by estrogen and progesterone. That is why, although all the hormones named so far are present during pregnancy, secretion of milk is negligible.

Secretion and Ejection of Milk

During parturition, the placenta is also expelled. Expulsion of the placenta removes from the body a major source of estrogen and progesterone. Therefore the estrogen and progesterone levels decrease markedly after birth. As mentioned above, these hormones inhibit the secretion of milk. Therefore a decrease in the level of these hormones removes the inhibition, and the action of prolactin now results in secretion of milk.

However, secretion of milk is not enough. It has to be ejected from the alveoli. This results from the action of oxytocin. Oxytocin produces contraction of myoepithelial cells surrounding the alveoli, leading to ejection of milk into the ductal system.

Milk Ejection Reflex

When the baby suckles the mother's breast, sensory stimuli arising from the nipple and areola lead to the milk ejection reflex. The effects of the reflex are release of prolactin and oxytocin. Oxytocin leads to ejection of milk. Prolactin is also important because unless secretion of milk continues, lactation will be impossible. Not only stimulation of the nipple or areola but even fondling the baby or hearing the baby's cry for milk can evoke the milk ejection reflex.

Lactational Amenorrhea

Amenorrhea is absence of menstrual cycles. Amenorrhea is seen not only during pregnancy but also during lactation. During lactation, amenorrhea is due to secretion of prolactin during every feed. Prolactin inhibits secretion of GnRH from the hypothalamus. Inhibition of GnRH secretion inhibits release of FSH and LH from the pituitary. Inhibition of FSH and LH keeps ovaries inactive. When gonadotropins as well as ovarian hormones are depressed, neither ovulation nor menstruation are possible. After lactation, when the menstrual cycles start again, they are without ovulation (anovulatory) for about 6 months. Lactational amenorrhea is nature's method of preventing another pregnancy during lactation. Therefore if the child is breastfed, besides the other advantages of breastfeeding (Chapter 9), there is also spacing between two children even without the use of any contraceptive.

CONTRACEPTION

Explosive growth of population in developing countries like India in the recent past is a major problem because it neutralizes to a large extent the increase in productivity. The increase in population is primarily due to a marked decrease in death rate which has resulted from improved public health measures. The birth rate, on the other hand, has not fallen much in spite of a vigorous family planning policy.

Contraception means preventing conception. The surest and safest method of contraception is **abstinence**. But its acceptibility is very poor among young couples who need contraception the most. A better accepted method is the **rhythm method**. This method involves abstinence only around the time of ovulation so that conception is unlikely. Since ovulation takes place about 14 days before the onset of menstruation, its date can be guessed provided the cycle length is fairly constant in a woman. An indication about ovulation is also provided by a rise in basal body temperature on the day of ovulation by about 1°C, and by a progressive decrease in viscosity (and therefore an increase in stretchability) of the cervical mucus as the day of ovulation approaches. By avoiding sexual intercourse for a couple of days before and after ovulation, conception can be prevented. While the acceptance of the method is good, its rate of failure is fairly high. Hence, there is a need for other methods of birth control. Contraceptive methods may be divided into those to be used by men, and those which are suitable for women (Figs 12.16A and B).

Contraceptives for Men

The male contribution to the reproductive process may be blocked by either preventing normal spermatogenesis, or by blocking the transport of spermatozoa at some point in the male genital tract.

Inhibiting Spermatogenesis

Gossypol, a substance found in cotton seed oil, inhibits spermatogenesis. However, its side effects have prevented it from becoming popular.

Vasectomy

Vasectomy is a surgical procedure in which the continuity of vas deferens is disturbed by cutting it. Therefore vasectomy prevents sperms from being transported towards the urethra. It is a simple, essentially harmless procedure and completely reliable. Once done, it provides contraception permanently unless the procedure is reversed surgically.

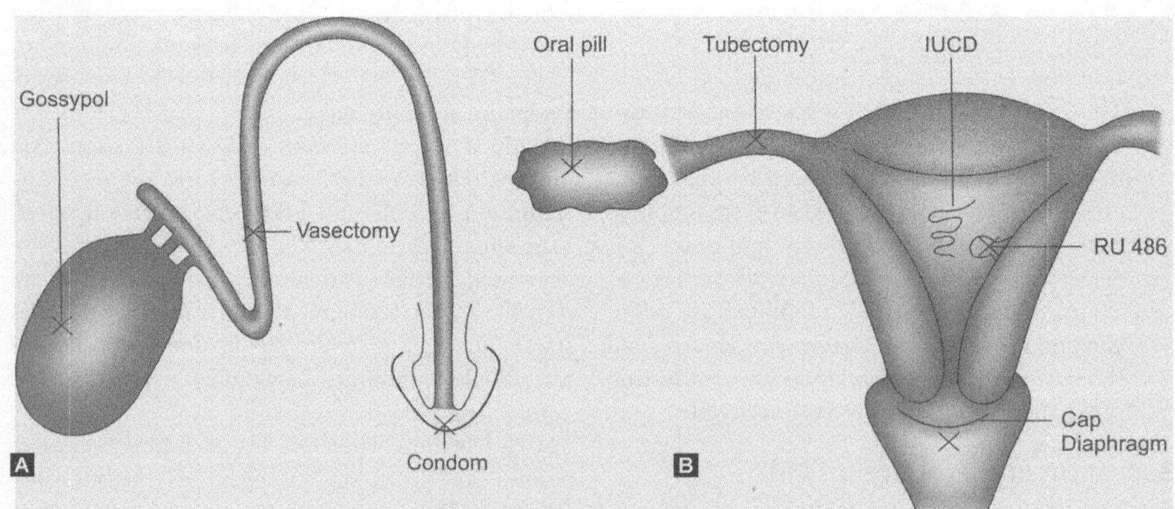

Figs 12.16A and B Physiological basis of contraception in males (A) and females (B)

Condom

Condom is a simple device to prevent the ejaculated semen from reaching the vagina. It is essentially a cap for the penis which holds the ejaculate during sexual intercourse. However, its efficacy is not very reliable; hence conception due to condom failure is quite high.

Contraceptives for Women

In women, there are at least three alternative approaches for achieving contraception: to inhibit ovulation, to prevent ovum transport, and to prevent fertilization. To these may be added a fourth approach which does not prevent conception but prevents implantation or development of the embryo at a very early age.

Inhibiting Ovulation

The oral pill acts by inhibiting ovulation. The commonest and most successful pill has a combination of estrogen and progesterone. It is used during the first 21 days of the menstrual cycle. By maintaining a high blood level of estrogen and progesterone, this pill inhibits the FSH and LH surge, and thereby prevents ovulation. After the 21st day of the cycle, when the pill is stopped, hormonal withdrawal leads to menstruation. Thus a superficial resemblance to the normal cycle is maintained, but there is no ovulation.

A similar result may be achieved by a slow-release injection of estrogen and progesterone. This has the added convenience that the woman does not have to remember to take the pill every day.

Preventing Ovum Transport: Tubectomy

Tubectomy is a surgical procedure in which the Fallopian tubes are cut so that the ovum cannot be Fransported towards the uterus. Like vasectomy, tubectomy is also a permanent procedure. Laparoscopic surgery has made tubectomy far more convenient for the patient.

Diaphragm and Cervical Cap

These are devices comparable to the condom for use by the female. They create a mechanical barrier between the sperm and the ovum. Their efficacy may be improved by using a spermicidal jelly.

Intrauterine Contraceptive Devices

Lippe's loop and copper-T are two popular intrauterine contraceptive devices (IUCDs). Their mechanism of action is not clearly understood. One plausible mechanism is that, being a foreign body, an IUCD induces inflammatory reaction in the uterus. The inflammatory response is associated with leukocytic infiltration. Leukocytes possibly release chemicals which are toxic to sperms.

Preventing Growth and Development of the Zygote

An embryo starts producing hCG at a very early stage of development. If hCG can be neutralized by using an antibody against it, progress of pregnancy can be arrested.

Progesterone is necessary for making the uterus suitable for implantation. An anti-progestin such as RU 486 arrests progress of pregnancy by preventing implantation.

QUESTIONS

1. Why is spermatogenesis markedly reduced in undescended testes?
2. Why does the menstrual blood not clot?
3. During menstruation, the protective epithelial lining of the uterus breaks down, and blood, which is a good medium for growth of bacteria, is available. Still, uterine infection as a result of menstruation is very rare. Why?

ANSWERS

1. It is generally believed that optimum spermatogenesis requires a temperature about 3°C below the core body temperature. This is generally possible if the testes descend into the scrotum. But undescended testes are exposed to the abdominal, or core body temperature (about 37°C). Therefore spermatogenesis is very poor or absent in such testes.
2. Menstrual blood normally does not clot because of the presence of fibrinolysin derived from endometrial tissues.
3. During the secretory phase, the endometrium shows leukocytic inflitration. Therefore, during menstruation a large number of leukocytes are also released. Leukocytes, being phagocytic in nature, possibly help in preventing infection. There may be other anti-infective substances also in the menstrual blood or tissue debris.

CHAPTER

13 Physiology of Locomotion

"Going up and down the stairs – you cannot imagine how useful that can be from the point of view of physical culture, if you know how to make use of it. Instead of going up because you are going up and coming down because you are coming down, like any ordinary man, you go up with the consciousness of all the muscles which are working and of making them work harmoniously."

—THE MOTHER (of Sri Aurobindo Ashram)

Chapter Outline

- Functional Anatomy of Skeletal Muscle
- Resting Membrane Potential
- Two Steps to Activation
- Action Potential
- Neuromuscular Transmission
- Contraction of Skeletal Muscle
- Electromyography
- Smooth Muscle
- Physiology of Nerve Fibers

Locomotion is an important characteristic of all animals. Although it makes no direct contribution to homeostasis, it is essential for life. An animal cannot get food, escape from an enemy, or find a mate without moving. These functions are essential for the organism to stay alive and to reproduce.

Locomotion is achieved by skeletal muscles. Skeletal muscles are supplied by motor nerve fibers. The activity of skeletal muscles is entirely dependent on activity in these nerve fibers. Motor nerve fibers are actually axons of motor neurons. The cell bodies of motor neurons are located in the anterior column of the spinal cord (Fig. 13.1). Motor neurons are under the control of will power. Therefore skeletal muscle contraction is also under the control of will power. That is the reason why skeletal muscles are also called voluntary muscles. However, that does not mean that all skeletal muscle activity is voluntary. Reflex contraction of these muscles, e.g. withdrawal of the hand to escape a pin prick, is involuntary. Reflex actions will be dealt with in some detail in Chapter 14. In this chapter we shall start with a discussion of structure of the skeletal muscle.

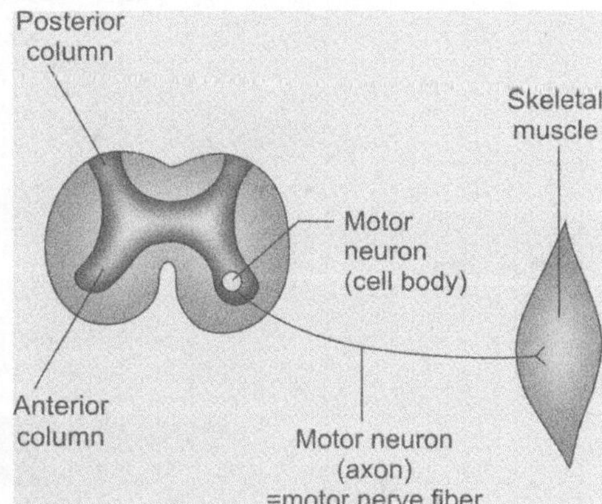

Fig. 13.1 Simplified view of the nerve supply of skeletal muscles. Each skeletal muscle is supplied by a large number of motor nerve fibers, only one of which has been shown in the diagram

FUNCTIONAL ANATOMY OF SKELETAL MUSCLE

A typical skeletal muscle consists of a bulky belly tapering into a tendon at either end. The two tendons are attached to two different bones, i.e. the muscle crosses a joint. That is why the muscle can bring about movement at the joint. A cross section of the muscle belly shows that it consists of a large number of muscle bundles. Further magnification shows that each muscle bundle consists of a large number of muscle *fibers*. A muscle fiber is equivalent to *a cell*.

Muscle Fiber

A muscle fiber is elongated in shape.

It is enclosed in a cell membrane which is called sarcolemma. The cytoplasm of a muscle fiber is called sarcoplasm. The sarcoplasm is packed with contractile proteins.

Organization of Contractile Elements

A muscle fiber consists of a large number of myofibrils. Myofibrils show a repeating pattern of lines and bands (Figs 13.2A to C). The portion of a myofibril between two Z lines is called a sarcomere.

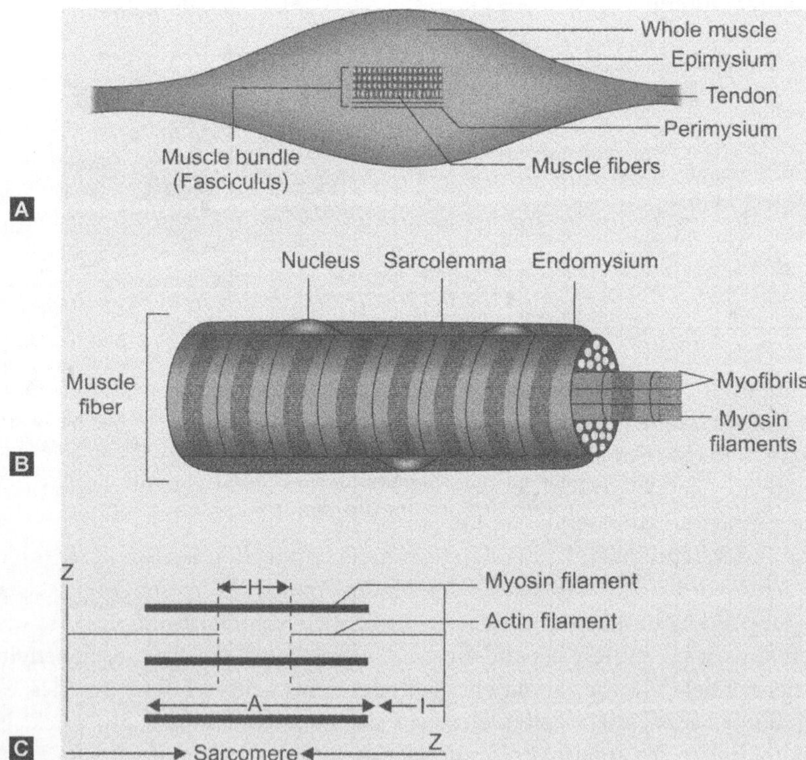

Figs 13.2A to C Structure of skeletal muscle. (A) A muscle belly is composed of several muscle bundles. Each muscle bundle has several muscle fibers; (B) Each muscle fiber (equivalent to a muscle cell) has several peripherally placed nuclei. It is made up of several myofibrils; (C) Each myofibril has myofilaments arranged as shown here. Sarcomere is considered a unit of contraction

A sarcomere is the functional unit of contraction. The nomenclature of lines and bands is best understood in terms of the arrangement of contractile proteins. Contractile proteins are mainly arranged in the form of two types of myofilaments: thick and thin.

The thick filament forms the A band. It is made up of the protein called myosin. The thin filament forms the I band and also extends partly into the A band. The thin filament is made up primarily of the protein called actin. H band represents the region where there is no overlap between actin and myosin filaments.

Under a light microscope, A band is darkly stained and I band is lightly stained giving a striped appearance. Further, all the myofibrils in a muscle fiber are so arranged that the A and I bands of all myofibrils are at the same level. This gives a striped appearance to the whole muscle fiber. That is why skeletal muscle is also known as striped or striated.

When a muscle contracts, the length of the A band does not change but the I band shortens. This has been explained by proposing that during contraction actin filaments slide between myosin filaments towards the center of the sarcomere. We shall study this process in more detail a little later.

Sarcoplasmic Reticulum

Sarcoplasmic reticulum is a very prominent structure in the muscle fiber. It consists of a network of tubular structures (Fig. 13.3). The network divides the muscle fiber into myofibrils. At the junctions of A and I bands, the sarcoplasmic reticulum forms ring-like enlargements known as terminal cisterns or sacs. Terminal sacs can store calcium and release it at an appropriate time.

At the A-I junctions, the sarcolemma also dips deep into the sarcoplasm, forming transverse or T-tubules. A T-tubule and the two terminal sacs near it together form a triad. As you can see, T-tubules are essentially an extension of the extracellular space, and their wall is a continuation of the sarcolemma. Therefore an action potential on the sarcolemma is propagated along the walls of T-tubules. When the action potential reaches the triad zone, calcium is released from terminal sacs. Release of calcium into the sarcoplasm leads to contraction.

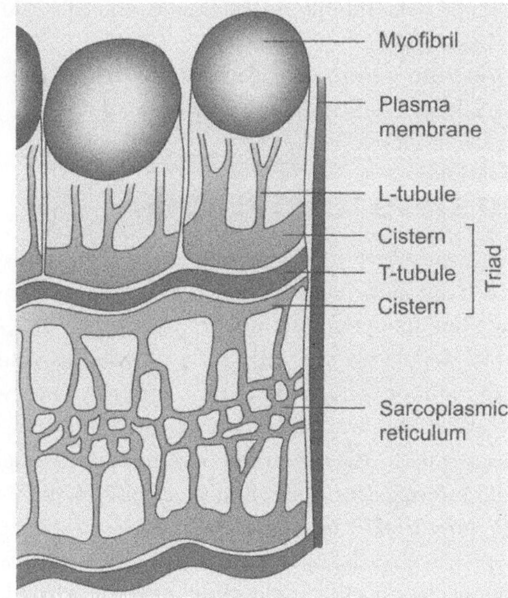

Fig. 13.3 The sarcoplasmic reticulum

RESTING MEMBRANE POTENTIAL

The factors responsible for genesis of resting membrane potential (RMP) in skeletal muscles are similar to those discussed in case of cardiac muscle (Chapter 5).[1] To recapitulate, the RMP is about –80 mV, the potential being negative inside the cell as compared to the outside.

RMP is the result of:

a. The intracellular potassium concentration being higher than the extracellular potassium concentration,
b. Impermeability of the membrane to intracellular proteins, which are negatively charged,

[1]The student is strongly urged to revise the electrophysiology of cardiac muscle. Since there is a lot in common between the electrophysiology of all excitable tissues, the fundamentals have not been repeated anywhere else in the book.

c. Poor permeability of the membrane to sodium ions, and
d. Sodium pump, which maintains a high extracellular sodium concentration as well as electrical gradient.

TWO STEPS TO ACTIVATION

If you again refer to Chapter 5, you would observe that activation, or depolarization, takes place in two steps. First, there is a slow and graded depolarization. If this depolarization crosses a threshold value, an all-or-none action potential is fired. The two depolarizations are clearly demarcated in case of skeletal muscle. The message of activation brought by the motor nerve fibers first gives rise to the **end plate potential**. End plate potential is a graded, non-propagated depolarization. When the end plate potential crosses a threshold value, an action potential is fired and is propagated along the cell membrane.

ACTION POTENTIAL

Action potential is a brief depolarization. Because of their brief duration and relatively large magnitude, action potentials are also referred to as 'impulses' or 'spikes'.

The action potential consists of a sharp depolarization followed by repolarization (Fig. 13.4). The depolarization involves a change in the membrane potential from about –90 mV to +30 mV. Repolarization implies a return to the resting membrane potential, i.e. about –90 mV.

Ionic Basis of Action Potential

You might have observed that the action potential of skeletal muscle (Fig. 13.4) is somewhat different from that of cardiac muscle (refer to Fig. 5.10). The action potential of skeletal muscle does not have a plateau phase. Accordingly, the ionic basis of skeletal muscle action potential is also simpler. The depolarization phase of skeletal muscle action potential is due to an increase in permeability to sodium ions (Figs 13.5A and B). The concentration gradient as well as the electrical gradient favor the entry of sodium ions into the cell. Hence the increase in permeability leads to a rapid entry of sodium ions. Since the inside of a resting cell is negative as compared to the outside, entry of positively charged sodium ions leads to depolarization. The duration of increase in permeability to sodium is very short. When the sodium permeability starts declining, the membrane permeability to potassium starts increasing. The concentration of potassium is higher inside the cell. And, the outside of the cell is negative at the peak of the action potential. Therefore both the concentration and electrical gradients favor exit of potassium ions. Exit of positively charged potassium ions and decrease in permeability to sodium ions together bring about repolarization.

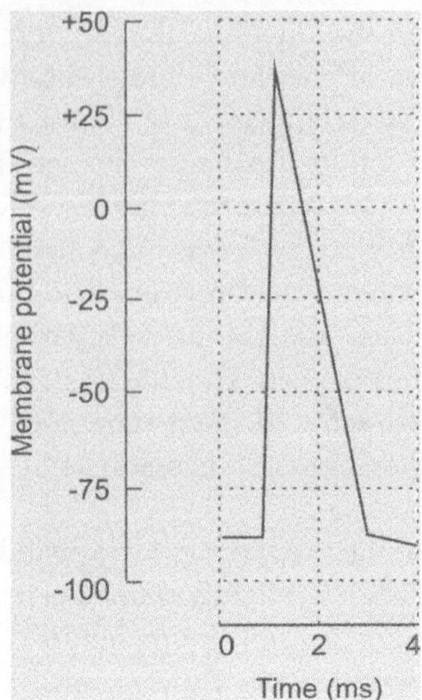

Fig. 13.4 Action potential in a skeletal muscle

NEUROMUSCULAR TRANSMISSION

A skeletal muscle is supplied by a group of motor nerve fibers. Each motor nerve fiber is the axon of a motor neuron (Fig. 13.1). After entering the muscle, each motor nerve fiber divides into several branches. Each branch of the nerve fiber innervates one muscle fiber. The junction between the nerve fiber and the muscle fiber is called the **neuromuscular junction** or **motor end plate**.

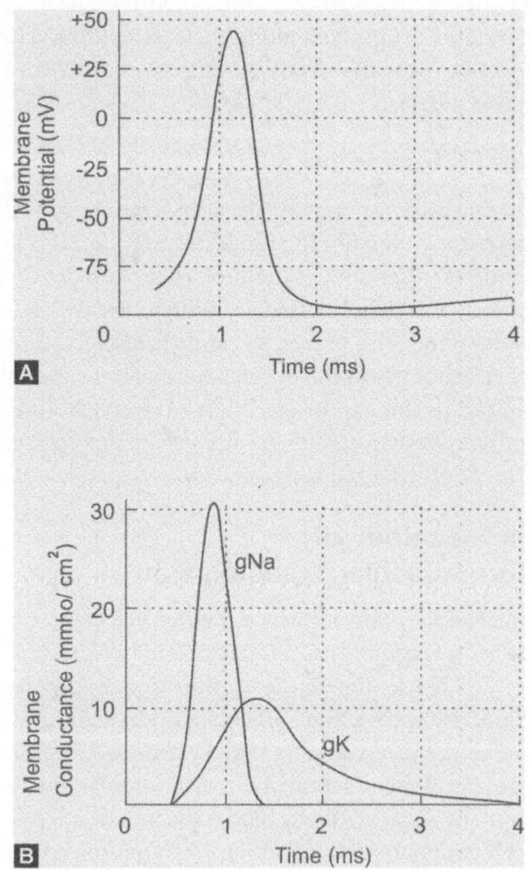

Figs 13.5A and B Ionic basis of action potential. (A) Action potential; (B) Change in membrane conductance (which corresponds to permeability) for sodium and potassium. gNa, sodium conductance; gK, potassium conductance. Note that depolarization is due to increase in sodium permeability, which leads to sodium influx. Repolarization is due to an increase in potassium permeability, which leads to potassium efflux (The time relations are somewhat different from those in Figure 13.4 because here the action potential illustrated is that of a nerve fiber. The ionic basis of action potential is, however, similar for both nerve and skeletal muscle)

Functional Anatomy of the Neuromuscular Junction

The nerve fiber branches still further at the neuromuscular junction. Each branch ends in a rounded or flattened terminal which fits into a depression on the surface of the muscle fiber (Fig. 13.6). The neuronal membrane participating in the junction is called the presynaptic membrane. The muscle fiber membrane at the junction is called the postsynaptic membrane. The gap between the presynaptic membrane and post-synaptic membrane is called the synaptic cleft.

The axon terminal has a large number of mitochondria, indicating that it is a region of high metabolic activity. It also has vesicles containing the neurotransmitter which, in case of skeletal muscle, is acetylcholine. The synaptic cleft contains an enzyme acetylcholinesterase, which can break down acetylcholine. The postsynaptic membrane is thrown into folds which increase its surface area. The postsynaptic membrane has receptors for acetylcholine. These receptors are specialized areas in the membrane into which acetylcholine molecules can fit as a key fits into a lock.

Physiology of Neuromuscular Transmission

Let us start with a summary of the process. A convenient point to begin is the action potential propagated along the motor nerve fiber. When this action potential reaches the axon terminal, acetylcholine is released into the synaptic cleft. Acetylcholine leads to graded depolarization of

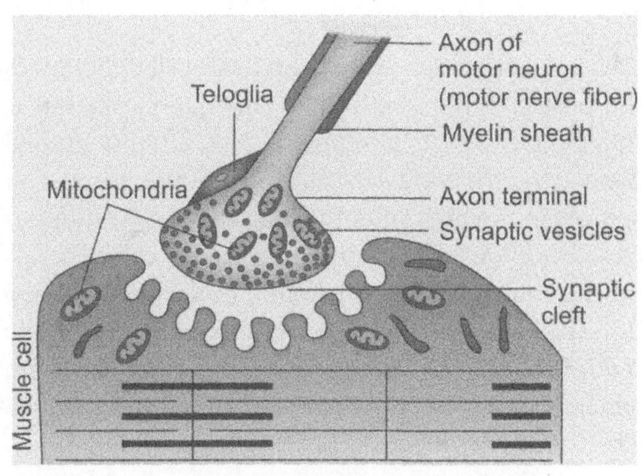

Fig. 13.6 Schematic representation of microscopic structure of a neuromuscular junction in skeletal muscle

the postsynaptic membrane. This depolarization is called the end plate potential. When the magnitude of the end plate potential crosses a threshold value, an action potential is fired and propagated along the sarcolemma in both directions. In this way the whole muscle fiber gets excited. By this process the excitation of the motor nerve fiber is transmitted (i.e. passed on) to the muscle fiber. Now we shall study the process in some detail, step by step.

Release of Acetylcholine

When an action potential arrives at the axon terminal, it opens up calcium channels in the axon terminal membrane. As a result calcium ions enter the terminal. Calcium ions make the acetylcholine vesicles move towards the presynaptic membrane. Then the vesicles release acetylcholine into the synaptic cleft.

Effect of Acetylcholine on the Postsynaptic Membrane

Acetylcholine diffuses through the synaptic cleft to reach the postsynaptic membrane. Then acetylcholine molecules attach themselves to acetylcholine receptors on the postsynaptic membrane. As a result, sodium channels open up in the postsynaptic membrane. Sodium ions rush in from the extracellular fluid into the muscle cell.

End Plate Potential

Entry of sodium ions into the muscle cell depolarizes the postsynaptic membrane. This depolarization is called the end plate potential (EPP). EPP is a graded depolarization because it depends on the number of sodium ions which enter the muscle cell. The number of sodium ions which enter the muscle cell depends on the number of acetylcholine molecules released into the synaptic cleft. The number of acetylcholine molecules released depends on the *frequency* with which action potentials arrive at the axon terminal. The frequency of action potentials depends on how strongly the central nervous system has decided that the muscle should contract.

Coming back to the EPP, the EPP may cross the threshold for the firing of an action potential. In that case, the EPP leads to an action potential. The action potential is propagated along the sarcolemma. How the action potential leads to muscle contraction is discussed later.

Fate of Acetylcholine

The duration of action of acetylcholine on the postsynaptic membrane is extremely brief. The reason is that the synaptic cleft contains an enzyme, acetylcholinesterase, which breaks down acetylcholine. This prevents unduly prolonged action of acetylcholine on the postsynaptic membrane. But if undue prolongation of action of acetylcholine is required, we can use those drugs which block the action of acetylcholinesterase.

Pharmacology of Neuromuscular Transmission

Drugs which can influence neuromuscular transmission are required most frequently in two situations: first, to block transmission during surgery; and second, to improve transmission in myasthenia gravis. Some of the drugs used in both situations are similar because prolonged action of a neuromuscular junction 'stimulant' also eventually blocks the junction.

During surgery, blocking the neuromuscular transmission is useful. It is useful because it paralyses the skeletal muscles. Paralysis, or relaxation, of muscles facilitates surgery, specially abdominal surgery. However, when skeletal muscles are paralysed, artificial respiration becomes essential.[2]

Neuromuscular blocking agents are of two types: the depolarizing type and non-depolarizing type (Figs 13.7A and B).

Depolarizing Type Blockers

These agents act like acetylcholine (ACh) but cannot be broken down by acetylcholinesterase (AChE). Therefore their action is long-lasting. These agents initially act like ACh. They depolarize the muscle

[2]Respiratory muscles are also skeletal muscles. Paralysis of respiratory muscles leads to death within minutes unless artificial respiration is given.

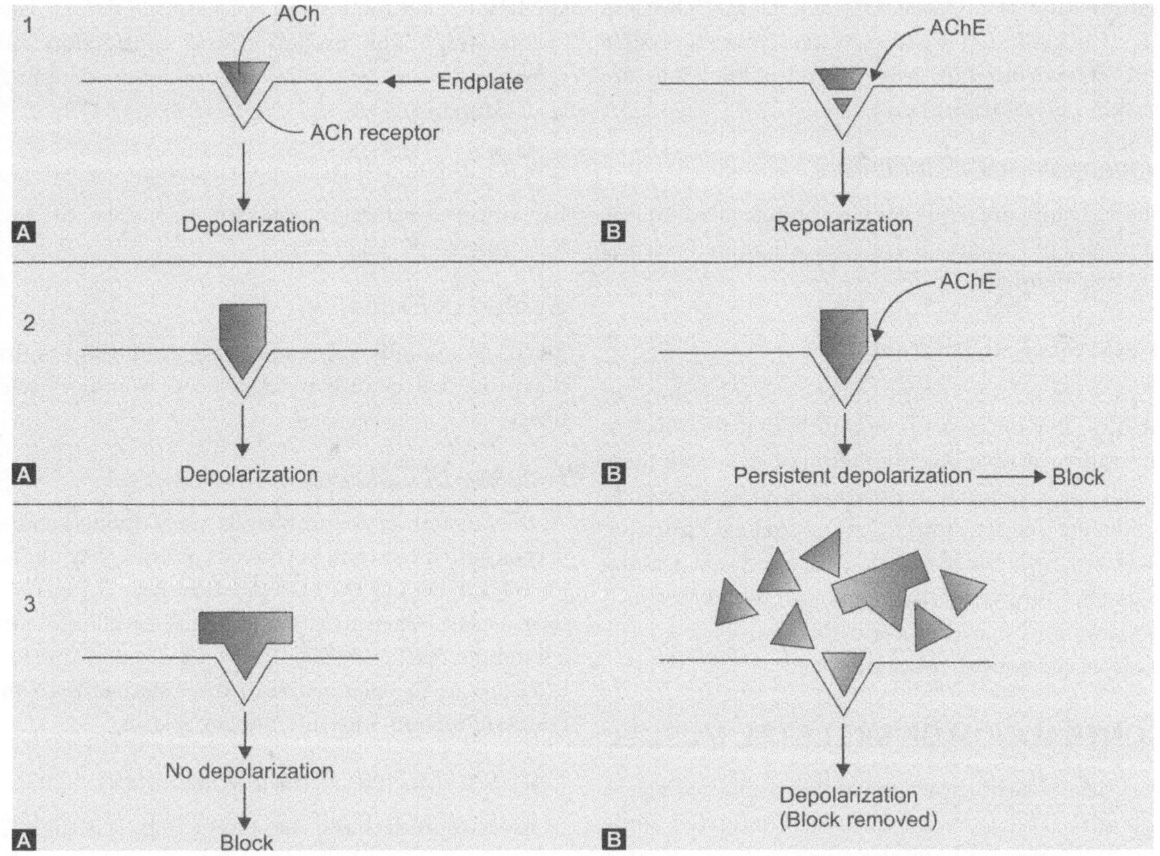

Figs 13.7A and B Depolarizing and non-depolarizing type of neuromuscular blocking agents.

1. Acetylcholine (ACh) produces short-lasting depolarization (A) because it is hydrolyzed by acetylcholinesterase (AChE) (B).
2. Depolarizing type of blockers act like acetylcholine and produce depolarization (A). But this depolarization is persistent because these blockers are resistant to the effects of AChE (B). Persistent depolarization blocks the neuromuscular junction.
3. Non-depolarizing type of blockers occupy ACh receptors but do not produce depolarization. Therefore they block neuromuscular transmission (A). The effect of these blockers can be reversed by excess of acetylcholine (B).

membrane (sarcolemma) and induce muscle contraction. But later, prolonged depolarization leads to paralysis of the muscle. An example of this type of drug is succinylcholine.

Nondepolarizing Type Blockers

These agents compete with ACh for ACh receptors. They block ACh receptors but do not have the biological activity of ACh. By preventing ACh from attaching to its receptors, these drugs block neuromuscular transmission. However, since the block is competitive, it can be overcome by an excess of ACh. Examples of this group of drugs are gallamine (Flaxedil) and curare.

In myasthenia gravis[3], the type of drugs which are useful are AChE inhibitors. AChE inhibitors do not let AChE destroy ACh. Therefore ACh released at the neuromuscular junction can accumulate. Excess ACh can overcome the poor neuromuscular

[3]Myasthenia gravis is a disease in which there is weakness of muscles due to poor neuromuscular transmission. Excess ACh can overcome the effects of poor transmission.

transmission of myasthenia gravis (Figs 13.8A and B). ACh inhibitors are also of two types: reversible and irreversible, but only the reversible ones are useful in myasthenia gravis.

Reversible AChE Inhibitors

These agents are competitive inhibitors of AChE. Examples of this group are physostigmine (eserine) and neostigmine.

Irreversible AChE Inhibitors

These agents are non-competitive inhibitors of AChE. They bind AChE so tightly that the block is almost irreversible. Accumulation of ACh with these agents leads to initial stimulation of skeletal muscles producing convulsions. Later, skeletal muscles, including respiratory muscles, are paralysed, leading to death. Examples of this group are insecticides such as parathion, malathion and Baygon. That is why these insecticides are poisonous.

CONTRACTION OF SKELETAL MUSCLE

We have learnt how the EPP leads to action potential. The action potential is conducted along the sarcolemma in both directions. Action potential is an electrical phenomenon, and is sometimes called excitation. Contraction is a mechanical process. The events which link excitation and contraction are together known as excitation-contraction coupling (E-C coupling).

Excitation–Contraction Coupling

Excitation-contraction coupling consists of the following steps (Fig. 13.9).

Spread of Excitation

Electrical excitation spreads along the T-tubules. In that process, excitation reaches the interior of muscle fibers.

Release of Calcium

At the junction of A and I bands, the T-tubules come very close to the cisternae of the sarcoplasmic reticulum. One T-tubule and the two cisternae near it together form a triad. When an action potential travelling along a T-tubule reaches a triad, the depolarization spreads to cisternae. Depolarization of the cisternae leads to release of calcium ions into the sarcoplasm.

Calcium–Muscle Protein Interaction

In order to understand this interaction, it is important to learn something about four muscle proteins: myosin, actin, tropomyosin and troponin.

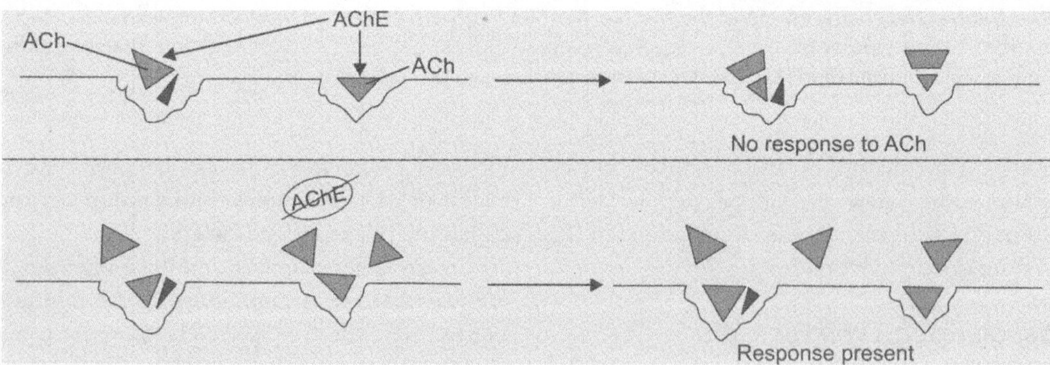

Figs 13.8A and B Utility of acetylcholinesterase (AChE) inhibitors in myasthenia gravis. (A) Due to a defect at the neuromuscular junction, normal quantity of acetylcholine (ACh) staying for the normal duration does not lead to neuromuscular transmission; (B) If destruction of ACh is prevented by inhibiting the action of AChE, ACh accumulates and continues to act at the neuromuscular junction for a longer time. That results in neuromuscular transmission in spite of the defect at the junction. The small black filled-in triangle represents AChE

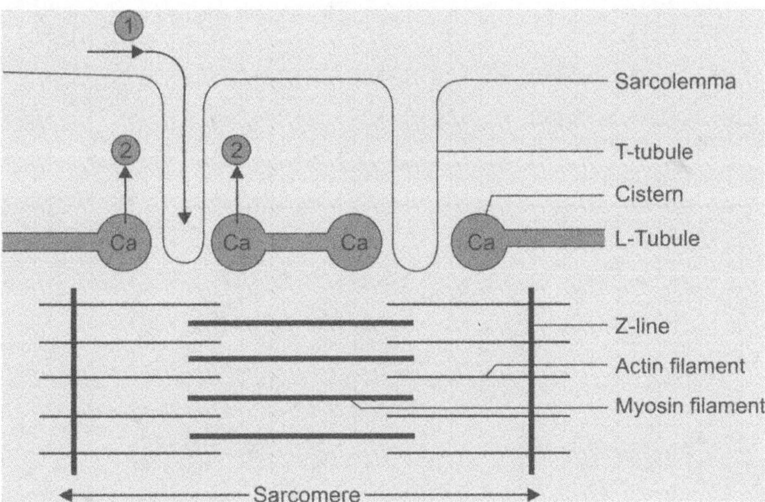

Fig. 13.9 Excitation-contraction coupling. The wave of excitation spreads along the sarcolemma to its invaginations known as transverse (T) tubules (1). That leads to release of calcium ions from the terminal cisterns of longitudinal (L) tubules of the sarcoplasmic reticulum (2). Increase in sarcoplasmic calcium ion concentration triggers the contractile process leading to sliding of actin filaments (Fig. 13.14)

Myosin forms the thick filaments. Each thick filament is made up of more than 200 myosin molecules. Each myosin molecule consists of a long tail, a short arm and a head (Figs 13.10A and B). The arms and heads together form the cross bridges which play an important role in contraction. Each cross bridge can bend at two points or 'hinges'. One hinge is at the junction of the arm and the tail; the other is at the junction of the arm and the head. Myosin not only participates in the contractile mechanism but also acts as an ATPase, i.e. it breaks down ATP to release energy.

Actin is the major protein of thin filaments (Fig. 13.11). Actin filaments carry ADP molecules at regular intervals. ADP molecules are thought to be the active sites which interact with myosin cross bridges during the process of contraction.

Tropomyosin is also a part of the thin filaments. Tropomyosin is wrapped spirally around the actin filament. Tropomyosin covers the active sites on the actin filament. But if tropomyosin sinks deeper in the grooves between the actin coils, the active sites may be exposed.

Troponin is also associated with thin filaments. Troponin is a globular protein having three subunits: TnI, which has a strong affinity for actin (the major protein of the I band): TnT, which has a strong affinity for tropomyosin; and TnC, which has a strong affinity for calcium.

Let us go back to the calcium-muscle protein interaction. We have seen how release of calcium from the cisternae increases the calcium ion concentration in the muscle fiber. Calcium ions combine with TnC. The combination alters the shape of the troponin molecule. Since troponin is attached to tropomyosin, alteration in the shape of troponin shifts tropomyosin. Shifting of tropomyosin exposes the active sites on actin. Exposure of the active sites leads to an interaction between actin and myosin (Figs 13.12A and B).

Actin–myosin Interaction

The interaction is energized by hydrolysis of ATP, which is catalyzed by myosin. The interaction has features of a ratchet mechanism (Figs 13.13A to C), and leads to movement of actin filaments towards

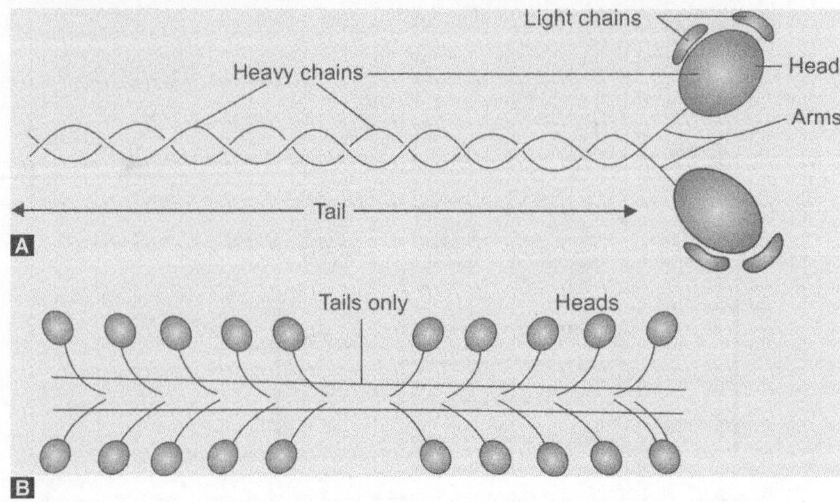

Figs 13.10A and B (A) Diagrammatic representation of structure of the myosin molecule; (B) Diagrammatic representation of arrangement of myosin molecules in the myosin filament

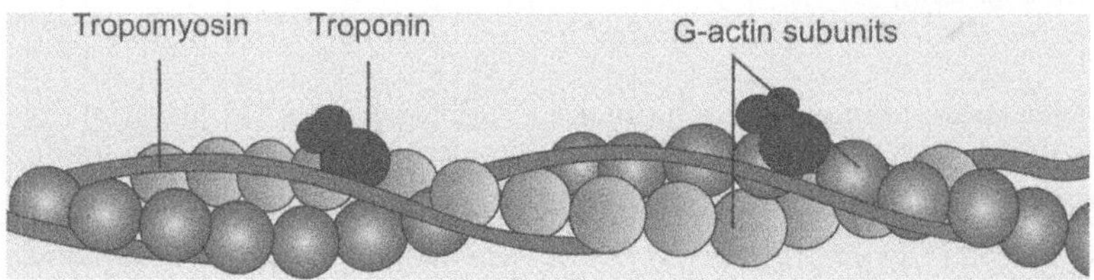

Fig. 13.11 Diagrammatic representation of the molecular arrangement in a thin filament. G-actin, globular actin

the center of the sarcomere. Since the process involves sliding of actin filaments between the myosin filaments, it is called the sliding filament mechanism (Figs 13.14A and B).

Stimulus–response Relationship in Skeletal Muscle

If an isolated muscle is stimulated experimentally, the strength of contraction depends on the strength of the stimulus (Fig. 13.15). But this relationship has limits. If the stimulus is below threshold, no contraction is obtained. If the stimulus is stronger than the maximal stimulus, there is no further increase in the strength of contraction.

The increase in strength of contraction with increasing strength of the stimulus seems, at first, to violate the all or none law. In fact, skeletal muscle also follows all or none law *at cellular level.* Each muscle fiber either contracts with full force or not at all. But the *number* of muscle fibers contracting at a time can be altered. Larger the number of muscle fibers which contract, stronger is the contraction.

Effect of Frequency of Stimulation on Contraction

The contractile response of a skeletal muscle to a single brief stimulus is called a simple muscle twitch (Figs 13.16A to C). If the muscle is stimulated repeatedly at a low frequency, each stimulus gives an individual response. At a higher frequency, the individual responses are partly fused: the phenomenon is called incomplete tetanus. At a still higher frequency, individual responses are fused completely: the phenomenon is called complete

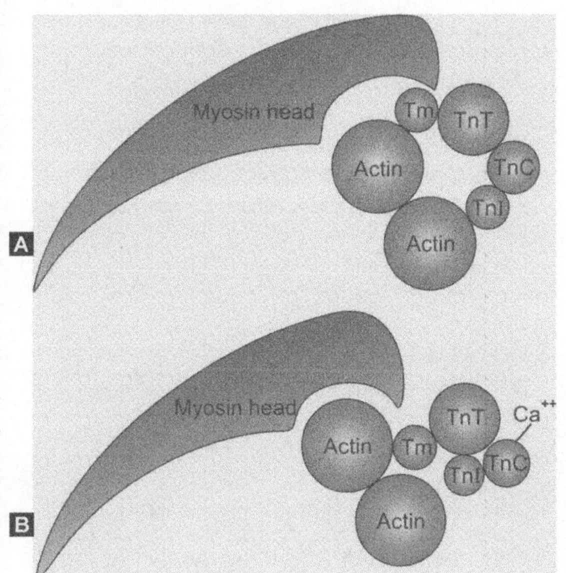

Figs 13.12A and B Calcium-muscle protein interaction. (A) Resting state. Tropomyosin (Tm) blocks the interaction between actin and myosin; (B) Active state. In the presence of calcium ions, the three subunits of troponin (TnT, TnC and TnI) bind to each other more tightly. As a result, tropomyosin (Tm) sinks deeper in the groove between the two actin strands. Hence the block is removed, and the actin and myosin can interact with each other. (Adapted from Cohen C. The protein switch of muscle contraction. Sc Am 1975; 233 (5): 36-45)

tetanus. The maximum tension generated during a tetanus is greater than during a twitch. One reason for this may be that calcium ions are released from the cisternae in response to each stimulus. If the interval between stimuli is small, there is not enough time between responses for the calcium ions to return to the cisternae completely. Therefore calcium concentration in the muscle increases with successive stimuli. Higher levels of calcium may lead to greater interaction between actin and myosin, and hence greater force of contraction.

Regulation of Force of Contraction in the Body

In the intact body also, the force of muscular contraction is regulated by two mechanisms similar to those outlined above. *First*, the force may be increased by increasing the number of muscle fibers activated. This is done by increasing the number of motor units activated.[4] *Second*, the force may be increased by increasing the frequency of activation of motor units. However, even at low frequencies of activation, contraction in the intact muscles is not jerky as seen experimentally (Figs 13.16A to C). The smoothness in the intact body is due to the fact that different motor units are activated at slightly different times, i.e. asynchronously. Asynchronous jerky contractions of a large number of motor units together produce a contraction which seems smooth (Figs 13.17A and B).

Isometric and Isotonic Contraction

Isometric contraction means contraction in which there is no change in length of the muscle but there is increase in tension. As an example, isometric contraction takes place in muscles of the upper limb when we try to push a wall.

Isotonic contraction means contraction in which there is a change of length but tension remains constant. The tension is equal to the weight lifted by the muscle during contraction. Isotonic contraction is very common in everyday life, and takes place whenever we lift a weight.

Length–tension Relationship in Isometric Contraction

The tension developed during isometric contraction depends on the initial length of the muscle.

1. If a muscle is removed from the body, it becomes slightly shorter. This shorter length is called its resting length. It means that a muscle is fixed to its bony attachments in a slightly stretched state.
2. If a muscle is stretched beyond its resting length, it develops some tension, which is called resting tension. As the muscle is stretched more and more, the resting tension increases.
3. If the muscle is stimulated under isometric conditions, it develops contractile tension, also

[4]A motor unit consists of a motor neuron and all the muscle fibers which it innervates.

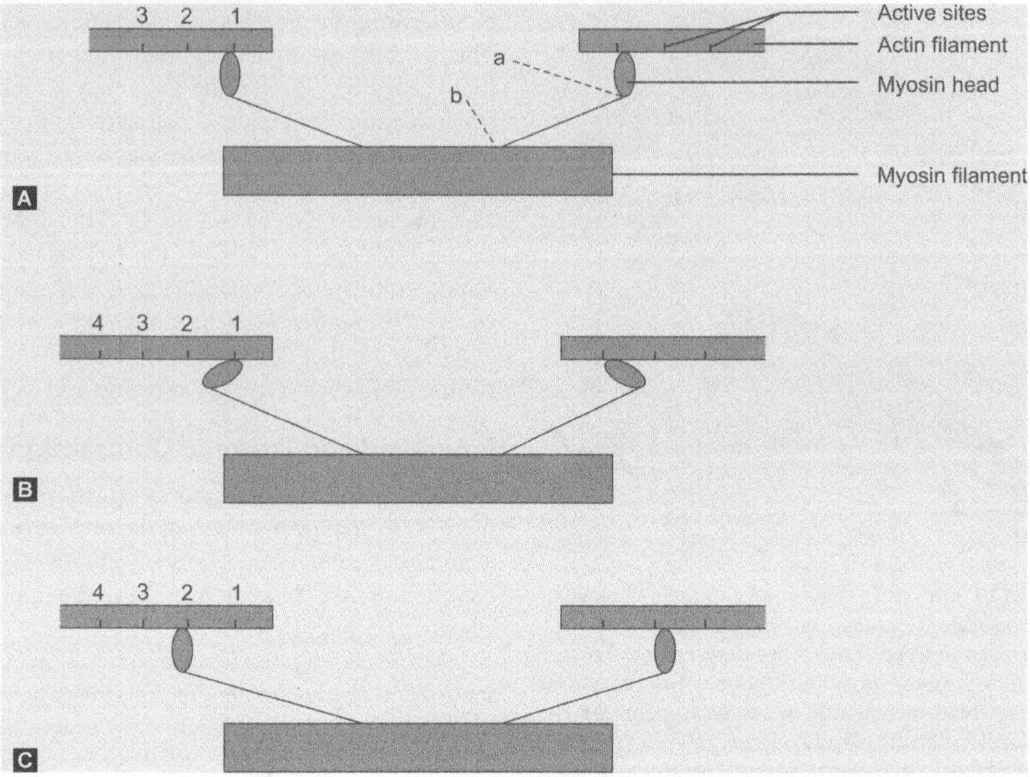

Figs 13.13A to C The ratchet mechanism of contraction. (A) Relaxed state; (B) The actin filaments slide closer to each other as a result of actin-myosin interaction. During the interaction, the myosin molecule bends at the hinges, a and b; (C) The myosin molecule is restored to its original shape but now it is attached to active site '2' on the actin filament (instead of '1'). By a repetition of the process the actin filaments can move still closer to each other

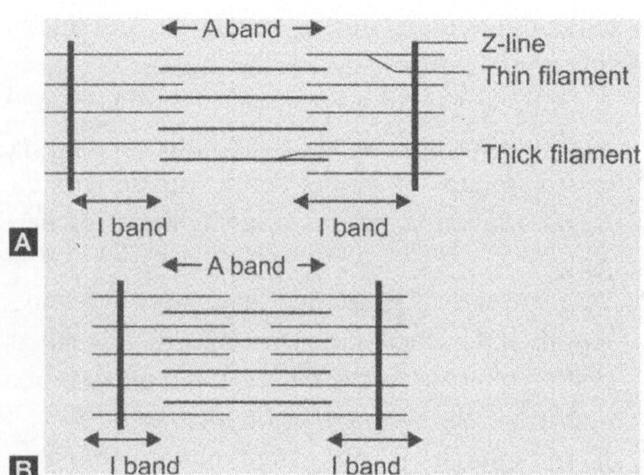

Figs 13.14A and B Diagrammatic representation of a sarcomere to illustrate the sliding filament mechanism of contraction. (A) Relaxed state; (B) Contracted state

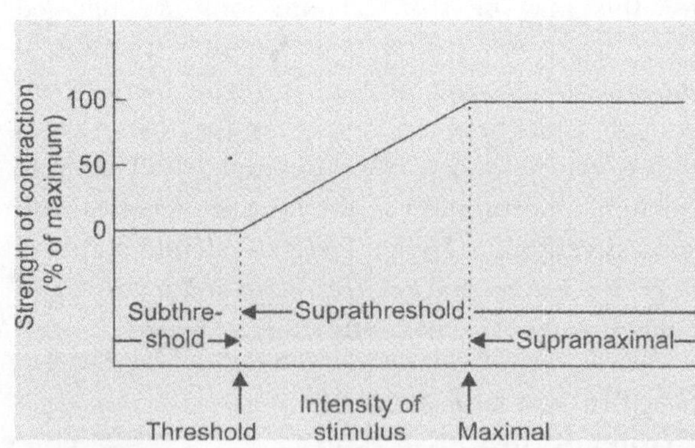

Fig. 13.15 Stimulus-response relationship in skeletal muscle. For stimulus intensities between the threshold and maximal, the strength of contraction shows a continuous gradation due to progressive recruitment of additional muscle fibers

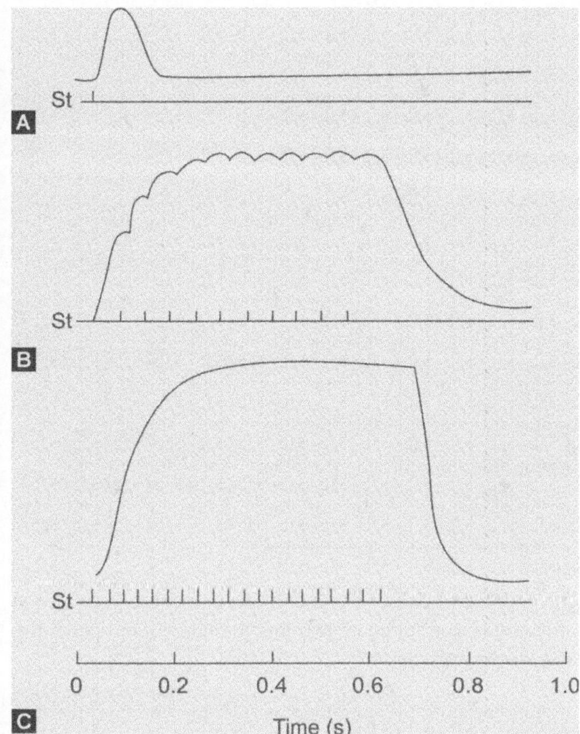

Figs 13.16A to C Response of a skeletal muscle to single and repetitive stimuli. (A) Response to a single stimulus: the simple muscle twitch; (B) Response to repetitive stimuli at low frequency: incomplete tetanus; (C) Response to repetitive stimuli at high frequency: complete tetanus. St, stimulus signals

called active tension. The recorded tension (total tension) is equal to the sum of the resting tension and active tension.

4. Active tension depends on the initial length of the muscle. It is observed that maximum active tension develops at a length slightly longer than the resting length (Fig. 13.18). Since the initial length in the body is also slightly longer than the resting length, it means that the muscle is fixed in the body at a length which is just right for maximum contractile force.

ELECTROMYOGRAPHY

Electromyography (EMG) is a technique for recording gross electrical activity in a muscle (Fig. 13.19). It may be recorded by electrodes placed on the surface of the body or by fine needle electrodes inserted into the muscle.

EMG activity consists fundamentally of motor unit potentials.

Motor Unit

A motor unit consists of a motor neuron together with all the muscle fibers which it innervates (Fig. 13.20). The muscle fibers belonging to a motor unit are scattered throughout the muscle. The number of muscle fibers in a motor unit is highly variable. Muscles with finely regulated contractions (e.g. finger muscles) have a smaller number of muscle fibers in each motor unit than muscles which show gross movements (e.g. leg muscles).

SMOOTH MUSCLE

Hollow internal organs such as the stomach, urinary bladder or blood vessels undergo alteration in shape and size. The alteration is brought about by contraction of smooth muscle. Smooth muscle activity is not under the control of will power.

Structure of Smooth Muscle

Smooth muscle lacks the striations seen in skeletal muscle. That is why it is called smooth (Figs 13.21A and B). The basic structural unit of smooth muscle is called a muscle fiber. Smooth muscle fibers are spindle shaped. Adjacent muscle fibers are connected to each other by gap junctions which allow ionic movement between cells. Smooth muscle fibers contain actin and myosin filaments but their arrangement is not as well organized as in skeletal muscle (Fig. 13.22). The sarcoplasmic reticulum of smooth muscles is also rudimentary as compared to that of skeletal muscle.

Smooth muscle is supplied by sympathetic and parasympathetic nerve fibers. Besides these nerves, smooth muscle activity may also be regulated by an intrinsic nerve plexus, hormones and several other physical or chemical factors.

Classification

Smooth muscle may be of the single unit or multi-unit type.

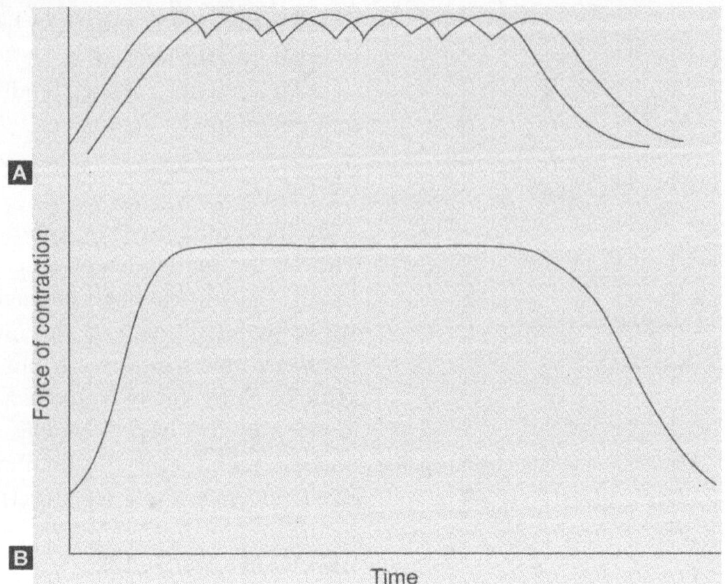

Figs 13.17A and B Diagrammatic representation of how asynchronous contraction of several motor units in incomplete tetanus results in a smooth contraction of the muscle. (A) Asynchronous contraction of two motor units; (B) Fusion of the asynchronous contractions to produce a smooth contraction of the whole muscle

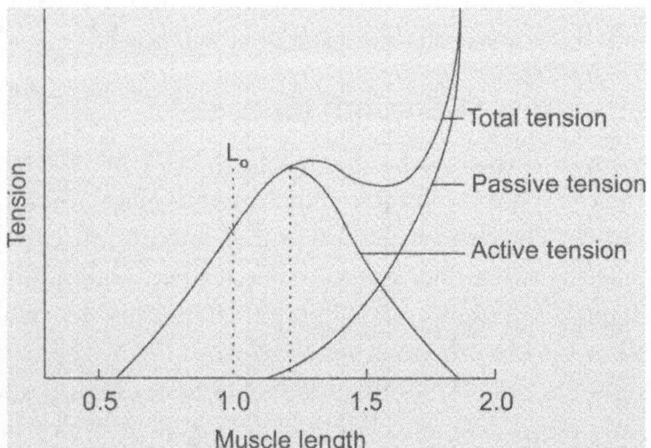

Fig. 13.18 Length-tension relationship. Relationship between muscle length and contracite tension developed during isometric contraction. Muscle length has been indicated in terms of Lo, the resting length. Maximum active tension develops at a length about 1.2 times the resting length, i.e. when the muscle is slightly stretched

Single unit type of smooth muscle behaves as if the entire muscle mass is a single functional unit. The gap junctions between fibers ensure rapid spread of activity throughout the muscle. Such an arrangement is also called a functional syncytium. Although single-unit smooth muscle has a nerve supply, the nerve supply only serves to increase or decrease the activity. Even after denervation the muscle retains its activity, which can still be increased or decreased by hormones. Smooth muscle of the gut, ureters and uterus is of the single-unit type.

Multi-unit type of smooth muscle has independent nerve supply for each muscle fiber. Activation of one muscle fiber does not by itself lead to activation of neighboring muscle fibers. Examples of multi-unit type of smooth muscle are found in ciliary muscles of the eye and in vas deferens.

Electrophysiology

The electrophysiology of smooth muscle is more complex than that of skeletal muscle but the general principles remain the same.

Resting Membrane Potential

Smooth muscle membrane is quite permeable to ions even while at rest. Hence the resting membrane

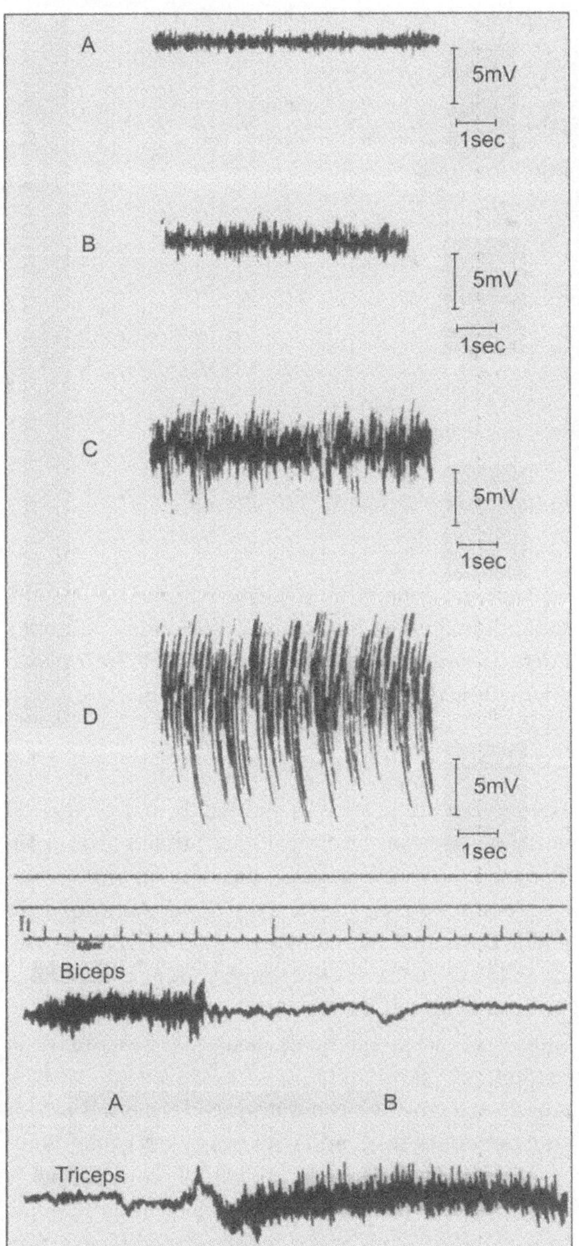

Fig. 13.19 Electromyography (EMG). Above EMG of the biceps muscle recorded during progressively stronger contractions from A-D. Below EMG of biceps and triceps muscles recorded during flexion A and extension B of the arm. (*Courtesy:* Department of Physiology, All India Institute of Medical Sciences, New Delhi)

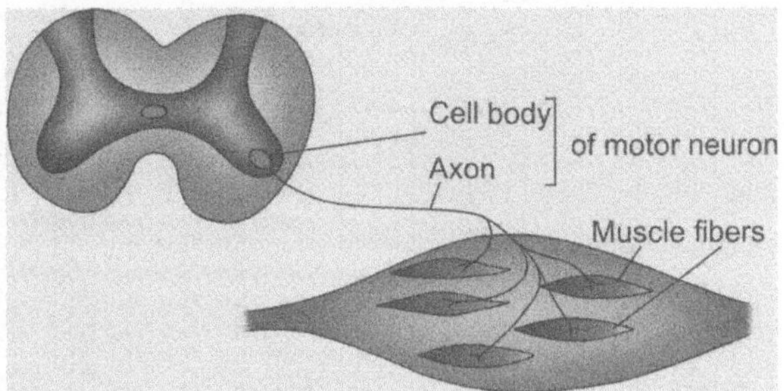

Fig. 13.20 A motor unit consists of a motor neuron together with the muscle fibers which it innervates. The motor unit illustrated here has only five muscle fibers

potential (RMP) of smooth muscle is only about –60 mV. Further, it is unstable, i.e. it may change 'spontaneously'. The change may be quite rhythmic, and may periodically cross the threshold of excitation, leading to 'spontaneous' contractions. Alternatively, there may be rhythmic variations in muscle tone synchronous with variations in RMP (Figs 13.23A to D).

Action Potential

Action potentials of smooth muscle may resemble the 'spikes' observed in skeletal muscle, or the prolonged action potential seen in cardiac muscle. A burst of action potentials may occur rhythmically in association with a cyclic change in RMP.

Modes of Stimulation of Smooth Muscle

Depending on the site, smooth muscle may be stimulated by one or more of the following factors:

a. Sympathetic or parasympathetic nerves
b. Stretch
c. Changes in PO_2 or PCO_2
d. Chemicals, such as histamine, serotonin, prostaglandins or adenosine.

Excitation–Contraction Coupling

As in skeletal muscle, excitation–contraction coupling is mediated by calcium ions. Following excitation, there is an increase in the sarcoplasmic concentration of calcium ions. Calcium ion concentration increases as a result of:

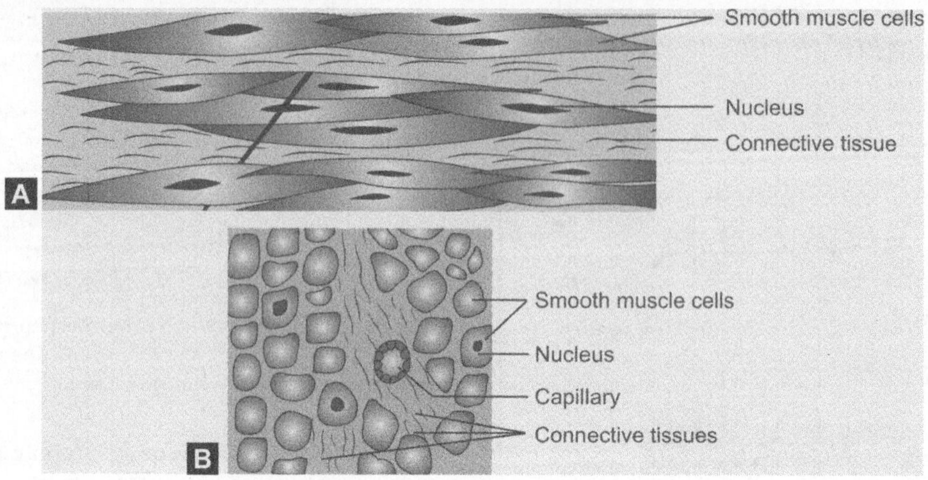

Figs 13.21A and B Histology of smooth muscle. (A) Longitudinal section; (B) Transverse section

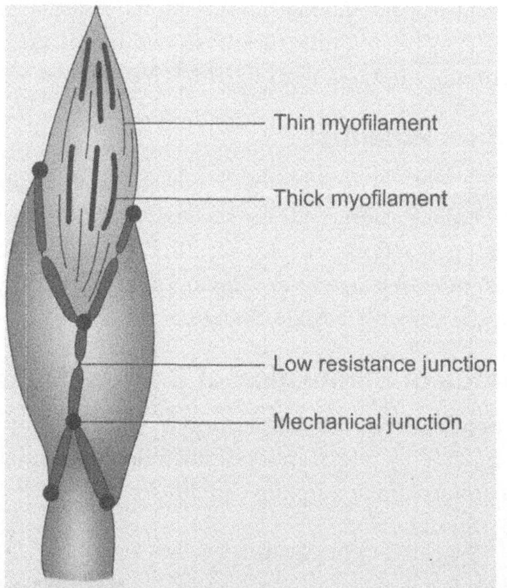

Fig. 13.22 Diagrammatic representation of the organization of cytoskeleton and myofilaments in smooth muscle. Note the similarity between the organization of thick and thin filaments here and in skeletal muscle. Adjacent cells are coupled mechanically as well as electrically

a. Release of calcium ions from the sarcoplasmic reticulum, and
b. Entry of calcium ions from the extracellular fluid.

Calcium ions bind to a smooth muscle protein, calmodulin. The calcium-calmodulin complex interacts with myosin, and initiates an actin-myosin interaction similar to that in skeletal muscle.

Contractile Process

The contractile process is similar to that of skeletal muscle. Myosin cross-bridges attach to actin filaments. Myosin heads, besides having cross-bridge function, also serve as ATPase. Actin-myosin interaction activates ATPase. Hydrolysis of ATP by ATPase releases the energy for cross-bridge movement which leads to sliding of actin filaments. Sliding of actin filaments leads to generation of tension, or shortening. As compared to skeletal muscle, the tension in smooth muscle is sustained for long periods of time, and with much less expenditure of energy. However, the speed of contraction is much slower than in case of skeletal muscle. Slow and sustained contraction is the type of contraction required in hollow viscera, and the function of smooth muscle is admirably suited to the requirements.

PHYSIOLOGY OF NERVE FIBERS

All peripheral nerves are bundles of nerve fibers. Nerve fibers are parts of nerve cells. Mammalian

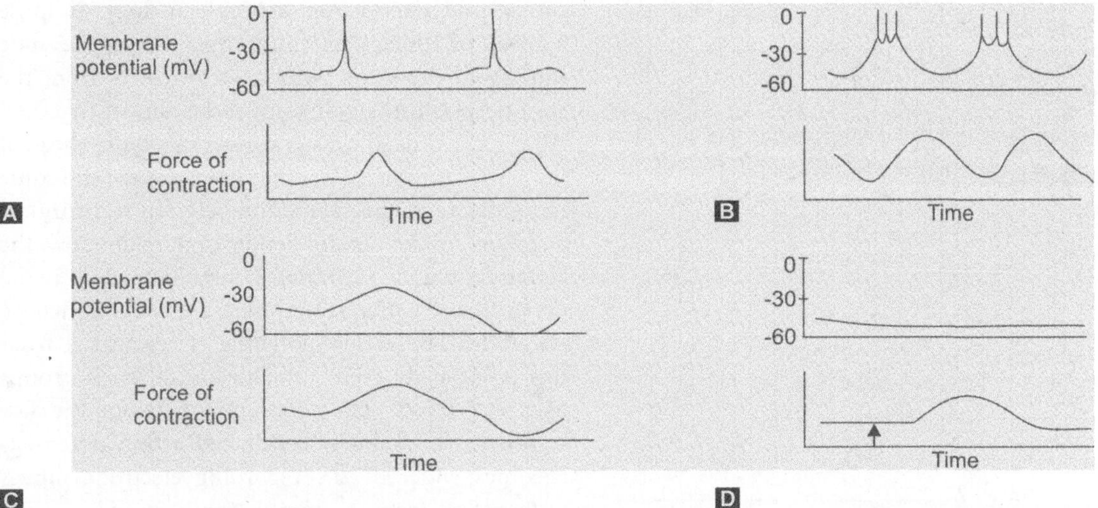

Figs 13.23A to D Diversity of relationship between membrane potential and force of contraction in smooth muscle. (A) Each action potential is followed by a mechanical response. The relationship is similar to that seen in skeletal muscle; (B) The membrane potential shows rhythmic changes. During the depolarization phase, there is a burst of action potentials. Each burst of action potentials is followed by a mechanical response; (C) The membrane potential shows slow fluctuations, which are associated with synchronous fluctuations in tone; (D) Addition of a neurohumor at the point indicated by the arrow leads to a mechanical response without any associated change in membrane potential

nerve fibers vary from less than one micron to about 20 microns in diameter.

Conduction of the Nerve Impulse

Impulse is a word commonly used for the action potential. Action potential at one point in a nerve fiber induces an action potential at the next point. Thus the action potential is conducted (or propagated) from point to point along a nerve fiber. In case of myelinated nerve fibers, the conduction of impulse is from one node of Ranvier to the next (Fig. 13.24). This happens because myelin is an insulator. An action potential can be induced much more easily in the unmyelinated gap, i.e. the node. Conduction in a myelinated nerve fiber is called **saltatory conduction** (*saltare*, to dance) because the impulse seems to jump from node to node. Saltatory conduction increases the velocity of conduction. Therefore myelinated fibers have a higher velocity of

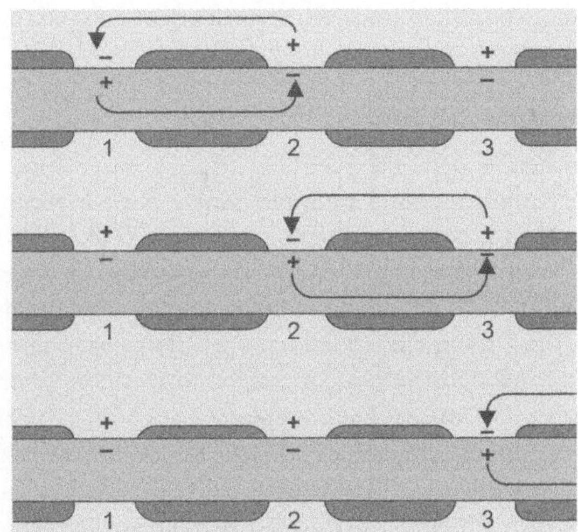

Fig. 13.24 Saltatory conduction. In a myelinated nerve fiber the action potential 'jumps' from node to node (e.g. from 1 to 2, and from 2 to 3, in this diagram)

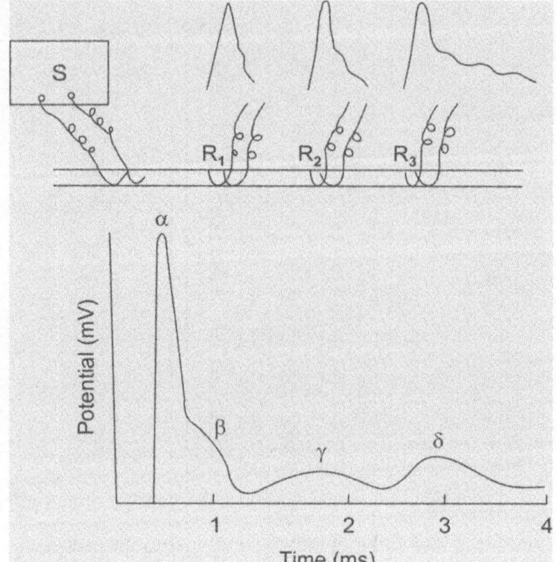

Fig. 13.25 Compound action potential. If a mixed nerve is stimulated, the potentials recorded at points R_1, R_2 and R_3 are different due to progressively wider separation of components travelling at different speeds. An idealized diagram showing several of the components of a compound action potential is also shown. S, stimulator

conduction than unmyelinated fibers of comparable diameter.

Compound Action Potential

An action potential recorded from a nerve (not a nerve fiber)[5] shows multiple peaks. Such a record is called a compound action potential (Fig. 13.25). As seen in the figure, the peaks separate out more and more as the distance between the stimulating and recording electrode increases. This observation indicates that the peaks correspond to nerve fibers with different conduction velocities. The first peak corresponds to the fibers with the fastest conduction velocity.

How different conduction velocities give rise to multiple peaks, and why the peaks separate out more at longer distances from the stimulating electrode can be understood from a simple analogy. Suppose a group of athletes start running a race at the same time from the same point. A few meters from the starting point, they all seem to be almost together. After some time, the faster runners are quite ahead of the slower runners. After they have covered still some more distance, the separation between fast runners and slow runners is still better. In the same way, the action potential is initiated simultaneously in all nerve fibers at the same point, i.e. the stimulating electrode. The action potential is conducted from this point at different velocities in different groups of nerve fibers. The separation between the fast conducted and slowly conducted action potentials becomes wider as the recording electrode moves farther away from the stimulating electrode.

Nerve fibers which differ in conduction velocity also differ in some other respects. This forms the basis of their classification.

Classification of Nerve Fibers

There are two commonly used classifications of nerve fibers: one originally proposed by Erlanger and Gasser, and the other by Lloyd and Hunt. The former covers all nerve fibers and divides them into groups A, B and C. The latter classifies only sensory fibers and divides them into groups I, II, III and IV. We shall consider primarily Erlanger and Gasser's classification and mention the roughly equivalent group in Lloyd and Hunt's classification. Group A fibers are further classified into subgroups A alpha, A beta, A gamma and A delta.

A Alpha

This group of nerve fibers are myelinated, 13-20 microns in diameter, with a conduction velocity of 70-120 m/s. It is helpful to keep in mind that for myelinated nerve fibers, the conduction velocity in m/s is approximately 6 times the diameter in microns. A alpha fibers include sensory fibers which convey proprioceptive inpulses and also somatic motor nerve fibers which supply skeletal muscles. In Lloyd's classification A alpha fibers of the sensory type are designated group I fibers.

[5]A nerve is made up of thousands of nerve fibers. A nerve fiber corresponds to one excitable cell.

A Beta

This group of nerve fibers are also myelinated but smaller in diameter (4-13 microns). If you know the diameter, you can calculate the conduction velocity. A beta fibers are sensory nerve fibers conveying touch, pressure and kinesthetic sense. In Lloyd's classification, A beta fibers correspond to group II.

A Gamma

This group of nerve fibers are also myelinated and their diameter is 3-6 microns. They are motor fibers supplying intrafusal (within the muscle spindle; Chapter 15) muscle fibers. Since A gamma fibers are motor fibers, they are ignored by Lloyd's classification.

A Delta

This group of nerve fibers are also myelinated but still thinner, being 1-5 microns in diameter. They convey the sensations of sharp pricking pain, temperature and fine pressure. In Lloyd's classification, A delta fibers are designated group III fibers.

You might have observed that all group A fibers are myelinated. Further, conduction through all these fibers can be most easily blocked by pressure. That is why when your finger gets hurt, you instinctively press it hard. That relieves the sharp pricking pain which is conveyed by A delta fibers.

Group B

Group B fibers are also myelinated but still thinner, being 1-3 microns in diameter. These fibers constitute the preganglionic autonomic fibers of both the sympathetic and parasympathetic divisions. Conduction through group B fibers can be most easily blocked by hypoxia. Since group B fibers are motor fibers, they are not considered in Lloyd's classification.

Group C

Group C fibers are the only ones that are unmyelinated. Their diameter is also the smallest, 0.2-1.0 micron. Lack of myelination and small diameter account for their low conduction velocity of only 0.2-2 m/s. But still the velocity is quite sufficient for most purposes. That is why C fibers are the most numerous in peripheral nerves. The advantage in getting most of the jobs done by C fibers is that the diameter of the nerves can stay within reasonable limits. If all nerve fibers were of type A, peripheral nerves would look like thick ropes. Group C fibers convey the sensations of burning and dull aching pain, temperature and crude pressure. All postganglionic autonomic fibers also belong to group C. The sensory fibers of group C are designated group IV in Lloyd's classification.

Conduction through group C fibers can be most easily blocked by local anesthetics. That is why after local anesthesia the more agonizing burning pain is blocked but the sharp pricking pain and touch conveyed by group A fibers may not be completely blocked. Hence the patient may complain that he can feel the knife, there is some sharp pain also along the incision, but the pain is not very agonizing.

The salient features of different groups of nerve fibers have been summarised in Table 13.1

Response of Nerve Fibers to Injury

If a nerve fiber is cut, both ends of the fiber undergo degeneration. The degeneration of the distal end is called Wallerian degeneration. But a few days after degeneration, regeneration beings. The proximal stump grows about 50 sprouts. One of these is generally able to find its way into the hollow endoneurial tube which is still available in the distal stump. The sprout grows 1-3 mm per day, and finally reaches the target organ to reinnervate it. Reinnervation is not perfect, but is better than total loss. Reinnervation is possible only if (a) the endoneurial sheath survives, and (b) the gap between the proximal and distal cut ends is less than 3 mm. Suturing can help in reducing the gap. If the gap is large, or if the distal end is not viable, the sprouts from the proximal end form a confused mass of fibers called a neuroma. In case of sensory fibers a neuroma can be very painful and is a dreaded complication of amputations.

Table 13.1 Classification of mammalian nerve fibers

Group						
Erlanger and Gasser	*Lloyd and Hunt**	*Myelination***	*Diameter (microns)*	*Conduction velocity (m/s)*	*Function*	*Agent to which conduction is most susceptible*
A alpha	I	M	13-20	70-120	Proprioception Motor supply to skeletal muscles	Pressure
A beta	II	M	4-13	25-70	Touch, kinesthetic sense, pressure	Pressure
A gamma	–	M	3-6	15-30	Motor supply to intrafusal muscle fibers	Pressure
A delta	III	M	1-5	5-30	Pain, temperature, pressure, touch	Pressure
B	–	M	1-3	3-14	Preganlionic autonomic fibers	Hypoxia
C	IV	UM	0.2-1.0	0.2-2	Pain, temperature, pressure Postganglionic autonomic fibers	Local anesthetics

* Considers only sensory fibers
** M, myelinated; UM, unmyelinated

QUESTIONS

1. Give an example of isometric contraction.
2. Discuss the type of muscle contraction involved in lifting up a suitcase.
3. Explain briefly why strong muscles of the back and abdomen help in preventing backache.

ANSWERS

1. Trying to push a wall is an example of isometric contraction.
2. To start with, the handle is held, muscles get stretched but their length remains constant. Therefore, the contraction is isometric. The muscles contract, but the suitcase does not move. Thus the length of muscles does not change, but the contraction of muscles leads to an increase in tension. The muscles continue to contract isometrically more and more strongly, and the tension keeps increasing. As soon as the tension exceeds the weight of the suitcase, the suitcase moves up. From now on, the tension is equal to the weight of the suitcase. The tension remains constant at this level, but the muscles continue to contract. Therefore, now the contraction is isotonic. The isotonic contraction leads to flexion of the forearm, which in turn lifts up the suitcase. In short, the contraction is isometric till the suitcase moves. After that, the contraction is isotonic.
   It is also clear from the above discussion that trying to lift up a suitcase which is too heavy to move will lead to only isometric contraction.
3. Because contraction of these muscles makes the chest and abdomen behave like a rigid cylinder which shares the weight on the spine. Thus the weight imposed remaining the same, the pressure per unit area on the intervertebral discs is much less if the back and abdominal muscles are strong.

CHAPTER

14 Nervous System: General Concepts

"Then mark the cloven sphere that holds, All thought in its mysterious folds, That feels sensation's faintest thrill And flashes forth the sovereign will; Think on the stormy world that dwells, Locked in its dim and clustering cells! The lightning gleams of power it shreds Along its slender glassy threads!"

—OLIVER WENDELL HOLMES

Chapter Outline

- Coordination Needs Communication
- Reflex Arc and Reflexes
- Cerebrospinal Fluid
- Synaptic Transmission

The study of nervous system is of great interest to us because it promises to provide us answers to questions such as 'what is intelligence', 'how do we learn' and 'how do we remember.' Before we come to these fascinating questions, however, we should understand the basic function of the nervous system. The nervous system co-ordinates the activity of all other systems of the body.[1] For example, when we take exercise, the skeletal muscles need more nutrients. These are supplied by enhanced blood flow. Increase in blood flow needs vasodilatation and also increase in heart rate and stroke volume. In order to keep pace with increased oxygen consumption and carbon dioxide production of exercising muscles, the rate and depth of respiration have to increase. All these changes in cardiovascular and respiratory system take place at the right time due to the coordinating activity of the nervous system.

[1]The same function is also performed by the endocrine system. Nervous system and endocrine system work hand-in hand.

COORDINATION NEEDS COMMUNICATION

Communication is essential for coordination. For example, in case of exercise, the nervous system should know that the muscles are exercising. That needs communication from muscles to the nervous system. Then the heart should know that it should beat faster during exercise. That needs communication from nervous system to the heart (Fig. 14.1). The structural units of nervous system are ideal for communication. These units are called neurons (Fig. 14.2). A nerve cell, or neuron, has long thread-like processes or extensions for carrying messages. The messages are carried by these extensions in the form of nerve impulses. Extensions which carry messages to the cell body of the neuron are called **dendrites**. Extensions which carry messages from the cell body of the neuron are called **axons**. Neurons communicate not only with structures such as muscles or heart, but also with each other. The elaborate coordination seen in the body is made possible by complex networks in which several neurons talk to each other (Figs 14.3A to C). However, the basic model on which these networks are designed is illustrated by a reflex arc.

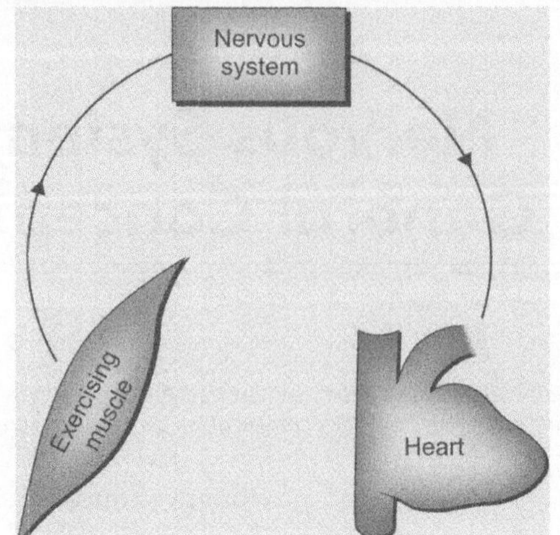

Fig. 14.1 Coordination needs communication. When the exercising muscles send a message to the nervous system, the nervous system tells the heart to beat faster

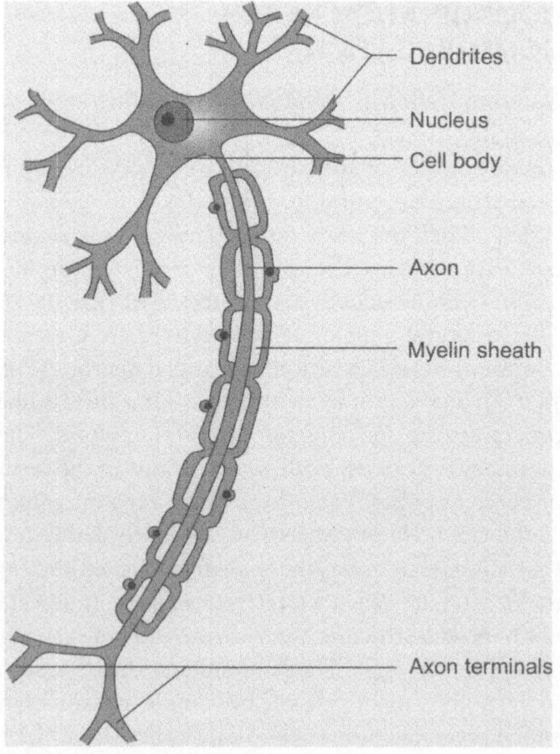

Fig. 14.2 A typical neuron

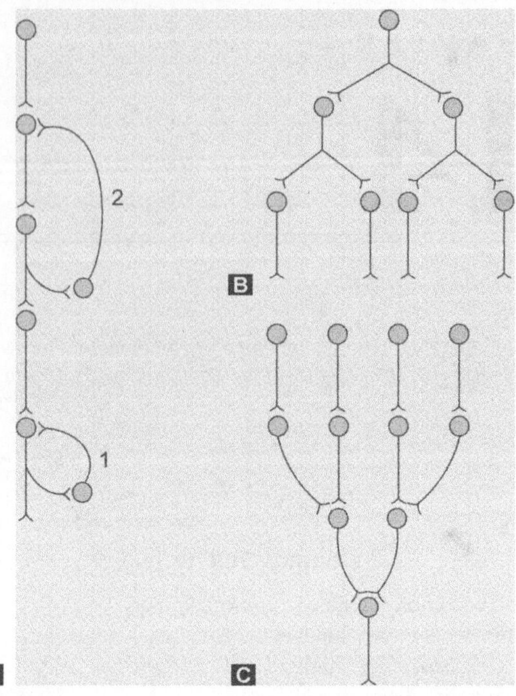

Figs 14.3A to C Three simple neuronal networks. (A) Neurons 1 and 2 are providing feedback signals to the chain of neurons; (B) A divergent network of neurons; (C) A convergent network of neurons

REFLEX ARC AND REFLEXES

A reflex arc (Figs 14.4A and B) consists of a sensory neuron, generally one or more neurons in the spinal cord or brain,[2] and a motor neuron. The reflex arc neurons in the central nervous system (CNS) are called interneurons.

The sensory neuron receives information from a receptor and conveys it to the CNS (Fig. 14.5). Interneurons in the CNS process the information. As a result of the processing, a 'decision' is arrived at. The decision is conveyed to the motor neuron. The motor neuron delivers the message to the effector organ, which is either a muscle or a gland.

[2]Spinal cord and brain are together called the central nervous system.

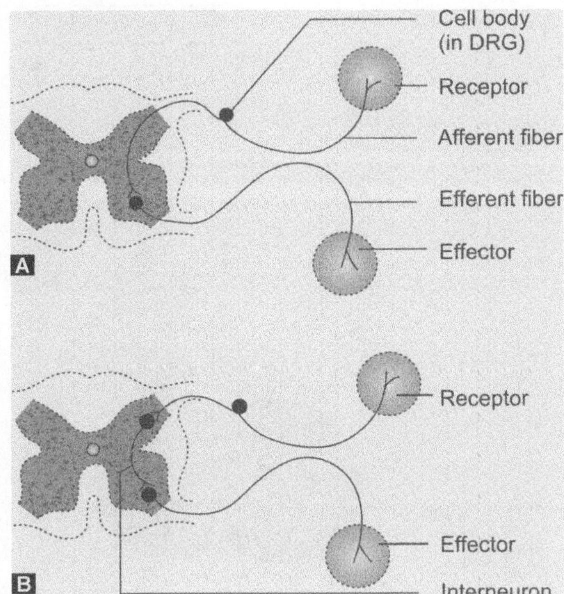

Figs 14.4A and B A reflex arc. (A) The simplest reflex arc involving only one synapse (monosynaptic); (B) A reflex arc which includes an interneuron, and therefore involves an additional synapse. DRG, dorsal root ganglion

An example may make the process clearer. Suppose the finger touches a sharp pin accidentally (Fig. 14.6). The pin prick activates a sensory neuron. Information about the pin prick is conveyed to the spinal cord. Processing of the information by interneurons leads to the 'decision' that the hand should be moved away (i.e. withdrawn) from the pin. This is conveyed to motor neurons supplying the biceps muscle. As a result, the biceps contracts, leading to withdrawal of the hand. The entire process takes place so quickly that the hand is withdrawn almost as soon as it touches the pin. The hand is withdrawn even before the person becomes aware of the pin prick. Awareness of the pin prick needs the message to be conveyed to the 'highest' part of the brain, the cerebral cortex (Fig. 14.7). Since the reflex withdrawal of the hand takes place before the conscious awareness of the pin prick, we can say that it takes place without needing our will power. We do not consciously decide to withdraw the hand. The 'decision' by the interneurons in the spinal cord does not need will power. We do not have to think and say in our mind 'I will withdraw the hand'. Such an action, which does not need will power, is called involuntary.

The above example illustrates many features of a reflex, which have been summarized below.

A reflex:

a. Is an involuntary action,
b. Is mediated by a reflex arc, and
c. Needs processing in the CNS below the level of the cerebral cortex.

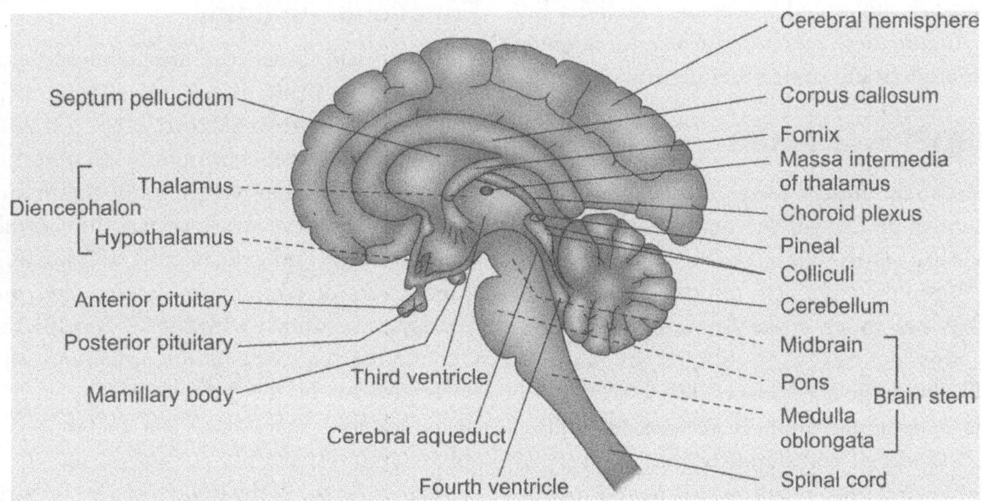

Fig. 14.5 A simplified view of sagittal section of the human brain, showing the major anatomical features

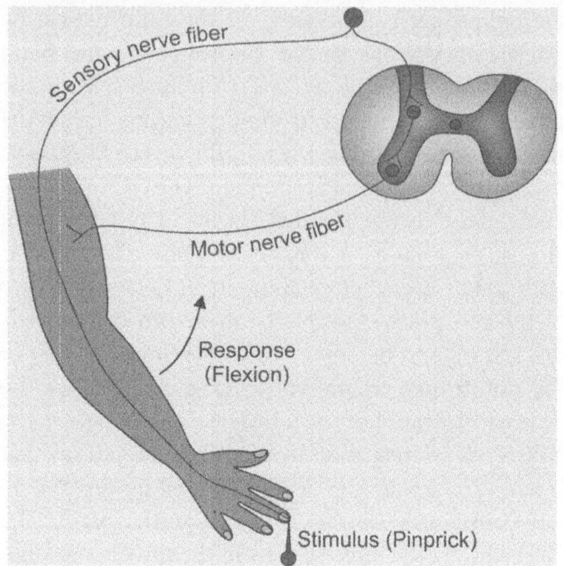

Fig. 14.6 Diagrammatic representation of the neuronal pathway of reflex response to a pinprick. The information about the pinprick is conveyed to the spinal cord by the sensory nerve fiber. That leads to activation of the motor neurons supplying the biceps muscle. Contraction of the biceps muscle leads to flexion of the forearm

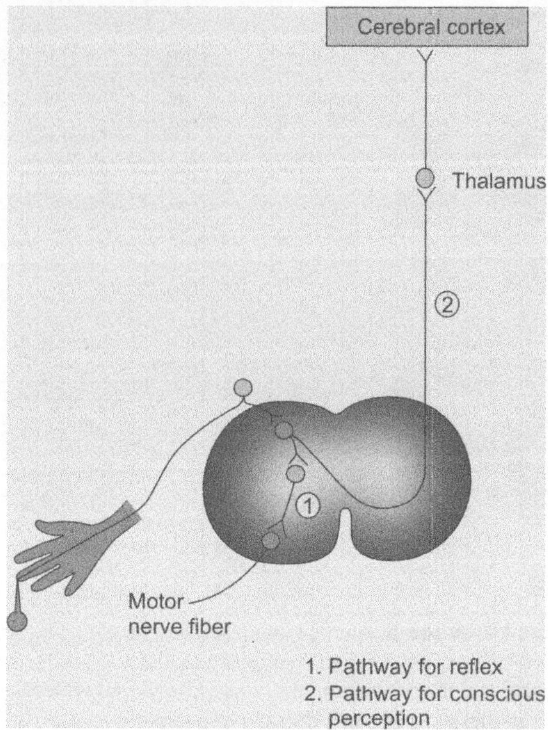

Fig. 14.7 Reflex withdrawal of the hand in response to a pinprick involves only a relatively short pathway (1) at the level of the spinal cord. On the other hand, awareness, or conscious perception of the painful stimulus depends on a longer path (2) and needs the message to reach the cerebral cortex

Since the reflex arc provides the basic model for the functional organization of the nervous system, the physiology of the nervous system may be studied in terms of sensory, motor and processing functions. But before we discuss these functional divisions, it would be useful to understand some other general concepts.

CEREBROSPINAL FLUID

The interstitial fluid forms the immediate environment of all cells of the body. Its constancy, i.e. homeostasis, is the basic goal of all systems of the body. But in the CNS, cells are so closely packed that there is not much space for interstitial fluid. However, this deficiency is fulfilled by another extracellular fluid, the cerebrospinal fluid (CSF).

CSF is a dynamic fluid. It is formed continuously and absorbed continuously into the venous system. Some structural relationships would help in understanding the circulation of CSF.

Functional Anatomy

The brain and spinal cord are hollow structures. The hollow spaces in the brain are called ventricles. The hollow space in the spinal cord is the central canal. The ventricular system is continuous with the central canal (Fig. 14.8). The four ventricles of the brain contain bunches of blood vessels known as the choroid plexus.

The brain and spinal cord are surrounded by three layers of connective tissue called **meninges**. The layer in contact with the CNS is the pia mater. Outside the pia mater is the arachnoid mater. The outermost layer is the dura mater. The space between the arachnoid mater and pia mater is called the subarachnoid space.

CSF is found in the hollow spaces (ventricles and central canal) as well as in the subarachroid space.

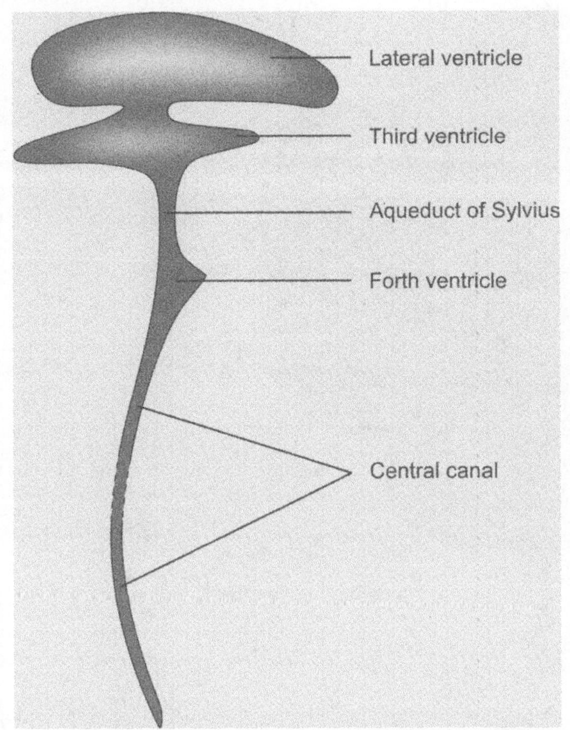

Fig. 14.8 Hollow spaces of the brain and spinal cord

The ventricular system communicates with the subarachroid space through openings in the fourth ventricle. The subarachroid space also communicates with the venous system.

Formation of CSF

CSF is formed by a combination of filtration, secretion and reabsorption. These three terms might remind you of the kidney. In fact, the process is similar. Just as renal glomeruli filter the plasma, the blood vessels of the choroid plexus also filter the plasma. In both cases, the composition of the filtrate is modified by secretion and reabsorption.

Circulation of CSF

Choroid plexus delivers CSF to the ventricles. CSF moves down towards the fourth ventricle. There it leaves through the openings in the fourth ventricle to enter the subarachnoid space. In the subarachroid space, CSF moves upwards towards the brain as well as downwards in the subarachnoid space around the spinal cord. The CSF in the spinal subarachnoid space again moves up towards the cerebral subarachnoid space (Fig. 14.9).

Absorption of CSF

CSF is absorbed from the subarachroid space around the brain into subdural venous sinuses. Thus the CSF finally returns to the blood.

Functions of CSF

The functions of CSF are:

Providing Optimum Environment to Neurons

As mentioned earlier, CSF serves as the interstitial fluid of the CNS. It provides a constant optimum environment to the neurons.

Homeostatic Role

An increase in hydrogen ion concentration in the CSF stimulates chemosensitive cells in the brain, thereby leading to increased respiratory activity. CSF also transmits changes in PCO_2 to cerebral blood vessels. An increase in PCO_2 leads to cerebral vasodilation, and a decrease leads to vasoconstriction.

Removal of Proteins

As in other tissues, a small amount of protein leaks out of cerebral capillaries. In other tissues, the protein is removed by the lymphatics. In the brain, the protein enters the CSF, which returns it to the blood. Brain has no lymphatics but the function of lymphatics is performed by the CSF.

Protection

CSF protects the brain from injury. It acts as a cushion around the brain.

Clinical Physiology of CSF

CSF examination is of great importance in several clinical conditions.

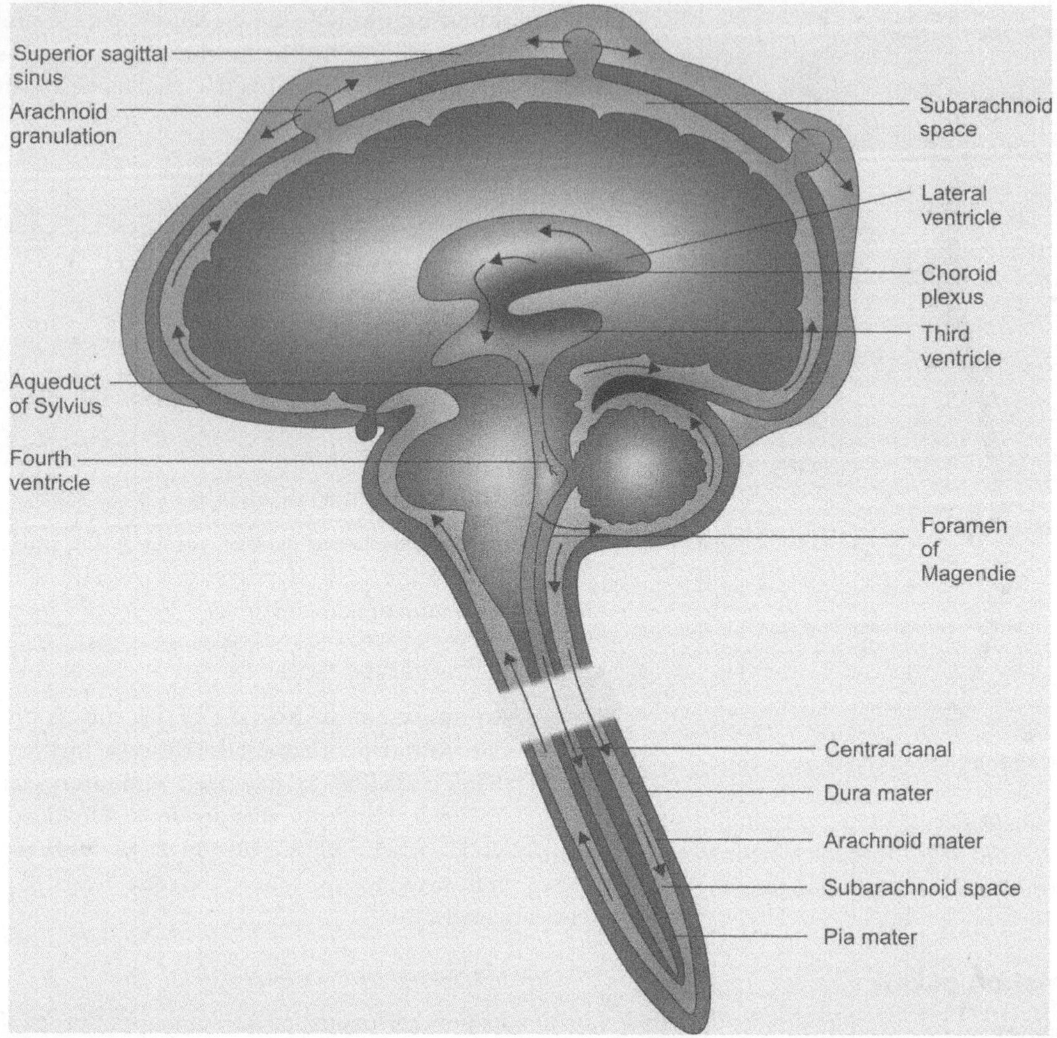

Fig. 14.9 Circulation of cerebrospinal fluid. The gap between the brain and the spinal cord represents the long segment of spinal cord which has been omitted to save space. CSF leaves the ventricular system to enter the subarachnoid space through the foramen of Magendie (shown) and foramina of Luschka (not shown). It is absorbed through the arachnoid granulations into the venous blood

Examination of CSF

A sample of the CSF may be obtained by lumbar puncture. During lumbar puncture, a needle is introduced between the third and the fourth, or between the fourth and the fifth lumbar vertebra. This level is safe because the spinal cord extends only up to the first lumbar vertebra. Examination of the CSF includes:

a. Measurement of CSF pressure (normal: 65-200 mm CSF or water, or 5-15 mmHg, in the lying down posture),
b. Visual examination for turbidity,
c. Microscopic examination for cells, and
d. Chemical examination for concentration of glucose and proteins.

Raised CSF Pressure

Rise in CSF pressure can be detected by examination of the fundus of the eye. When the CSF pressure is raised the fundus shows papilledema (swelling of veins around the optic disc).

Fundus examination should always be done before lumbar puncture because lumbar puncture is dangerous when the CSF pressure is high. When the CSF pressure is high, lumbar puncture may suck the brain stem downwards.

Brain stem has vital cardiorespiratory centers. Therefore downward movement of the brain stem may cause death. The phenomenon is also known as herniation of the medulla oblongata or coning. This serious accident can be prevented by doing a fundus examination before doing a lumbar puncture. If papilledema is present, lumbar puncture should not be done.

Blood Brain Barrier

Many substances present in the blood do not reach the brain because they are unable to enter the CSF. Thus there is a 'blood-brain barrier'. The barrier protects the brain from many harmful substances. The blood brain barrier is weak in infants. That is why, if an infant has jaundice, bilirubin may enter the brain. The parts of the brain most affected are the basal ganglia, brain stem and cerebellum, perhaps because these regions have a higher affinity for bilirubin. The condition is known as kernicterus.

SYNAPTIC TRANSMISSION

Synapse is a junction between two neuorns. Synaptic transmission is the process by which a message passes across the junction. The message is passed on only in one direction, i.e. from the axon of one neuron to the dendrites or cell body of the other. There is great similarity between synaptic transmission and neuromusclar transmission (Chapter 13).

Structure of a Synapse

Synapse is usually between the axon of one neuron and dendrites of the other (axo-dendritic) or between the axon of the neuron and cell body of the other (axo-somatic). The axon participating in a synapse belongs to the presynaptic neuron. Dendrites or cell body participating in the synpase belong to the postsynaptic neuron.

The presynaptic axon terminal has vesicles containing the neurotransmitter (Fig. 14.10). The postsynaptic membrane bears a prominent structure called the postsynaptic density. There is a 20-50 nm wide gap between the presynaptic and postsynaptic membrane. The gap is called synaptic cleft.

The Process of Synaptic Transmission

Synaptic transmission takes only about 1 msec. But it consists of several steps as outlined below (Fig. 14.11).

Arrival of the Message

The message arrives in the form of action potentials conducted along the presynaptic axon. When action potentials reach the presynaptic terminal, calcium channels there open up. As a result, calcium ions enter the presynaptic terminal.

Release of Neurotransmitter

Entry of calcium ions into the presynaptic terminals leads to release of the neurotransmitter from synaptic vesicles into the synaptic cleft. There is a large variety of neurotransmitters in the CNS.

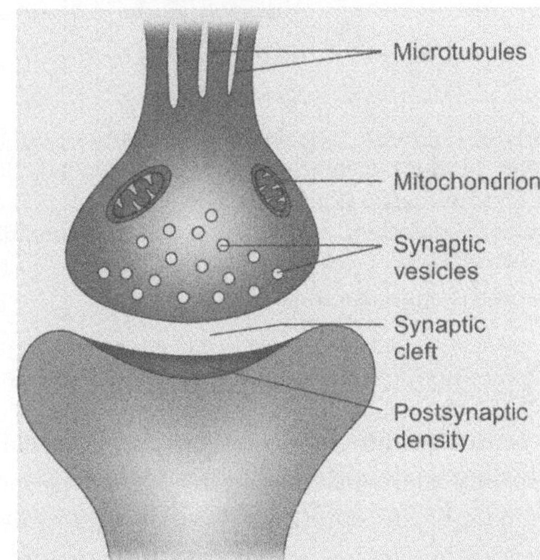

Fig. 14.10 Schematic diagram of the structure of a synapse

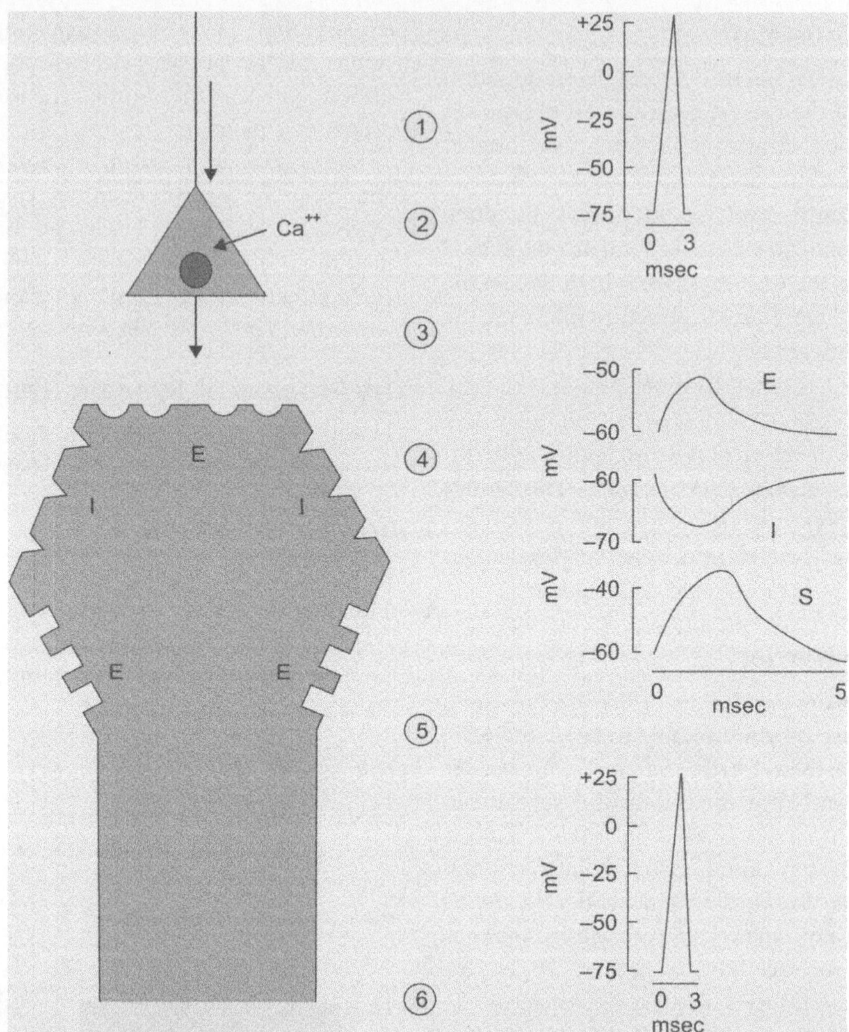

Fig. 14.11 The major steps in synaptic transmission. (1) Arrival of the message. The message is in the form of action potential, as shown diagrammatically on the right. (2) Influx of calcium ions. (3) Release of neurotransmitter. (4) Development of postsynaptic potential. Several excitatory (E) and inhibitory (I) neurotransmitters may act on the postsynaptic membrane simultaneously. (5) The postsynaptic potentials are integrated at the axon hillock. If the summated postsynaptic potential (S) crosses a threshold depolarization, the postsynaptic membrane is ready to fire. (6) Action potential in the axon of the postsynaptic neuron

Development of Postsynaptic Potentials

The neurotransmitter diffuses across the synaptic cleft to the postsynaptic membrane. The postsynaptic membrane has receptors for the neurotransmitter. Neurotransmitter molecules fit into the receptors as a key fits into a lock. Combination of neurotransmitter molecules with their receptors leads to opening up of certain ionic channels in the postsynaptic membrane. Opening up of these channels brings about a change in the postsynaptic resting membrane potential. The new potential is called the postsynaptic potential (PSP). The exact channels opened and the direction of the PSP depend on the neurotransmitter.

If the neurotransmitter is an excitatory one, it opens up sodium and potassium channels in the postsynaptic membrane (Fig. 14.12). Opening up of these channels leads to sodium influx (entry) and potassium efflux (exit). The net result of these ionic movements is hypopolarization. Since hypopolarization makes the postsynaptic neuron more excitable, it is called excitatory postsynaptic potential (EPSP).

If the neurotransmitter is an inhibitory one, it opens up chloride channels, or potassium channels, or both (Fig. 14.13). That leads to chloride influx or potassium efflux. The net result of these ionic movements is hyperpolarization. Since hyperpolarization makes the postsynaptic neuron less excitable, it is called inhibitory postsynaptic potential (IPSP).

EPSP as well as IPSP are graded, nonpropogated changes in membrane potential. That is, their magnitude is variable. The magnitude depends on the amount of neurotransmitter released at the synapse. Further, EPSP and IPSP are not conducted from point to point. You would recognize that EPSP and IPSP closely resemble the end plate potential in their characteristics.

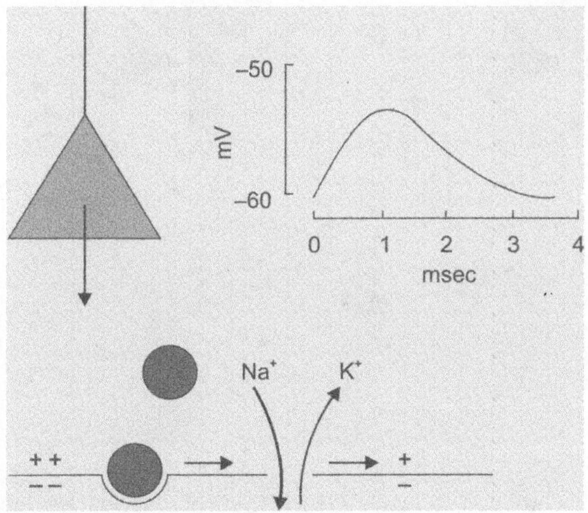

Fig. 14.12 Excitatory postsynaptic potential. The release of neurotransmitter in the synaptic cleft leads to an increase in permeability of the postsynaptic membrane to sodium and potassium. As a result, the postsynaptic neuron shows a depolarization known as excitatory postsynaptic potential (EPSP)

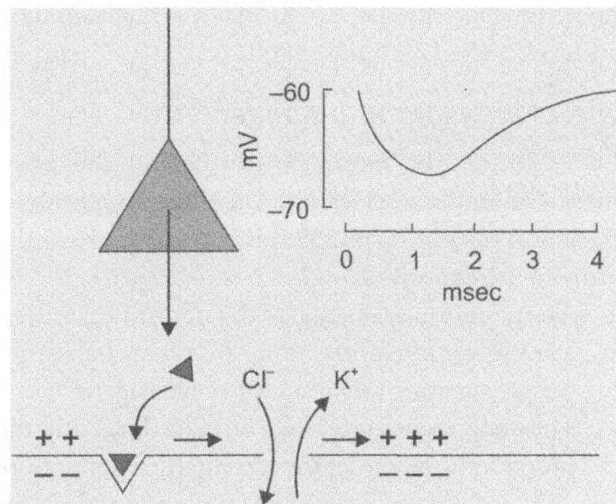

Fig. 14.13 Inhibitory postsynaptic potential. The release of neurotransmitter in the synaptic cleft leads to an increase in the permeability of the postsynaptic membrane to either chloride or potassium. As a result, the postsynaptic membrane shows a hyperpolarization known as inhibitory postsynaptic potential (IPSP)

Summation of Postsynaptic Potentials

Each postsynaptic neuron may receive messages from thousands of presynaptic neurons. Some of these presynaptic neurons may be excitatory and others inhibitory. Accordingly, some EPSPs and some IPSPs may be generated simultaneously. The EPSPs and IPSPs summate along with postsynaptic membrane. The summated potential at the axon hillock (the beginning of the axon) determines whether an action potential will be fired. If the summated potential is of the excitatory type (i.e. hypopolarization) and crosses the threshold for excitation, an action potential is fired (Figs 14.14A to C).

Generation and Conduction of Action Potential

An action potential is generated by depolarization which should be of at least threshold value. The site where this threshold is the lowest is the axon hillock. Therefore if the depolarization is greater than the threshold for generation of action potential at the axon hillock, an action potential is generated there.

The action potential is an all or none phenomenon and is conducted along the axon from point to point.

Fate of the Neurotransmitter

The action of the neurotransmitter on the postsynaptic membrane does not continue indefinitely. The action may be terminated by one or more of the following mechanisms:

a. An enzyme may inactivate the neurotransmitter,
b. The neurotransmitter may be taken back into the presynaptic terminal for recycling, or
c. The neurotransmitter may be taken back into the presynaptic terminal for enzymatic inactivation.

Central Neurotransmitters

The molecules employed as neurotransmitters in the CNS are either small molecules or large molecule peptides.

The small molecule neurotransmitters are acetylcholine, norepinephrine, dopamine, serotonin, gamma-amino butyric acid (GABA) and glycine.

More than 30 large molecule peptides are thought to affect synaptic function. All of them may not be classical neurotransmitters. Many of them perhaps only increase or decrease the sensitivity of a synapse for long periods of time (several minutes to days).

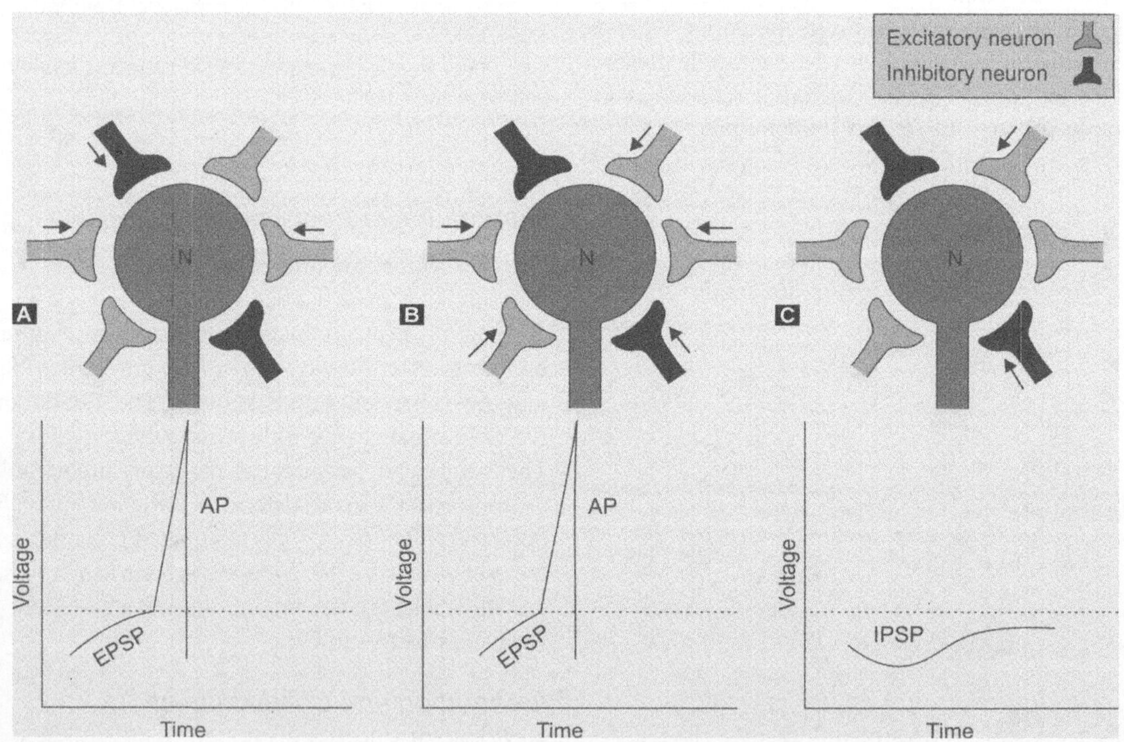

Figs 14.14A to C Summation of postsynaptic potentials. Three hypothetical situations (A, B and C) in a postsynaptic neuron with six presynaptic neurons influencing it (In practice, there may be a thousand of them, not just six). Arrows indicate the presynaptic neurons which are active in the three situations. When active, each excitatory neuron generates an EPSP, and each inhibitory neuron generates an IPSP. The summated EPSP or IPSP has been shown in each case. The PSP near the axon hillock is more effective than that farther away on the postsynaptic membrane. If the summated PSP is excitatory, and crosses a certain threshold value (indicated by the dotted line), an action potential (AP) is fired, and propagated along the axon

At one synapse, a number of large molecule peptides may be released, or, at some synapses, a large molecule peptide and a small molecular neurotransmitter may be released together.

Thus complexity of the neurotransmitter profile adds to the complexity of the neuronal connections to determine the function of the nervous system. This complexity is necessary because the nervous system has to take care of so many factors simultaneously to ensure homeostasis.

QUESTIONS

1. Are all reflexes present at birth?
2. Compare and contrast the brain and computers.

ANSWERS

1. No, some reflexes appear, or get modified as a result of further development of the nervous system which takes place after birth. But reflexes are inborn, which means that they do not have to be learnt. This is true of classical reflexes, but conditioned reflexes have to be learnt (Chapter 18).
2. Brain and computers can perform some of the same tasks, e.g. calculations. But it is quite possible that they may be doing similar jobs using very dissimilar methods. The principal features of the brain and computers have been compared in Table 14.1.
   However, some of the newer advanced programs have made computer responses quite flexible and functions bearing a superficial resemblance to creativity are also now possible with computers.

Table 14.1 Brain compared with early computers

Feature	*Brain*	*Computers*
Input	Sensory information	Data
Processing	In the brain. Nature of processing depends on neuronal connections	In the central processing unit. Nature of processing depends on the program
Output	Motor response	Data
Flexibility of output	Present	Absent
Speed	Generally relatively slow	Fast
Originality	Present	Absent
Abstract thought and creativity	Present	Absent

CHAPTER

15 Nervous System: Sensory Functions

"See how you beam of seeming white, Is braided out of seven-hued light, Yet in those lucid globes no ray, By any chance shall break astray. Hark how the rolling surge of sound, Arches and spirals circling round, Wakes the hushed spirit through thine ear with music it is heaven to hear."

—OLIVER WENDELL HOLMES

Chapter Outline

- Skin
- Transduction
- Action Potential
- Adaptation
- From Periphery to Center
- Descending Fibers of the Sensory System
- Pain
- Vision
- Hearing
- Taste
- Smell

Sensory functions of the nervous system enable us to gain knowledge about our surroundings, or the state of affairs within the body. The first step in the process is detection of stimuli by sensory receptors. Receptors which provide information about our surroundings are called **exteroceptors**. Receptors which provide information about blood pressure, pH of body fluids and other aspects of the interior of the body are called **interoceptors**. In addition, there are also receptors in joints, muscles and tendons, which provide information about position or posture of the body; these receptors are called **proprioceptors**. The general principles of action of all receptors are the same. In this chapter, we shall discuss only exteroceptors, viz. skin, eyes, ears, nose and tongue. Information provided by these receptors reaches consciousness, and enables us to form an image of the world around us.

SKIN

Receptors present in the skin are responsible for the sensations of touch, pain, temperature and pressure. The skin has a wide variety of sensory end organs: Meissner's corpuscles, Pacinian corpuscles, Merkel's disks, Ruffini's nerve endings and free nerve endings. It is now believed that all the specialized end organs detect different forms of touch and pressure, while free nerve endings detect pain and temperature.

The general process of sensory perception (Figs 15.1A and B) consists of the following steps:

a. Conversion of the sensory stimulus into the electrical language of the nervous system (transduction).
b. Transmission of nerve impulses from the periphery to the central nervous system.
c. Transmission of nerve impulses along a specific pathway in the central nervous system. The pathway passes through the thalamus and terminates in the cerebral cortex in case of sensory stimuli which reach consciousness. That the information should reach the cerebral

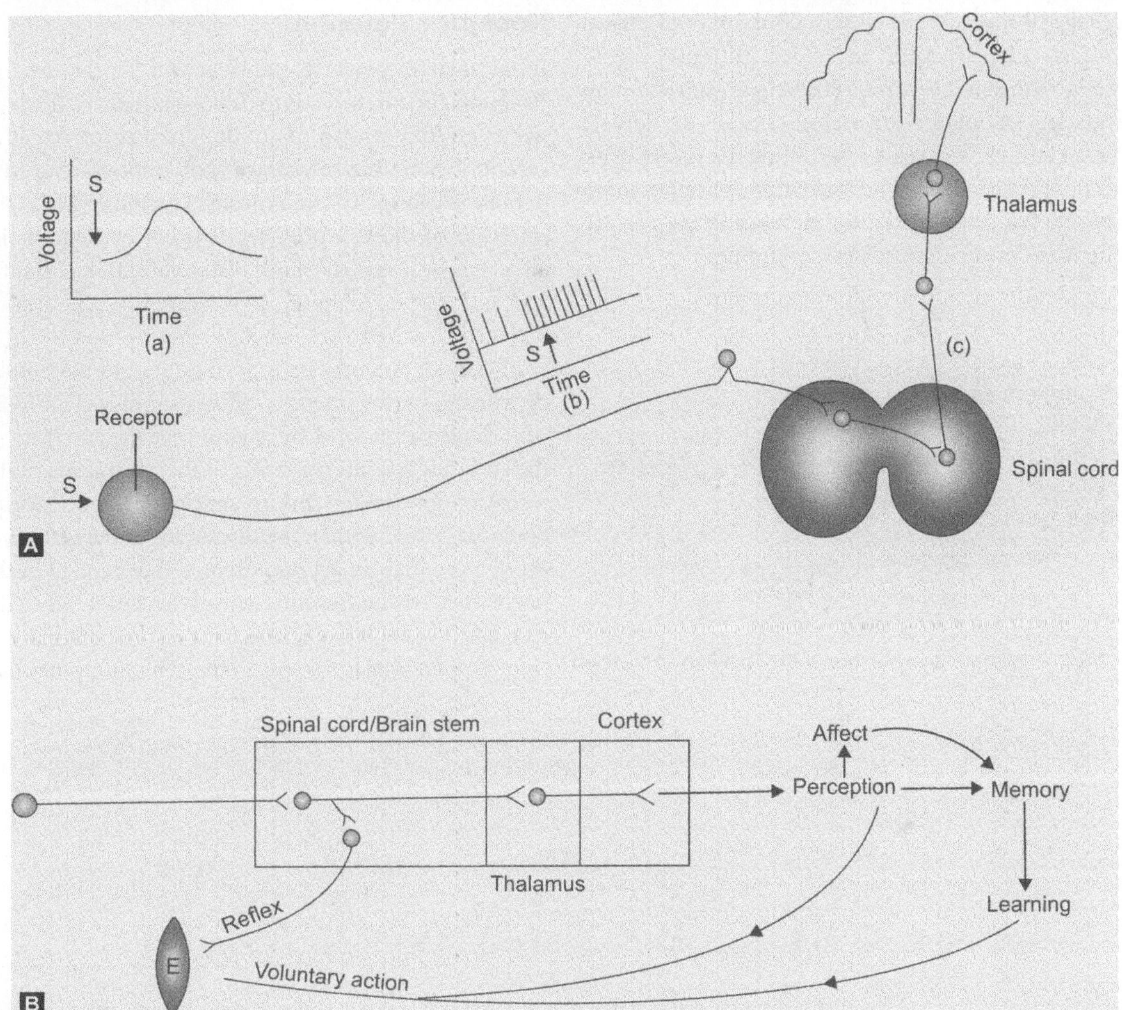

Figs 15.1A and B The general process of sensory perception. (A) Conscious perception involves (a) transduction, which leads to the generation of receptor potential, (b) transmission of nerve impulses (action potentials) by the sensory nerve fiber, and (c) transmission of nerve impulses along a specific pathway in the central nervous system. The pathway terminates in the cerebral cortex; (B) For all sensory stimuli, including those reaching consciousness, some processing takes place in the spinal cord or brain stem leading to reflexes. Once a stimulus is consciously perceived, it may lead to a feeling (affect), it may be stored in the memory, it may modify future behavior (learning) and may lead to a voluntary action. Thus sensory, motivational and motor systems are interconnected. They are studied separately only for convenience

cortex seems to be an essential requirement for conscious perception. In case of sensory stimuli which do not reach consciousness, the pathway terminates in the central nervous system below the level of the cerebral cortex.

TRANSDUCTION

Transduction means conversion of one form of energy into another. In the present context, it refers to conversion of the stimulus energy (mechanical, thermal, etc.) into electrical energy, because the language of the nervous system consists of electrical impulses. The receptor in which the process of transduction has been best studied is the Pacinian corpuscle. Pacinian corpuscles consist of several layers of connective tissue resembling the layers of an onion peel (Fig. 15.2). The structure of the Pacinian corpuscle is ideally suited for transmitting pressure to the bare (unmyelinated) nerve ending.

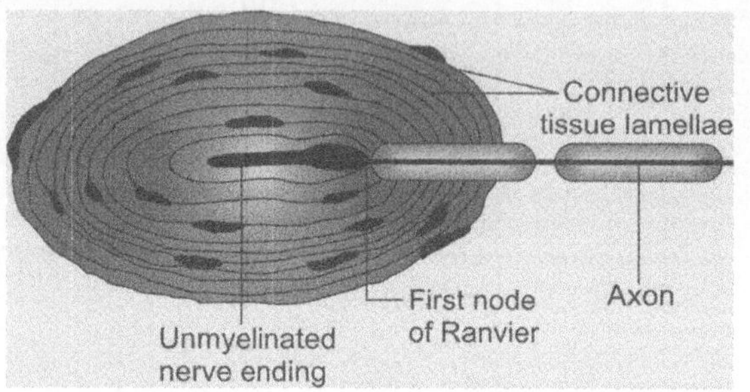

Fig. 15.2 Diagrammatic structure of the Pacinian corpuscle

Receptor Potential

It has been observed that application of pressure to a Pacinain corpuscle leads to depolarization of the bare nerve ending within. This depolarization is called receptor potential. Receptor potential is a graded depolarization, its magnitude varying with the intensity of the stimulus. In its other characteristics also it resembles the end plate potential (Chapter 13) and EPSP (Chapter 14). Receptor potential is believed to arise from influx of sodium ions.

Receptor potential is a graded change. Its magnitude depends upon the intensity of the stimulus (Fig. 15.3). This is also expressed by saying that the intensity of the stimulus is coded in terms of the magnitude of the receptor potential. If the magnitude of the receptor potential is greater than the threshold for the genesis of action potential, an action potential is generated in the nerve fiber arising from the sensory receptor. Since the receptor potential may generate the action potential, the receptor potential is also called the generator potential.

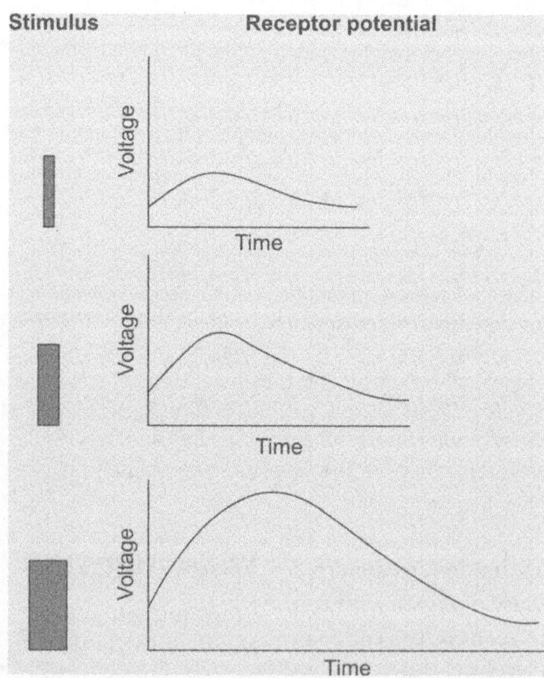

Fig. 15.3 Receptor potential is a graded change. As the intensity of the stimulus increases, the amplitude of the receptor potential increases

ACTION POTENTIAL

The action potential is a brief all or none depolarization propagated along the sensory nerve fiber. Larger the amplitude of the receptor potential, higher the frequency of action potentials.

Now the mechanism of coding of the intensity of the stimulus may be summarized. Intensity of the stimulus is coded in terms of:

a. Amplitude of the receptor potential,
b. Frequency of the action potentials, and
c. Number of the receptors stimulated.

That is why a strong stimulus affecting a small area of the skin can be distinguished from a weak stimulus spread over a large area of the skin (Figs 15.4A and B).

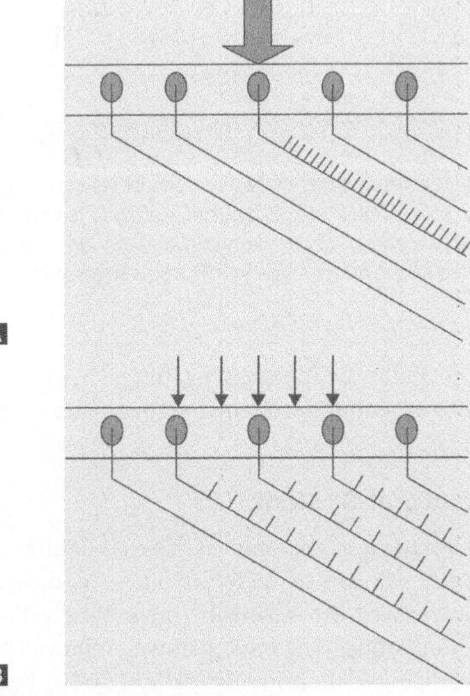

Figs 15.4A and B Coding of stimulus intensity: distinguishing a strong stimulus acting on a small area of the skin (A) from a weak stimulus acting on a large area of the skin (B). The frequency of nerve impulses in afferent nerve fibers is higher in A but the number of receptors stimulated is greater in B

ADAPTATION

If a stimulus is prolonged, the receptor response decreases after some time. The phenomenon is called adaptation because the receptor seems to have adapted (or got used to) the stimulus. The rate of adaptation varies with the receptor (Fig. 15.5). Rapidly adapting receptors are good for detecting the onset, termination, and change in the intensity of a stimulus. Slowly adapting receptors are good when continuous information about a steady stimulus is important. Now try to think why rapid adaptation of touch receptors and near absence of adaptation in muscle spindles is good for us.[1]

FROM PERIPHERY TO CENTER

The nerve fiber arising from a sensory receptor is part of a neuron. The cell body of this neuron lies in the dorsal root ganglion (Fig. 15.1). Dorsal root ganglia (DRG) are located near the spinal cord, but outside it, i.e. at 'the periphery'. The DRG axon continues further to enter the spinal cord, which is a part of the central nervous system, or 'the center'. Thus the DRG cell conveys the signal generated by the stimulus from the periphery to the center.

After entering the spinal cord, the central axons of the DRG cells give branches which are distributed along three routes (Fig. 15.6). First, a few branches synapse with motor neurons in the anterior column of the spinal cord, directly or through interneurons, to complete the reflex arcs for spinal reflexes. Second, they ascend up towards the brain stem in specific tracts, resulting in conscious perception. Third, they relay in reticular formation and nonspecific thalamic nuclei, resulting in general arousal.

We shall concentrate here only on the specific pathways which are responsible for conscious per-

[1]It is due to rapid adaptation of touch receptors that we are normally not aware of our clothes. On the other hand, slow adaptation of muscle spindles ensures continuous supply of information about the position of the body, which is important for maintenance of posture (Chapter 16).

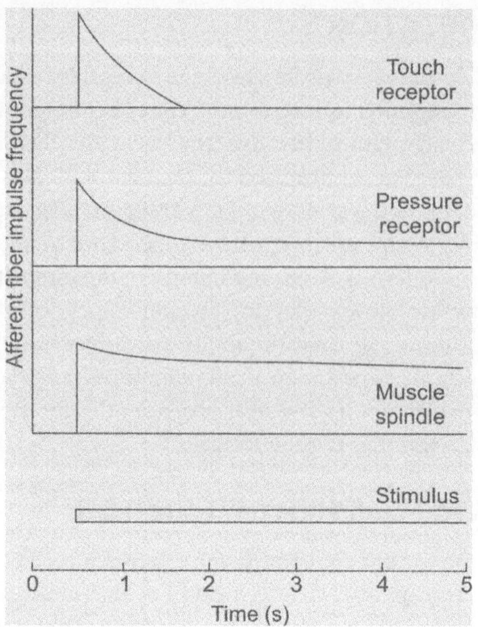

Fig. 15.5 Adaptation of sensory receptors. The diagram shows the frequency of impulses in afferent nerve fibers in response to a sustained stimulus. The frequency rises promptly at the onset of the stimulus in all receptors. But the frequency is sustained only in very slowly adapting receptors such as the muscle spindle. Touch receptors adapt extremely rapidly to a sustained stimulus

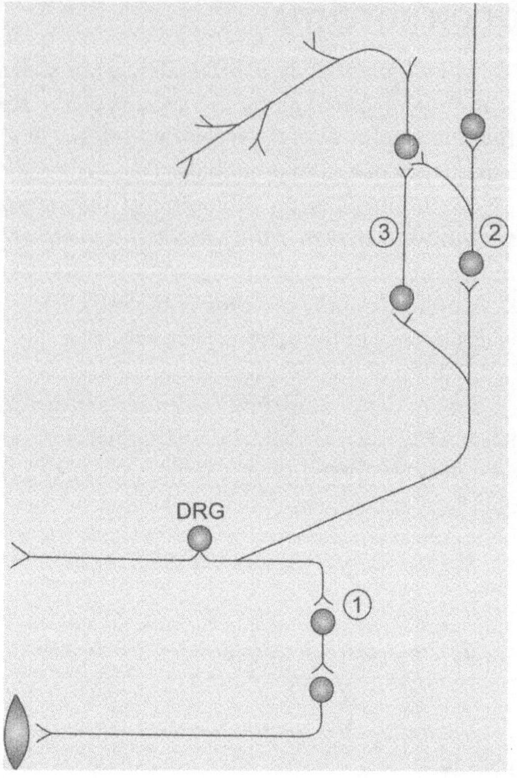

Fig. 15.6 The three types of destinations of sensory nerve fibers. (1) Spinal reflex arc; (2) Specific pathway leading to conscious perception of the stimulus; and (3) Nonspecific pathway leading to general arousal. DRG, dorsal root ganglion

ception.[2] Depending on the modality, the specific ascending fibers travel in the dorsal column or the anterolateral column of the spinal cord.

Dorsal Column System

The dorsal column system conveys the modalities of fine touch, and position (proprioception). These modalities are localized with great precision. For example, we know accurately which part of the body is being touched. These modalities are also characterized by precise discriminative ability. For example, we can distinguish between two positions of the thumb which may be only slightly different.

[2]We shall discuss some spinal reflexes in Chapter 16. The role of nonspecific pathways will figure with the physiology of sleep in Chapter 18.

The basic pathway followed by fibers belonging to the dorsal column system has been shown in Figure 15.7.

Anterolateral System

The anterolateral system conveys the modalities of crude touch, pain and temperature. These modalities are characterized by relatively poor localization and discrimination. The basic pathway followed by fibers belonging to the anterolateral system has been shown in Figure 15.8.

Thalamus

Sensory fibers of the dorsal column system as well as the anterolateral system relay in the thalamus. As we

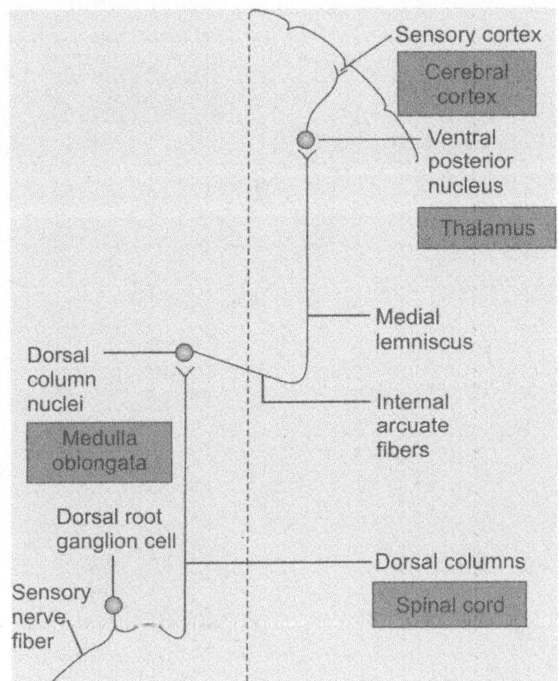

Fig. 15.7 The dorsal column system for transmitting sensory signals. The dotted line represents the midline

shall see later, afferent fibers from special senses also relay in the thalamus. Thus all sensory information reaches the thalamus where it can be integrated. In addition, the thalamus also has motor functions, motivational functions, and an important role in sleep and wakefulness.

Sensory information from all parts of the body relays in the contralateral thalamus, i.e. on the opposite side. For example, information from the right side of the body relays in the left side of the thalamus (Figs 15.7 and 15.8).

The Cerebral Cortex

The cerebral cortex is organized into six layers (Fig. 15.9) which have fairly distinct functions (Table 15.1). The specific sensory information is received from the thalamus by layer IV of the cerebral cortex. The area of the cerebral cortex to which the thalamic fibers project depends on the nature of the stimulus. General somatic sensations project to the somatic sensory cortex which is located predominantly in the postcentral gyrus (Brodmann's areas 3, 1 and 2). These areas constitute the primary sensory area SI *(S-One)*. Area SI has a complete and orderly representation of the body, with the feet up and the head down. The representation is not only upside down but also grossly distorted, with the face and fingers taking up a disproportionately large area (Fig. 15.10). The area dedicated to a part of the body seems to be related to the precision with which stimuli there are perceived. There is also a complete representation of the body in the superior wall of the Sylvian fissure, in an area called SII *(S-Two)*. Visual, auditory, olfactory and gustatory stimuli project to specific circumscribed areas of the cortex as described later in the chapter.

Having received the signals in layer IV, granule cells of layer III convey the information to association areas. In the association areas sensory signals from multiple points on the body are put together to arrive at a meaningful interpretation of signals.

The *function* of sensory cortex has been inferred from several types of studies. In *animals*, stimulation of skin receptors leads to change in the activity of neurons in the cerebral cortex. Thus stimulation of the foot leads to a change in the neuronal activity in the top part of area SI. From this we may infer that the foot is represented there. In this way the representation of the whole body in the cerebral cortex can be mapped out. In *human beings*, we can study the effect of stimulation of a part of the body on regional blood flow in the brain. An area of the brain which is more active shows an increase in blood flow. These studies can be interpreted in the same way as the animal experiments.

Some of the most interesting human studies, however, were performed by Penfield and Rasmussen on neurosurgical patients whose cerebral cortex had been exposed under local anesthesia. Stimulation of discrete points in the sensory cortex led to sensory experiences referred to specific parts of the body. For example, stimulation of what is now known as the 'foot area' of SI led to a feeling of tingling in the foot. In this way the topographic representation of the entire body in the sensory cortex could be mapped,

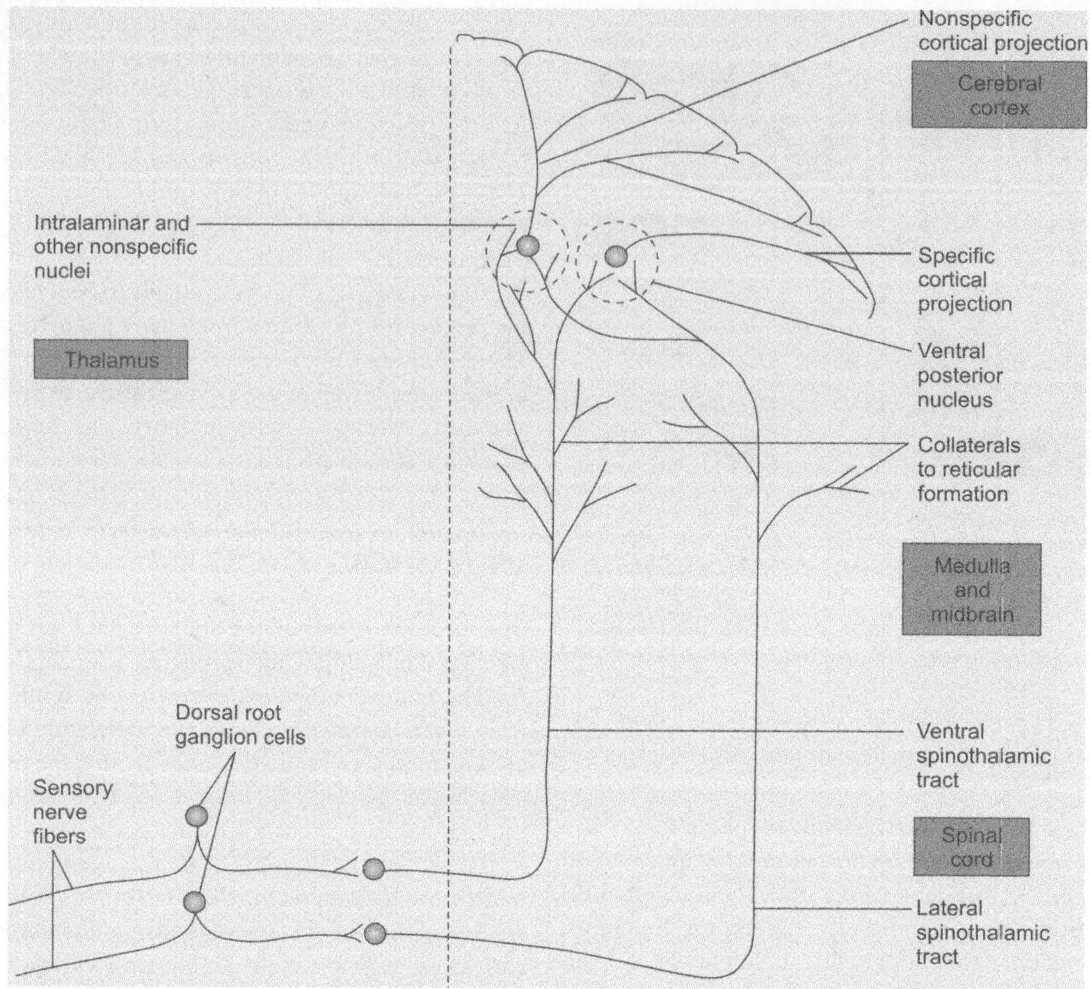

Fig. 15.8 The anterolateral system for transmitting sensory signals. The dotted line represents the midline

and a homunculus of the type illustrated in Figure 15.10 was constructed.

Although some crude awareness may exist at the thalamic level, it is almost certain that conscious awareness of a sensory stimulus is achieved only at the cortical level. When information about a sensory stimulus reaches area SI, the individual becomes aware of the modality of the stimulus (e.g. touch), and its localization. But that much is not enough. Further elaboration is made possible by the connections of area SI with neighboring areas, association areas, motor areas, and contralateral cortex. These connections relate the stimulus to other stimuli simultaneously present, and other stimuli experienced in the past. The result of this processing is that (a) the stimulus acquires a meaning (e.g. the stimulus is a 'pen'), and (b) a motor response, if warranted by the stimulus, is executed. In addition, there may also be an emotional reaction to the stimulus; that is mediated by the connections between the cortex and the limbic system (Chapter 17).

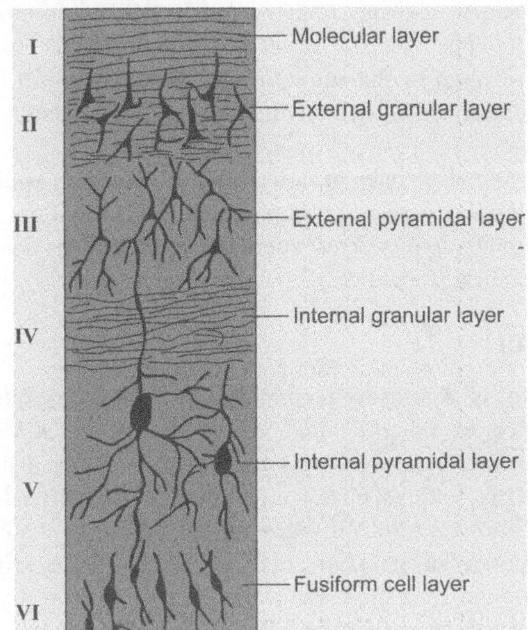

Fig. 15.9 Diagrammatic representation of microscopic structure of the cerebral cortex showing its six layers

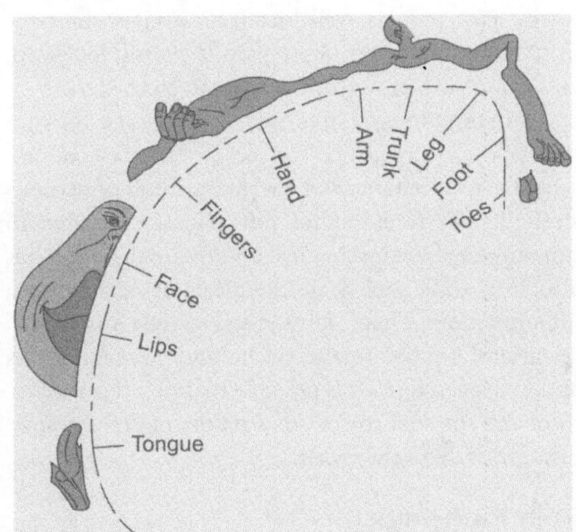

Fig. 15.10 Representation of different parts of the body in the primary sensory area (SI) of the cerebral cortex, as deduced by Penfield and Rasmussen from their studies on neurosurgical patients

Table 15.1 Functional organization of the cerebral cortex

Layer	*Predominant element*	*Function*
I	Nerve fibers	Receives diffuse nonspecific sensory input
II	Nerve fibers and granule cells	Receives diffuse, non-specific sensory input Sends axons to related areas of the cortex
III	Granule cells and small pyramidal cells	Sends axons to related areas of the cortex
IV	Nerve fibers	Receives specific sensory input
V	Large pyramidal cells and spinal cord	Sends axons to brain stem
VI	Fusiform cells	Sends axons to thalamus

Cognition, Conation and Affect

Awareness of a stimulus and its interpretation is called cognition. The motor response to the stimulus is called conation, and the emotional reaction to the stimulus is called affect. For example, when a mouse is faced with a cat, identification of the cat is cognition. Running away from the cat is conation. And, the feeling of fear experienced by the mouse is the affect.

Labeled Line Code

It was once considered a point of debate whether the perceived modality of a stimulus depends on the receptor or the pathway in the central nervous system. It is now reasonably certain that it depends on the pathway. The receptor only makes it easier for a particular type of stimulus to activate the pathway. To give an extreme and impractical example, if the retina were connected to the auditory nerve, stimulation of the retina by light would evoke a sensation of sound. That is, we would be able to 'hear' a candle! This concept of the modality being dependent on the pathway has been termed the labeled line code. That is, the pathways (or lines) are labeled as touch lines, temperature lines, etc. The labeling of lines takes place early during development of the nervous system.

Weber–Fechner Law

This law gives the relationship between how strong we think a stimulus is, and how strong it actually is. As a stimulus gets stronger, it is also felt to be stronger, but the feeling grows at a much slower rate than the stimulus. Mathematically, the interpreted (felt) strength is proportional to the logarithm of the absolute (actual) strength.

The law may be illustrated by an example. A sound which is 100 times louder in terms of the amplitude of the sound waves is perceived as only three times louder (log 100 = 3). As a result, the ability to distinguish between different grades of stimuli diminishes as the absolute intensity increases. For example, if one is just able to distinguish a 30 g weight from 31 g, it will not be possible to distinguish a 300 g weight from 301 g. But it will be just possible to distinguish a 300 g weight from 310 g. Thus the just noticeable difference (JND) bears a constant ratio to the stimulus intensity. In the above example, the ratio is 1/30 or 10/300, i.e. 0.03.

Weber–Fechner law does not hold good for all stimuli over the entire range of intensities. But it is a good working concept.

DESCENDING FIBERS OF THE SENSORY SYSTEM

The sensory pathways consist of not just the fibers which ascend from the spinal cord to the cortex. There are also descending fibers from the cortex to the spinal cord which follow a route quite similar to the ascending fibers. Therefore every region of the nervous system has some control over the information that goes to it. The ultimate impact of the descending fibers of the sensory system is that the sensory signal is modulated in the dorsal horn of the spinal cord. Hence, the way a stimulus is perceived depends not only on the nature of the stimulus itself but also on the nature of the descending influences. Since the descending fiber activity may be affected by accompanying sensory stimuli other than the one under consideration, the perception of a stimulus is affected by associated stimuli. For example, the intensity of a painful stimulus may be reduced by touch, specially a loving touch. It is a common experience that the sensitivity to a stimulus may be affected by the attention paid to it. The effect of attention is likely to be mediated by the descending fibers.

We shall refer to descending fibers again while discussing perception of pain and the perception of sound — two systems where descending fibers have been best studied.

PAIN

Pain is a sensory experience of special significance to doctors and nurses because it is the commonest presenting symptom of patients. Pain has two features. First, it is an unpleasant experience. Secondly, it results from a stimulus which is actually or potentially damaging to living tissues. That is why, although it is unpleasant, pain serves a protective function by making us aware of actual or possible harm to the body.

From a physiological point of view, there are two types of pain. One, 'fast pain', is conducted by fast-conducting myelinated fibers. The other, 'slow pain', is conducted by slow-conducting unmyelinated fibers. Fast pain is well localized, and is sharp or pricking in character. Slow pain is poorly localized, and is burning or dull and aching in character.

Pain receptors are 'free' nerve endings, i.e. they are not enclosed in a capsule. The receptors for fast pain are sensitive to mechanical or thermal stimuli of noxious strength. The receptors for slow pain are sensitive to not only noxious mechanical and thermal stimuli but also to a wide variety of chemicals associated with inflammation. These substances include histamine, serotonin, bradykinin, acetylcholine, potassium ions and hydrogen ions. It is possible that noxious mechanical and thermal stimuli also act through the release of some of these chemicals.

Pain Pathways

Fast pain is conducted to the spinal cord by A-delta type of nerve fibers, which have a conduction velocity of 6-30 m/s. The course of these fibers in the central nervous system has been

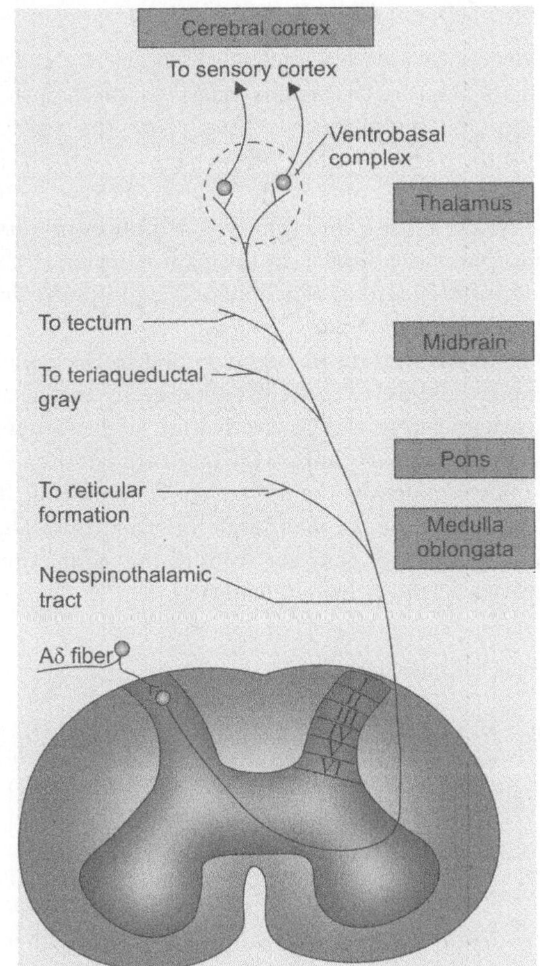

Fig. 15.11 Pathway by which fast pain is conveyed to the central nervous system. I-VI, laminae of the dorsal horn of the spinal cord

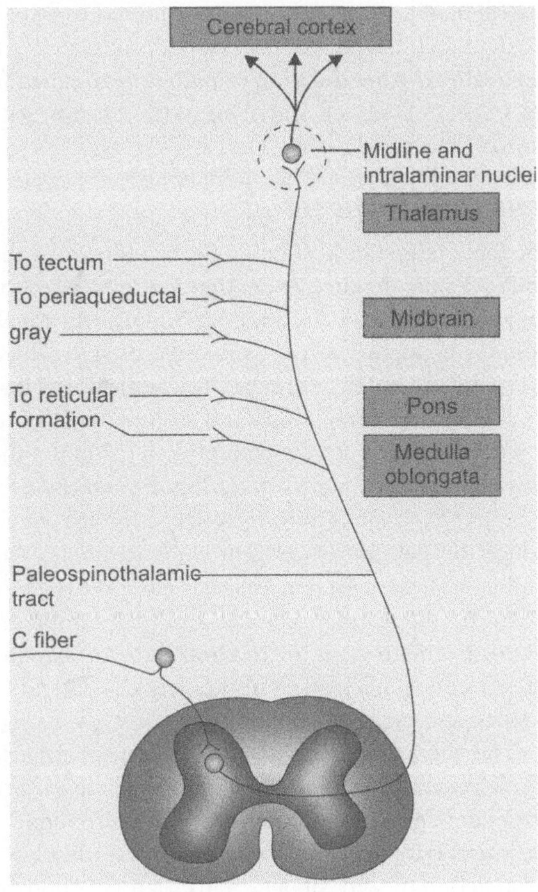

Fig. 15.12 Pathway by which slow pain is conveyed to the central nervous system

shown in Figure 15.11. *Slow pain* is conducted to the spinal cord by C type of nerve fibers, which have a conduction velocity of 0.5-2 m/s. The slow pain pathway has been shown in Figure 15.12. Note in the fast as well as slow pain pathway the collaterals. Some of these are involved in mediating reflex responses to painful stimuli, some join the nonspecific sensory pathway which keeps us awake, and some project to the endogenous pain relief system. Also note that the slow pain pathway relays in the nonspecific midline and intralaminar thalamic nuclei. That is why slow pain is more likely to keep us awake.[3]

Modulation of Pain

Noxious stimuli of comparable intensity may produce varying degrees of pain in the same individual under different circumstances. For example, an injury acquired by an athlete in the sports field or by a soldier in the battlefield is less

[3]This will become clearer when you reach the physiology of sleep in Chapter 18.

painful than a comparable injury suffered in a road accident. In other words, pain can be modulated. An explanation for modulation of pain was *proposed* in the 1960s by Melzack and Wall in the form of gate control theory.

Gate Control Theory

The theory explains how pain may be reduced by the simultaneous presence of another stimulus which is not painful (e.g. a touch stimulus). Suppose the touch stimulus is applied to the same area of skin which has received a painful stimulus. It was proposed that the touch fiber gave a collateral in the dorsal horn of the spinal cord. The collateral then inhibited the pain pathway through an inhibitory interneuron (Fig. 15.13). That is how a touch stimulus could reduce the painfulness of a noxious stimulus. The inhibitory interneuron acts as a gate. When it is activated, the gate is closed, and pain impulses cannot ascend towards the cerebral cortex. When the gate neuron is inactive, pain impulses can ascend to make us conscious of the pain.

The theory appeals to commonsense because it is a general experience that touch or any other stimulus (e.g. a counterirritant ointment) reduces the intensity of pain. But experimental studies have failed to find the type of neuronal circuitry proposed by the theory. But research based on the theory contributed to the discovery of an endogenous pain relief system.

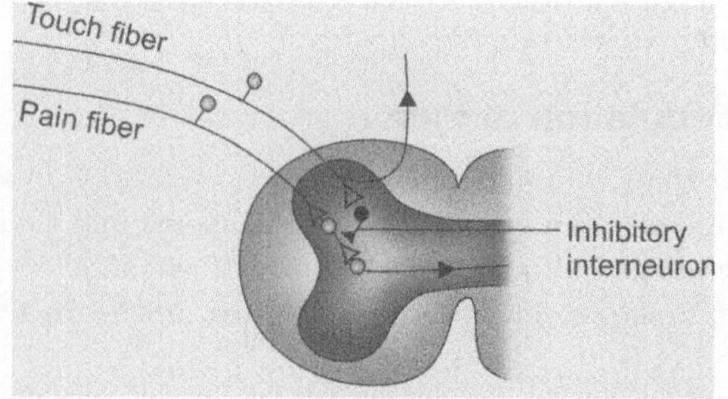

Fig. 15.13 Gate control theory. Activation of the inhibitory interneuron in the substantia gelatinosa 'closes the gate' through which the sensation of pain may be conveyed

Endogenous Pain Relief System

Endogenous means within the body. Hence endogenous pain relief system refers to mechanisms within the body which relieve pain. The system depends on descending fibers (Fig. 15.14). It is interesting that some of the neurons belonging to the system release endorphins as neurotransmitters: endorphins are similar to the pain-relieving drug, morphine. Neurons which release endorphins are called enkephalinergic.

The descending fibers belonging to the endogenous pain relief system converge in the periaqueductal gray (PAG). Activation of PAG neurons releases serotonin as a neurotransmitter in the dorsal horn of the spinal cord. Serotonin, in turn, activates enkephalinergic interneurons. The enkephalinergic neurons inhibit the projection neurons of the pain pathway (Fig. 15.15). That is

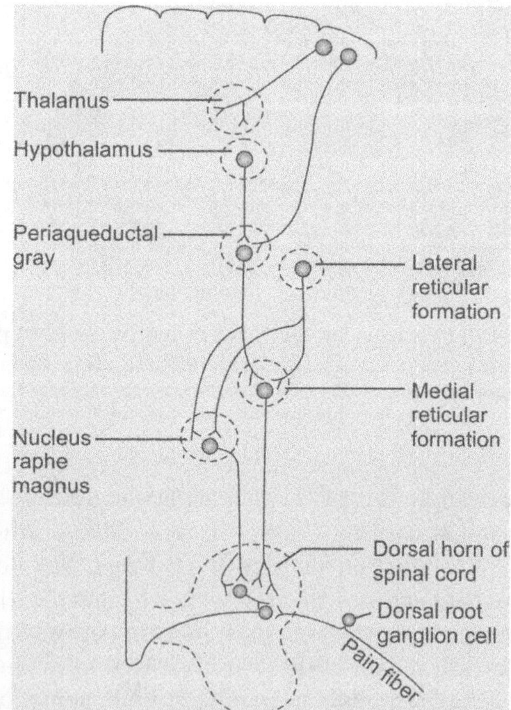

Fig. 15.14 Descending fiber tracts which influence the transmission of pain to the central nervous system

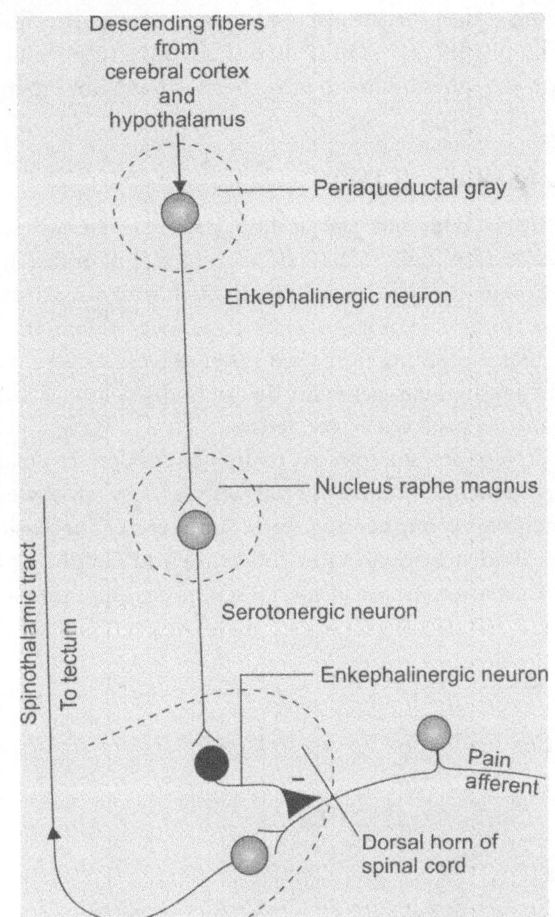

Fig. 15.15 Endogenous pain relief system. Details in text

how descending fibers can modulate the intensity of pain. The endogenous pain relief system is activated by any form of stress, including the stress of severe pain. The great Urdu poet, Ghalib, rightly said, "*Ishrat-e-katra hai dariya mein fana ho jana/ Dard ka had se guzarna hai dava ho jana*" (Just as a drop of water gets lost in a river, when pain crosses a limit, it cures itself). Physiologically, intense pleasure is as much a stress as intense pain. Norman Cousins found through his own experience that ten minutes of laughter induced by watching comedies relieved his pain for about two hours.

Revaluation of the Gate Control Theory

The interneurons which inhibit projection neurons of the pain system do exist in the spinal cord. But these inhibitory interneurons are not activated by touch and other primary afferents, as postulated by the gate control theory. Instead, the inhibitory interneurons seem to be activated by fibers descending from PAG and related areas. How, then, can we explain the modulation of pain by touch and other competing stimuli? The dorsal column fibers, while ascending to the thalamus, give off collaterals to the reticular formation. These collaterals could activate the descending fibers of the endogenous analgesic system. Thus a touch stimulus can still close the gate, although indirectly (Fig. 15.16). Supporting this concept is the observation that dorsal column

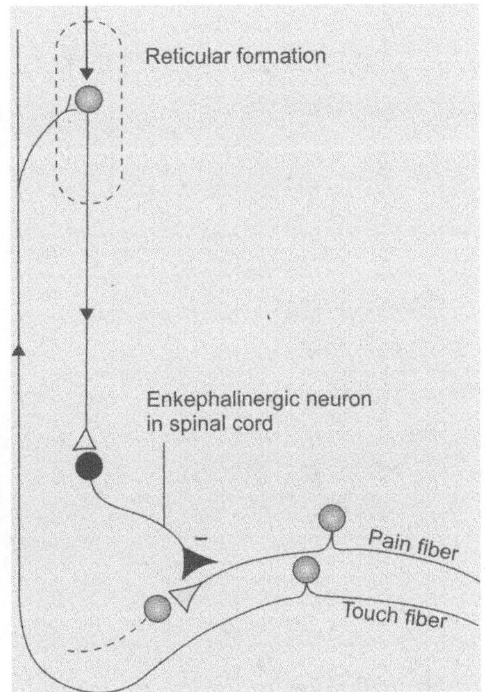

Fig. 15.16 Revaluation of the gate control theory. The highly simplified neuronal circuitry in this diagram shows how stimulation of a touch fiber might indirectly activate the inhibitory enkephalinergic interneuron in the spinal cord

stimulation often produces analgesia. The effect is sometimes made use of by neurosurgeons to provide therapeutic pain relief.

Referred Pain

It is sometimes observed that disease of a deep organ gives rise to superficial pain in some part of the body, not necessarily overlying the deep organ. For example, inflammation of the appendix usually produces pain around the umbilicus, and disease of the gallbladder often produces pain at the right shoulder. Such pain is called referred pain. The common point between the site of referred pain and the diseased organ is that both are innervated by the same segment of the spinal cord. Since the brain is normally accustomed to receiving information about painful stimuli only from superficial parts of the body, it interprets an occasional painful stimulus from a deep organ also as originating superficially. The possible types of neuronal circuitry responsible for the phenomenon have been shown in Figure 15.17.

Life Without Pain

Pain is bad, but not feeling pain can be worse. Some rare individuals who cannot feel pain due to a congenital defect are known. Such individuals are very poor at avoiding accidental injuries. Often, they inflict mutilating injuries on themselves. As a result such individuals generally do not live very long. Thus pain is a protective experience.

Now we shall go on to the discussion of what are generally called special senses. Special senses include vision, hearing, taste and smell. The basic mechanisms involved in collection and handling of information in case of special senses are quite similar

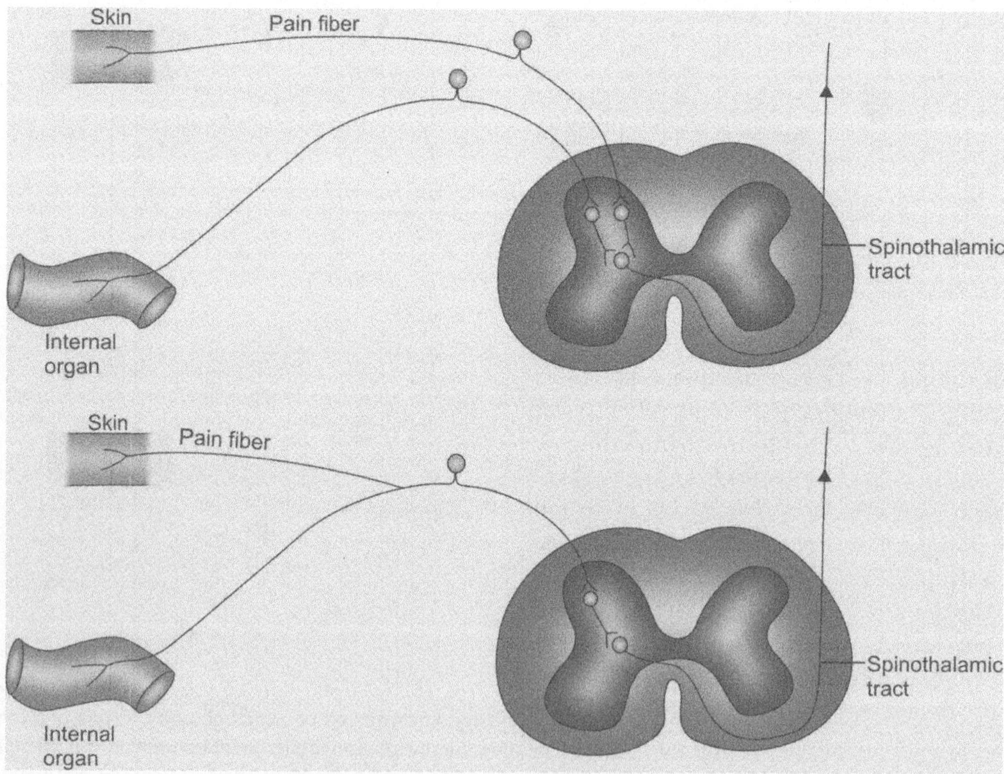

Fig. 15.17 Two types of neuronal circuitry which may be responsible for the phenomenon of referred pain

to those employed by the 'not-so-special' senses discussed above.

VISION

Seeing is a sensory experience, the receptors for which are in the eyes. The eyes consist of an optical system which generates an image, or a visual message. As in other sensory systems, the message is converted by the receptors into neural impulses and then transmitted to the brain (Fig. 15.18).

Functional Anatomy

The eye has a rounded structure, and is hence commonly called the eyeball. The wall of the eyeball is made up of three layers (Fig. 15.19). The outermost layer is the tough and white **sclera**, which continues anteriorly as the transparent and more convex **cornea**. The middle layer is the vascular **choroid**, which forms the **iris** and **ciliary body** anteriorly. The color of the eye depends on the color of the iris. The iris has a small circular adjustable gap in the front, called the **pupil**. The innermost layer is the light-sensitive **retina**. The central part of the retina is responsible for more sharp vision and is called the **macula lutea**. The central part of the macula lutea is the region of maximum visual acuity, and is called **fovea centralis**.

The exposed part of the eye is kept moist by a thin film of tears. Tears are secreted by the **lacrimal glands** (Fig. 15.20). Tears have important protective functions. If any particulate matter falls in the eye, a

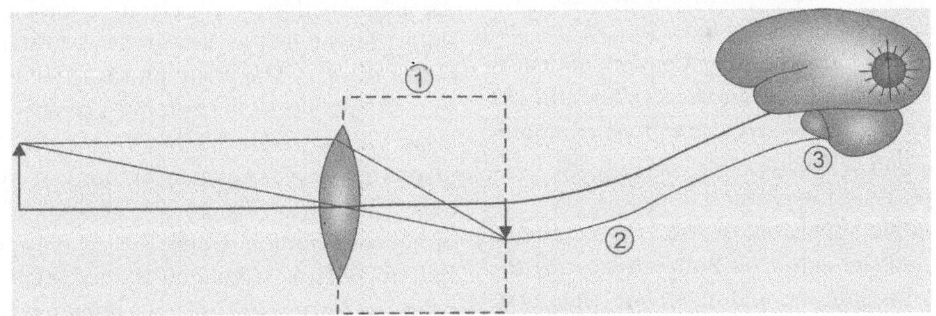

Fig. 15.18 The visual process involves formation of an image (1) and its transmission (2) to the brain (3). In the body, 1 corresponds to the eye, 2 to the visual pathways, and 3 to the visual areas of the brain

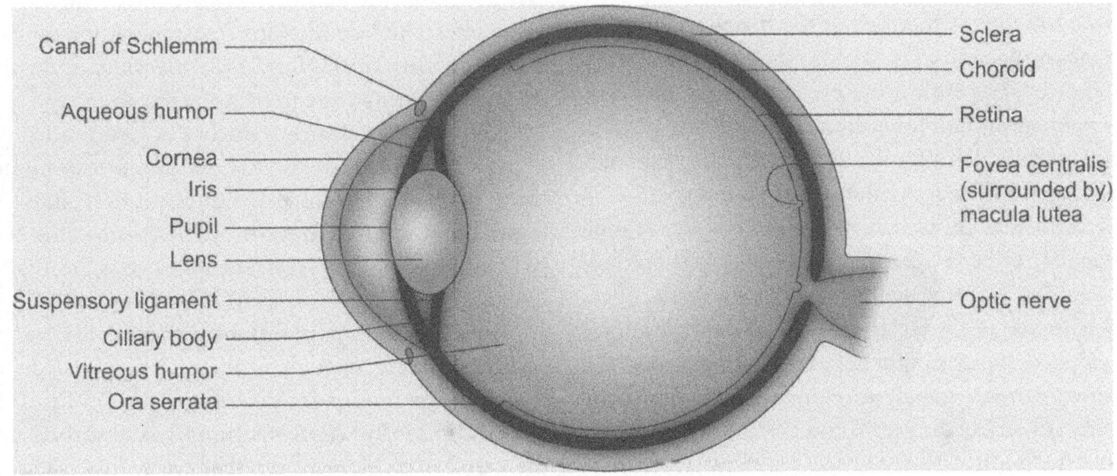

Fig. 15.19 Diagrammatic representation of a horizontal section of the eyeball

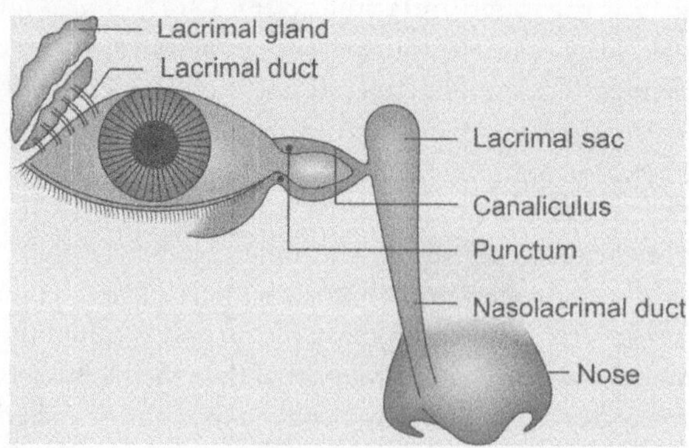

Fig. 15.20 The lacrimal apparatus

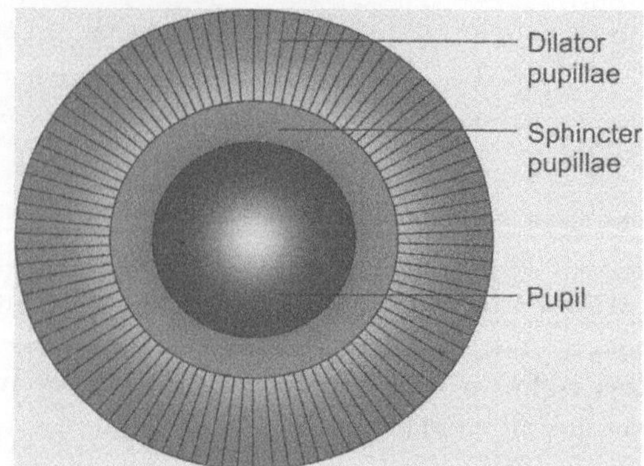

Fig. 15.21 Diagrammatic representation of the muscles of the iris which constrict and dilate the pupil

reflex increases tear secretion, and tears rinse away the particles. Tears contain bactericidal enzymes. Besides, tears protect the eyes from drying up, and thereby improve its optical properties. Further, tears reduce friction between the eyelids and the eyeball during blinking. Tears also express emotions, specially in women. Whether this function also has a protective role is for the reader to judge.

The **dioptric apparatus** of the eye consists of the cornea and the lens. The hollow spaces in the eyeball are the anterior and posterior chambers, and the **vitreous**. The anterior and posterior chambers contain a clear fluid, the **aqueous humor**. The vitreous contains a jelly like substance, the vitreous. Vitreous is also perfectly transparent.

Movements of the eyeball are brought about by six **extraocular muscles**. Besides these muscles, there are also muscles within the eyeball: **ciliary muscles**, which are important for accommodation (see below), and muscles which alter the diameter of the pupil, viz. **sphincter pupillae** and **dilator pupillae** (Fig. 15.21).

Extraocular muscles are supplied by cranial nerves III, IV and VI. Ciliary muscles and sphincter pupillae are supplied by parasympathetic fibers which travel in cranial nerve III. Dilator pupillae is supplied by sympathetic nerve fibers from the superior cervical ganglion. Hence parasympathetic activity constricts the pupil, and sympathetic activity dilates the pupil.

Aqueous Humor

As mentioned above, aqueous humor is the clear fluid present in the anterior and posterior chamber of the eye. The posterior chamber is 'posterior' only in relation to the anterior chamber; otherwise, even the posterior chamber is quite 'anteriorly' placed in the eye. Aqueous humor is secreted by the ciliary processes (Fig. 15.22). The rate of formation of aqueous humor is only 2-5 cu mm per minute. But since its total volume is very small, there is a complete turnover of aqueous humor every hour.

Aqueous humor is not a simple filtrate of the plasma. Its formation involves active secretion of sodium ions. Since sodium ions are positively charged, chloride and bicarbonate ions follow them passively. The accumulation of these ions raises the osmolarity of the fluid, which results in passive transport of water due to osmotic forces.

The concentration of glucose is lower, and that of pyruvate and lactate higher, in the aqueous humor than in plasma. Glucose concentration may be lower because of utilization by the cornea and lens; pyruvate and lactate concentration may be higher due to anaerobic glycolysis in these structures.

Aqueous humor is formed continuously but its volume remains constant. From this it may be deduced that aqueous humor is also being removed from the eye continuously. Aqueous humor is absorbed into the **canal of Schlemm**, a rather wide duct arranged

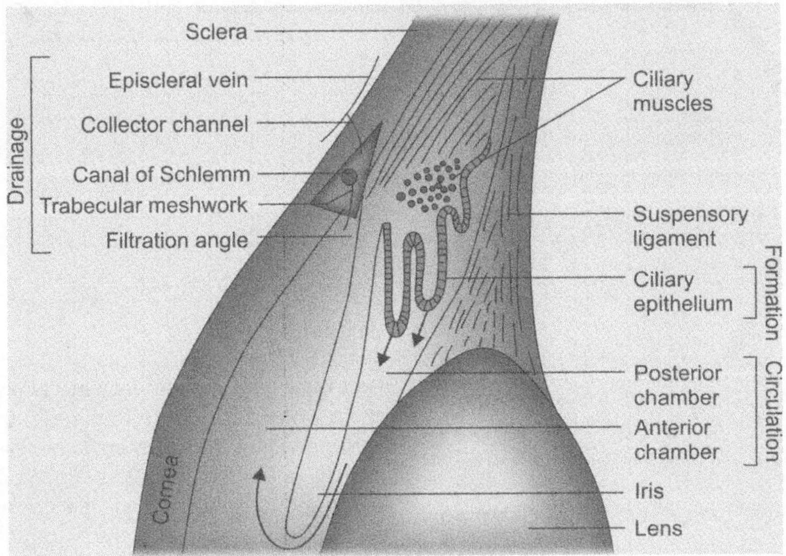

Fig. 15.22 Formation, circulation and drainage of aqueous humor. After being secreted by the ciliary epithelium, the aqueous humor enters the posterior chamber and flows towards the anterior chamber. It leaves the anterior chamber through the filtration angle. Then it negotiates the trabecular meshwork to enter the canal of Schlemm. From the canal of Schlemm it passes into the collector channels of the sclera before finally draining into the episcleral venous system

like a ring at the corneo-scleral junction (Fig. 15.22). Thus the route taken by the aqueous humor is from the posterior chamber to the anterior chamber, and from there into the canal of Schlemm.

Aqueous humor is the principal determinant of the intraocular pressure (IOP). The normal pressure, or tension, within the eyeball is about 15 mm Hg. The tension is useful in maintaining the spherical shape of the eyeball. But if it becomes too high, it can exert undue pressure on the retina and damage it. Hence rise in IOP, called **glaucoma**, is a serious condition. Glaucoma can be precipitated by drugs which dilate the pupil, and conversely it may be relieved by drugs which constrict the pupil.

You might have observed many similarities between the CSF (Chapter 14) and aqueous humor. Here is yet one more similarity. Just as there is a blood-brain barrier, there is also a blood-aqueous barrier, with characteristics quite similar to it. The elements of the retina are also organized like neurons in the brain. Truly, the eye is essentially an extension of the brain.

Optics of Vision

The eye is, in many respects, comparable to a camera. Its optical system behaves like a convex lens which forms a real inverted image on the retina. The amount of light entering the eye can be altered by varying the diameter of the pupil.

Refraction in the Eye

The refraction first takes place as the light passes through the cornea. The cornea, together with the aqueous humor behind it, behaves like a plano-convex lens of about 40 diopters (Fig. 15.23). After passing through the cornea, the rays of light pass through the lens. The lens has an effective power of about 20 diopters. The reason why the fat-bodied lens contributes much less to the refractive power of the eye than the cornea lies in the surroundings of the two structures. Cornea has air (refractive index 1.0) on one side and aqueous humor (refractive index 1.33) on the other. Therefore rays of light coming from outside pass from a rarer to a denser medium

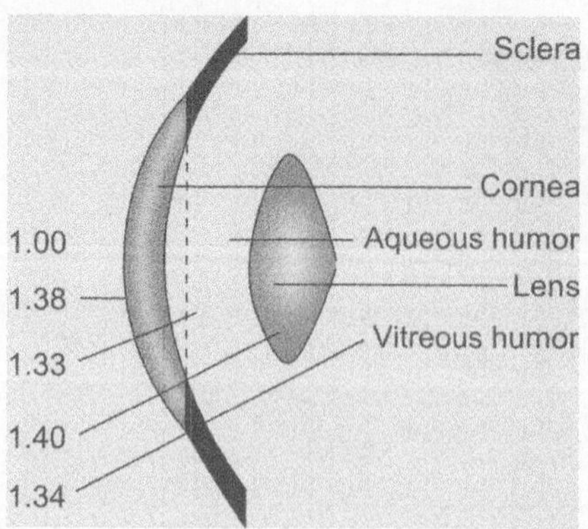

Fig. 15.23 The cornea, together with the aqueous humor, behaves like a plano-convex lens, as indicated by the dotted line. The refractive indices of different media and structures are indicated on the left

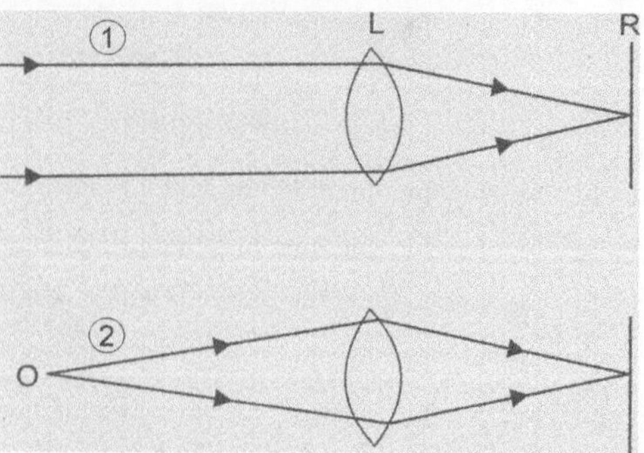

Fig. 15.24 The unaccommodated eye (1) forms a sharp and clear image of distant objects on the retina (R). But if the object (O) is close to the eye, the image is blurred. Accommodation involves an increase in the dioptic power of the lens (L) of the eye. The accommodated eye (2) forms a sharp and clear image of an object close to the eye. As seen in the figure, the lens of the accommodated eye is more globular, chiefly due to an increase in the convexity of the anterior surface

as they pass through the cornea. But the lens has on either side a fluid having a refractive index not very different from the lens itself. Hence light undergoes very little refraction as it passes through the lens. If the lens were surrounded by air, its power would be 150 diopters. A better example of the influence of surroundings on abilities would be difficult to find.

Although the contribution of the lens to the refractive power of the eye is small, its importance lies in the fact that it is adjustable. Normally, when a person shifts his sight from a distant object to a near object, there is an involuntary increase in the dioptic power of the lens. The process is called **accommodation**. Accommodation enables the person to obtain a sharp image of the near object (Fig. 15.24). Accommodation is due to contraction of ciliary muscles that reduces the stretching effect of suspensory ligaments on the lens. That, in turn, allows the lens to become more globular (Fig. 15.25).

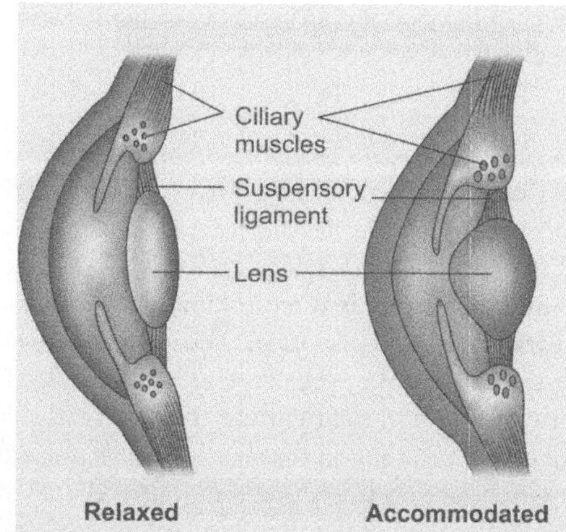

Fig. 15.25 Schematic diagram showing how contraction of ciliary muscles reduces the tension in suspensory ligaments, thereby making the lens more convex

Reduced Eye

The eye, with its multiple surfaces of refraction, is too complex for schematic construction of the image. However, if we consider the eye to have only a single convex lens of 59 D with its optical center (here called the **nodal point**) 17 mm in front of the retina, we get a situation which is optically almost identical with the normal eye. Such a theoretical eye is called **reduced eye**. The principal plane of the reduced eye is 1.5 mm behind the anterior surface of the cornea. In such an eye, the image can be easily constructed using the basic principles of optics (Fig. 15.26).

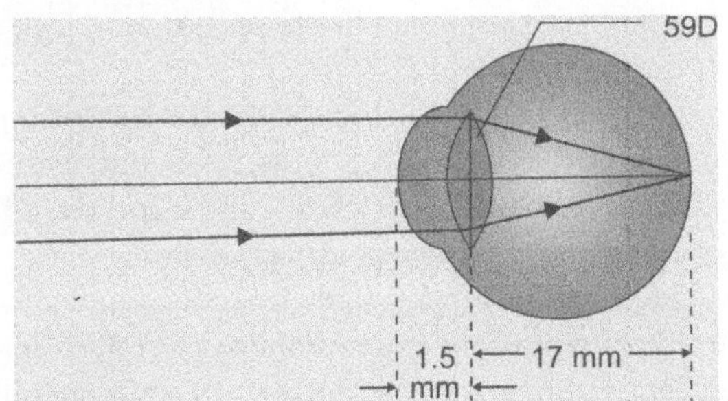

Fig. 15.26 The reduced eye. Observe that the rays of light which are parallel to the principal axis are coming to a focus exactly on the retina, i.e. 17 mm behind the optical center (or nodal point). Calculate whether the power of a lens having a focal length of 17 mm is actually 59 diopters as indicated in the diagram

Errors of Refraction

The common errors of refraction are described below:

1. *Myopia:* In this error, refraction is a little too strong, or the eyeball a bit too long. The result is that the well-focussed image of distant objects is formed a little in front of the retina. Hence the image on the retina is blurred. Howevever, if the object is nearer than a certain point, the image on the retina is well-focussed. This point is called the far point. By using an appropriate concave lens, the additional dioptic power of the myopic eye can be neutralized, and the error can be corrected (Fig. 15.27).
2. *Hypermetropia:* In this error, refraction is a little too weak, or the eyeball is a little too short. The result is that the well-focussed image of near objects is formed a little behind the retina. Hence the image on the retina is blurred. However,if the object is farther than a certain point, the image on the retina is well-focussed. This point is called the near point. By using appropriate convex lens, the deficient dioptic power of the hypermetropic eye can be corrected (Fig. 15.28).
3. *Presbyopia:* This error is generally seen after the age of forty, and becomes progressively worse with age. It is due to the failure of the eye to accommodate adequately. Presbyopia is at least partly due to hardening of the lens material. As a result, the shape of the lens does not change sufficiently in spite of the contraction of ciliary

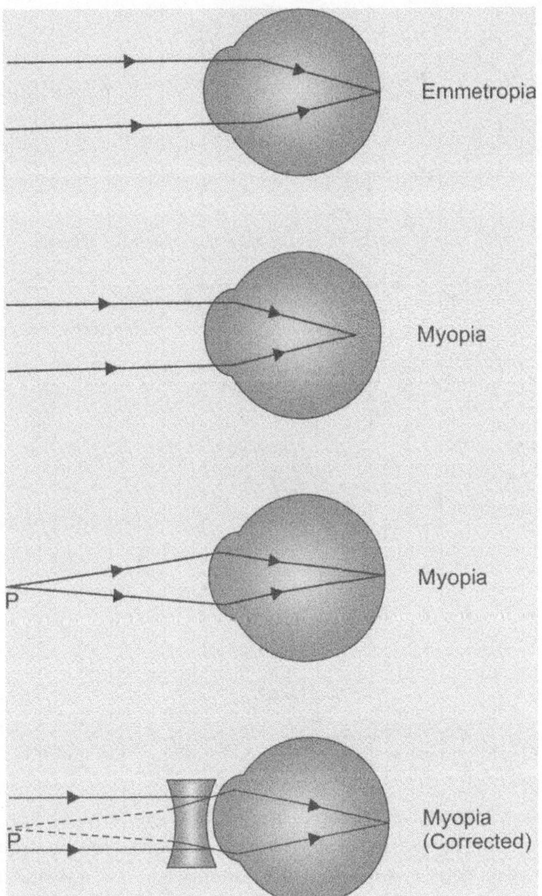

Fig. 15.27 Myopia. In a normal eye (emmetropic), rays of light coming from a distant object are focussed exactly on the retina. In myopia, which may be due to the eyeball being too long, such rays of light are focussed in front of the retina. But rays of light coming from objects at point P, or nearer than that, are focussed exactly on the retina, and therefore such objects are seen clearly. If an appropriate concave lens is placed in front of the myopic eye, rays of light coming from a distant object seem to come from the point P, and are therefore focussed exactly on the retina. Therefore distant objects are seen clearly by the corrected myopic eye

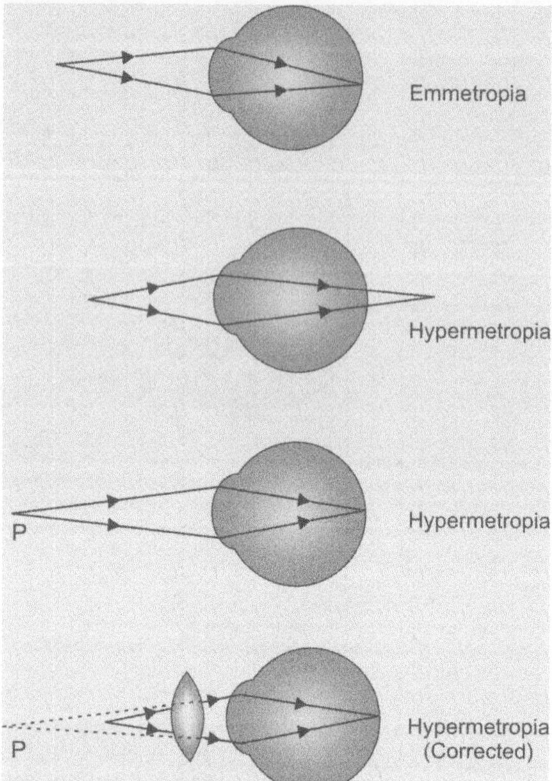

Fig. 15.28 Hypermetropia. In a normal eye (emmetropic), accommodation ensures that rays of light coming from a near object are focussed exactly on the retina. In hypermetropia, which may be due to a weak lens, such rays of light are focussed behind the retina. But, rays of light coming from objects at a distant point P, or farther away than that, are focussed exactly on the retina, and therefore such objects are seen clearly. If an appropriate convex lens is placed in front of the hypermetropic eye, rays of light from a near object seem to come from the point P, and are therefore focussed exactly on the retina. Therefore near objects are seen clearly by the corrected hypermetropic eye

muscles. As a result, accommodation, which involves an increase in dioptic power of the eye, is inadequate. Since the lens does not become as convex as it should when the person is trying to look at a near object, the net effect is as if the dioptic power of the eye is deficient, or similar to hypermetropia. Hence this error is also corrected by use of appropriate convex lenses whenever the person has to see a near object, as during reading.

4. *Astigmatism:* This error is due to lack of uniformity of refracting power of the eye in different planes. The error can be corrected by using appropriate cylindrical lenses.

The capacity of man-made lenses to supplement the lens system of the eye to achieve perfection is an excellent example of what doctors do so frequently: they mimic nature to assist nature correct itself.

Retinal Function

Retina has the receptors of the eye. Receptors transduce visual stimuli into changes in electrical potential. Retina also has neurons which can process the transduced stimuli. The processed signals are transmitted to the brain.

Structure of the Retina

Retina consists of several layers of cells which have been shown in a simplified form in Figure 15.29. The number of rods is about 20 times the number of cones. But the central retina has more cones than rods. At the fovea centralis, cones are the only type of receptors. Rods provide some vision in dim light, while cones provide high acuity vision in bright light and also detect color. The differences between the peripheral and central retina have been enumerated in Table 15.2. The structure of rods and cones has been shown in Figure 15.30.

Rods and cones communicate their message to bipolar cells. Bipolar cells, in turn, pass on the message to ganglion cells. The axons of ganglion cells form the optic nerve.

Excitation of Retina

Retina is excited when light reaches the rods and cones. Light brings about a chemical change in the pigment present in the outer segment of rods and cones. The pigment in rods is rhodopsin. Cone pigment is of three types, and accordingly there are three types of cones. Rhodopsin and the three cone pigments differ primarily in the wavelength of light to which they are maximally sensitive. But the basic

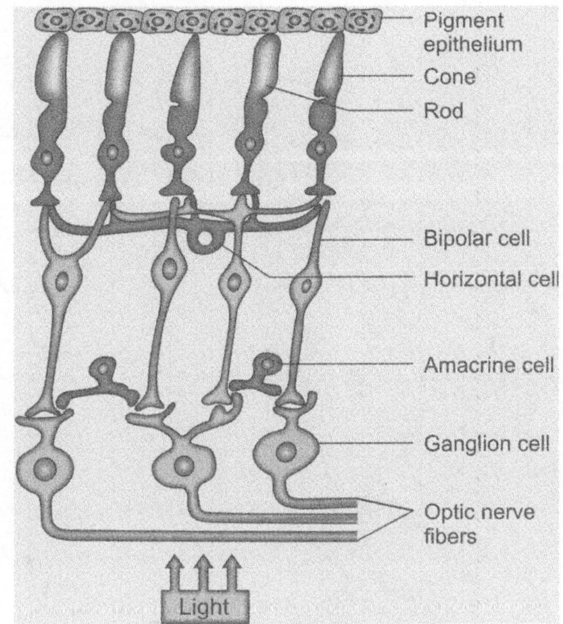

Fig. 15.29 Schematic diagram of the structure of the retina. Note that the chain essentially consists of rods/cones, bipolar cells and ganglion cells. Horizontal cells and amacrine cells possibly achieve horizontal integration of information

Table 15.2 Difference between peripheral and central retina

Peripheral retina	*Central retina*
1. Receptors are mainly rods (diameter, 2-5 microns) and some cones (diameter, 5-8 microns).	Receptors are mainly cones (diameter, 1.5 microns) and some rods. At the fovea, there are no rods
2. Light passes through ganglion and bipolar cells before reaching the receptors	Ganglion and bipolar cells pushed aside to reduce barriers between light and receptors. At the fovea, the displacement is so complete that light reaches the cones directly
3. Marked convergence, resulting in large receptive fields for bipolar and ganglion cells	Convergence much less, resulting in small receptive fields for bipolar and ganglion cells
4. Sensitivity to light high, but visual acuity low	Sensitivity to light low, but visual acuity high

reactions are the same for all pigments. Rhodopsin has been used for illustrating the reactions in Figure 15.31. Retinal is a vitamin A derivative, while opsin is a protein. Light breaks down the pigment, and hence reduces its quantity in the rods and cones. The pigment is resynthesized in darkness.

When a person has stayed in bright light for a long time, almost all the rhodopsin in his rods is in the decomposed state. Secondly, the rods, like other receptors, undergo adaptation. Therefore, if this person now enters a darkroom, he can see almost nothing. But gradually he can see even in the dark. The phenomenon is called **dark adaptation**. Most of us have experienced dark adaptation upon entering a dark cinema hall. Dark adaptation has two distinct phases (Fig. 15.32). The first phase is rapid. During this phase, there is a small improvement in vision within ten minutes. This phase is neural in origin. Rods, which had adapted to a prolonged strong stimulus get 'deadapted', or recover their sensitivity. The second phase is slow. During this phase, there is a marked improvement in vision in about one hour. This phase is chemical in origin. During this phase, rhodopsin is resynthesized. Since retinal is a vitamin A derivative, replenishment of rhodopsin may be inadequate in vitamin A deficiency. Hence impaired dark adaptation is one of the earliest symptoms of vitamin A deficiency.

Transduction: Activation of visual pigments by light leads to a change in the membrane potential of the visual receptors (rods and cones). Visual receptors are unique in undergoing hyperpolarization when stimulated. This hyperpolarization response has all the features of a receptor potential. Rods and cones release a neurotransmitter (glutamate) at rest. The light stimulus, and the resulting hyperpolarization, leads to a decrease in the rate of release of the neurotransmitter (Fig. 15.33).

Signal processing: A visual stimulus leads to a change in the amount of neurotransmitter released by visual receptors. Change in the amount of neurotransmitter released leads to a change in the activity of bipolar cells, which in turn affects the activity of ganglion cells. Bipolar and ganglion cells do not simply transmit

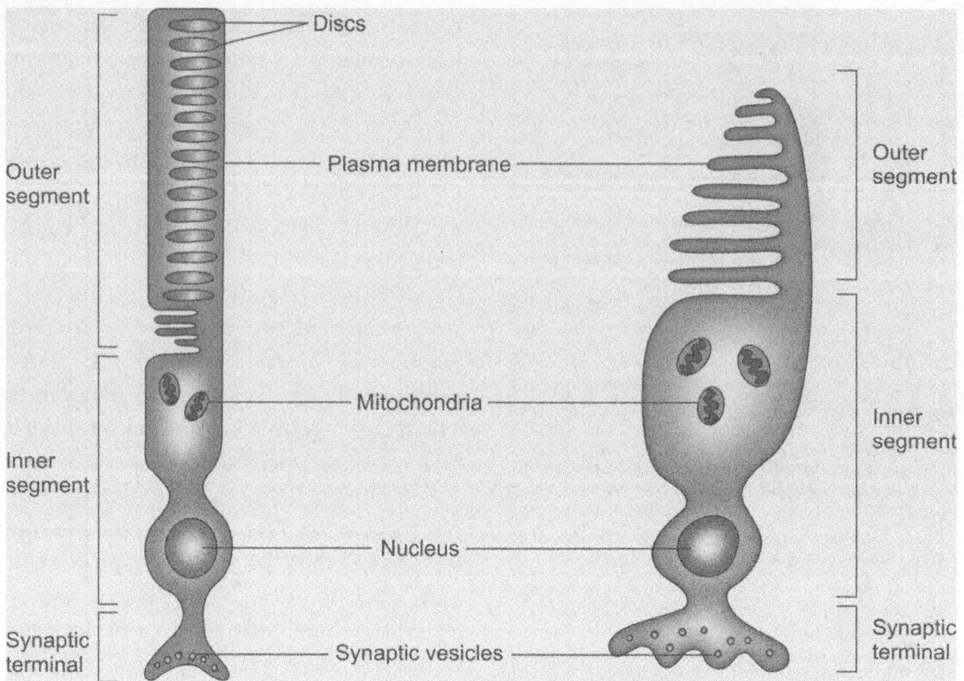

Fig. 15.30 Structure of rods and cones

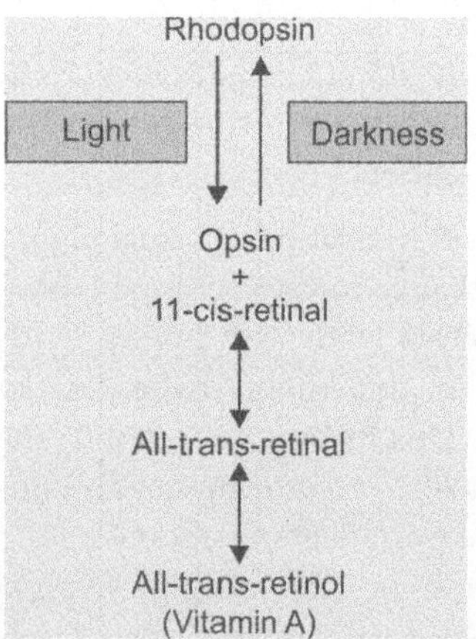

Fig. 15.31 Photochemical reactions involved in stimulation of visual receptors and regeneration of the visual pigment, rhodopsin

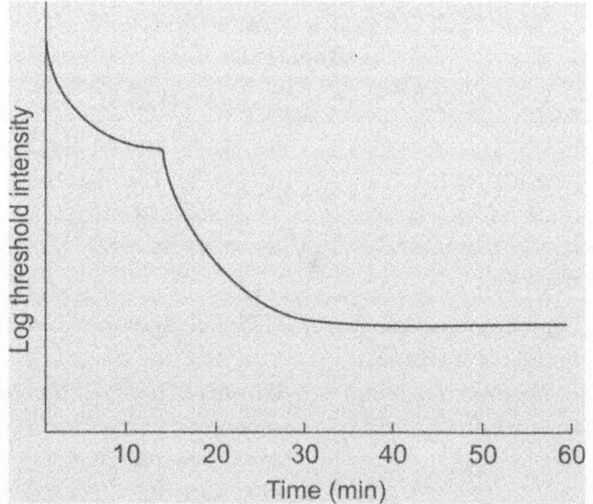

Fig. 15.32 Time course of dark adaptation. The threshold for visual perception declines in two phases after a person is exposed to darkness

the signal generated by the visual receptors; they also process the signal. As a result, impulses carried by the optic nerve fibers undergo maximum change in response to a visual stimulus characterized by contrast. That is perhaps the reason why we can appreciate the borders of objects much better than the objects. This is useful because appreciation of borders is more important for perception of form as well as movement.

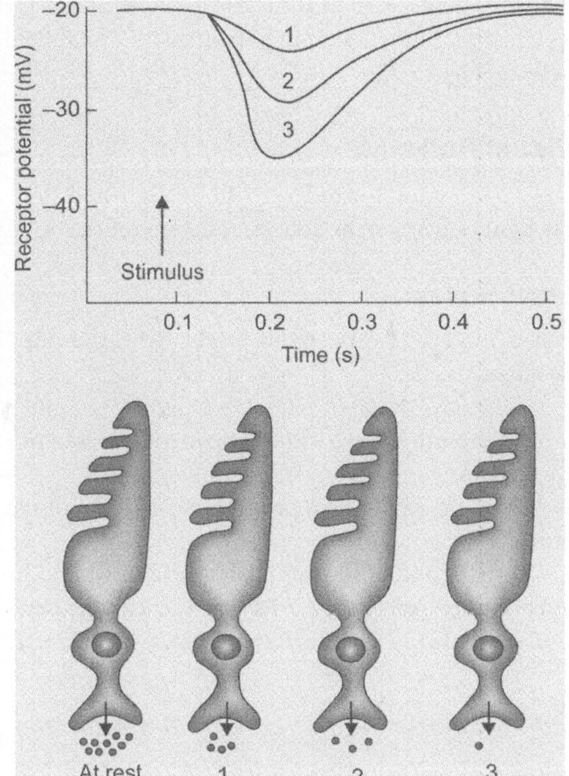

Fig. 15.33 Activation of photoreceptors. (Above) The resting membrane potential of photoreceptors is about –20 mV. Application of a stimulus, such as a flash of light, results in hyperpolarization, the magnitude of which is proportional to the intensity of the stimulus. 1, 2 and 3 represent responses to progressively stronger stimuli. (Below) A 'resting' photoreceptor (rod or cone) releases its neurotransmitter at a certain steady rate. A stimulus, such as a flash of light, reduces the rate of release of the neurotransmitter. 1, 2 and 3 represent responses to progressively stronger stimuli

Visual Pathways

The visual message travels from the eyes towards the brain in the optic nerves.

The two optic nerves converge and meet at the optic chiasma. From the optic chiasma, the visual fibers again emerge in two groups known as the optic tracts. If we look at the distribution of fibers in the optic nerves and optic tracts, we find that an orderly rearrangement of optic nerve fibers takes place in the optic chiasma. The fibers of the optic nerve originating in the temporal half of the retina continue in the optic tract on the same side. But optic nerve fibers originating in the nasal half of the retina cross over to the contralateral optic tract. The result is that information from the right visual field travels in the left optic tract, and *vice versa* (Fig. 15.34). The situation is similar to that in case of other sensory modalities where too, in general, the right side of the body sends information to the left side of the brain.

The two optic tracts give some collaterals to superior colliculi, pretectal area and the hypothalamus. But the major destination of each optic tract is the lateral geniculate nucleus (LGN) of the thalamus.

The chief efferent tracts originating in the superior colliculi are the tectospinal and tectopontine tracts. The superior colliculi are the integrating centers for the head and neck movements associated

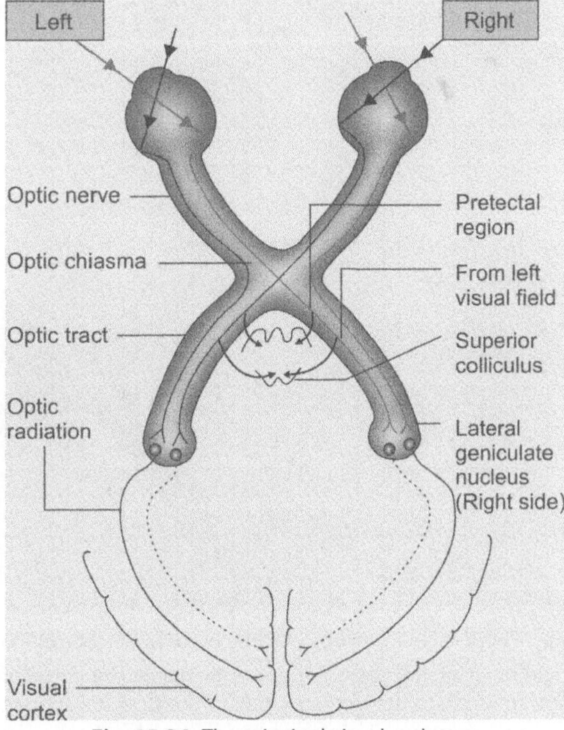

Fig. 15.34 The principal visual pathways

with visual stimuli (e.g. when you turn your head to see something interesting). These head and neck movements are executed via the tectospinal tract. The tectopontine tracts project to the cerebellum where visual information is added to proprioceptive information to achieve better motor control.

Let us now resume the journey of the conscious visual pathway from the LGN onwards. LGN neurons fan out to form the optic radiation which terminates in the visual cortex. The primary visual cortex (or Brodmann's area 17) is in the occipital lobe. The areas surrounding it (areas 18 and 19) are the visual association areas. Although the visual cortex is a long distance away from the retina, the journey is very orderly indeed. There is a clear retinotopic organization in the LGN as well as visual cortex. Not only is the organization retinotopic, the central portions of the retina have a much bigger representation in the LGN as well as cortex than the peripheral portions. Detailed knowledge of the retinotopic map at different levels is useful for localization of the lesion in patients with visual field defects (Fig. 15.35).

Visual Reflexes

Only two important reflexes will be discussed here: the light reflex and the accommodation reflex.

Light Reflex

When the eye is exposed to bright light, the pupil becomes smaller.

Clinically, the light relex is elicited by shining a torch light into the eye while the patient is seated in a dark room.

The light results in a prompt constriction of the pupil.

Constriction of the pupil of the eye in which the light is shone is called the *direct* light reflex. The pupil constricts also in the other eye which is not directly

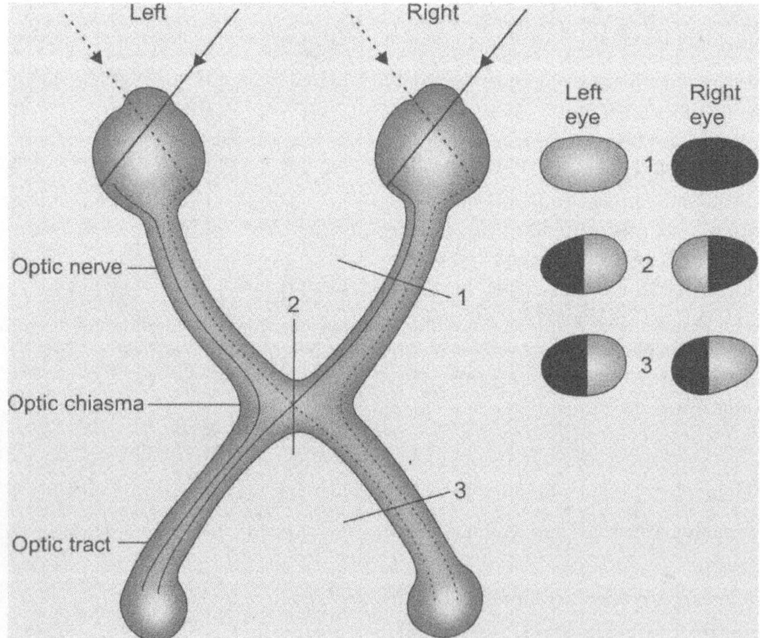

Fig. 15.35 Schematic diagram to show how the site of lesion may be deduced from the nature of the defect in the field of vision. (1) Lesion of the optic nerve: the corresponding eye is blind; (2) Lesion of the optic chiasma: there is loss of vision in the temporal half of the field of vision in both eyes (bitemporal hemianopia); (3) Lesion of the optic tract: there is loss of vision in the controlateral half of the field of vision in both eyes (homonymous hemianopia)

stimulated by light; this is called the *consensual* light reflex.

Both the direct and consensual light reflexes can be understood in light of the pathays involved (Fig. 15.36). The collaterals from the optic tract to the superior colliculi and pretectal area are given off to both sides from either tract. After processing in these midbrain centers, the efferents originate in the parasympathetic part of the oculomotor nucleus (Edinger–Westphal nucleus).

Preganglionic neurons from the Edinger–Westphal nucleus project to the ciliary ganglion, from where postganglionic fibers travel to the sphincter pupillae. That is how stimulation by bright light results in constriction of the pupil.

Accommodation Reflex

When we shift our attention from a distant object to a near object, there is a reflex increase in the dioptic power of the lens, constriction of the pupil, and covergence of the two eyes. The phenomenon is called accommodation reflex. The response has three

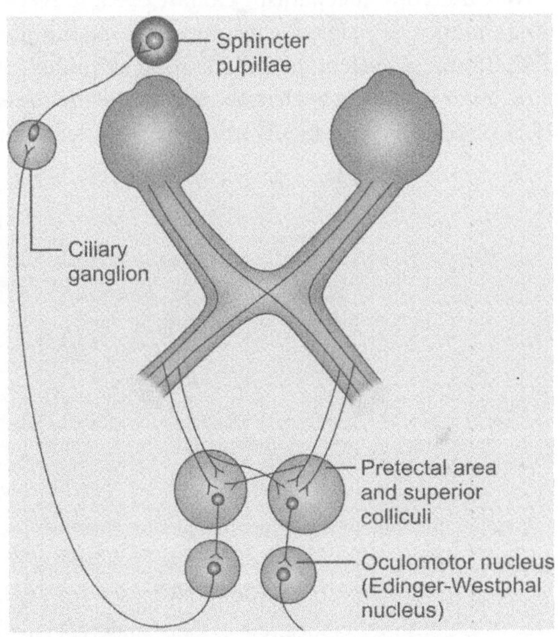

Fig. 15.36 Pathway for the light reflex

components, and all three help in better appreciation of the near object.

It is easy to understand from the principles of optics how a change in the dioptic power of the lens will help in forming a clear image of the near object.

Suppose the distant object is at infinity, the distance between the dioptic apparatus and the retina is v, and the focal length of the dioptic apparatus is f_1 and its power D_1.

Then $$\frac{1}{\infty} + \frac{1}{v} = \frac{1}{f_1}$$

or $$\frac{1}{v} = \frac{1}{f_1}$$

or $$\frac{1}{v} = D_1 \ldots\ldots\ldots\ldots\ldots \text{(i)}$$

Suppose accommodation involves visualizing an object at a distance of 25 cm (0.25 m) from the eye, and a change in focal length to f_2 or the dioptic power to D_2.

Then

$$\frac{1}{0.25} + \frac{1}{v} = \frac{1}{f_2}$$

Substituting the value of 1/v from (i),

or $$\frac{1}{0.25} + D_1 = D_2$$

$$= D_1 + 4 \text{ Diopters}$$

Thus an increase of 4 diopters is required in the convergence power of the eye when the attention is shifted from a distant object to an object at a distance of 25 cm. Children have a capacity to increase the dioptic power of the eye by more than 10 D. But the capacity declines with age. That is why presbyopia is universal after the age of about 40 years.

Increase in the dioptric power of the lens during accommodation is due to a change in the shape of the lens. The lens of the accommodated eye is more globular (see Fig. 15.25).

The neural pathways responsible for the accommodation reflex involve the cerebral cortex. This is so because the decision to focus on a near object is a conscious decision. The efferent fibers arise in the oculomotor nerve nucleus and supply the ciliary muscle, sphincter pupillae muscle and medial rectus muscle. Contraction of the three sets of muscles is responsible for the three components of the accommodation reflex.

Argyll Robertson Pupil

In neurological lesions around the cerebral aqueduct at the level of the superior colliculi, the fibers mediating light reflex are damaged. Such lesions may be seen in neurosyphilis, but are rare now because syphilis can be treated effectively at an early stage these days. However, if such a lesion is present, light reflex is absent. However, since accommodation reflex involves the cortex rather than superior colliculi, accommodation reflex is still present. This condition in which light reflex is absent but accommodation reflex is present is called Argyll Robertson pupil. In this condition, the pupil constricts in response to accommodation but not in response to light.

Eye Movements

Each eyeball has six muscles of the voluntary variety attached to it on the outer surface. These muscles, called extraocular muscles, can move the eyes in different directions. The muscles, their innervation and actions have been shown in Table 15.3.

Table 15.3 Extraocular muscles

Muscle	*Innervation (Cranial nerve)*	*Action*
Medial rectus	III	Adduction
Lateral rectus	VI	Abduction
Superior rectus	III	Upward movement with adduction and intorsion
Inferior rectus	III	Downward movement with adduction and extorsion
Superior oblique	IV	Intorsion, abduction and downward movement
Inferior oblique	III	Extorsion, abduction and upward movement

Visual Perception

The visual message is processed into a more and more elaborate form at successive levels of the visual pathway (Fig. 15.34) till finally it is perceived at the cortical level. Peception involves awareness of the stimulus and its attributes such as form, color, movement and depth.

Color Vision

A partial but clear basis for color vision lies in the three types of cones. The three types of pigments present in the three types of cones have different absorption spectra (Fig. 15.37). The peak absorption of the three pigments is at the wavelengths of 420 nm (blue), 530 nm (green) and 560 nm (red) respectively. Since there is considerable overlap between the absorption spectra of the three pigments, most colors would affect at least two, if not all the three types of cones. The color perceived depends on the ratio of excitation of the three types of cones. In this way, hundreds of different patterns of excitation are possible, and hence a very large number of colors can be distinguished from one another.

But the cone mechanism cannot explain everything about color vision. For example, a weak stimulus of optimum wavelength, or a strong stimulus of some other suitable wavelength, may excite the same set of cones. Such problems are sorted out by color

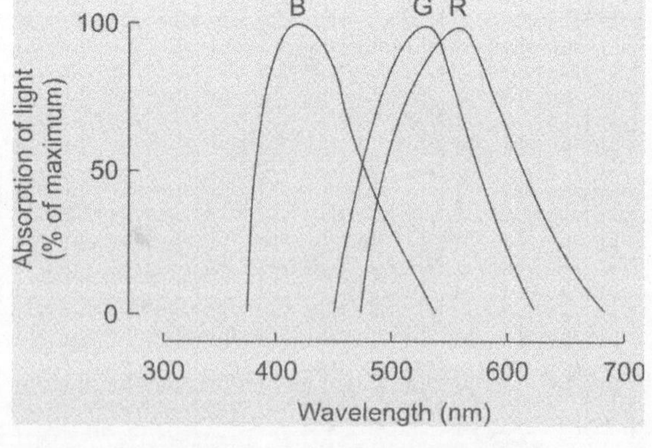

Fig. 15.37 Absorption spectrum of the pigments of blue (B), green (G) and red (R) cones

sensitive cells among the ganglion cells, LGN cells and cortical cells.

Color Blindness

Total color blindness is extremely rare. But some degree of genetically inherited color blindness affects about 10 percent of males. There are three broad categories of genetic color blindness.

1. *Trichromats:* A normal person whose color vision is based on three types of cones is also called a trichromat. But there are some trichromats with color weakness in whom one type of cones are fewer or defective. If the deficiency is that of 'red cones', the defect is called *protanomaly*, if that of 'green cones', it is called *deuteranomaly*, and if that of 'blue cones', it is called *tritanomaly*. Such individuals make minor mistakes in color identification. The mistakes may become serious if the individual happens to be an engine driver or a pilot, and is operating under bad weather conditions.
2. *Dichromats:* Dichromats have only two type of cones in the retina. Depending on whether the 'red', 'green' or 'blue cones' are absent, the condition is called protanopia, deuteranopia, or tritanopia respectively. Such individuals make gross mistakes in identification of colors.
3. *Monochromats:* Monochromats have only one type of cones. Such individuals are totally color blind. Fortunately this defect is very rare.

Color blindness affects males but it is almost absent in females. This is because the genes for 'red' and 'green cones' are recessive and are present on the X chromosome. That is why females, with two X chromosomes, are generally only the carriers of the defect. The gene for 'blue cones' is, however, present on an autosome. The most common form of color blindness is deuteranomaly, which affects about 5 percent of the males.

HEARING

The organ of hearing is the ear. The ear has one more function, viz. maintenance of balance, about which we shall talk in Chapter 16. The quality of a sound stimulus is measured in terms of its intensity and frequency. The intensity of sound is measured in decibels (dB). The intensity of some familiar sounds is given in Figure 15.38 to help you form a mental picture of what a sound of 40 dB or 80 dB means. The frequency of sound corresponds roughly to its pitch. It is measured in cycles per second, or Hertz (Hz). The human ear can detect sounds having frequencies between 20 and 20,000 Hz. But most of the common sounds that we hear fall between 200 and 4,500 Hz.

The visible part of the ear is only a part of what is called the external ear. The other parts of the ear are the middle ear and inner ear (Fig. 15.39).

The External Ear

The visible part of the external ear is called the **pinna**. It is commonly thought to collect the sound waves and funnel them into the ear canal. But at least in human beings, where the pinna is rather small, it is unlikely that this function is significant. Sound is conveyed from the pinna to the ear drum by the **ear canal**. The peak resonance frequency of the ear canal is 2000-5000 Hz. Therefore sounds in this frequency range get a boost of about 15 dB while passing through the ear canal. Since most of the audible sounds belong to this frequency range, the ear canal not only conveys sound but also magnifies it.

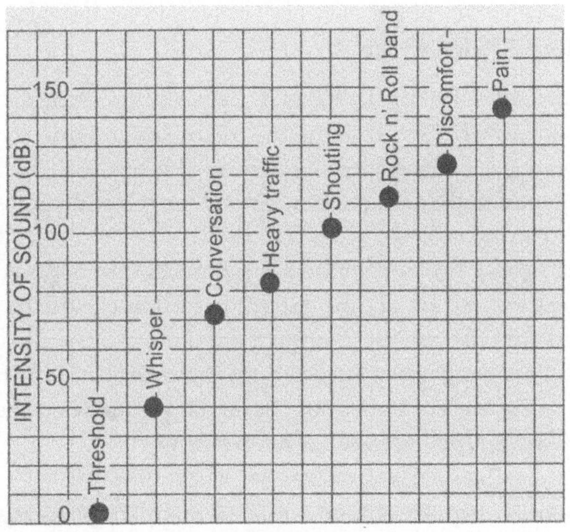

Fig. 15.38 Intensity of a few familiar sounds, and the intensity of sound which evokes discomfort or pain in the ear

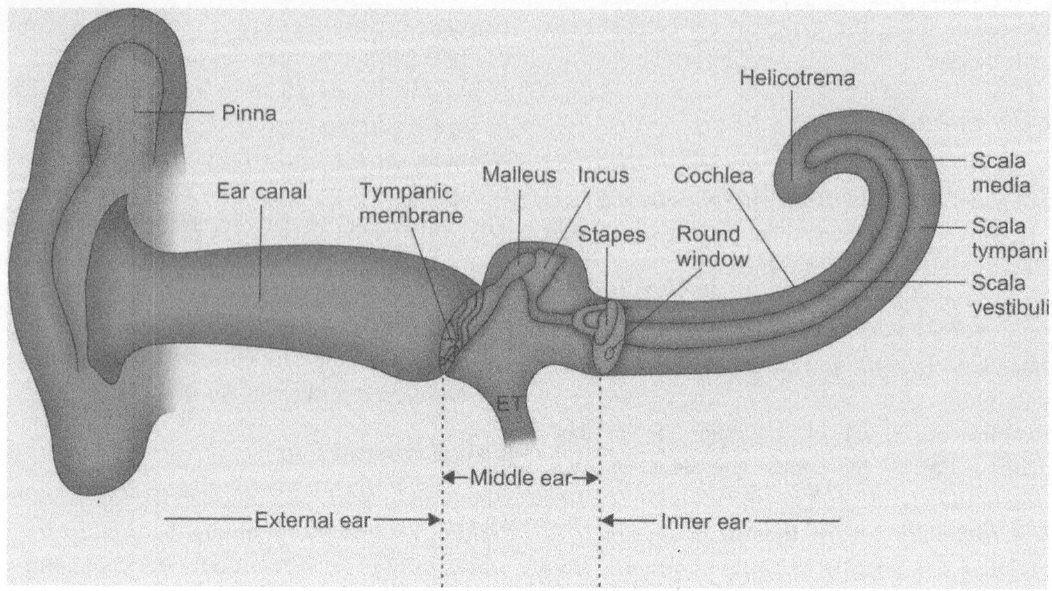

Fig. 15.39 The external, middle and inner ear. ET, eustachian tube

The ear drum, or **tympanic membrane**, separates the external ear from the middle ear. As a result of sounds conveyed by the ear canal, the tympanic membrane is thrown into tiny vibrations. The sensitivity of the ear may be imagined from the fact that threshold sounds produce in the tympanic membrane a movement of only 10^{-8} mm.

The Middle Ear

The middle ear is located between the external and inner ear. It contains three interconnected bones, called ossicles, named on the basis of their shapes: **malleus** (hammer), **incus** (anvil) and **stapes** (stirrup).[4]

These bones provide a mechanical link between the eardrum and the inner ear. The middle ear also has two minute muscles, tensor tympani and stapedius. Tensor tympani is supplied by the trigeminal (fifth cranial) nerve. Stapedius, the smallest muscle in the body, is supplied by the seventh cranial (facial) nerve.

[4]Anvil is the platform on which an ironsmith beats the iron. Stirrup is the characteristic piece of iron on which a horse rider rests his foot.

The middle ear cavity is connected to the pharynx by the eustachian tube. The major function of the middle ear is to transmit the disturbance caused by movements of the tympanic membrane to the inner ear. However, it is more than simple transmission. The external and middle ear contain air, whereas the inner ear contains fluids. Fluids offer much greater impedance (which is comparable to resistance) to sound than air. The middle ear amplifies the pressure of the sound waves which it transmits, so that the inner ear can be stimulated in spite of its higher impedance. That is why the middle ear is said to match the impedance of the external ear to that of the middle ear.

Now let us see how the middle ear magnifies the pressure of the sound stimulus. The area of the tympanic membrane is about 200 times the area of the footplate of stapes. Since force = pressure × area, when a sound impinging on the tympanic membrane with a given force is transmitted to the stapes, its pressure is much higher at the stapes. And, the ability of the stimulus to move the cochlear fluid depends on the pressure rather than force. This fact may be visualized from a simple analogy. A person lying down on sand does not sink as deep as when standing on sand. This is so because although the force is the same in both cases, while standing the force is exerted over a much smaller area and hence the pressure is much higher.

Besides impedance matching, the middle ear also has some other functions. The tensor tympani and stapedius muscles possibly play a role in protecting the ear from the damaging effects of very loud sounds, and in protecting our mind from the disturbing effects of our own voice. Stimulation of the ear by intense sounds produces contraction of the stapedius and tensor tympani muscles; this is known as the **acoustic reflex.** Stapedius pulls the stapes medially while the tensor tympani pulls the malleus anteromedially. The overall effect of the actions of these muscles is to press the ossicles against one another, thereby increasing the rigidity of the ossicular lever system. That makes the system more stable while at the same time reducing the efficiency with which the sound signal would be transmitted to the inner ear. The protective effect of the acoustic reflex is, however, doubtful. The reflex is too slow to be useful in protecting the ear from damage due to loud sounds. Further, the ear is rarely exposed to sounds loud enough to evoke the reflex. A more likely benefit of the reflex is attenuation of internal sounds. Acoustic reflex attenuates low frequency sounds the best, and most of the internal sounds have low frequencies. Attenuation of internal sounds would reduce their masking effect, thereby improving the sensitivity of the ear to external sounds which need to be heard.

At this juncture, it is pertinent to introduce the eustachian tube which joins the middle ear to the nasopharynx. This tube is about 4 cm long, and its diameter is three times larger at its middle ear opening than at its nasopharyngeal opening. In fact, the nasopharyngeal end of the tube is normally closed, and opens only during swallowing, yawning, sneezing or shouting. The opening up of the tube particularly during swallowing serves to keep the middle ear pressure equal to the pressure in the nasopharynx, which in turn is equal to the atmospheric pressure. The presssure in the external ear is also, quite obviously, equal to the atmospheric pressure. Thus the eustachian tube keeps the pressure on the two sides of the tympanic membrane equal. This is important to prevent the tympanic membrane from bulging on either side. Bulging would impair its function, and bulging beyond a certain limit could damage the tympanic membrane. Another function of the eustachian tube is to prevent any fluid from collecting in the middle ear. It drains the fluid into the nasopharynx. If this drainage mechanism was absent, any fluid collecting as a result of inflammation or extravasation would tear through the tympanic membrane.

The Inner Ear

The inner ear consists of two parts : one concerned with equilibrium, the **vestibule**; and another concerned with hearing, the **cochlea**. The delicate neural structures constituting the vestibule and cochlea are called the membranous labyrinth. The membranous labyrinth is encased in a closely fitting bony shell called the bony labyrinth. The membranous labyrinth is separated from the bony labyrinth by a fluid known as the **perilymph**.

The cochlea is lodged in the hardest bone of the body, the temporal bone. The bony shell of the cochlea resembles a snail, and consists of two and a half turns. The cochlea is a tubular structure coiled in the same manner as its bony shell. The cochlear tube is divided along its length into three compartments: **scala vestibuli, scala media** and **scala tympani** (Figs 15.39 and 15.40). Scala media is an independent compartment throughout the length of the cochlea. But scala vestibuli and scala tympani communicate with each other at the apex of the cochlea through an opening known as the **helicotrema**. Scala media is separated from the scala vestibuli by the Reissner's membrane and from the scala tympani by the basilar membrane. Scala vestibuli and scala tympani contain a fluid known as the **perilimph**, which resembles the extracellular fluid elsewhere in having a high sodium and low potassium concentration. As noted earlier, perilymph is also present between the bony and

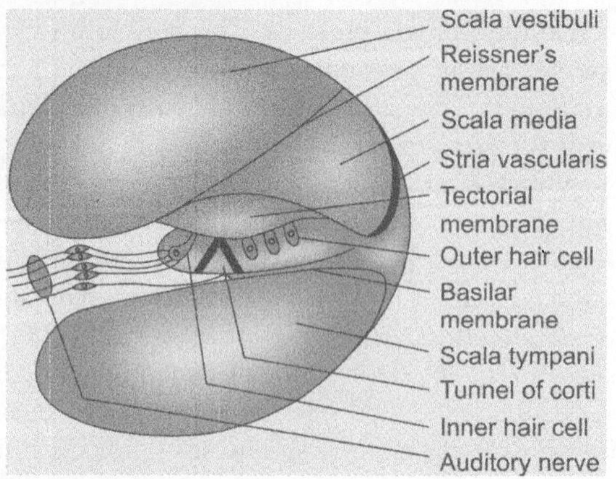

Fig. 15.40 Schematic representation of a cross section of the cochlea showing its three major compartments

membranous labyrinth. Perilymph appears to be a filtrate formed under capiliary pressure. Scala media or the cochlear duct contains another fluid known as the **endolymph**, which has a high potassium and low sodium concentration. The origin of endolymph is not fully understood. But **stria vascularis**, a highly vascular structure along the outer side of the cochlear duct, seems to play an important role in maintaining the high potassium concentration of endolymph.

The sensory cells responsible for hearing are located on the basilar membrane within a structure known as the **organ of Corti**. The organ of Corti is partitioned by two rows of peculiar shaped cells known as pillar cells. The pillar cells enclose the tunnel of Corti. Outside the tunnel, on its outer side are three rows of **outer hair cells** (OHC), and on its inner side is a single row of **inner hair cells** (IHC). Interspersed between hair cells are also some supporting cells. The hair cells and supporting cells are connected to one another at their apices by tight junctions forming a surface known as the **reticular lamina**. The hair of the hair cells seem to project out of the reticular lamina. Overlying the hair is an acellular flap called the **tectorial membrane**. The tectorial membrane consists of fibrils embedded in a gelatinous matrix. The fluid in the space between the tectorial membrane and reticular lamina is endolymph. Thus endolymph bathes the stereocilia of hair cells. But the body of the hair cells, which lies below the reticular lamina, is bathed by perilymph. Hence there is a potential difference between the upper and lower surfaces of reticular lamina. The importance of this difference in transduction will be discussed later.

Ultrastructure of Hair Cells

OHC are test-tube shaped while IHC are flask shaped. At the apex, both bear the fibrous cuticular plate from which project neatly arranged stereocilia. The OHC have three rows of stereocilia arranged like a W. The three rows of cilia are neatly graded in length. The tips of the tallest cilia are attached to the underside of the tectorial membrane. The IHC have three or more rows of stereocilia arranged linearly. There is no evidence that any of the IHC cilia are attached to the tectorial membrane (Fig. 15.41).

Rows of cilia on a hair cell are linked laterally. The tips of short cilia are attached to the sides of adjacent long cilia by structures bearing the vividly descriptive name, tip-to-side links (Fig. 15.42).

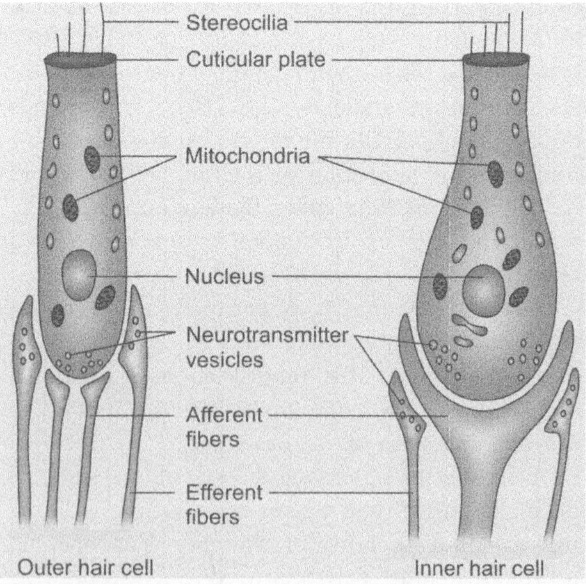

Fig. 15.41 Ultrastructure of auditory receptors, the outer and inner hair cells

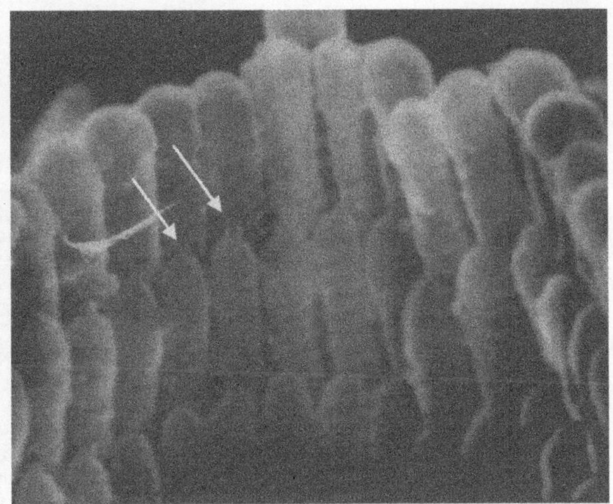

Fig. 15.42 Scanning electron microscopic view of the stereocilia seen from the top. Observe the tip-to-side links indicated by the arrows. (Reproduced, with permission, from Scott-Brown's Otolaryngology, Volume 1, 5th edition, 1987, Fig. 2.14, p. 68, Courtesy: Butterworth-Heinemann, Surrey, UK)

Innervation of the Cochlea

The cochlea is innervated by the cochlear nerve, which is a part of the VIIIth cranial nerve. The signals generated in hair cells are transmitted to the central nervous system by *afferent* nerve fibers.

Besides afferent nerve fibers, the hair cells are also innervated by *efferent* fibers which originate in the superior olivary complex and travel to the cochlea in the olivocochlear bundle.

Function of the Inner Ear

We left middle ear function at the point where the sound stimulus results in movement of the stapes. The footplate of the stapes is adjacent to the oval window of the inner ear. The stapes footplate moves in and out like a piston in response to sound stimuli. Since the footplate is adjacent to the oval window of the inner ear, its movements produce pressure variations in cochlear fluids. These variations result in movements of the basilar membrane (BM). Since the organ of Corti rests on the BM, movements of the BM result in movements of hair cells. Hair cell movement displaces their stereocilia, which in turn, enhances or depresses hair cell excitability. Altered excitability of hair cells is conveyed by afferent nerve fibers to the central nervous system (Fig. 15.43). In short, the inner ear transducts a vibratory stimulus into a form suitable for the central nervous system. But the inner ear is more than a transducer. It also performs a preliminary analysis of the sound stimulus in terms of its frequency and amplitude characteristics. The BM plays an important role in this analysis, specially the frequency analysis. We shall first examine this role of the BM in some detail before going into the hair cell function.

Basilar membrane function: If we look at the entire length of the BM, we observe a graded change in its physical characteristics as we proceed from the base (near the stapes) to the apex (near the helicotrema). The differences between the two ends of the BM may be summarized as follows:

Base	**Apex**
Narrow	Wide
Thick	Thin
Stiff	Relatively flaccid

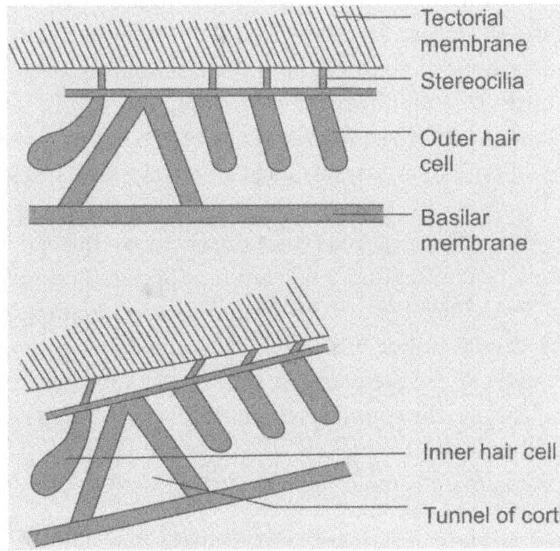

Fig. 15.43 Schematic diagram showing how movements of the basilar membrane result in displacement of stereocilia of the hair cells

Try to form a mental picture of a series of coupled resonators with the above gradation. Even if you are not very familiar with musical instruments, you would be able to imagine that high frequency pressure oscillations would make the base of the BM vibrate most strongly while low frequencies would affect the apical regions most strongly. A series of observations have confirmed these theoretical predictions. High frequency sounds make the BM oscillate mainly near the base of the cochlea. On the other hand, low frequency sounds trigger oscillations in the BM which extend right upto the apical region, where the oscillations are also the maximum. The fact that a specific region of the BM responds maximally to a specific stimulus frequency is spoken of as *tuning* of the BM. The pattern of vibration of the BM is also worth noticing. Every stimulus, irrespective of its frequency, triggers waveform motion at the base. The amplitude of movement increases till the wave reaches the spot on the BM which is best tuned for the frequency of the stimulus. After that, the vibratory wave dies down rather abruptly. The pattern for a few frequencies has been shown in Figure 15.44. It would be observed that each stimulus affects maximally a specific region, and to some extent also the regions tuned for frequencies higher than that of the stimulus,. Thus low frequency sounds affect a much longer length of the BM than high frequency sounds. The vibratory wave affecting the BM is also called a travelling wave. A series of travelling waves in response to a stimulus form an envelope as shown in Figure 15.45.

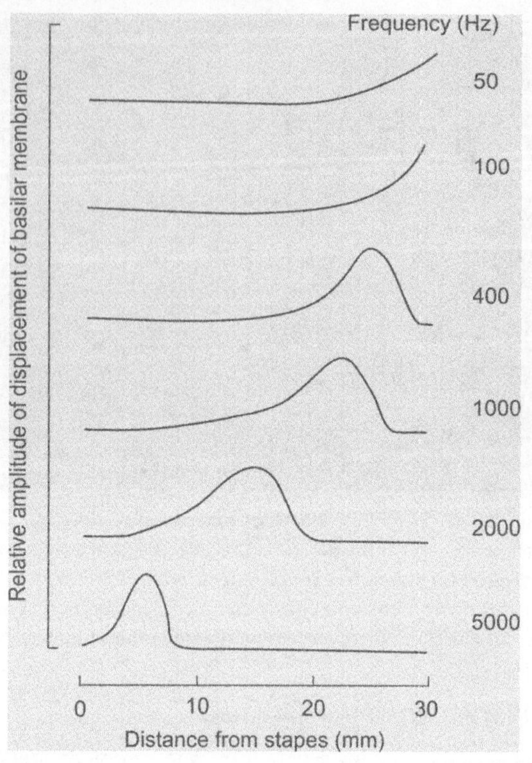

Fig. 15.44 Relative amplitude of displacement and pattern of vibration of the basilar membrane in response to sound stimuli of different frequencies

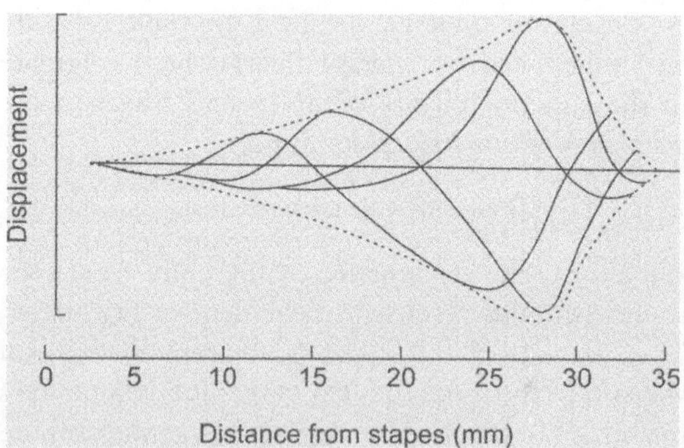

Fig. 15.45 A series of travelling waves in the basilar membrane form an envelope. The pattern depicted in the figure is in response to a sound stimulus of about 400 Hz

BM vibrations were first observed by Bekesy in human cadavers and a few animal species. Recently, the sound level (in dB) required to give a constant BM displacement has been determined for sounds of varying frequencies. If the results are plotted graphically, the sound level required shows a marked decline at the frequency to which the spot on BM being studied is most sensitive (Fig. 15.46).

Hair cell function: It was mentioned earlier that BM movement moves the hair cells, which displaces the stereocilia, which in turn generates an electrical signal in the hair cells. This is no longer just a conjecture. It is possible to culture hair cells in an organ culture medium. Stereocilia of these cultured hair cells are not shielded by the tectorial membrane. Experiments

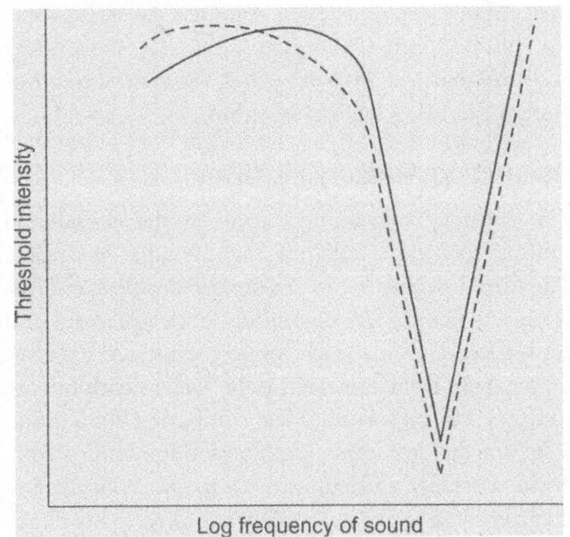

Fig. 15.46 Threshold sound intensity required to give a certain constant displacement of the basilar membrane (continuous line) and to elicit a response in the auditory nerve fibers originating from that area of the basement membrane. (Based on Wilson JP. Br Med Bull 1987;43:821-37)

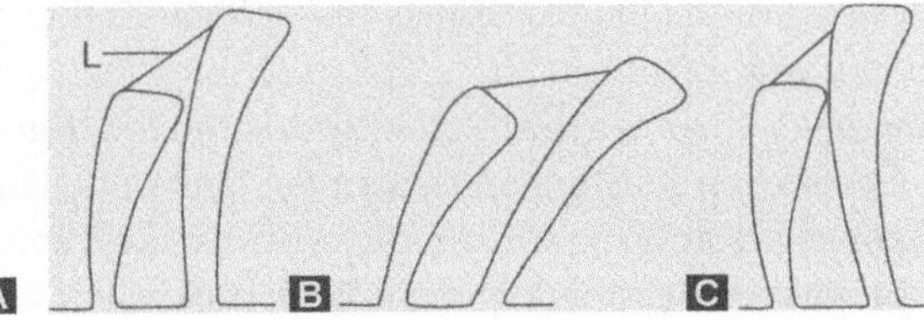

Figs 15.47A to C Hudspeth's model for mechanoelectrical transduction by hair cells. In this diagrammatic illustration, only two adjacent stereocilia are shown, together with their tip-to-side link (L). (A) Resting position, in which part of the time is spent with the ionic gates open, and part with the gates closed; (B) Stereocilia bent in such a way that the fraction of the time spent with the ionic gates open increases, resulting in depolarization; (C) Stereocilia bent in a direction opposite to that in (B). Now the fraction of time spent with the ionic gates open decreases, resulting in hyperpolarization

have been performed in which the sterocilia of such cultured cells have been displaced with the tip of a fine glass probe, and the electrical responses of hair cells recorded simultaneously. Displacement of the stereocilia in cultured mouse cochlea gives an electrical response. Displacement in one direction leads to hypopolarization while displacement in the opposite direction gives hyperpolarization.

It is tempting to enquire how displacement of stereocilia evokes an electrical response in hair cells. A model which explains all these observations has been proposed by Hudspeth (Figs 15.47A to C). According to this model, there are a few regulated ionic gates at the tip of each stereocilium. In the resting position, each gate swings back and forth between its closed and open positions as a result of random molecular motion. It has been estimated that each gate is open about 20 percent of the time. The duration for which a gate is open can be influenced by the position of a transduction linkage which connects a stereocilium to its neighboring stereocilium. Displacement of the stereocilium in a specific direction keeps the channels open for a longer time, leading to depolarization. Displacement in the opposite direction keeps the channels open for a shorter time, leading to hyperpolarization. Electron microscopy has demonstrated that the tip of each stereocilium is linked to the flank of the adjacent longer stereocilium by a fine filament, the tip-to-side link (Fig. 15.42). Although it has not been proven, it is tempting to assume that the linking filament is the anatomical counterpart of the transduction linkage in Hudspeth's model.

In the model of mechanoelectric transduction described above, the ions that move have not been identified. It is believed that open ionic channels are reasonably large and non-selective, so that sodium, potassium and calcium ions can pass through them with equal ease. But the ions that actually pass would depend on the electrochemical gradient. The apical surface of hair cells is surrounded by the endolymph in the scala media, which displays an electrical potential of +80 mV with respect to the perilymph. This positive potential is due to the large concentration of potassium ions in the endolymph. The interior of the hair cells is negative with respect to the peirlymph, the resting level being –45 mV in case of inner hair cells, and –70 mV in case of outer hair cells. Thus the interior of the cells is strongly negative with respect to the endolymph. Hence the opening of the ionic channels results in an influx of potassium ions from the endolymph into the cells, for which there is a marked electrical gradient. Entry of potassium ions hypopolarizes the hair cells. This hypopolarization has the characteristics of a receptor potential. When the hypopolarization of a hair cell reaches a threshold value, it leads to an increase in the frequency of impulses in the auditory nerve fibers innervating it. A neurotransmitter (possibly glutamate) is thought to be involved in transmitting the message from the hair cell to the nerve fibers. Auditory nerve fibers show a finite resting discharge, which makes it possible to carry information about hypopolarization as well as hyperpolarization of hair cells. Hypopolarization tends to increase the frequency of discharge while hyperpolarization tends to decrease it.

To summarize, the inner ear analyzes the sound stimulus as well as transducts it into an electrical signal. The analysis is in terms of frequency and intensity. The frequency of the sound stimulus determines the area on the BM that vibrates the most, which in turn determines the specific hair cells that would be affected the most. Frequency remaining the same, if the intensity of the sound stimulus is increased, the point of maximum vibration of the BM remains the same, but neighboring regions of the BM get involved in the vibration to a greater extent. The greater the vibration of a particular point on the BM, greater is the depolarization of hair cells situated at that point on the BM. More the depolarization of the hair cells, higher is the frequency of discharge of auditory nerve fibers arising from these hair cells. That is how the inner ear sends information to the central nervous system in a reasonably well analyzed form.

Auditory Pathways

There exists a fairly distinct chain of neurons from the hair cells of the cochlea to the cerebral cortex. The path taken by this chain is the ascending auditory pathway. The fact that the path exists does not, however, mean that the whole of it is actually used everytime we receive a sound stimulus. The stimulus may merely evoke a reflex response involving only the brain stem. There exists also a descending auditory pathway through which the central nervous system can influence ear function.

Ascending Auditory Pathway

The auditory nerve fibers relay in the dorsal and ventral cochlear nuclei of the medulla oblongata. The fibers originating in the ventral cochlear nucleus project to the olivary complexes, both ipsilateral and contralateral. Thus each olivary complex receives inputs from both ears. Hence there is, in each olivary complex, an opportunity for comparing the stimuli affecting the two ears. The fibers originating in the dorsal cochlear nucleus project to the contralateral nucleus of the lateral lemniscus. The olivary complexes also project to the nuclei of the lateral lemniscus. From the nuclei of the lateral lemniscus, the auditory tract relays to the inferior colliculus, medial geniculate body of the thalamus, and finally the auditory cortex. The primary auditory cortex is located in Brodmann's areas 41 and 42 in the superior temporal gyrus. Surrounding the primary auditory cortex are auditory association areas, which receive inputs from the primary auditory cortex as well as the thalamus. As seen in Figure 15.48 information from either ear is projected to the auditory cortex on both sides but the projection is heavier on the contralateral side. The main auditory pathway described above gives collaterals along its route by which it interacts with pathways conveying other sensory inputs to the brain.

Each *auditory nerve* fiber innervates one or more hair cells at a specific place on the basilar membrane. Since the place of maximum vibration on the basilar membrane is related to the frequency of the acoustic stimulus, each auditory nerve fiber gets maximally stimulated by a particular frequency. In other words, the threshold stimulus for an auditory nerve fiber varies with the frequency of the stimulus. The graphic representation of the relationship between the threshold stimulus and the frequency of the stimulus for a given auditory nerve fiber is called the tuning curve of the fiber (Fig. 15.49). As seen in the figure, the threshold is minimal for a specific frequency : this

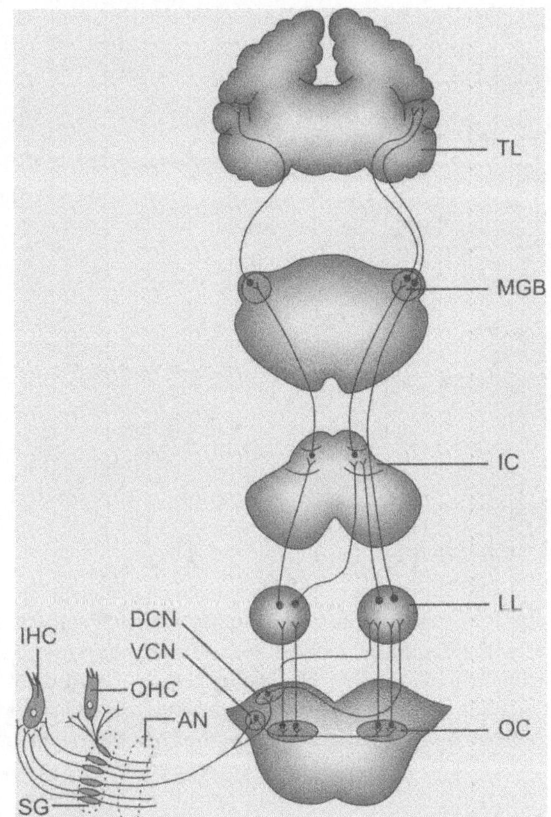

Fig. 15.48 The ascending auditory pathways. Only the major pathways are shown. The collaterals to cerebellum and ascending reticular activating system are not shown. OHC, outer hair cells; IHC, inner hair cells; SG, spiral ganglion; AN, auditory nerve; DCN, dorsal cochlear nucleus; VCN, ventral cochlear nucleus; OC, olivary complex; LL, nucleus of lateral lemniscus; MGB, medial geniculate body; TL, temporal lobe

frequency is known as the characteristic frequency (CF) of the nerve fiber. The threshold rises sharply as the frequency increases above the CF. But at frequencies below the CF, the threshold does not rise so steeply. Can you explain why?[5]

[5]If you consider any point on the basilar membrane, it vibrates maximally in response to a particular frequency, considerably in response to almost all frequencies below it, but not much in response to frequencies even moderately above it (Fig. 15.44). This fact is reflected also in the tuning curves of auditory nerve fibers (Fig. 15.49)

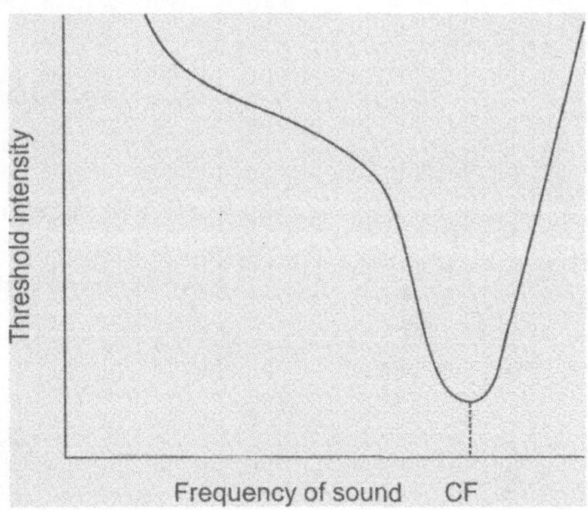

Fig. 15.49 The tuning curve of an auditory nerve fiber, CF, characteristic frequency. Note that the threshold does not rise as steeply for frequencies below CF as for frequencies above it. If you cannot think of the reason for the shape of the curve, read the explanation in the text

Besides frequency, there is also coding of intensity of the acoustic stimulus in the auditory nerve fibers. The intensity is coded by the following mechanisms:

i. As the intensity of acoustic stimulus increases, the frequency of impulses in the auditory nerve fiber(s) stimulated increases (Figs 15.50A and B).
ii. As the intensity of the acoustic stimulus increases, additional auditory nerve fibers are stimulated. Recruitment of additional nerve fibers is brought about by two mechanisms:
   a. As the intensity of the stimulus increases, not only the nerve fiber with a CF matching that of the stimulus but also nerve fibers with neighboring CF are stimulated (Fig. 15.51A).
   b. Different auditory nerve fibers with the same CF also have different threshold. Hence an increase in the intensity of the stimulus brings about recruitment of additional fibers having a CF equal to the frequency of the stimulus (Fig. 15.51B).

The orderly gradation of sensitivity to the frequency of sound seen in the cochlea continues throughout the auditory pathway.

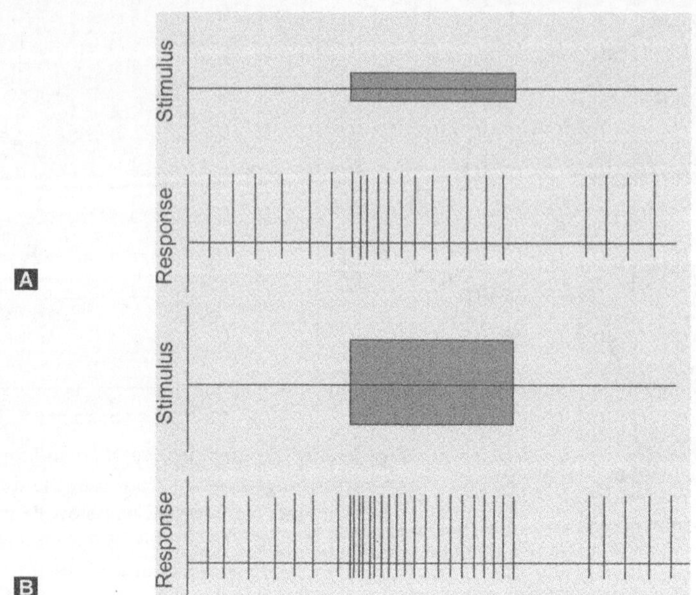

Figs 15.50A and B Diagrammatic representation of one mechanism for coding of intensity in auditory nerve fibers. For a sound of a given frequency, as the intensity of the stimulus increases, the frequency of nerve fiber discharge increases. (A) Weak stimulus; (B) Strong stimulus. Note that the frequency of firing in the auditory nerve fiber is higher than in A. Also note that there is a resting nerve discharge even in the absence of the stimulus. This provides scope for inhibition in addition to excitation. As seen in the figure, a temporary inhibition of resting discharge is seen immediately after the end of the stimulus

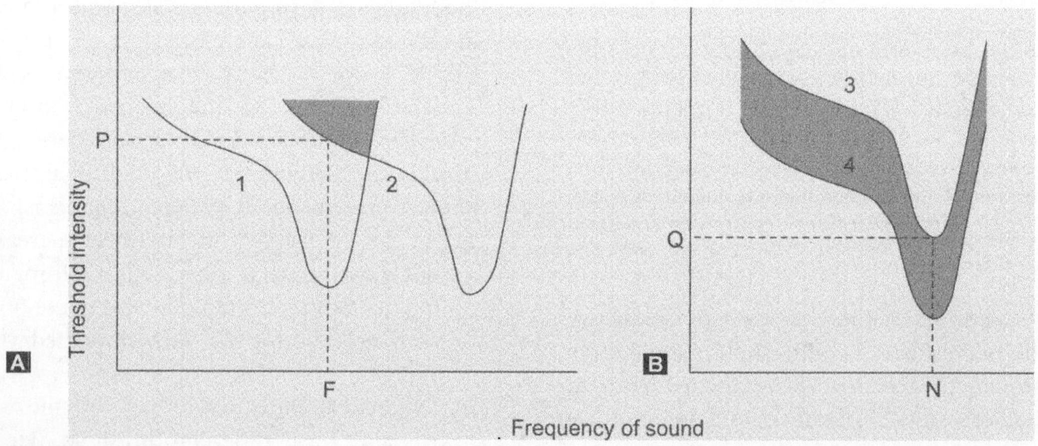

Figs 15.51A and B Coding of intensity of stimulus in auditory nerve fibers by recruitment of additional fibers; (A) Auditory nerve fibers 1 and 2 have different characteristic frequencies (CF). Let the frequency of the acoustic stimulus be F, which is the CF of fiber 1. Then, if intensity < P, only fiber 1 will be stimulated. But if intensity > P, fiber 2 will also be stimulated. The cross-hatched area defines the stimulus characteristics which would result in stimulation of both fibers 1 and 2; (B) Auditory nerve fibers 3 and 4 have the same CF, i.e. N. Let the frequency of the acoustic stimulus be N. Then, if intensity < Q, only fiber 4 will be stimulated. But if intensity > Q, fiber 3 will also be stimulated. Note that 4 is a more sensitive fiber than 3. Any stimulus which activates fiber 3 will also activate fiber 4. But a stimulus which activates fiber 4 will activate fiber 3 only if its intensity exceeds that represented by the cross-hatched area

Neurons sensitive to high frequencies are located in one area, neurons sensitive to low frequencies are located in another area, and neurons sensitive to intermediate frequencies are located between them in a proper order. This orderly organiation is called tonotopic organization.

One feature which distinguishes auditory pathway responses from those of the auditory nerve fibers is that the auditory neurons of the central nervous system do not necessarily respond to an acoustic stimulus by simple excitation. At levels as low as the *cochlear nucleus*, there are some neurons which respond only to the onset of a stimulus, some which respond after a long latency, and some in which the excitatory response decays at an exponential rate or builds up slowly. Superior olivary complex is the lowest level in the auditory pathway which receives input from both ears on either side. Hence olivary neurons are in a position to compare the input to the two ears, which is an exercise important for localization of a sound. The comparison seems to be accomplished by two types of neurons. One type of neurons, found in the medial superior olive, are sensitive to interaural time difference (ITD). The other type of neurons, found in the lateral superior olive, are sensitive to interaural intensity difference (IID).

The unique feature of *cortical* neuronal response to acoustic stimuli is the brief duration of response. The response is seen at the onset and at the termination of the stimulus but is not sustained throughout the stimulus. Other features, viz. tonotopic organization, and sensitivity to IID and ITD are seen also in the auditory cortex.

The electrical responses of cortical neurons suggest their special contribution in perception of a change in stimulus characteristics, and it is true that points of change are more important for interpreting a stimulus. Secondly, lack of sustained response to a prolonged stimulus correlates well with the observation that a monotonous stimulus may be ignored. In fact, ignoring a persistent sound, such as background noise, is necessary for proper adaptation to the enviroment. The most important functions of the cortex in hearing are localization of sound and discrimination based on the sequence of sounds in a composite stimulus.

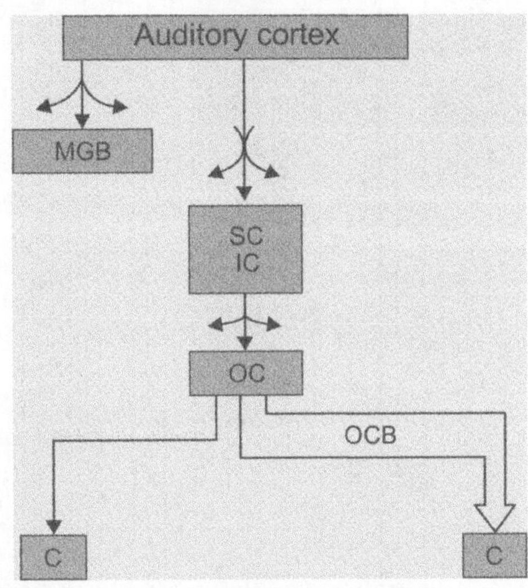

Fig. 15.52 The descending auditory pathway. The fibers to the cerebellum are not shown. MGB, medial geniculate body; SC, superior colliculus; IC, inferior colliculus; OC, olivary complex; OCB, olivo-cochlear bundle; C, cochlea

Descending Auditory Pathways

The descending pathway of the auditory system parallels the ascending pathways (Fig. 15.52). The olivocochlear bundle, which descends from the olive to the cochlea, is the best known descending tract of the auditory system. The efferent fibers end on the hair cells of the cochlea. The interaction between the ascending and descending pathways is not restricted to the hair cells. They influence each other's activity at all the stations between the cortex and the cochlea. Further, they also interact with a lot of other traffic in the central nervous system through lateral connections (Fig. 15.53). To complicate matters further, there is considerable interaction between different sensory modalities. For example, the projection from auditory cortex to superior colliculi possibly means an interaction with visual stimuli, and the projection from the auditory cortex to the cerebellum possibly means an interaction with the vestibular stimuli. No wonder then, that the fate of

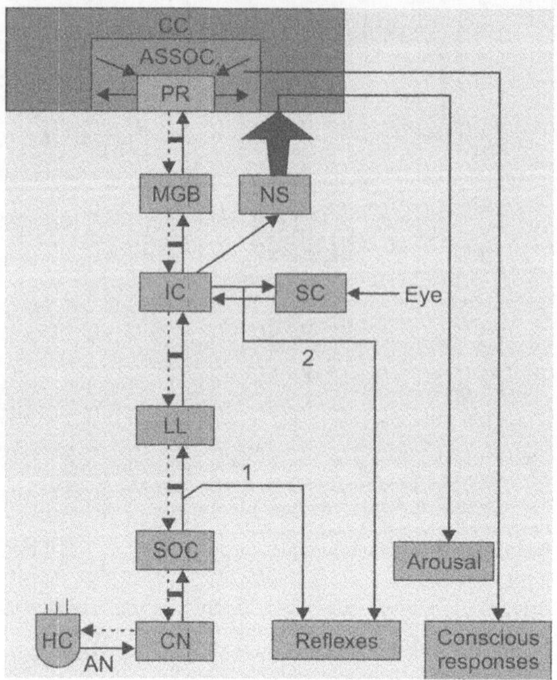

Fig. 15.53 The interaction between the ascending and the descending auditory pathway extends throughout the two pathways. The descending pathway has been shown by dotted lines, and its connections with the ascending pathway by heavy black lines. An acoustic stimulus may result in a reflex, a conscious behavioral response or arousal. The responses involve interaction with other sensory inputs, from among which only the visual input has been shown. HC, hair cell; AN, auditory nerve; CN, cochlear nucleus; SOC, superior olivary complex; LL, nucleus of lateral lemniscus; IC, inferior colliculus; SC, superior colliculus; MGB, medial geniculate body; NS, nonspecific nuclei of thalamus; PR, primary auditory cortex; ASSOC, association auditory cortex; CC, cerebral cortex. 1, short loop pathway for a reflex; 2, long loop pathway

a sound stimulus is so uncertain even when the ears are normal. Normal ears do not ensure hearing, and hearing does not guarantee listening. It is perhaps the descending tracts which help in selecting stimuli which are heard. The stimuli which receive maximum attention are non-monotonous stimuli which do not face competition from other simultaneous stimuli. Most important of all, it is only if the individual considers the stimulus important will it be listened to carefully.

Perception of Different Characteristics of Sound

Frequency

As seen earlier, dissection of sound stimuli in terms of frequency takes place as early as the basilar membrane. A slight sharpening of the frequency analysis may occur at the hair cells. Tonotopic organization continues throughout the auditory pathway. Final perception of frequency may therefore be considered to reside in the auditory cortex.

Intensity

Coding for intensity begins at the receptor level. Since the outer hair cells (OHC) are farther away from the hinge-point of the basilar membrane as compared to inner hair cells (IHC), the OHC are stimulated even by weaker stimuli. In the auditory nerve fibers, as in other sense organs, the frequency of nerve impulses is related to the intensity of the stimulus. In the auditory cortex, neurons maximally sensitive to a specific intensity have been described (Fig. 15.54), and these possibly are involved in perception of intensity of sound, or the loudness.

Direction

The direction from which a sound is coming is judged from the difference in the time at which the

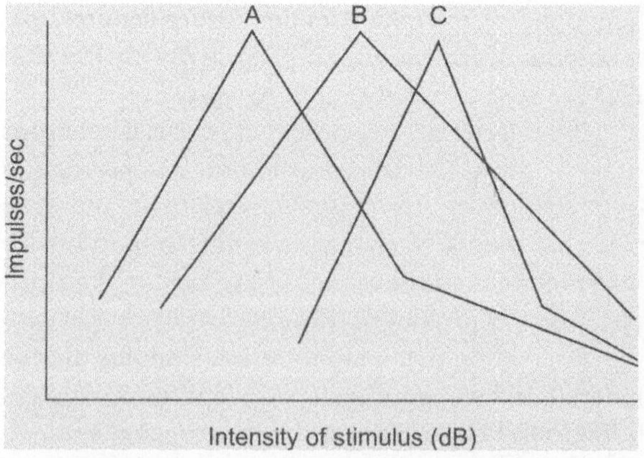

Fig. 15.54 Intensity-sensitive neurons of the auditory cortex. (Based on Moore DR, Br Med Bull 1987;43:856-70)

sound arrives at the two ears, and the difference in the intensity of the sound at the two ears (Figs 15.55A to C). Although neurons sensitive to inter-aural time difference (ITD) and inter-aural intensity difference (IID) are present in the superior olivary nucleus, auditory cortex is essential for perception of direction of sound. It is believed that depending on the magnitude of ITD and IID, different sets of neurons are activated in the superior olivary nucleus. The specific spatial orientation of the neurons stimulated is maintained all the way up to the auditory cortex. The area of the auditory cortex stimulated for discrimination of direction is different from that stimulated for perception of the existence of the sound. The cortical area for discrimination of direction also has a tonotopic organization.

Pattern

Pattern of a sound means the sequence in which different components of the sound appear. Recognition of the pattern of a sound is entirely a cortical function. Animals whose auditory cortex has been removed lose the ability to recognize the pattern of a sound completely although they can still detect sounds and react to them in a crude manner.

Interpretation of Speech

Interpretation of speech or any other meaningful stimulus is a complex phenomenon. To consider it a simple combination of the perception of frequency, intensity and pattern would be rather naive. Observations on patients suggest that in man perception of speech is possible even if only the primary auditory cortex is intact. But understanding the meaning of the spoken word needs also the association areas of auditory cortex. For meaningful listening, besides the mechanisms of perception, a contribution from previous learning is necessary. This contribution is possibly made by the association cortex.

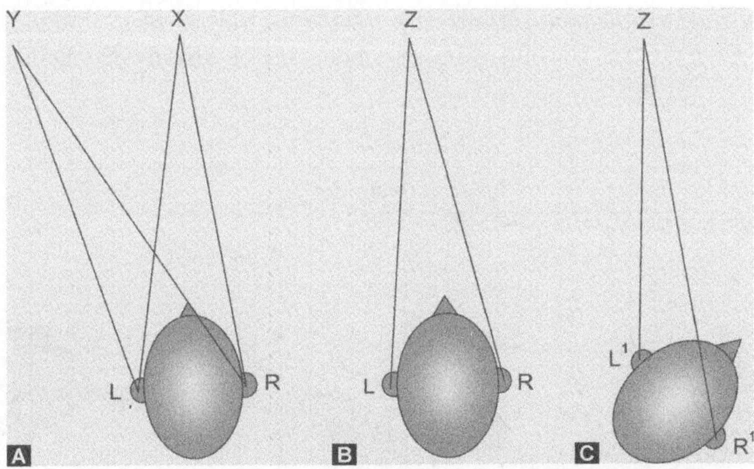

Figs 15.55A to C Localization of sound. (A) A sound coming from the midline (X) reaches both the left ear (L) and right ear (R) at the same time, and with the same intensity. Therefore inter-aural time difference (ITD) and inter-aural intensity difference (IID) are zero. But for a sound from the left hand side (Y), YR > YL. Therefore it reaches the left ear before reaching the right ear, and stimulates the left ear with greater intensity. Neuronal mechanisms sensitive to ITD and IID presumably help localize the sound as coming from the left; (B) If the sound is only slightly to the left of the midline (Z), ITD and IID will be very small. Therefore it may be difficult or confusing to localize the sound; (C) In order to localize a sound which is only slightly off the midline, we often turn our head. Now $ZR^1 > ZL^1$; and hence ITD and IID will be quite large. Therefore the central nervous system will easily perceive the sound as coming from the left. Animals who have mobile pinnae achieve the same end by moving these. Since man cannot move the external ear, better localization of sounds is achieved by turning the head which bears the external ears

Hearing Defects

From a physiological point of view, impairment of hearing, or deafness, is of two types (Fig. 15.56).

Conduction Deafness

In conduction deafness, sound cannot be conducted to the cochlear receptors (hair cells) efficiently. It could be due to a defect either in the external or the middle ear. Common causes of conduction deafness are wax in the ear canal, perforation of the tympanic membrane, inflammatory disease of the middle ear (otitis media), or immobility of ossicles (otosclerosis).

Sensorineural Deafness or Nerve Deafness

Nerve deafness is due to an injury to hair cells or the auditory nerve or the auditory pathways. Very loud sounds can cause a temporary shift in threshold of hearing due to reversible hair cell damage. With repeated exposure to loud sounds, the damage can become permanent.

Gradually progressive nerve deafness is normally seen as a part of the aging process. Starting with very mild hearing impairment at 30 years of age, the loss becomes a handicap in old age. The hearing loss associated with aging is called presbyacusis, and is particularly marked for higher frequencies.

Evaluation of Auditory Function

Preliminary evaluation of hearing can be carried out simply by finding the maximum distance from which the patient can hear the ticking of a watch. The distance is then compared with the corresponding distance for a normal person. Better evaluation of hearing may be carried out by tuning fork tests and audiometry.

Tuning Fork Tests

These tests are based on the principle that although normally sound is conducted to the ear by air (air conduction), it is also possible to stimulate the ear by applying the base of a tuning fork to a part of the skull. The vibrations of the tuning fork are then conducted by the skull to the temporal bone enclosing the cochlea. Vibrations of the temporal bone travel directly to the cochlear fluids. This

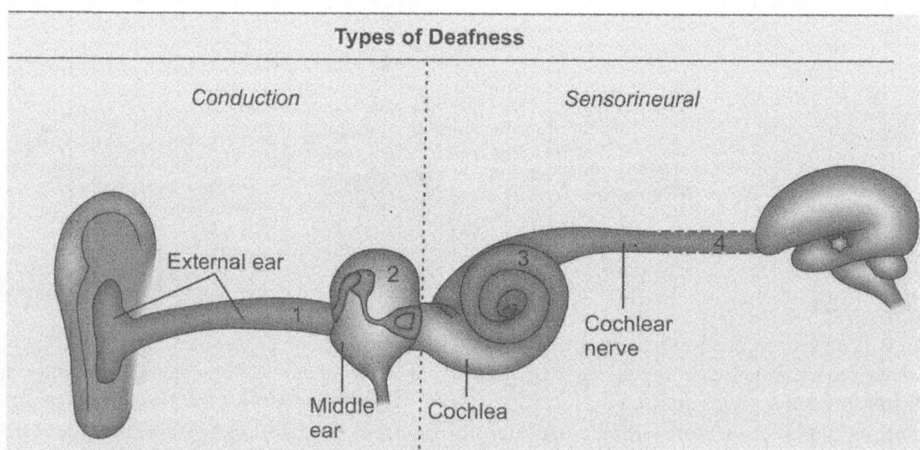

Fig. 15.56 The process of hearing involves conduction of the stimulus through the external and middle ear, its transduction in the cochlea and transmission to the brain. Hence impairment of hearing may be due to a defect on either side of the dotted line; accordingly, deafness is classified as conduction deafness or sensorineural deafness. Common causes of conduction deafness include wax or some other obstruction in the ear canal (1) or middle ear disease (2). Possible causes of sensorineural deafness include a defect in the cochlea (3) or in the auditory pathways (4)

mode of stimulation is called bone conduction. Normally air conduction is more efficient than bone conduction. But in conduction deafness the normal mode of conduction, i.e. air conduction, is impaired. However, conduction deafness does not impair bone conduction because that does not require the participation of the external or middle ear. Therefore, in an ear having conduction deafness, bone conduction may be better than air conduction. Moreover, in unilateral conduction deafness, bone conduction in the diseased ear is better than in the normal ear. This is because on the normal side the sound transmitted by bone conduction is masked by other sounds reaching the ear by air conduction. But on the diseased side, the masking effect is less or absent, thereby improving the relative efficiency of bone conduction.

The commonly performed tuning fork tests are:

i. *Weber's test:* Strike the tuning fork to make it vibrate. Place the base of the tuning fork on the vertex of the skull or the forehead in the midline. Normally the sound is heard equally well on both sides. Since nerve deafness affects air conduction as well as bone conduction adversely, in nerve deafness the sound is heard better on the healthy side (Fig. 15.57). But in conduction deafness, the sound is heard better on the diseased side.[6]

ii. *Rinne's test:* The vibrating tuning fork is placed on the mastoid process to allow bone conduction till it can be heard. Then it is placed close to the ear to allow air conduction. In a normal ear or an ear with nerve deafness it should be possible to hear the tuning fork for some more time because air conduction is better than bone conduction. In the ear with conduction deafness, bone conduction is better than air conduction, and hence the tuning fork can be heard longer over the mastoid than close to the ear (Fig. 15.58).

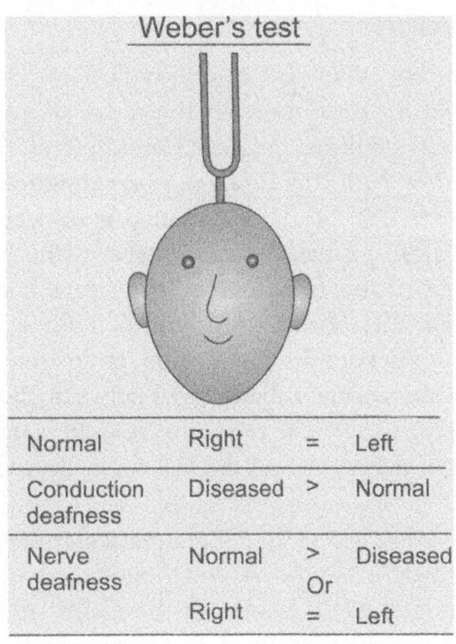

Normal	Right	=	Left
Conduction deafness	Diseased	>	Normal
Nerve deafness	Normal	>	Diseased
		Or	
	Right	=	Left

Fig. 15.57 Weber's test. The common findings have been tabulated. Right, right ear; Left, left ear; Diseased, diseased ear; Normal, normal ear; =, equally well heard; >, heard better/longer than

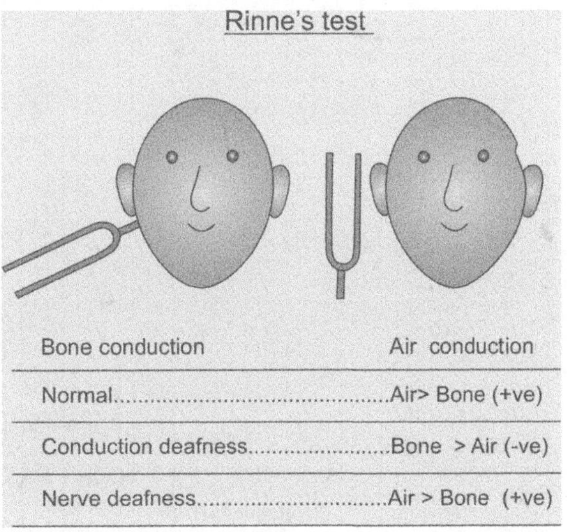

Bone conduction	Air conduction
Normal	Air> Bone (+ve)
Conduction deafness	Bone > Air (-ve)
Nerve deafness	Air > Bone (+ve)

Fig. 15.58 Rinne's Test. The common findings have been tabulated. When the findings are as in a normal person, the test is said to be positive. Air, air conduction; Bone, bone conduction, >, heard better/longer than

[6]If you do not understand why the sound is heard better on the diseased side, read the explanation above, viz. the masking of the healthy ear.

Audiometry

Audiometry involves determination of hearing threshold for pure tones in the range of 125-8000 Hz. The sounds are presented one by one, to both ears and by both routes (air or bone conduction) in succession. The results are plotted graphically in a standardized format. The graph shows the hearing threshold of the subject in relation to the normal threshold. The normal threshold is defined on the basis of observations made on a large number of otologically normal subjects aged between 18 and 30 years (Fig. 15.59). The normal threshold is depicted as 0 dB in the graph and the loss for each frequency plotted.

A hearing loss of 20 dB at a particular frequency means that the sound at that frequency had to be made at least 20 dB louder for the patient to hear it than for normal persons. A few sample audiograms are shown in Figures 15.60A to C. The interpretation of findings is as for tuning fork tests.

The results of bone conduction tests may be misleading in case of unilateral deafness because when the vibrator is placed on the mastoid on the diseased side, sound may be conducted around

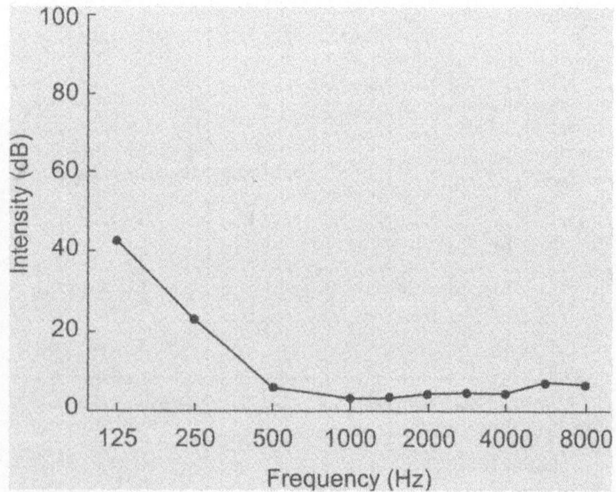

Fig. 15.59 Normal hearing threshold for sounds of different frequency. The normal threshold intensity for each frequency is considered the 'zero' hearing level in conventional audiograms (Based on data from Gelfand, 1981)

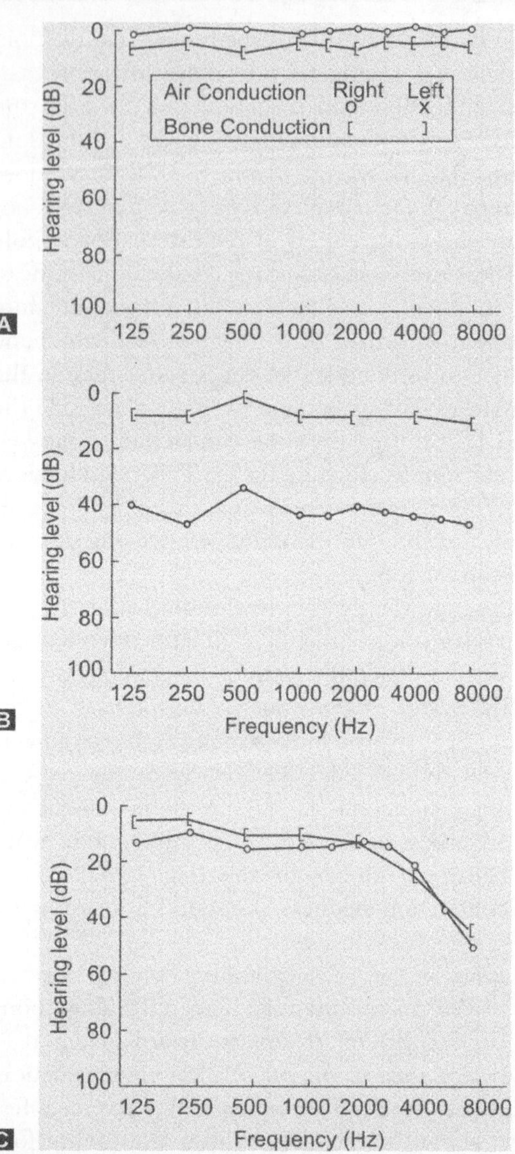

Figs 15.60A to C Sample audiograms. The 'zero' hearing level corresponds to the normal threshold. Hence the hearing level indicates the hearing loss in the subject. Only the right ear plots have been depicted in the figures. (A) Normal audiogram. Note that air conduction is better than bone conduction; (B) Audiogram suggesting conduction deafness. Symbols have the same connotation as in A; (C) Audiogram suggesting sensorineural deafness. Note that deafness is especially marked for higher frequencies, as happens in presbyacusis. Symbols have the same connotation as in A

the head to the healthy ear giving a near normal threshold. This fallacy may be overcome by providing a masking sound to the healthy ear. Since the contralateral effect of masking is minimal, the diseased ear's bone conduction can still be evaluated. But the masking sound will prevent the healthy ear from contributing to the perception of the sound presented to the diseased ear.

TASTE

Modern man uses the sense of taste mainly to derive pleasure. But its original significance possibly was to provide a warning against harmful foods. Poisonous plants are frequently bitter or unpleasant to taste. Taste may also occasionally guide us towards the foods we need. Definite evidence in support of this concept is available only for salt. An adrenalectomized animal loses large amounts of salt in the urine, and therefore needs more salt. It also shows a marked preference for salty solutions, indicating that it likes their taste.

Taste Receptors

Receptors for taste are located on the tongue in taste buds (Fig. 15.61). Taste buds are grouped in structures called papillae (*papilla,* nipple). There are three types of papillae (Fig. 15.62) with a characteristic distribution over the surface of the tongue (Fig. 15.63). As their names indicate, fungiform papillae resemble a mushroom, which is a fungus; foliate papillae resemble a leaf; and circumvallate papillae resemble a well, or rather a moat.

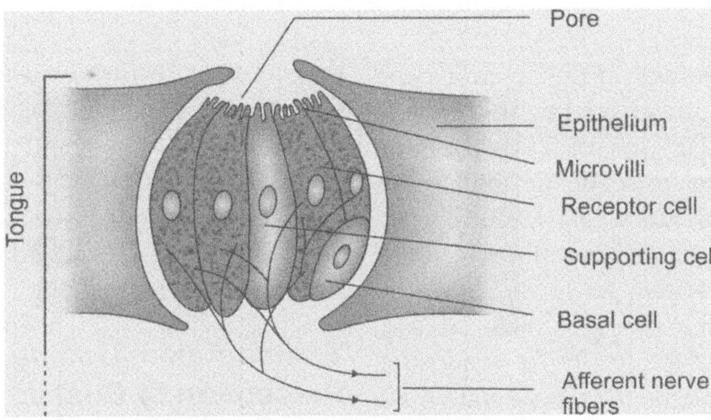

Fig. 15.61 Structure of a taste bud

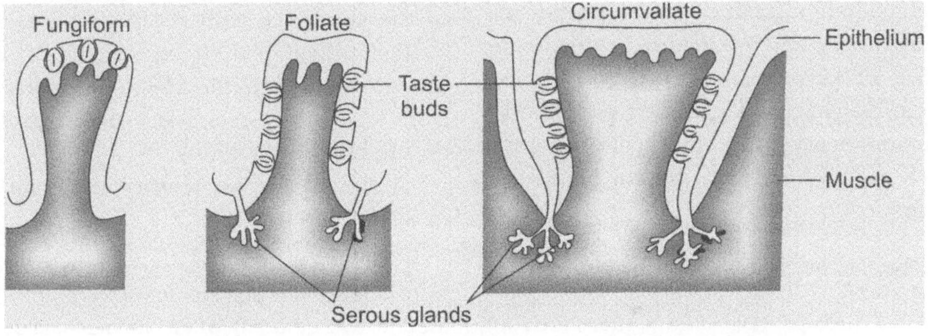

Fig. 15.62 The three types of papillae seen in the tongue

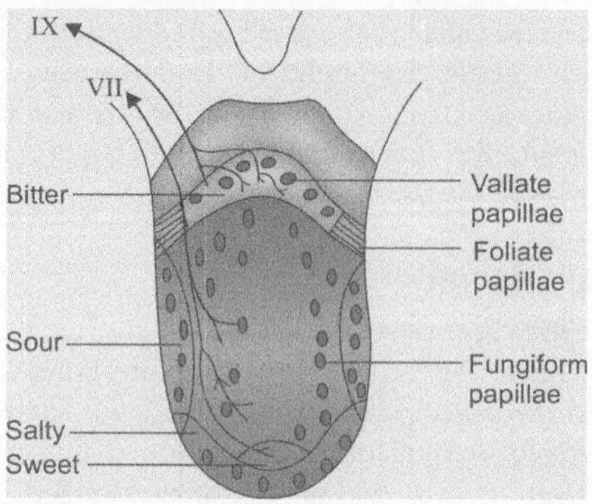

Fig. 15.63 Distribution of the three types of papillae on the surface of the tongue. Also shown are the regional distribution of sensitivity of the tongue to the four basic tastes, and the innervation of the taste receptors in the anterior two-thirds and the posterior one-third of the tongue

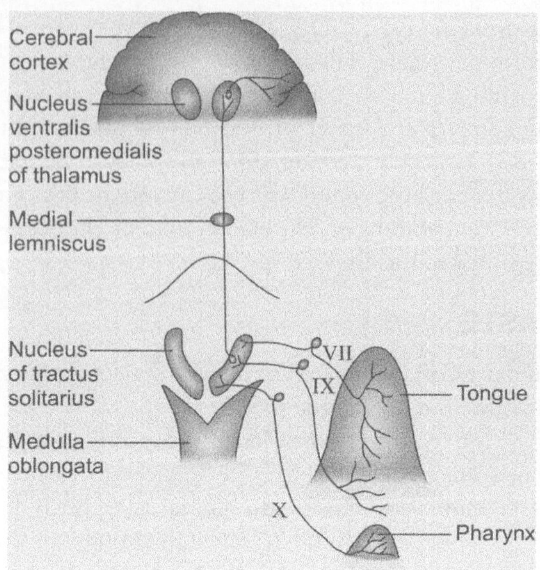

Fig. 15.64 The major taste pathway

Taste Pathways

Sensory cells for taste located in the anterior two-thirds of the tongue are innervated by the seventh cranial (facial) nerve (Fig. 15.63). Taste receptor cells in the posterior one-third of the tongue are innervated by the ninth cranial (glossopharyngeal) nerve. The path taken by the afferent fibers for taste in the central nervous system has been shown in Figure 15.64. In the cerebral cortex, there are two taste areas. Taste area I is located in the postcentral gyrus, close to the somesthetic representation of the tongue (i.e. where general sensations like touch, pain, pressure or temperature project). Taste area II lies buried in the insular cortex.

The interaction of taste fibers in the tractus solitarius with salivatory and vagal nuclei explains the reflex increase in salivary and gastric secretion in response to a food having a pleasant taste. Similar other interactions may explain other reflex responses to taste, such as vomiting following an unpleasant taste stimulus.

The Four Basic Tastes

Just as there are three primary colors, there are four basic tastes: sweet, sour, salty and bitter. Parts of the tongue differ in their sensitivity to different tastes (Fig. 15.64). The tip of the tongue is most sensitive to sweet, edges to sour, and the back is most sensitive to bitter. That is why if we have to swallow a bitter pill, we avoid letting it touch the back of the tongue. Senstivity to salty taste is fairly widely distributed over the tongue.

Transduction, Coding and Perception of Gustatory Stimuli

When a substance having a taste is put in the mouth, it interacts with the sensory cells. The interaction involves a combination of the molecules of the substance with receptor (recognition sites) on the surface of the receptor (sensory) cells.[7] The interaction leads to the release of a neurotransmitter from the sensory cell. The neurotransmitter excites the afferent nerve ending.

Although a given sensory cell is most sensitive to a specific taste, it shows some response to other

[7]It is unfortunate that the word 'receptor' is commonly used in two different ways. Its meaning at a particular place is judged from the context in which it is used.

tastes also. The situation is similar to vision where a cone is most sensitive to a specific color but shows some response to other colors also. Just as the perceived color depends on the pattern of stimulation of a large number of cones, the perceived taste also depends on the pattern of stimulation of a large number of sensory cells. That is why, just as we have a continuous spectrum of colors, we also have a continuous spectrum of tastes.

Like other senses, perception of taste also involves the cerebral cortex. But a part of the taste pathway terminates also in the limbic system. The cortex is possibly concerned with conscious perception while the limbic system is concerned with the emotional reaction to taste. The overall influence of civilization is to dissociate the two aspects, so that awareness of taste is possible without the accompanying emotional response, specially if the taste is unpleasant. When Mahatma Gandhi was in England, his commitment to vegetarianism and simplicity made him turn to foods like boiled spinach (without condiments or spices). But his commitment was so strong that he relished even such insipid dishes. While quoting these details in his autobiography, he wrote, "Many such experiments taught me that the real seat of taste was not the tongue but the mind". Now we have a plausible neurophysiological basis for his statement.

SMELL

Man's sense of smell falls far short of that of some animals such as dogs, but is still quite impressive. Man can distinguish hundreds of substances on the basis of smell. But smell does not have much survival value for the modern man; for him it is basically a luxury or a nuisance, depending on the nature of the stimulus. For animals, smell is important in detection of food, mate and enemy, which gives it enormous survival value.

Olfactory Receptors

Olfactory receptors are situated in the nasal cavity on the olfactory mucosa. Olfactory mucosa is restricted to the superior and middle conchae and adjacent areas of the nasal septum (Fig. 15.65). The rest of the nasal mucosa is considered respiratory in function, but has free nerve endings belonging to the trigeminal (fifth cranial) nerve which gets stimulated by strong smells and evoke a feeling of irritation.

Olfactory mucosa has cilia bearing receptors (recognition sites) for odoriferous chemicals (Fig. 15.66). The cilia are a part of sensory cells. The sensory cells have a life span of only 60 days. They are renewed by proliferation of basal cells. Olfactory receptor cells are the only neurons in the body known to be replenished by cell division.

Olfactory Pathways

The axons of olfactory sensory cells travel through the cribriform plate (*cribrum*, sieve; *forma*, shape) of the ethmoid bone to join the olfactory bulb. Olfactory bulb is an extension of the brain, and has complex neuronal circuitry (Fig. 15.67). Olfactory bulb is connected to the brain by the olfactory tract. Olfactory tract contains the axons of mitral cells. Like the taste fibers, olfactory tract also projects to the primitive parts of the brain (limbic system) as well as the neocortex (Fig. 15.68).

The Primary Odors

The primary odors, if any, are not known with certainty. One of the better known schemes proposes seven primary odors: camphoraceous, musky, floral, peppermint, ethereal, pungent and putrid.

Transduction, Coding and Perception of Olfactory Stimuli

Odoriferous substances are volatile. That is why their vapors can travel long distances. In the olfactory mucosa they combine with the specific receptor (recognition site) on the cilia of the sensory cells. This interaction leads to depolarization of the sensory cells. The depolarization has the characters of a receptor potential. The axons of the olfactory sensory cells also show action potentials. The frequency of the action potentials depends on the magnitude of the receptor potential, which in turn depends on the intensity of the olfactory stimulus.

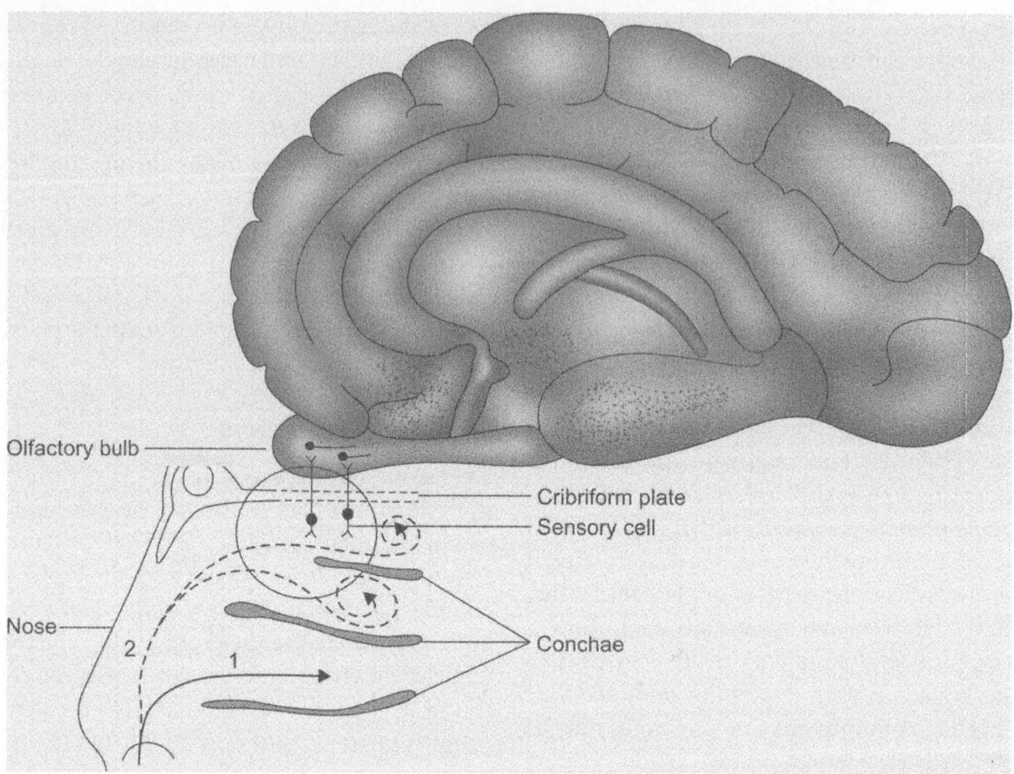

Fig. 15.65 Major structures associated with perception of smell. The olfactory mucosa (shaded area) is restricted to the superior and middle conchae and adjacent areas of the septum. Therefore a quiet inspiration (1) does not bring the inspired air in contact with the olfactory mucosa. It needs a forceful breath (2), which sets up eddy currents in the nasal cavity, to smell properly. The olfactory sensory cell axons pass through the cribriform plate of the skull to reach the olfactory bulb. The shaded areas in the brain show roughly the regions intimately involved in perception of smell. Note that these areas belong to the primitive parts of the brain, which are principally hidden behind the medial and basal surface of the human brain because of the enormous overgrowth of the phylogenetically more recent parts of the cerebral cortex. For details of olfactory mucosa, olfactory bulb and its central projections, see subsequent figures

There are about 1000 different types of receptor sites on olfactory sensory cells. The actual smell perceived depends on the proportion in which different types of receptors are activated by a particular stimulus. As in case of taste, the neocortical pathway is possibly concerned with conscious perception of smell, while the limbic pathway is responsible for the emotional responses to smell and integration of olfactory stimuli with feeding and reproductive behavior.

Here a difference between smell and other senses may be pointed out. In case of other senses, the cortical representation is generally related to the localization of the stimulus. But in case of smell, neighboring areas of the olfactory cortex represent different types of smell. That is why smell cannot be localized except by turning the head and finding what orientation of the nose results in the strongest smell.

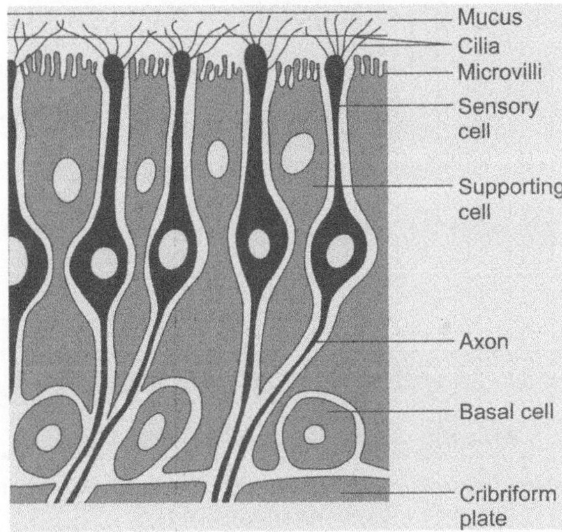

Fig. 15.66 Diagrammatic representation of histological structure of the olfactory mucosa

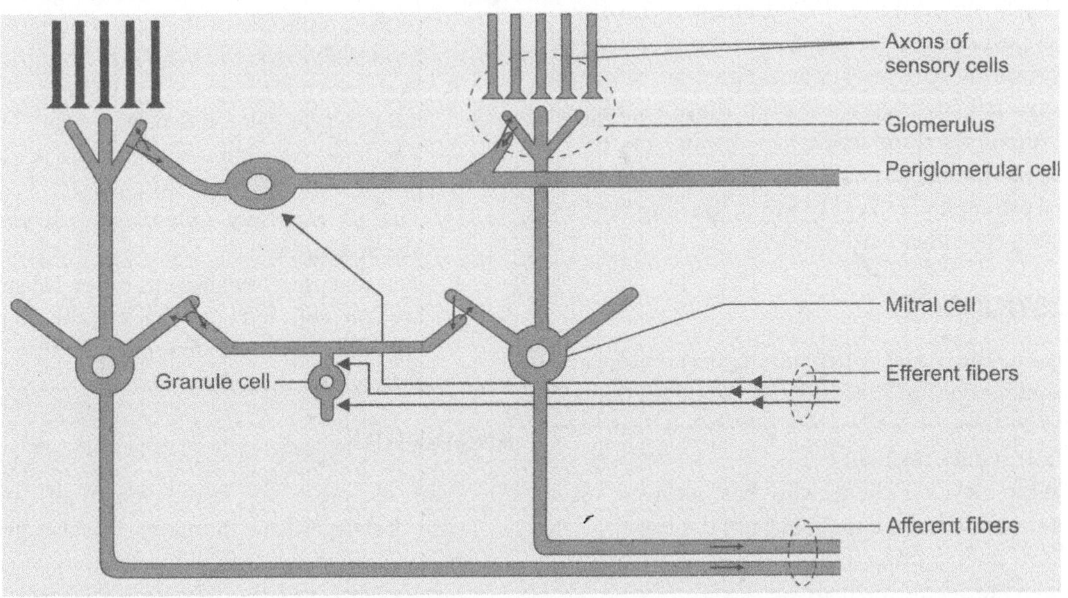

Fig. 15.67 A highly simplified diagrammatic representation of neuronal circuitry in the olfactory bulb

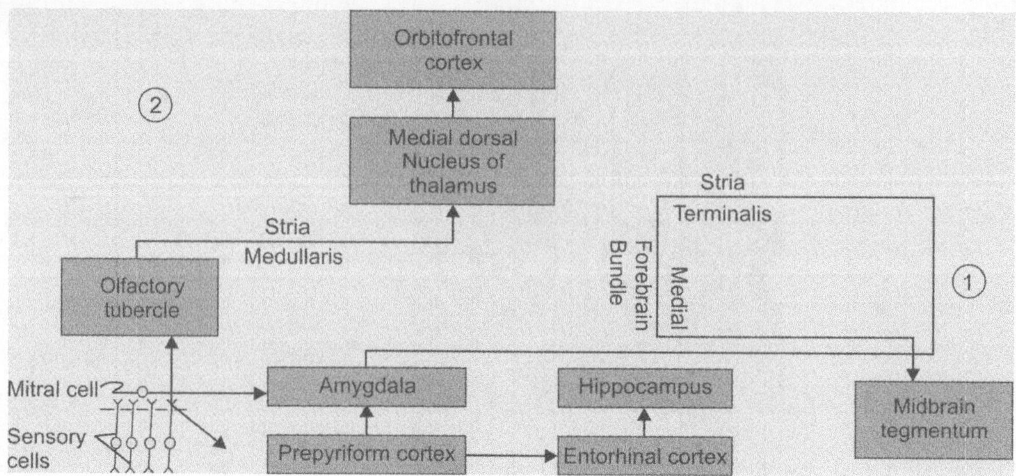

Fig. 15.68 Schematic representation of major olfactory pathways. 1. Projection to the limbic system and paleocortex. 2. Projection to the neocortex

CONCLUSION

A study of general and special senses shows a remarkable similarity in the mechanisms involved. Each stimulus is transducted, coded and conveyed to the central nervous system. The central neural pathways fall in three categories: those leading to reflex responses, those leading to affective reactions, and those leading to conscious perception. If these general principles are kept in mind, learning sensory physiology becomes very simple.

QUESTIONS

1. Name the tissues which have pain receptors and some inportant sites which do not have them.
2. Why does pressing a toe which has just been hurt reduce the pain ?
3. Why may a patient who has received local anesthesia feel the knife but not the pain ?
4. How does sniffing (taking a short sharp breath) help the act of smelling?
5. Conscious perception of a sensory stimulus takes place after information about the stimulus reaches the:
   A. Medulla
   B. Midbrain
   C. Thalamus
   D. Cerebral cortex
6. For each of the following statements, indicate whether it is true or false:
   A. The intensity of a stimulus is coded in terms of the amplitude of the action potentials in the sensory nerve fibers.
   B. Rods are the receptors for vision in bright light and for color vision.
   C. The lens contributes more to the refractive power of the eye than the cornea.
   D. The ear canal not only conveys sound but also magnifies it.
   E. The receptors sensitive to bitter substances are concentrated at the back of the tongue.
   F. Olfactory receptors are uniformly distributed throughout the nasal mucosa.

ANSWERS

1. Pain receptors are found maximally in the skin, but significant numbers are also present in the periosteum, arterial walls, joint surfaces, falx cerebri and the tentorium. Deep viscera are rather poorly supplied by pain receptors. Brain has no pain receptors. That is why a neurosurgeon can work on the brain after infiltration of the extracranial tissues with a local anesthetic. It is paradoxical that the organ which perceives pain cannot detect any painful stimulus.

2. Pressing the toe reduces the pain because pressure blocks conduction in fast fibers and hence blocks fast pain which appears immediately after injury. However, since pressure does not block slow fibers very effectively, dull aching slow pain may appear after a few minutes in spite of keeping on the pressure.
3. Local anesthetics are more effective in blocking slow fibers. Therefore, they block the slow pain completely. But since fast fibers may not be blocked completely, the patient may feel a pricking sensation along the line of the incision.
4. Sniffing helps because olfactory mucosa is confined to the upper parts of the nasal cavity. During quiet breathing, air does not reach as high as the olfactory mucosa.
5. D
6. A. False
   B. False
   C. False
   D. True
   E. True
   F. False

CHAPTER

16 Nervous System: Motor Functions

"But warmed with that unchanging flame, Behold the outward moving frame, Its living marbles jointed strong, With glistening band and silvery throng, And linked to reason's guiding reins by myriad rings in trembling chains, Each graven with the threaded zone, Which claims it as the master's own."

—OLIVER WENDELL HOLMES

Chapter Outline

- Spinal Motor Mechanisms
- Brain Stem Motor Mechanisms
- Cortical Motor Mechanisms
- The Cerebellum
- Basal Ganglia

Motor functions of the nervous system generally refer to control of skeletal muscle activity by the nervous system. We have already learnt that skeletal muscles are supplied by nerve fibers originating in the anterior column of the spinal cord (Chapter 13). The anterior column motor cells, also called alpha motor neurons, are the final common pathway for mediating neural influences to skeletal muscle. In this chapter we shall examine what those influences are, and how they operate.

Normal skeletal muscle activity always has a purpose. The purpose may be locomotion, communication (speech or gestures), reading (eye movements), temperature regulation (shivering) or maintenance of balance or posture. The simplest of these activities are reflexes (e.g. maintenance of balance and posture, shivering). The most complex muscular activities are voluntary throughout (e.g. playing a musical instrument). Several rhythmic activities lie between these two extremes. For example, walking, running or chewing start and stop voluntarily, but between the beginning and end they become mechanical, almost like a reflex. The mechanisms underlying these various activities are also accordingly different.

The lowest level of the central nervous system from where skeletal muscle activity is controlled is the spinal cord. Spinal cord mechanisms are subject to influences from the brain stem. Still higher influences arise from the cerebral cortex which affects spinal cord mechanisms directly, and also indirectly via the brain stem. In addition, basal ganglia and cerebellum also affect the brain stem and cortical motor mechanisms in very important ways (Fig. 16.1).

It is essential to keep in mind that motor functions cannot go on normally without inputs from the sensory system. For maintenance of balance and posture information about position and orientation of the body arising from muscle and joint receptors and the vestibular apparatus is essential. For smooth performance of voluntary movements also, sensory information about the environment as perceived by the eyes, ears and skin receptors is important, as is the continuous information about the degree of contraction of different muscles. For example, if

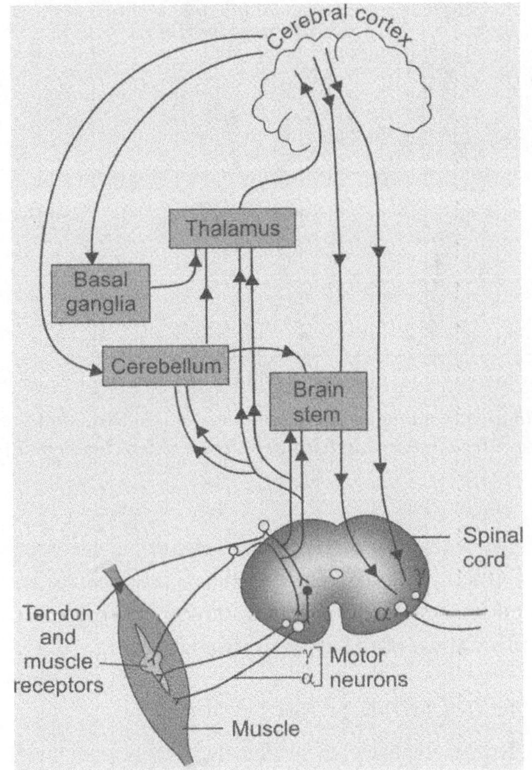

Fig. 16.1 Essential features of neural control of motor functions. All higher regions influence muscle activity by influencing the alpha and gamma motor neurons in the spinal cord. Note that all regions involved in motor function send information to the thalamus, and through the thalamus to the cerebral cortex. Also note that the basal ganglia receive sensory input only indirectly from the cerebral cortex. Further, the basal ganglia and thalamus do not influence the brain stem or spinal cord directly. They do so only indirectly through the cerebral cortex

we wish to pick up a pen, the eyes tell us where the pen is. That information is of obvious importance for moving the hand in the right direction. As the hand approaches the pen, continuous information from the muscles and joints involved tells the central nervous system how much of the necessary movement has been performed, and how much remains. Accordingly, there is a moment-to-moment change in the intensity of contraction of the muscles involved. That is why the hand approaches the pen smoothly and the pen is picked up without any difficulty. The information from muscles and joints is so reliable that once the pen has been seen and mental image of its position formed, the pen can be approached and picked up with amazing accuracy even with the eyes closed. You may try doing so just now to make sure that the book is right!

SPINAL MOTOR MECHANISMS

Spinal reflexes are the basic mechanisms involved in motor function. Higher control of these basic mechanisms leads to complex motor behavior. Stretch reflex is the simplest spinal reflex, and yet the most essential reflex for normal motor activity.

Stretch Reflex

If a skeletal muscle is stretched, it responds by contracting. In other words, if a muscle is stretched, it tends to become shorter and more stiff, thereby resisting the stretch. This is because of receptors sensitive to stretch within the muscle. Stretch receptors within a muscle are called **muscle spindles** (Figs 16.2A and B).

A muscle spindle consists of a bundle of specialized muscle fibers, called **intrafusal fibers** (because they are within the spindle). The central part of intrafusal fibers is non-contractile. It is the non-contractile central part of the spindle which is sensitive to stretch (Fig. 16.3). A muscle spindle has afferent as well as efferent nerve supply. The afferent nerve fibers innervate the central part of the spindle. The afferents are of two types: faster conducting group Ia fibers, and somewhat slower conducting group II fibers. The efferent nerve fibers originate in gamma motor neurons in the anterior column of the spinal cord. The efferents supply the contractile part of intrafusal fibers.

Reflex Arc for the Stretch Reflex

When a muscle is stretched, the spindles within it also get stretched. Stretching of the muscle spindles increases the afferent nerve activity from the muscle spindles. The increased activity is conveyed monosynaptically to alpha motor neurones supplying

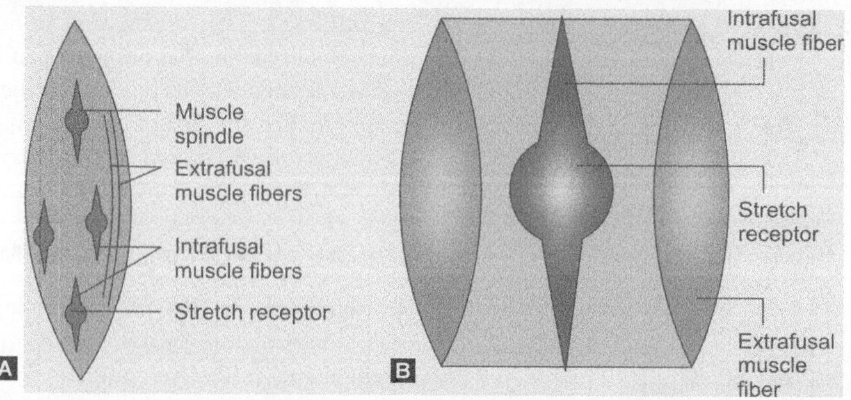

Figs 16.2A and B Schematic diagram showing the orientation of muscle spindles in a skeletal muscle (A) Note that the intrafusal muscle fibers are parallel to the extrafusal muscle fibers. This relationship has been shown more clearly in (B)

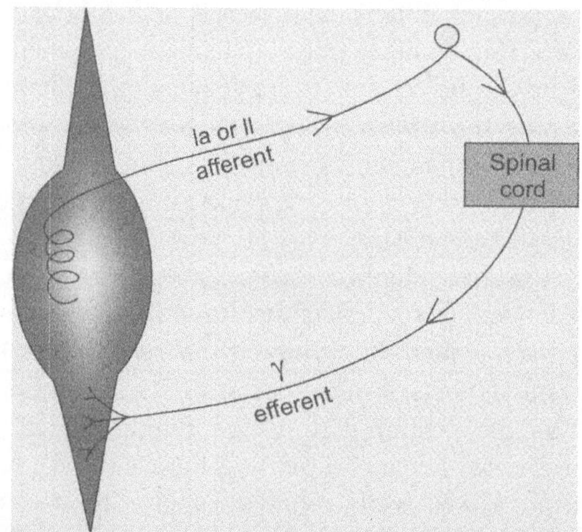

Fig. 16.3 Diagrammatic representation of the afferent and efferent nerve supply of muscle spindles

the muscle. Stimulation of the alpha motor neurone leads to contraction of the muscle (Fig. 16.4). *Stretch reflex is the only known example of a monosynaptic reflex.*

Depending on the type of afferent stimulated, stretch leads to two types of responses. One group of afferents respond primarily to the rate of change in the spindle length **(dynamic response).** The other group of afferents respond to the absolute length of the spindle **(static response).** The dynamic response makes the spindle very sensitive to even small changes in length. The static response ensures continuation of the afferent discharge (Fig. 16.5).

Role of Gamma Motor Neurons

As discussed above, the reflex arc for the stretch reflex involves only alpha motor neurons, which supply the ordinary extrafusal muscle fibers. The role of gamma motor neurons, which supply the intrafusal muscle fibers, will become clear once we realize a serious limitation of the spinal stretch reflex. Stretch of a muscle leads to its contraction. Contraction of the muscle relieves the stretch on the spindle (Figs 16.6A to C). The reflex is terminated, and the muscle relaxes. If the original stretch is continuing, the stretch reflex will be activated again, leading to a second contraction. Thus even a sustained stretch will produce only alternating contraction and relaxation. But this is not what the body needs. When we stand, the antigravity muscles get stretched. The stretch leads to a contraction of these muscles. Contraction of the antigravity muscles helps in maintaining the standing posture. But continuous standing is possible because contraction of antigravity muscles is continuous. Alternate contraction and relaxation of muscles will not be able to sustain a steady standing

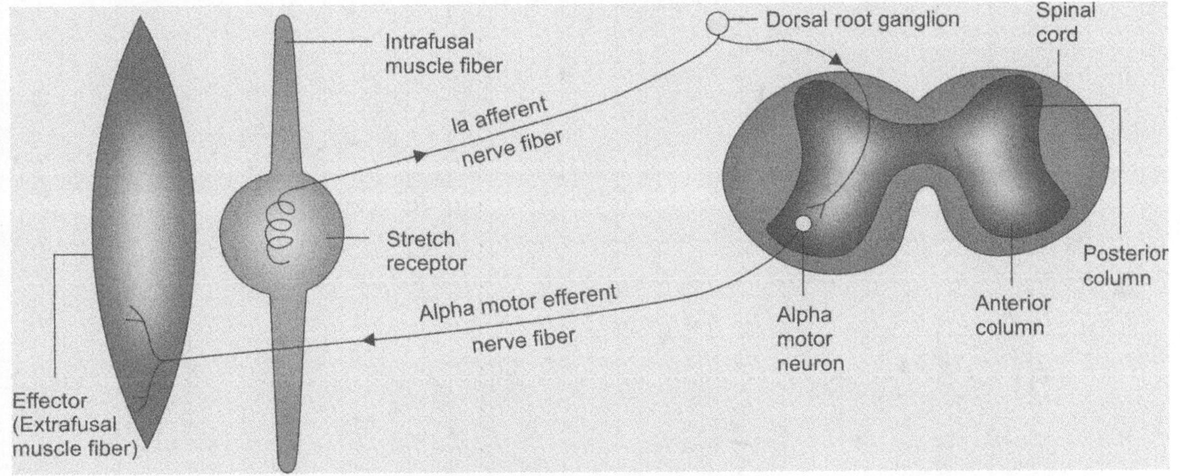

Fig. 16.4 Reflex arc for the stretch reflex

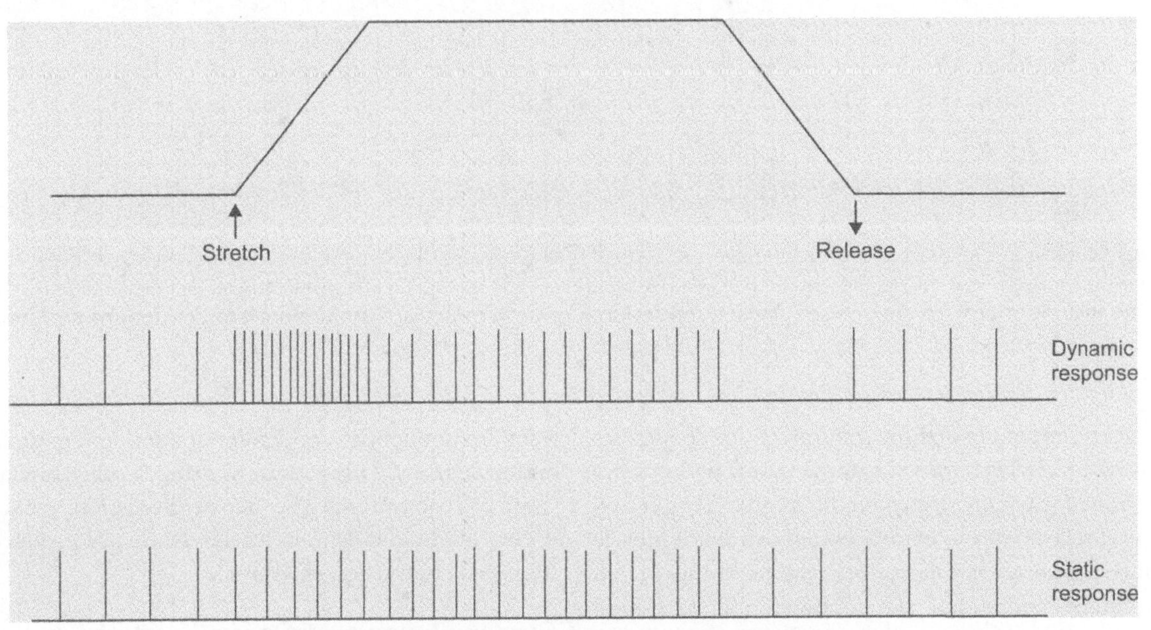

Fig. 16.5 Dynamic and static responses of afferent fibers to stretch and release of a muscle (Adapted from Matthews PBC. Physiol Rev 1964; 44: 219-88)

posture. Continuous contraction is made possible by activation of gamma motor neurons.[1]

[1]Contraction may not continue till the person is standing. After some time the set point of muscle length readjusts to the length required for standing.

Gamma motor neurons supply intrafusal muscle fibers. Activation of gamma motor neurons leads to a contraction of intrafusal muscle fibers. Contraction of these muscle fibers stretches the central region of the spindle. Thus the contraction of intrafusal muscle fibers has an effect on the spindle which is opposite

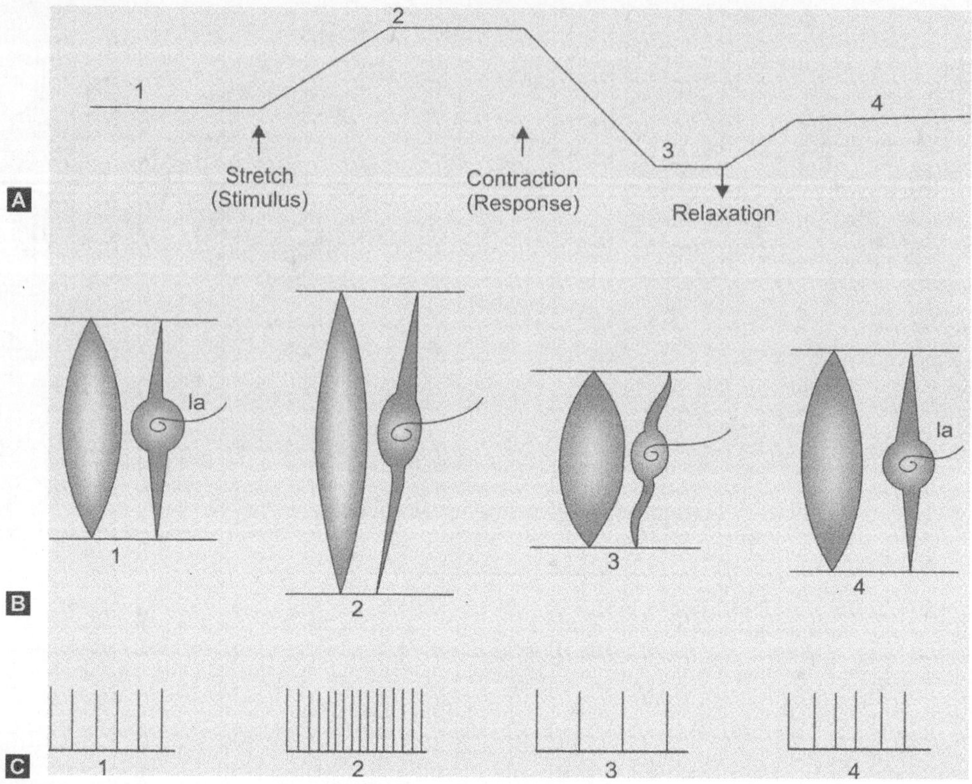

Figs 16.6A to C Limitation of the stretch reflex. (A) State of the muscle; (B) Diagrammatic representation of extrafusal and intrafusal muscle fibers; (C) Ia afferent discharge; (1) Muscle at resting length; (2) Stretched muscle; (3) Contracted muscle. Note that the stretch on the muscle spindle is relieved as a result of muscular contraction; (4) Muscle returns to resting length. To learn how this limitation of the stretch reflex is overcome in the body, see text and Figure 16.7

that of contraction of the extrafusal muscle fibers (Figs 16.7A to C). Therefore, if gamma motor neurons are activated when the stretch on the spindle is beginning to get relaxed due to contraction of extrafusal muscle fibers, the stretch will not get relaxed. If the stretch becomes continuous, the contraction of extrafusal muscle fibers becomes continuous.

The question then arises as to how the gamma motor neurons know when to get activated. The spinal stretch reflex activates only the alpha motor neurons (Fig. 16.4). But information from the muscle also travels simultaneously to higher regions of the nervous system which can influence gamma as well as alpha motor neurons. It has been found that stimulation of the motor cortex and other higher centers typically leads to simultaneous activation of alpha and gamma motor neurons. This pattern of firing is called alpha-gamma coactivation. The above discussion makes it clear that alpha-gamma coactivation can produce sustained contraction of a muscle.

Stretch Reflex as a Control System

Stretch reflex is a control system operating on the basis of negative feedback. Stretching a muscle increases its length. The increase in length is detected by muscle spindles. The muscle spindles convey this information to the spinal cord. The response is an increase in alpha motor neuron discharge, which leads to contraction of the muscle. Contraction is a decrease in the length. Thus the increase in length is corrected.

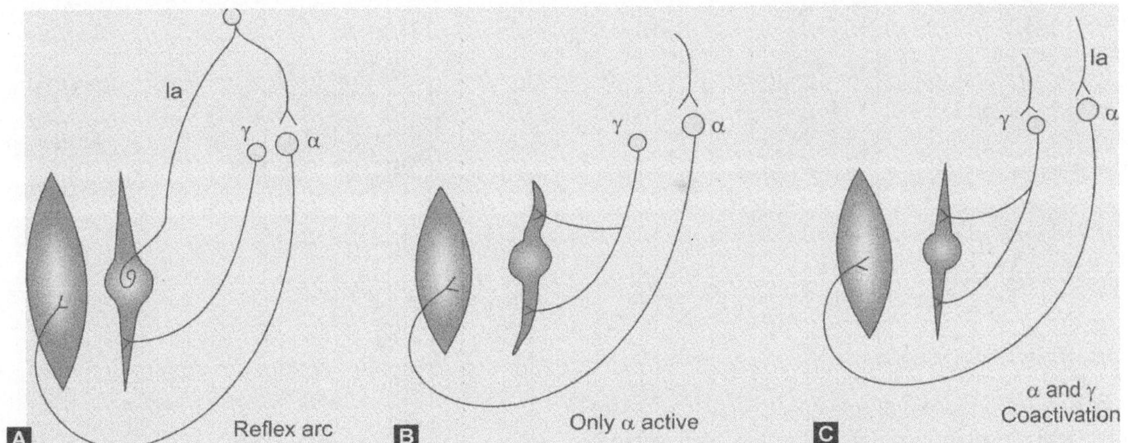

Figs 16.7A to C (A) Simplified view of the reflex arc for stretch reflex; (B) Response to stretch if only the alpha motor neuron is active. The extrafusal muscle contracts, relieving the stretch on the muscle spindle. But this is not what actually happens; (C) The actual response. Although the reflex arc activates only the alpha motor neuron, higher regions simultaneously activate also the gamma motor neuron. The result is that intrafusal muscle fibers also contract, leading to sustained stretch on the muscle spindle

But in practice stretch reflex is a more complex control system than this. *First*, its sensitivity (or gain) is not fixed. Activation of gamma motor neurons leads to contraction of intrafusal muscle fibers. Contraction of intrafusal muscle fibers stretches the central part of the spindle. The stretch makes the spindle more sensitive to further stretch. Thus gamma activation can increase the sensitivity (gain) of the control system. *Second*, the set point of the control system is also not fixed. The length which the control system may treat as the set point changes with the posture. In terms of mechanism, the desired muscle length (set point) of a muscle in a given posture is determined by the net facilitatory and inhibitory influences on the alpha motor neurons supplying the muscle. The facilitatory and inhibitory influences originate in higher regions of the central nervous system, about which we shall learn in the subsequent sections.

Functional Role of the Stretch Reflex

Stretch reflex has two principal functions:

a. To maintain muscle tone. Tone is the tendency of a muscle to resist being stretched. Muscle tone is not only important for maintaining posture but also facilitates locomotion and makes all voluntary movements smooth.
b. To make muscles respond to stretch and release. Stretch reflex makes a muscle respond to stretch by contraction and to release by relaxation. Both these responses, which oppose the triggering stimulus, help make voluntary movements smooth and graceful.

Inhibitory Interneurons

Muscles act to produce movement at joints. While one set of muscles produce flexion, another set produces extension. These two sets are said to be antagonistic (opposed) to each other. Contraction of a muscle cannot have its full effect unless its antagonistic muscle relaxes (Fig. 16.8). When a muscle contracts, simultaneous relaxation of its antagonist is ensured by inhibitory interneurons. This general principle has been illustrated by the action of inhibitory interneurons which relax antagonistic muscles during the stretch reflex (Fig. 16.9).

Golgi Tendon Organs

Golgi tendon organs are receptors sensitive to tension and are located in muscle tendons. When a muscle

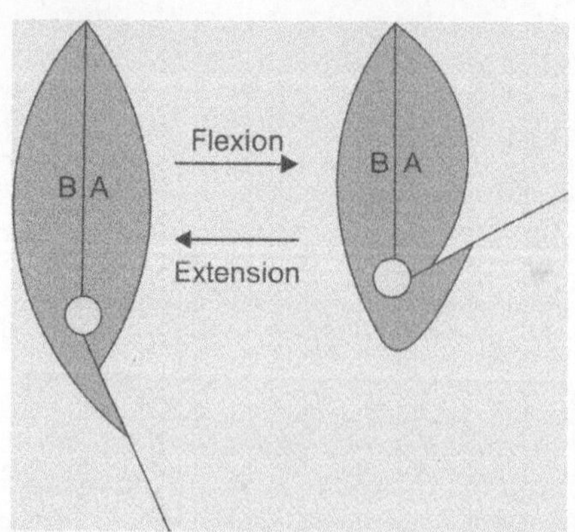

Fig. 16.8 In order to bend (flex) the limb, muscle A should contract and muscle B should relax. To straighten (extend) the limb, muscle B should contract and muscle A should relax. Muscles A and B are called antagonistic muscles

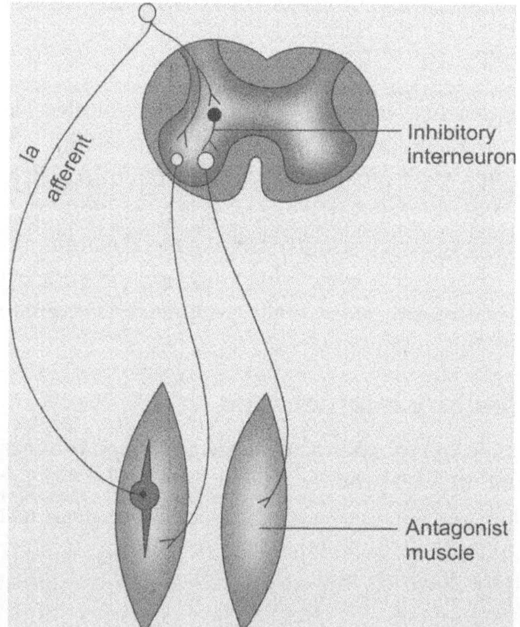

Fig. 16.9 When muscle A is stretched, the stretch reflex leads to its contraction. Simultaneously its antagonist muscle B relaxes due to activation of an inhibitory interneuron

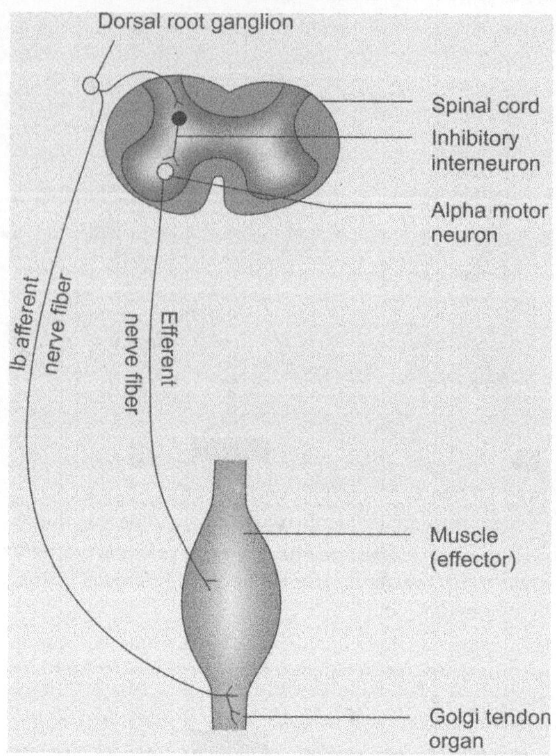

Fig. 16.10 Reflex arc for the Golgi tendon organ reflex

contracts, it pulls on the tendon. That increases the tension acting on Golgi tendon organs. As a result, the Golgi tendon afferents, which are innervated by Ib type of nerve fibers, get stimulated. Stimulation of Golgi tendon organs leads to relaxation of the contracting muscle. The relaxation is brought about by inhibitory interneurons (Fig. 16.10). In this way, Golgi tendon organs prevent a muscle from acting too strongly.

You might have observed two essential differences between muscle spindles and Golgi tendon organs:

a. Muscle spindles detect change in length of a muscle while Golgi tendon organs detect change in tension.
b. Stimulation of muscle spindles leads to contraction of the muscle whereas stimulation of Golgi tendon organs leads to relaxation of the muscle.

Although Golgi tendon organs seem to be opposed to the action of muscle spindles, it is not actually so. Stretching a muscle stretches mainly the muscle spindles. Conversely, contraction of a muscle makes the spindles lax but increases tension on the Golgi tendon organs (Fig. 16.11). Therefore the response to a change in muscle length or tension is similar from both types of receptors.

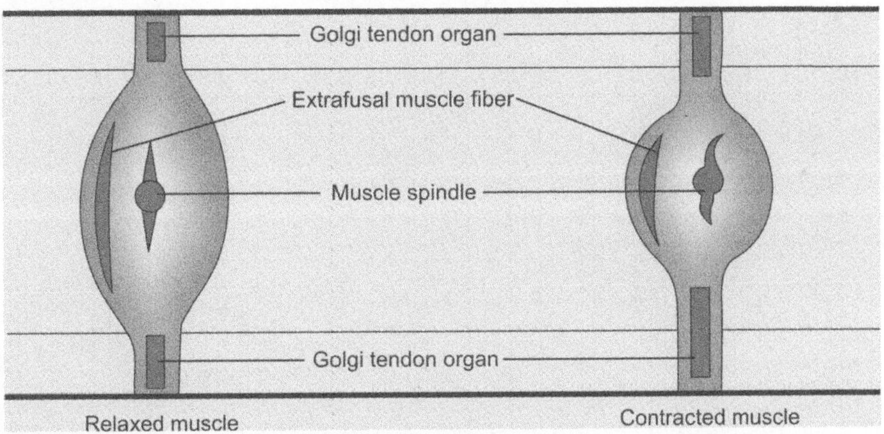

Fig. 16.11 Diagrammatic representation of the effect of contraction of a muscle on the muscle spindles and Golgi tendon organs. Note that muscle contraction reduces tension on the spindles but increases it on the Golgi tendon organs. This happens due to two factors: 1. In isometric contraction the origin and insertion of the muscle remain a fixed distance apart. Therefore the length of muscle + tendons does not change during contraction. Since the muscle contracts, the tendons get stretched and 2. The Golgi tendon organs are in series with, while muscle spindles are parallel to, the extrafusal muscle fibers

Renshaw Cells

Renshaw cells are inhibitory interneurons which are activated by collaterals from alpha motor neurons. They inhibit the same motor neuron which activates them (Fig. 16.12). Therefore when a motor neuron is activated, Renshaw cells prevent it from getting too active. Conversely, when the activity of a motor neuron is very low, Renshaw cells tend to activate it.

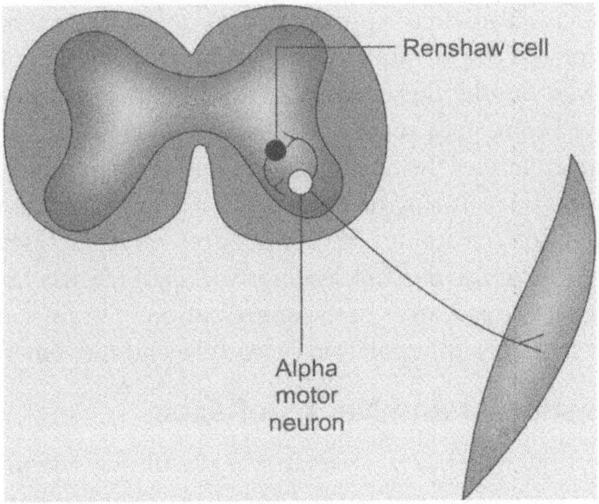

Fig. 16.12 Recurrent inhibition of a motor neuron by a Renshaw cell

This is a typical negative feedback control system. Thus Renshaw cells help stabilize the activity of motor neurons, and through them, the degree of contraction of muscles. Stabilization of muscle contraction, in turn, stabilizes the joints.

Flexion Reflex

Flexion reflex is a typical protective reflex. A painful stimulus applied to the hand or foot results in withdrawal of the limb. Withdrawal involves flexion of the limb. Therefore the reflex is called flexion reflex. Flexion results from contraction of flexor muscles and relaxation of extensor muscles. Simultaneous contraction of flexors and relaxation of extensors is brought about by reciprocal innervation (Fig. 16.13).

Crossed Extension Reflex

It is observed that whenever the flexion reflex is elicited in a limb, the other limb undergoes extension. This is called crossed extension reflex. The neuronal circuitry responsible for the crossed extension reflex is as shown in Figure 16.14. If you try to visualize a combination of flexion and crossed extension reflexes, you would realize that the latter tends to stabilize the posture.

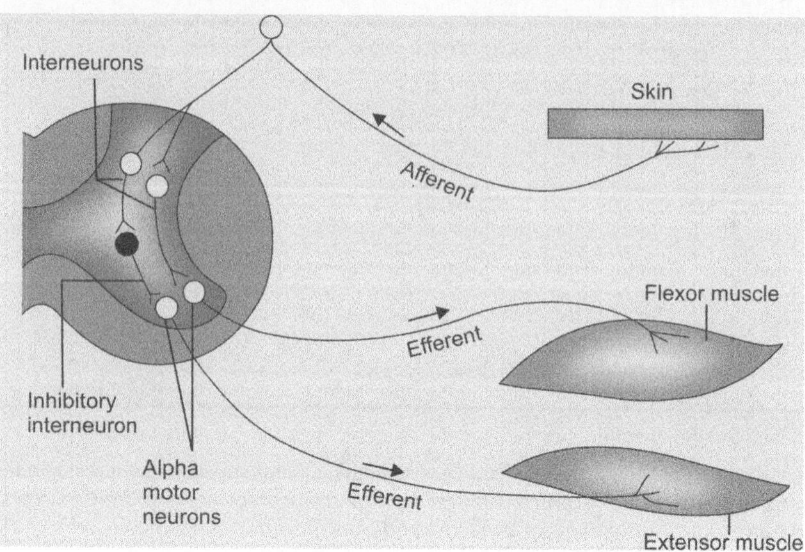

Fig. 16.13 Reflex arc for the flexion reflex. A noxious stimulus on the skin of a limb leads to contraction of the flexor and relaxation of the extensor of that limb

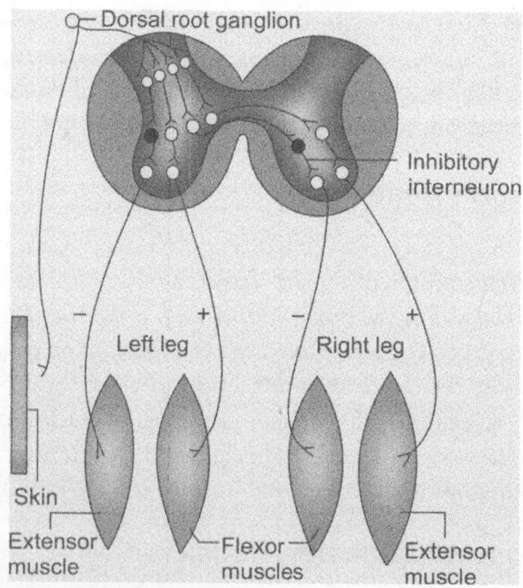

Fig. 16.14 Reflex arc for the crossed extension reflex. A noxious stimulus on the skin of the left leg leads to contraction of its flexor and relaxation of its extensor muscles (i.e. the left leg undergoes flexion). In the right leg, the extensor contracts and the flexor muscle relaxes (i.e. the right leg undergoes extension)

The neuronal circuitry employed for flexion and crossed extensor reflexes is not only used for the protective reflex but also for rhythmic movements such as walking. For that purpose, the spinal circuitry is further influenced by higher regions of the central nervous system.

BRAIN STEM MOTOR MECHANISMS

The higher regions of the central nervous system which influence spinal motor mechanisms are arranged in a roughly hierarchical fashion. The lowest among these higher regions is the brain stem. The brain stem mediates reflexes which coordinate movements of the head and eyes, and serve to stabilize the posture during movement. In addition, the brain stem also mediates the influences of still higher regions of the nervous system. We shall discuss here only a few examples of the contribution of brain stem mechanisms to regulation of posture and movement.

Vestibular and Neck Reflexes

Vestibular reflexes arise in the vestibular apparatus, which is a part of the inner ear. Neck reflexes originate in the muscle and joint receptors in the neck. Before going into these reflexes, we shall talk briefly about the vestibular apparatus.

Vestibular Apparatus

The inner ear consists of the organ of hearing (cochlea) and the vestibular apparatus. The cochlea has been discussed in Chapter 15. Here we shall restrict ourselves to the vestibular apparatus, often called just the vestibule. The vestibule consists of the otolith organs (saccule and utricle) and semicircular canals (Fig. 16.15). The sensory cells in the vestibule also are hair cells similar to those in the cochlea. The hair cells of the saccule and utricle respond to linear acceleration and to change in the position of the head, while those of semicircular canals respond to angular acceleration.

Vestibular Reflexes

Tilting the head forward without bending the neck leads to contraction of dorsal neck muscles. That stabilizes the neck and tends to keep the orientation of the head vertical.

During a free fall, vestibular reflexes ensure that upper limbs are extended and lower limbs are flexed. These responses reduce the chances of injury.

During linear or rotatory motion, vestibular reflexes lead to movement of the eyeballs so that an object can be followed for a reasonable distance. When it becomes impossible to follow that object, eyes suddenly shift their focus to a new object.

Neck Reflexes

Bending or rotating the neck towards one side leads to contraction of neck muscles on the other side. It also leads to extension of the arm and leg on the same side (ipsilateral limbs) and flexion of the arm and leg on the opposite side (contralateral limbs).

In humans, bending the neck backwards produces reflex extension of arms and legs. Bending the neck forwards produces flexion of arms and legs. In animals, the responses are somewhat different. However, to observe these reflexes, higher neural control has to be removed as can happen in injuries in humans, or can be done experimentally in animals.

Pathways for Vestibular and Neck Reflexes

Impulses from vestibular receptors or muscle and joint receptors in the neck reach the brain stem. After processing in the brain stem, descending pathways (vestibulospinal and reticulospinal tracts) convey the message to motor neurons in the spinal cord.

Although vestibular and neck reflexes have been described separately, in practice both may

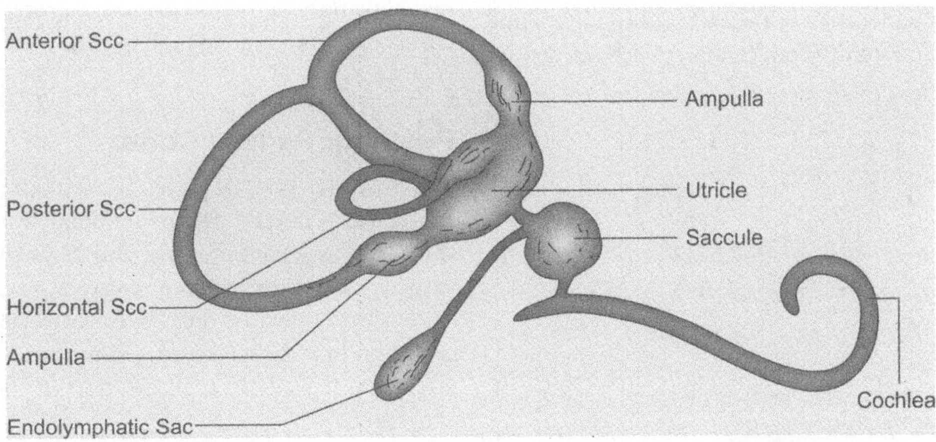

Fig. 16.15 A schematic diagram of the vestibular apparatus and cochlea. Only the membranous labyrinth has been shown. Scc, semicircular canal

be activated simultaneously. Further, in an intact animal, higher neural influences modify the basic brain stem reflexes.

Reticular Formation

The central core of the brain stem has a dense network of neurons called the reticular formation (RF). RF has both ascending and descending pathways. Here we are concerned primarily with the descending influences of RF.[2] The pontine RF is relatively medial and has a facilitatory influence on motor neurons. The medullary RF is relatively lateral and has a predominantly inhibitory influence on motor neurons.

Decerebrate Rigidity

Brain stem mechanisms have been studied experimentally in animals whose brain has been sectioned above the vestibular nuclei but below the red nucleus. Such a section can be achieved by making a cut between the superior and inferior colliculi (intercollicular transection). On making such a cut, the animal exhibits what is called decerebrate rigidity. Decerebrate rigidity was first described by Sherrington in 1896.

An animal with decerebrate rigidity has increase in muscle tone of the extensors of all limbs (Fig. 16.16). Such an animal can stand unsupported on a stable surface.

Human patients with decerebrate rigidity show an increase in extensor tone but not the characteristic posture.

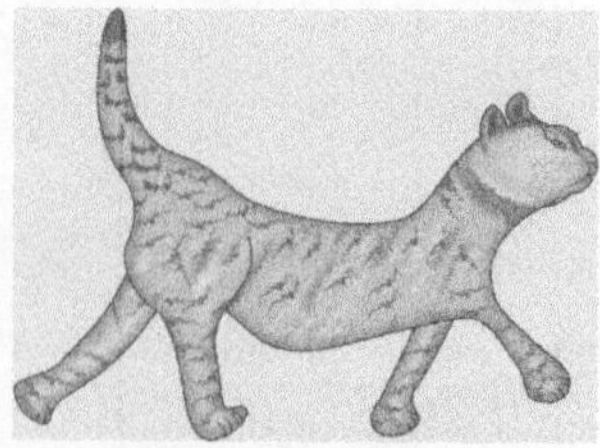

Fig. 16.16 The posture of a cat having decerebrate rigidity

[2]The ascending reticular formation will be discussed in Chapter 18.

Mechanism of Decerebrate Rigidity

Decerebrate rigidity is due to exaggerated stretch reflexes originating in the extensors. It is a combination of:

a. Uninhibited activity of vestibulospinal tract and pontine RF. Both these pathways have a facilitatory influence on alpha and gamma motor neurons of extensors.
b. Removal of the inhibition of extensor motor neurons by the higher centers, specially the red nucleus.

CORTICAL MOTOR MECHANISMS

Cortical motor mechanisms are involved in voluntary movements, i.e. movements which are under the control of will power. These movements involve a conscious decision, or a thought, that "I want to perform this movement". The thought may be triggered by an object which we wish to approach. Thus voluntary movements have up to three components:

A. Target identification, i.e. determining the goal or purpose of movement,
B. Plan of action, i.e. programming the sequence of movements, and
C. Execution, i.e. actually performing the movement.

These three components are handled by three neighboring areas of the cortex: the posterior parietal cortex, premotor areas and primary motor cortex (Fig. 16.17).

Posterior Parietal Cortex

The posterior parietal cortex receives afferents from the sensory cortex, from vestibular system, from the visual association cortex and from the auditory association cortex. Thus it receives a wide variety of sensory information. Its function is to direct attention to a chosen sensory stimulus. By directing attention, it leads to identification of the target of movement.

The posterior parietal cortex also receives afferents from the cingulate cortex, which is a part of the

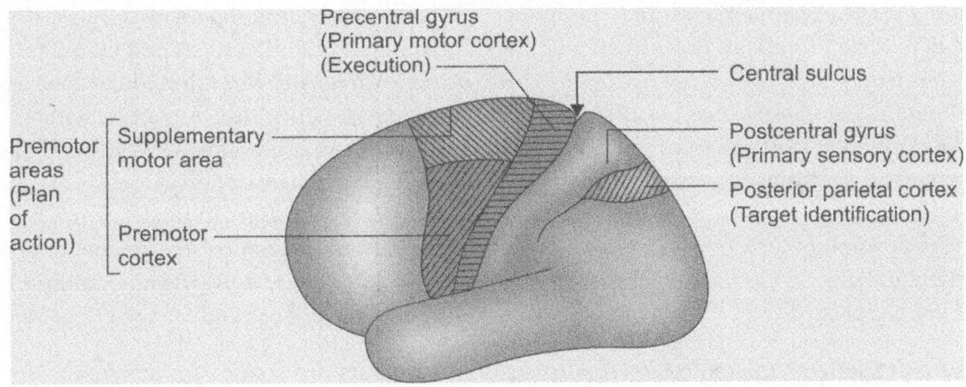

Fig. 16.17 The three principal areas of the cerebral cortex involved in motor functions

limbic system (Chapter 17). It is possibly through these connections that emotions or motivation affect voluntary movements.

The posterior parietal lobe sends efferents to the premotor cortex, which programs the movements. In turn, the posterior parietal lobe also receives afferents from the premotor cortex as feedback.

Premotor Cortical Areas

There are two premotor areas: first the supplementary motor area, also called the secondary motor cortex or M II; and second, the premotor cortex. Premotor areas receive afferents from the posterior lobe. On the basis of information about the target received from there, the premotor areas program the sequence of movements. Premotor cortical areas also coordinate movements of the two sides of the body.

The efferents from premtor areas project to the primary motor cortex and also to the brain stem and spinal cord.

Primary Motor Cortex

Primary motor cortex is located in the precentral gyrus. Stimulation of points in the primary motor cortex leads to movement of a well defined part of the body. On the basis of such experiments, a topographical map of the primary motor cortex has been worked out. The movements of jaws and other neighboring areas are initiated lower down while movements of legs are initiated in the upper

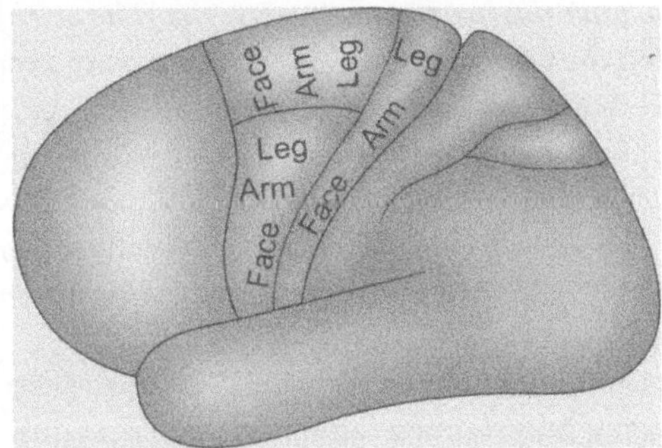

Fig. 16.18 Topographic representation of the body in primary motor area, supplementary motor area and premotor cortex

part of the primary motor cortex. Thus, as in the sensory cortex, in the motor cortex also, the body is represented upside down (Fig. 16.18). Also, as in the sensory cortex, parts with fine movements (e.g. fingers) have a much bigger representation than regions with coarse movements (e.g. trunk). Further, stimulation of the right motor cortex leads to movements on the left side of the body. Thus the control of movements by the cortex is contralateral. The posterior parietal lobe and premotor cortical areas also have a topographical representation (Fig. 16.17). Connections between the three cortical areas concerned with different aspects of motor function are predominantly between parts representing corresponding regions of the body. That is, the arm area of the posterior parietal lobe projects predominantly to the arm area of the premotor cortex which, in turn, projects to the arm area of the primary motor cortex.

The primary motor cortex receives afferents not only from the premotor cortical areas but also from the sensory cortex, thalamus, cerebellum and basal ganglia.

The primary motor cortex sends efferents to the brain stem and also to alpha and gamma motor neurons of the spinal cord.

Overview of Cortical Motor Mechanisms

Cortical motor mechanisms are concerned with voluntary movements. The process may be initiated by the intention to approach an object. The attention is fixed on the object, and its position with respect to the body is registered in the posterior parietal lobe. The information is transmitted to the premotor cortical areas.

Premotor cortex is the region where the sequence of motor activity is programmed. The program is transmitted to the primary motor cortex. The primary motor cortex executes the program by activating appropriate alpha motor neurons. As the movement continues, moment to moment information from muscles and joints is also provided to the motor cortex. On the basis of this information, the movement is guided accurately and terminated at the right moment.

THE CEREBELLUM

Once we have talked about the cortical mechanisms, the story of motor functions may seem to be complete. But there are still two more sets of structures which contribute major refinement to motor function: these are the cerebellum and the basal ganglia. When the function of these structures is impaired, movement is possible but becomes highly imperfect.

Functional Anatomy of the Cerebellum

The gross structure of the cerebellum is complex. But from the functional point of view, it is enough to know a few major divisions.

The cerebellum is divided by two transverse furrows, or grooves, into three lobes: anterior lobe, posterior lobe and flocculonodular lobe (Fig. 16.19). Similarly, longitudinal furrows divide it into the midline vermis (literally, a worm) and the left and right cerebellar hemispheres (Fig. 16.20). Buried deep into the cerebellum are its nuclei, which contain most of the output neurons of the cerebellum. The nuclei are (from outside towards the midline): dentate, emboliform, globose and fastigial (Fig. 16.21).

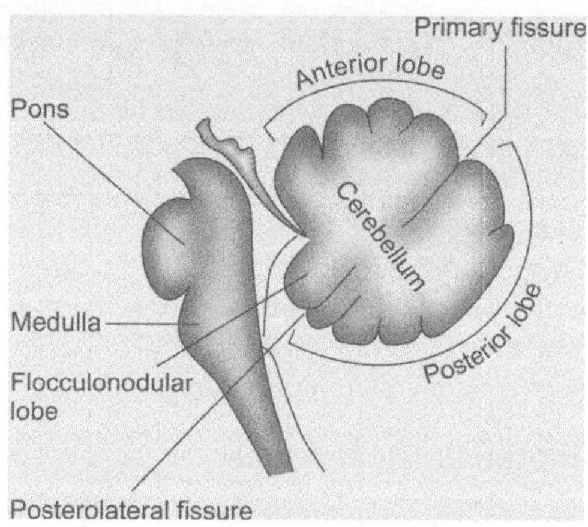

Fig. 16.19 The three lobes of the cerebellum

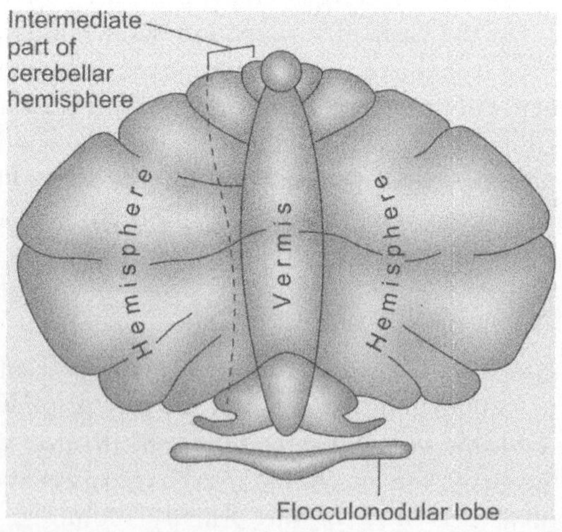

Fig. 16.20 The vermis and cerebellar hemispheres. Each hemisphere is further divided, from a functional point of view, into an intermediate part and a lateral part

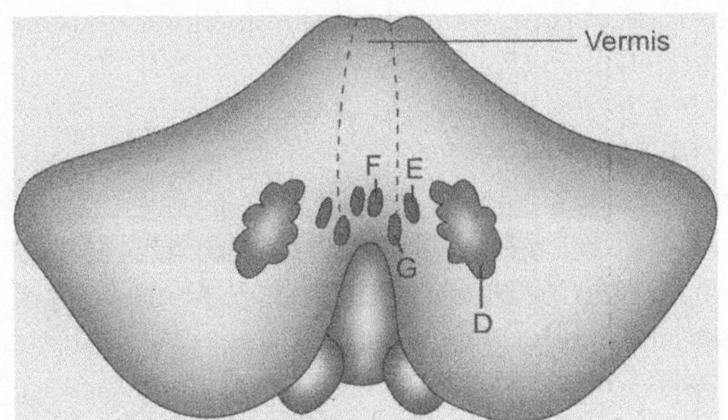

Fig. 16.21 The cerebellar nuclei. Dorsal view of the cerebellum with the deep nuclei shown as they would look if it was possible to see through the substance of the cerebellum. D, dentate nucleus; E, emboliform nucleus; G, globose nucleus; F, fastigial nucleus

The microscopic structure of the cerebellum is very neat and regular. It consists of a superficial cortex and underlying white matter. The cortex is arranged into three layers: molecular layer, Purkinje cell layer and granular layer (Fig. 16.22).

The white matter contains two types of afferent fibers. One of these are the climbing fibers, which bring information only from the inferior olivary nuclei, and establish excitatory synapses with Purkinje cells. All the other afferent input into the cerebellum is brought by the other type of afferent fibers, which are called mossy fibers. Mossy fibers establish excitatory synapses with granule cells in the granular cell layer. The axons of granule cells, called parallel fibers, stimulate the Purkinje cells. Thus

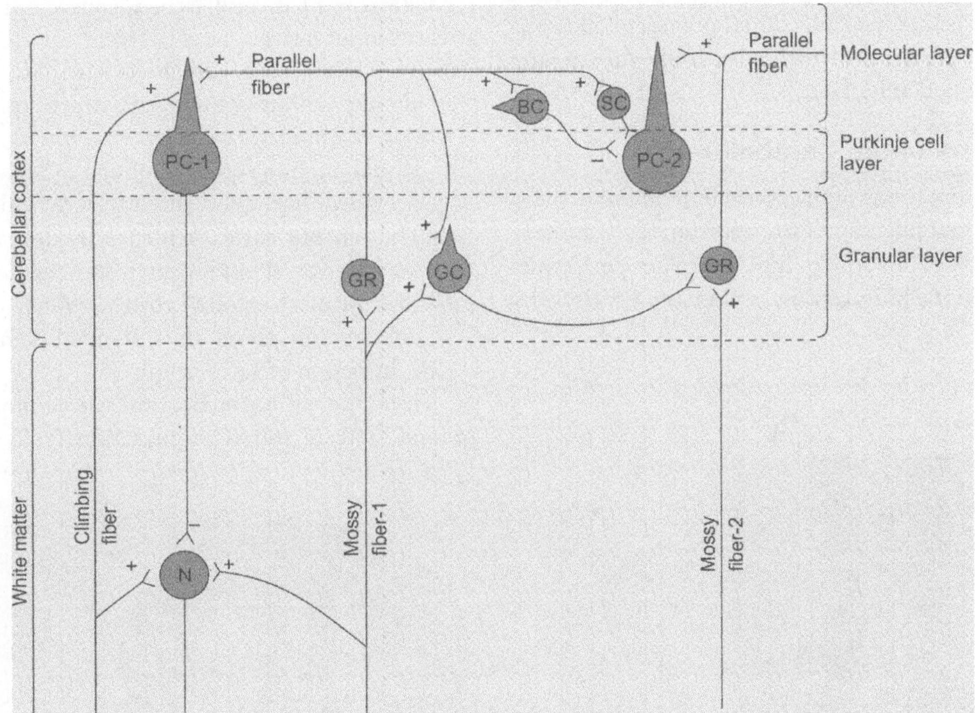

Fig. 16.22 Schematic diagram showing the neuronal circuitary of the cerebellum. The chief inputs into the cerebellum are the climbing and mossy fibers. The climbing fibers excite the Purkinje cells, as shown in case of PC-1. The mossy fibers excite Purkinje cells via granule cell (GR) axons, called parallel fibers. Note that mossy fiber-1 also excites Golgi cells (GC), basket cells (BC) and stellate cells (SC). GC, BC and SC inhibit the neighboring Purkinje cell, PC-2, directly or indirectly. Thus excitation of mossy fiber-1 not only stimulates PC-1 but also inhibits the neighboring cell PC-2. Besides affecting the activity of the chief output neurons of the cerebellar cortex, the Purkinje cells, the mossy and climbing fibers also directly stimulate the deep cerebellar nuclei (N). The layers of the cerebellum have also been indicated

mossy fibers, like the climbing fibers, also end up stimulating the Purkinje cells. The parallel fibers also stimulate three types of interneurons: stellate and basket cells in the molecular layer, and Golgi cells in the granular layer. These interneurons project to several neighboring Purkinje cells, and inhibit them.

Thus Purkinje cells are stimulated by climbing fibers and mossy fibers. But when a mossy fiber is excited, besides stimulating some Purkinje cells, it also inhibits their neighbors by stimulating the stellate, basket and Golgi cells. In this way the contrast between the stimulated Purkinje cells and the neighboring unstimulated cells is increased (Fig. 16.23).

Purkinje cells project to the deep cerebellar nuclei. Purkinje cells employ gamma-aminobutyric acid (GABA) as a neurotransmitter, and inhibit the neurons of the deep cerebellar nuclei. However, this inhibition is modulated by the stimulatory collaterals which the deep nuclei receive from mossy and climbing fibers (Fig. 16.22).

Functions of the Cerebellum

The main functions of the cerebellum are to achieve postural stability and to coordinate voluntary movements. How these functions are performed by the cerebellum can be understood better by considering one by one the three functional divisions of cerebellum (Fig. 16.24).

Vestibulocerebellum

This division consists of the flocculonodular lobe. It is essentially an extension of the vestibular apparatus. It receives afferents from the vestibular apparatus and sends efferents to the vestibular nuclei. It works with the vestibular apparatus to:

a. Modulate muscular activity so as to achieve postural equilibrium or balance, and
b. Coordinate movements of the eyes with movements of the head.

Spinocerebellum

This division consists of the vermis and the intermediate part of cerebellar hemispheres. It receives afferent input from:

a. The spinal cord, which provides information about position of limbs and degree of contraction of muscles,
b. Visual, auditory and vestibular systems, which provide information about the environment,
c. The sensory cortex, which provides still more information about the environment, and
d. The primary motor cortex, which provides information about the intended sequence of contraction of various muscles.

Thus the spinocerebellum can compare the present state of muscle contraction (achievement)

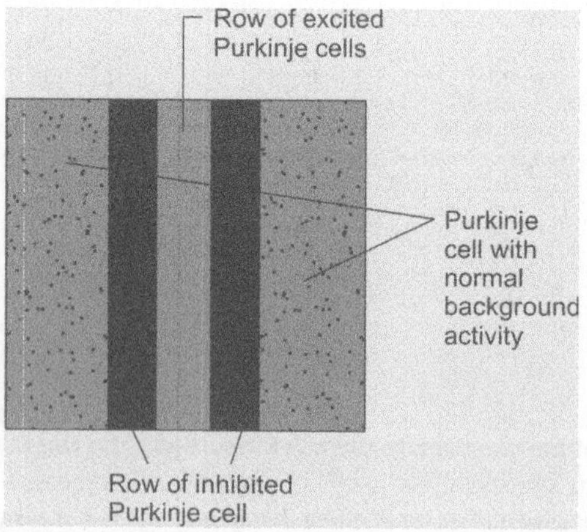

Fig. 16.23 Inhibition of neighboring Purkinje cells increases the contrast between the stimulated and unstimulated regions of the cerebellar cortex

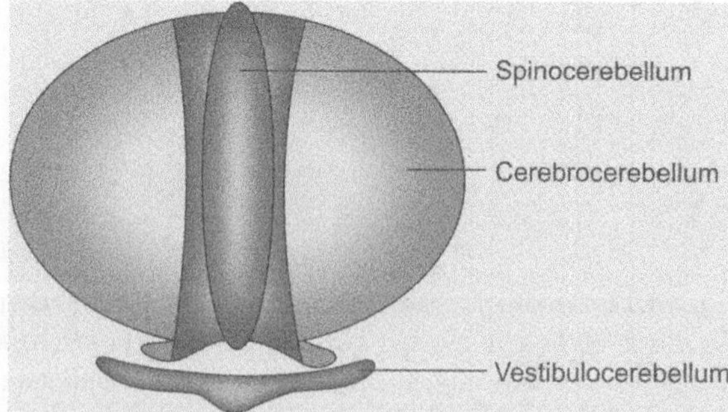

Fig. 16.24 The three functional divisions of cerebellum

with the desired muscle contraction (intention). By comparing the achievement with intention, the cerebellum can determine the error, and hence the correction to be applied so that the final achievement is exactly the same as the intention. Since the position of the moving limb changes from moment-to-moment, the cerebellar correction also changes continuously. That makes the movement smooth, or well coordinated. Further, information about the environment helps in making the muscular activity more accurate, for example, by directing the limb towards the target avoiding any obstruction.

These functions are performed by the cerebellum through its efferents which project to the motor cortex, reticular formation, red nucleus and vestibular nuclei. Through its projections specially to the reticular formation and red nucleus, the cerbellum also regulates muscle tone.

Cerebrocerebellum

This division consists of the lateral parts of the cerebellar hemispheres. It is essentially an extension of the cerebral cortex.

It receives afferents from the sensory cortex, primary motor cortex, premotor cortex, and the posterior parietal cortex. It sends efferents to the thalamus, premotor cortex and primary motor cortex.

The cerebrocerebellum is believed to process the information it receives, and accordingly it modulates the activity of the premotor and motor cortex. Thus it plays a role in planning and initiation of voluntary movements.

Role of Cerebellum in Motor Learning

There is evidence to indicate that cerebellar circuits can undergo sustained functional changes as a result of experience. The climbing fibers play an important role in this process. In a new situation, the climbing fiber activity is high, and it tends to reduce mossy fiber activity. On repeated exposure to the situation, the mossy fiber response gets stabilized at the low level without an increase in the climbing fiber activity.

Cerebellar learning may spare the cerebral cortex during learnt movements. That is probably why walking, swimming or typing need conscious effort while being learnt. But after learning, one can continue these activities mechanically without having to think about them. After learning, the responsibility for these activities seems to shift more and more to the cerebellum leaving the cerebral cortex free for other tasks. That is why a child who is learning to walk has to put all his mind into it. Any distraction may make him fall. But an adult can walk and perform many other mental activities while continuing to talk effortlessly.

Overview

The functions of the cerebellum may be summarized as follows:

a. Regulation of tone, posture and equilibrium.
b. Coordination of voluntary movements.
c. Coordination of eye movements.
d. Planning and initiation of movements.
e. Learning frequently performed voluntary movements.

Effects of Cerebellar Lesions

In view of the cerebellar functions discussed above, it is easy to explain the following clinical features which are observed in patients having cerebellar lesions:

a. Reduction in skeletal muscle tone (hypotonia).
b. Incoordination of voluntary movements (ataxia).
c. Tremors towards the end of a goal-oriented movement (Intention tremors).
d. Unstable posture.
e. Walking clumsily with feet widely separated to reduce instability (Wide-based ataxic gait).

BASAL GANGLIA

The basal ganglia seem to be a primitive version of the cerebral cortex and are richly connected with it. Like the cerebral cortex, basal ganglia have sensory, motor and motivational functions. But since it is the motor functions of basal ganglia which are most prominent, here we shall concentrate on those.

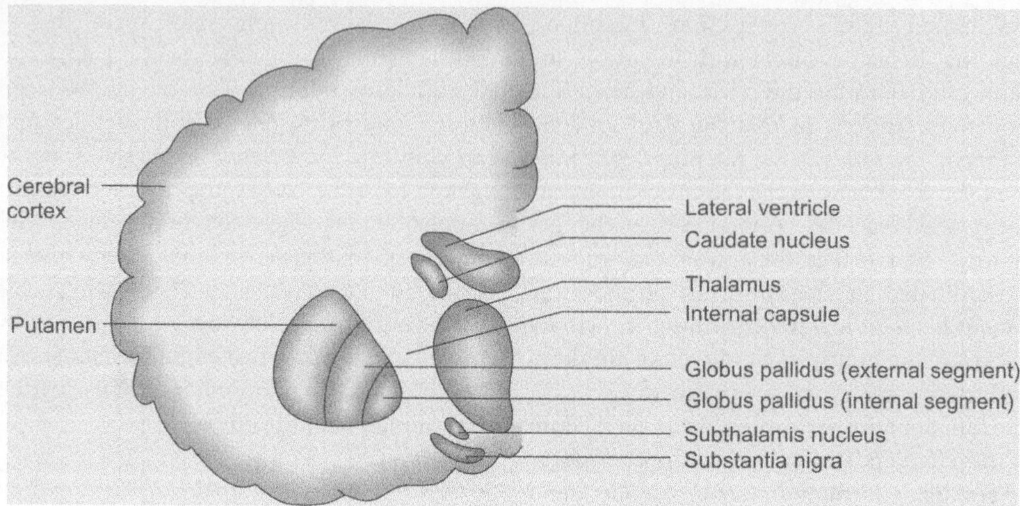

Fig. 16.25 The basal ganglia

Structure

The basal ganglia consist of (Fig. 16.25):

a. Caudate nucleus
b. Putamen
c. Globus pallidus
d. Subthalamic nucleus
e. Substantia nigra

Caudate and putamen are together called the straitum, and receive most of the afferent input coming to the basal ganglia. Globus pallidus and substantia nigra are the principal output nuclei, i.e. the efferents arise from these. From this it follows that different components of basal ganglia are extensively connected with one another.

Afferent Connections

The striatum (caudate and putamen) receives afferent fibers from all parts of the cerebral cortex (sensory, motor, association and limbic cortex). It also receives afferents from the thalamus (Fig. 16.26).

Internuclear Connections

Basal ganglia are richly connected with one another as shown in Figure 16.27.

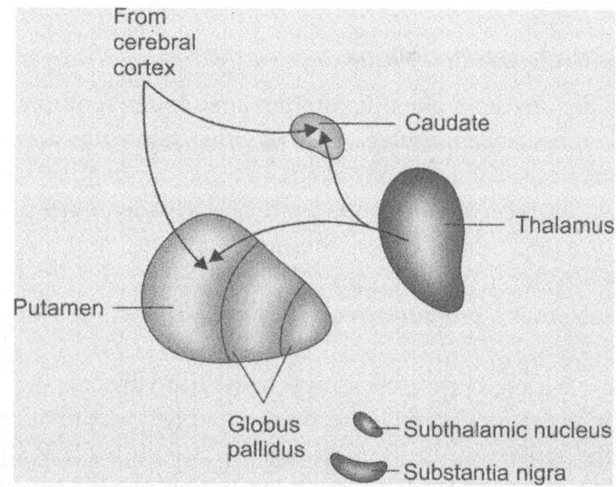

Fig. 16.26 Afferent connections of the basal ganglia

Efferent Connections

The efferents arise mainly from parts of globus pallidus and substantia nigra. The efferents project to the thalamus, and from there to the prefrontal cortex, premotor cortex, supplementary motor area and the primary motor cortex. Through the motor cortex, basal ganglia project to the brain stem and

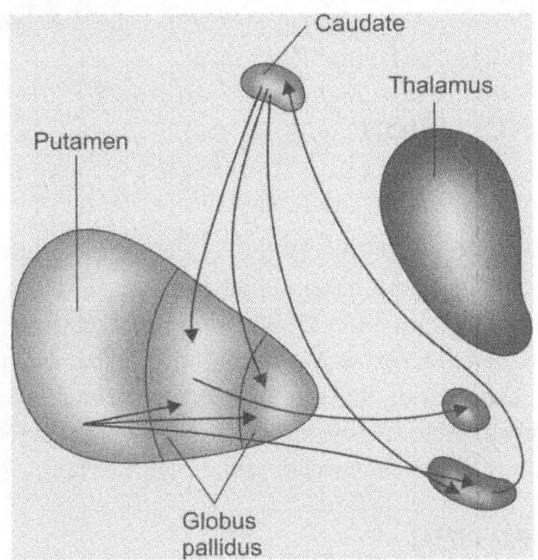

Fig. 16.27 Internuclear connections of the basal ganglia. Unlabeled structures are as in Figure 16.26

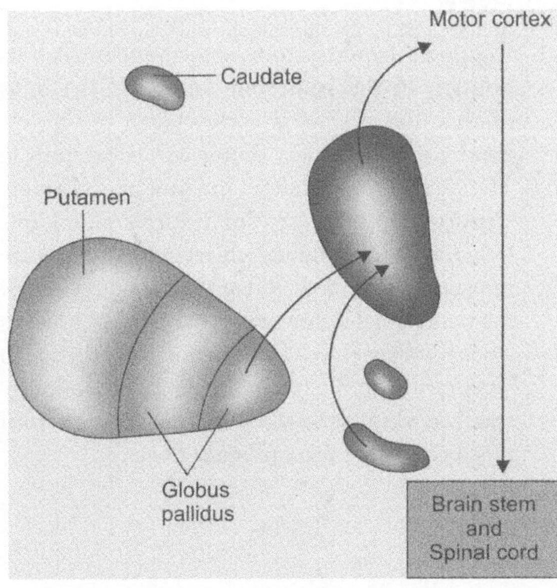

Fig. 16.28 Efferent connections of the basal ganglia. Unlabeled structures are as in Figure 16.26

spinal cord via corticobulbar and corticospinal tracts (Fig. 16.28). There are no direct connections between the brain stem or spinal cord and the basal ganglia.

Functions

The best known functions of basal ganglia are the motor functions.

Motor Functions

On the basis of their connections and also functional studies, the motor functions of basal ganglia are thought to be:

a. Selective facilitation of some movements and suppression of others.
b. Comparator function, similar to that of the cerebellum. Basal ganglia are also in a position to compare intentions of the cortex with achievements of the muscles and apply appropriate correction.
c. Regulation of muscle tone.
d. Initiation of movements generated by internal cues. In contrast with movements such as walking or picking up an object, there are movements such as scratching, moving the hands over the face, facial expression, etc. which apparently lack any motive. These movements are not conscious movements and can be easily observed in every member of a group assembled anywhere. You can verify this by observing your friends during a class without making them conscious of it. Before you conclude that such movements are funny, keep in mind that you make them too! Such internally generated movements are possibly initiated by the basal ganglia.[3]
e. Control of eye movements.

Other Functions

Although the connections of basal ganglia suggest that they possibly have sensory and motivational functions, these are not well understood. One function ascribed to them is that of geographical memory. This function is not entirely unrelated

[3]In contrast, voluntary movements generated by the external environment, such as walking or picking up an object, are initiated in the cerebral cortex.

to motor function. It is our memory of 'maps' that enables us to walk or drive effortlessly on familiar routes, without using our conscious mind (i.e. cerebral cortex). Birds can navigate long distances in a relatively featureless sky possibly because their basal ganglia are specially well developed.

Parkinson's Disease

The first lessons about basal ganglia were learnt from studies on patients having Parkinson's disease, named after James Parkinson, the physician who first described it in 1817. One thing common to all patients having the disease is a lesion in the basal ganglia. Now it is known that the primary defect is degeneration of the nerve fibers connecting substantia nigra to the striatum (nigrostriatal pathway). This pathway employs dopamine as the neurotransmitter.

The clinical features of Parkinson's disease are:

a. Age usually above 50 years.
b. Tremors at rest. The tremors are rhythmic (3-6 times/second) and present at rest but disappear when the patient starts performing a voluntary movement.[4]
c. Increase in muscle tone, characteristically called cogwheel rigidity.[5]
d. Lack of spontaneous, internally generated movements, called akinesia.
e. Slowness of voluntary movements, called bradykinesia.
f. Shuffling gait. The patient stoops forward and walks in small and rapid steps. He seems to be chasing his center of gravity.

The disease is often treated with L-DOPA, which generally gives favorable results.

CONCLUSION

The final common pathway for motor function is the alpha motor neuron. These neurons are influenced by a hierarchy of controls (Fig. 16.1). First, there are the stretch reflex and other spinal reflexes. Next are the brain stem controls. Still higher level control is exerted by the cerebral cortex. The cerebellum and basal ganglia join hands with the cerebral cortex to improve the quality of motor performance and to relieve the cerebral cortex of controlling well-learnt motor activities.

QUESTION

1. Explain how you can reach the tap in the bathroom even with your eyes closed.

ANSWER

1. Although the tap cannot be seen, memory of its position in the bathroom exists. On the basis of this, the premotor cortex plans the movement and the primary motor cortex executes it. The cerebellum monitors the minute-to-minute sensory information from muscles and joints to apply a continuous correction so that the movement is smooth and in the right direction. If the hand still does not reach the tap, but touches a neighboring object, information from the touch receptors helps the premotor cortex plan another small movement towards the tap. Execution of this movement makes us reach the tap.

---

[4]In contrast, a patient with cerebellar disease has no tremors at rest but gets tremors during a voluntary movement.

[5]Imagine the movement of a cogwheel to visualize the features of the rigidity.

CHAPTER

17 Nervous System: Visceral Functions and Motivation

"An old self lurks in the new self we are; Hardly we escape from what we once had been: In the dim gleam of habit's passages, In the subconscient's darkling corridors, All things are carried by the porter nerves and nothing checked by subterranean mind, Unstudied by the guardians of the doors and passed by a blind instinctive memory, The old gang dismissed, old cancelled passports serve, Nothing is wholly dead that once has lived."

—SRI AUROBINDO

(Savitri, Book 7, Canto 2, p. 483)

Chapter Outline

- Autonomic Functions
- Limbic System
- Hypothalamus

We have seen in the previous chapters that many sensory fibers in the ascending tracts terminate in the central nervous system at points below the cerebral cortex. Similarly, although voluntary motor activity is initiated in the cerebral cortex, considerable involuntary motor activity does not involve the cerebral cortex. In fact, much of living processes are regulated by levels of the nervous system below the cerebral cortex. These processes may be of two types. First, the activities of internal organs or viscera are regulated involuntarily without necessarily involving the cerebral cortex. That is why we do not have to make a voluntary or conscious effort to make the heart beat, or to make it beat faster during exercise. Second, some basic urges such as hunger, thirst or sex are satisfied without necessarily involving the cerebral cortex in reasoned planning. These needs are met, specially in animals, by the basic urge to seek pleasure and to avoid pain. In human beings and other higher animals, seeking food, water or a mate may seem to involve a lot of thinking, reasoning or planning. But these cortical activities are secondary to the basic motivations. If there were no basic motivation, the animal would not make the effort and take the risks involved in fulfilling these needs. Thus emotions are a fundamental force guiding the activities of all animals.

Visceral functions are also called autonomic functions. Behavioral responses to the basic emotions of pain and pleasure are also accompanied by marked changes in visceral activity. Thus visceral and motivational functions are closely related. Therefore, in the sections that follow, it will be difficult to separate them completely, and it is not at all necessary to do so.

AUTONOMIC FUNCTIONS

Autonomic functions are the functions which are not under the control of our will power, such as beating of the heart or movements of the stomach. These functions are regulated by the autonomic nervous system (ANS). ANS regulates these functions by controlling the activity of smooth muscle, cardiac muscle or glands.

The term autonomic refers to the fact that organs innervated by the ANS are not entirely dependent on nerve supply for their activity, i.e. they have an autonomous activity of their own. Innervation by the ANS only modulates (i.e. increases or decreases) the activity of these organs.

Both these facts, viz. that autonomic functions are not dependent on our will power, and that they are not entirely dependent on nerve supply, are very beneficial. If conscious effort were required to beat the heart, to breathe, and to digest food, we would have little time left to attend to anything else. And if, occasionally, we forgot to beat the heart for a few minutes, we would be no more! Further, if the nerve supply is interrupted, the function is impaired but does not stop altogether. This is a vital gain because some of the autonomic functions are essential for life.

Functional Anatomy

The effects of ANS are mediated by the preganglionic neurons, which are located in the intermediolateral column of the spinal cord, or corresponding group of neurons in the brain stem. Axons of preganglionic neurons synapse with postganglionic neurons in the ganglia, which are outside the central nervous system (Fig. 17.1).

ANS is further divided into two divisions: sympathetic and parasympathetic. The structural features of the two divisions have been depicted in Figure 17.2 and the two divisions have also been compared in Table 17.1. Note the similarities between the sympathetic division and adrenal medulla; both are generally activated together.

Neurotransmitters in ANS

In both sympathetic and parasympathetic system, the preganglionic neurons employ acetylcholine (ACh) as the neurotransmitter. The postganglionic parasympathetic neurons also employ ACh as the neurotransmitter. The postganglionic sympathetic neurons usually employ noradrenaline (NA) as the neurotransmitter (Fig. 17.3). But there are a few

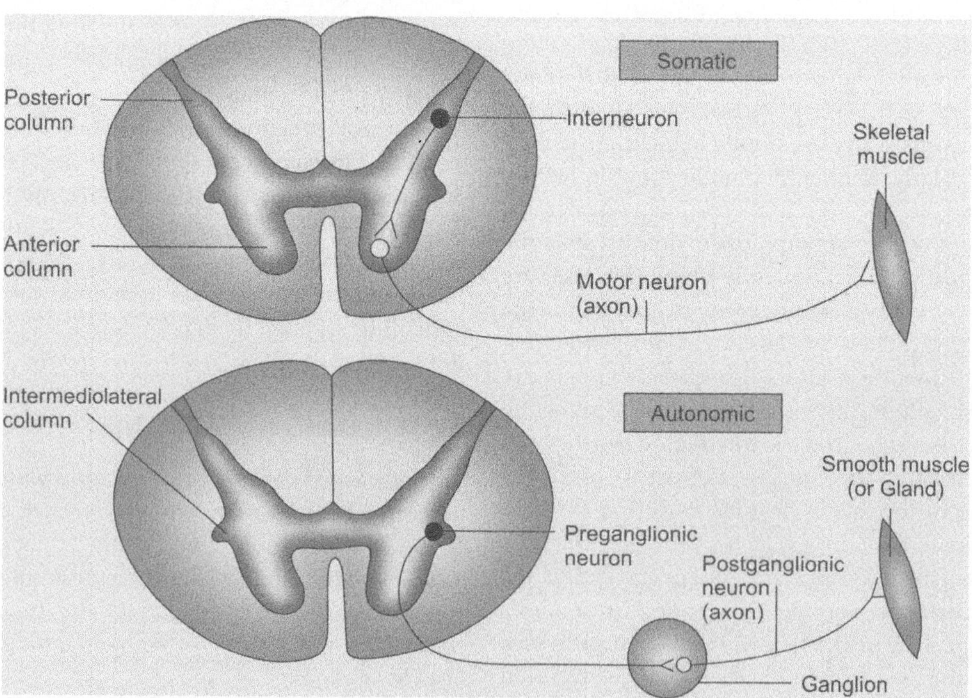

Fig. 17.1 Somatic and autonomic nervous systems compared

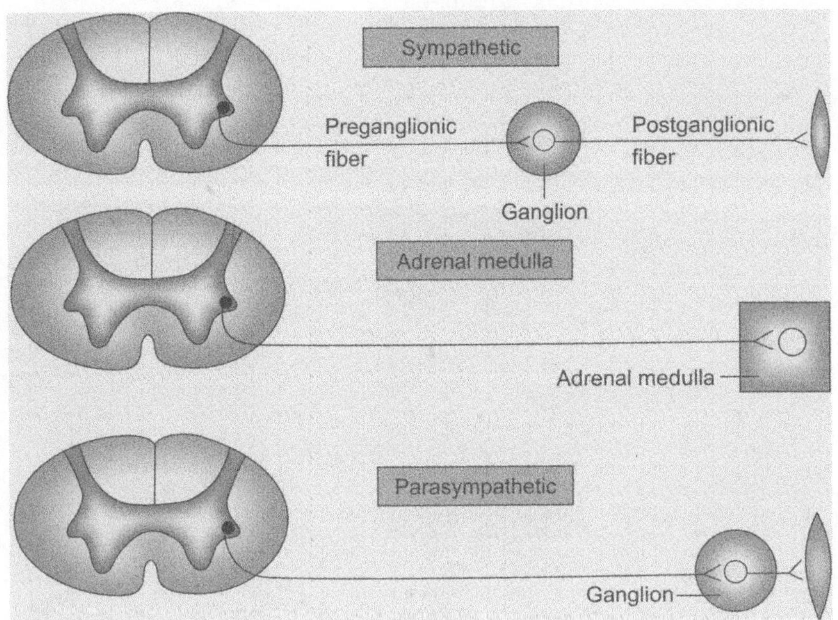

Fig. 17.2 The basic organization of the sympathetic nerves, adrenal medulla, and parasympathetic nerves

Table 17.1 Comparison between sympathetic and parasympathetic nervous system

	Sympathetic	*Parasympathetic*
Site of preganglionic neurons	Thoracolumbar (Segments T1-L3)	Craniosacral (Nuclei of cranial nerves III, VII, IX and X; Segments S2-4)
Site of ganglia	Paravertebral and prevertebral ganglia	Within or very close to the organ innervated
Preganglionic neurons	Cholinergic	Cholinergic
Postganglionic neurons	Adrenergic (Exceptions: In sweat glands and skeletal muscle, cholinergic)	Cholinergic
Activation	In emergencies, and in REM sleep	When relaxed, and in slow wave sleep
Effects	Useful in emergencies Substrates mobilized for providing energy Catabolic and thermogenic	Useful at rest Substrates deposited for storage Anabolic

notable exceptions. The postganglionic sympathetic neurons innervating sweat glands employ ACh as the neurotransmitter. The vasodilator fibers in skeletal muscles are also cholinergic.

The biologic effect of a neurotransmitter is the result of its interaction with the receptors in the target organ. For both ACh and NA, more than one type of receptors exist in the body.

Receptors for ACh are called *cholinergic receptors*. The cholinergic receptors in ganglia are called nicotinic. The cholinergic receptors at the targets of parasympathetic postganglionic nerve endings, and in sweat glands, are called muscarinic.

Receptors for NA and adrenaline are called adrenergic receptors. Adrenergic receptors also fall in two broad categories: alpha and beta. NA is primarily

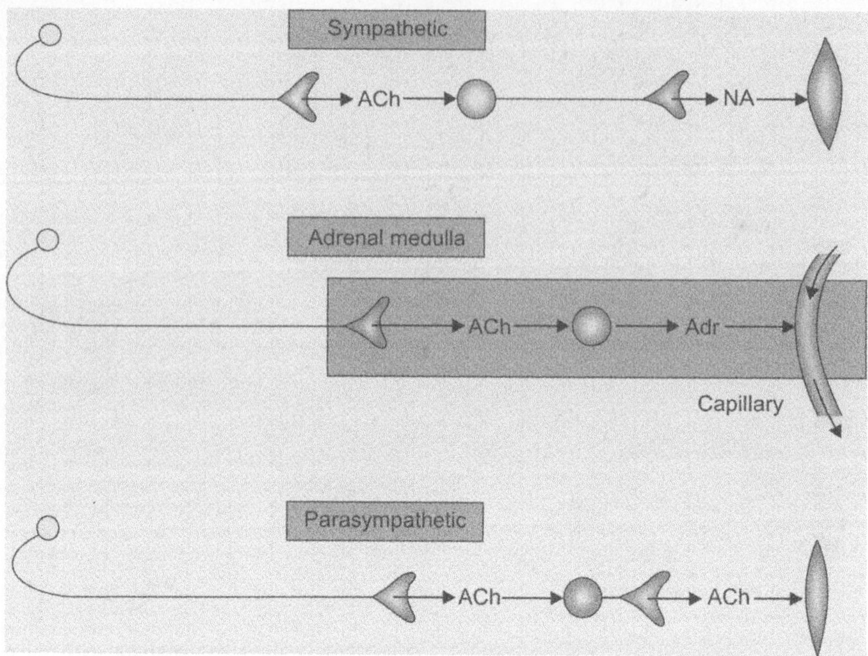

Fig. 17.3 Neurotransmitters employed by the autonomic nervous system. ACh, Acetylcholine; NA, noradrenaline; Adr, adrenaline

an alpha stimulator but does have a little beta receptor activity as well. Adrenaline stimulates alpha and beta receptors equally well. Postganglionic sympathetic nerve endings release only NA but adrenal medulla releases a mixture of adrenaline and NA.

Drugs which have effects similar to a neurotransmitter are called agonists. Drugs which block the action of neurotransmitters are called antagonists. Agonists and antagonists may be specific for a particular type of receptor. A few representative antagonists have been shown in Figure 17.4, and a few agonists and antagonists in Table 17.2.

Physiological Role of ANS

The physiological function of ANS is to modulate visceral and glandular activity in the body. Most organs innervated by ANS receive both sympathetic and parasympathetic supply, and the effect of activation of the two divisions of ANS on a given organ is opposite. What effect which division has on an organ can be best predicted in terms of its benefit to the body. The sympathetic division is called so because it 'sympathizes' with the body in an emergency. The types of effects it produces are useful in fighting an enemy or escaping a danger. On the other hand, parasympathetic division induces activities which are best performed in a relaxed state.

For example, while fighting or fleeing, the heart needs to beat harder and faster, and glucose and fatty acids should be mobilized from glycogen and triglycerides respectively, and these are all effects of sympathetic activation. Further, in such a situation, the bronchi should dilate so that breathing is facilitated, and pupils should dilate so that maximum possible light should enter the eyes: and that is what sympathetic activation does. On the other hand, when one is relaxed, one may eat, which should be followed by digestion. Accordingly, gastrointestinal secretion

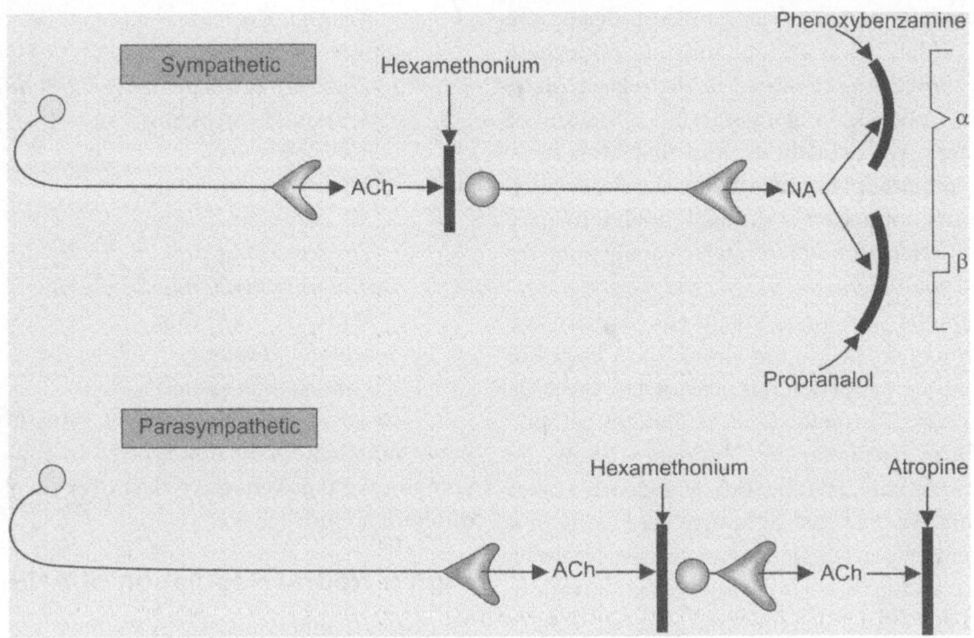

Fig. 17.4 Agents which may be employed to block the action of autonomic nerves at the level of the ganglia or the postganglionic fibers. ACh, acetylcholine; NA, noradrenaline

Table 17.2 Chemicals affecting autonomic function

Site	*Neurotransmitter*	*Agonist*	*Antagonist*
Ganglia	Acetylcholine	Nicotine, small doses Methacholine	Nicotine, large doses Hexamethonium
Postganglionic parasympathetic nerve endings	Acetylcholine	Muscarine, Pilocarpine Methacholine, Acetylcholinesterase inhibitors, e.g. Physostigmine, Neostigmine	Atropine
Postganglionic sympathetic nerve endings and adrenal medulla	Noradrenaline and Adrenaline	Alpha: Phenylephrine	Alpha: Phenoxybenzanine, Phentolamine
		Beta: Isoproterenol (Isoprenaline)	Beta: Propranalol
		Beta 2: Albuterol	Beta 1: Metoprolol

and motility are increased by parasympathetic activation. One would like to read a book also in the relaxed state. Reading needs a constricted pupil, which can be achieved by parasympathetic activation. The effects of sympathetic and parasympathetic are in terms of functional requirements rather than one always producing contraction and the other always producing relaxation. For example, sympathetic produces constriction of blood vessels but relaxes the gastrointestinal and bronchial musculature.

This principle is best illustrated by considering the functions of defecation and micturition. Both these functions should be performed in the relaxed state, and require contraction of a viscus but relaxation of its sphincters. We actually do find that both these functions require parasympathetic activity, which brings about contraction of the anal canal or urinary bladder but relaxation of the internal anal sphincter and vesical sphincter.

Sympathetic and parasympathetic activity are generally antagonistic but not always so. A beautiful example of their cooperation is provided by the male sex act. Erection is brought about by parasympathetic activity but ejaculation is brought about by sympathetic activity. Possibly this arrangement takes into account the fact that although sex begins in a relaxed atmosphere, it generates an excitement on its own, which in turn leads to sympathetic activation. Hence it is just as well that the 'final' part of the act is triggered by the sympathetic nervous system.

Another general principle of autonomic neural activity is that sympathetic activation is usually generalized while parasympathetic activity is relatively localized. This is partly because sympathetic activation is also associated with stimulation of the adrenal medulla which results in a systemic 'injection' of adrenaline. The arrangement is useful because cardiovascular, respiratory and other sympathetic effects are usually required simultaneously in an emergency whereas parasympathetic effects such as pupillary constriction, digestion or micturition are required only one at a time. However, there is one important exception to this generalization: thermal sweating is a sympathetic phenomenon but is not accompanied by other sympathetic effects. This is because sweating is required in isolation, and the isolated effect is perhaps made possible by the cholinergic innervation of sweat glands.

A beautiful description of the effects of sympathetic stimulation is available in the *Gita* (Chapter 1, verses 28-30). When Arjun stood up in his chariot in the battlefield, it suddenly dawned on him that he would have to fight those whom he loves and respects. He said:

Krishna, Krishna
Now as I look on
These my kinsmen arrayed for battle
My mouth is parching
My body trembles
My hair stands upright
My skin seems burning
The bow Gandiva
slips from my hand
My brain is whirling
round and round
I can stand no longer

A summary of the effects of sympathetic and parasympathetic activation is given in Table 17.3. As you go over these effects, reflect over their utility in different circumstances.

Higher Neural Regulation of ANS

The organs innervated by ANS have considerable autonomy. After denervation, they not only retain activity but can also modulate that activity to a considerable degree in response to changing conditions. For example, stretch leads to smooth muscle contraction. Hence even a denervated intestinal segment has a tendency to propel its contents. Secondly, some visceral organs, notably the gut, have a well developed plexus of neurons within their wall which can provide neural regulation in response to local stimuli. Therefore it may be considered quite enough to have some further modulation by autonomic nerves. But that is not so: the ANS activity itself is subject to modulation by higher neural structures.

First, ANS activity is directly influenced by sensory inputs which evoke autonomic reflexes.

Second, the intermediolateral column cells are subject to modulation by brain stem reticular formation.

Third, ANS activity is markedly affected by the hypothalamus. Generally speaking, posterior hypothalamus stimulates sympathetic activity whereas anterior hypothalamus evokes parasympathetic activity. But this is an oversimplification. Later experiments on awake, unrestrained animals, have

Table 17.3 Autonomic effects on various organs

Organ	Effects of: Sympathetic stimulation	Effects of: Parasympathetic stimulation
Heart	Increase in rate. Increase in force of contraction	Decrease in rate. Decrease in force of contraction
Lungs	Bronchodilation	Bronchoconstriction
Gastrointestinal tract	Decrease in motility, tone and secretion Contraction of sphincters	Increase in motility, tone and secretion Relaxation of sphincters
Bladder	Relaxation of detrusor Contraction of sphincter	Contraction of detrusor Relaxation of sphincter
Blood vessels	Splanchnic and cutaneous vasoconstriction Skeletal muscles: Constriction (adrenergic alpha), dilatation (adrenergic beta-2), dilatation (cholinergic)	None None
Eyes	Pupillary dilatation. Relaxaiton of ciliary muscles	Pupillary constriciton. Contraction of ciliary muscles
Sweat glands	Sweating (cholinergic)	Sweating on palms only
Metabolic effects	Glycogenolysis. Lipolysis	Not significant

shown that stimulation of the hypothalamus evokes a complete behavioral pattern. For example, stimulation of a specific area may lead to all the autonomic and somatic manifestations of anger. Thus the role of hypothalamic control of ANS is to weave different autonomic and somatic reflexes into a meaningful pattern. Hypothalamus is also an outlet for the influences of other still higher neural structures such as the limbic system and cerebral cortex on the ANS. That is why hypothalamus was called the head ganglion of the ANS by the renowned neurophysiologist, Sir Charles Sherrington.

The overall effect of higher influences is that not only autonomic activity manifests as a meaningful behavioral pattern but there are also emotions associated with it (ascribed to the limbic system), and the effects may anticipate body needs (ascribed to the cerebral cortex). For example, the increase in heart rate occurs on the mere thought of exercise, and salivary secretion occurs on the mere thought of food. These anticipatory effects are due to the influence of the cerebral cortex on ANS.

LIMBIC SYSTEM

The term limbic system has nothing to do with limbs. Limbic system (*limbus*, girdle or belt) is that part of the brain which encircles the corpus callosum and brain stem like a belt. Evolution of the limbic system added a strong emotional component to the basic drives which are important for preservation of self or the species. Emotions make an animal immensely more successful in the struggle for existence. For example, if food is a source of pleasure to an animal, the drive to pursue food is strengthened. In anticipation of this pleasure, the animal makes a vigorous search for food. If it is a carnivore, the animal becomes very aggressive when confronted with a potential source of food. On the other hand, looking at it from the point of view of the victim, the emotion of fear increases its speed of running, which is likely to facilitate safe escape. Thus in this brief example we have seen how the emotions of pleasure, aggression and fear aid survival. In reptiles the highest part of the neuraxis is essentially the limbic system. But in higher animals more and more neocortical control has been imposed on the limbic system. That is why the limbic system has very low *anatomical* visibility in the primate brain. It is only on cutting the cerebral hemispheres along the midline or by lifting the cerebral hemispheres up from the base of the skull that we can see the limbic system on the medial surface and undersurface of the brain. But even in the primate brain the limbic system has high *physiological* visibility. Strong emotions associated with food and sex are rather thinly veiled even in the most cultured of men.

Functional Anatomy

Given below is a list of structures on which there is general agreement about their inclusion in the limbic system (Fig. 17.5).

Neocortical Structures

Orbitofrontal cortex and part of the temporal lobe and parietal lobe.

Archicortical Structures

Subcallosal gyrus, cingulate gyrus, parahippocampal gyrus, hippocampus, dentate gyrus, subiculum, septum and parolfactory area.

Subcortical Structures

Anterior nuclei of thalamus, amygdala, nucleus accumbens (part of basal ganglia), hypothalamus.

There is some disagreement about the inclusion of hypothalamus in the limbic system. But hypothalamus is functionally so intimately related to the other limbic structures that it is impossible for a physiologist to think of the limbic system without the hypothalamus.

Connections

Limbic system is a link between the brain stem and the neocortex. Accordingly the limbic structures are richly connected by to and fro connections with each other, with the association cortex, and with the

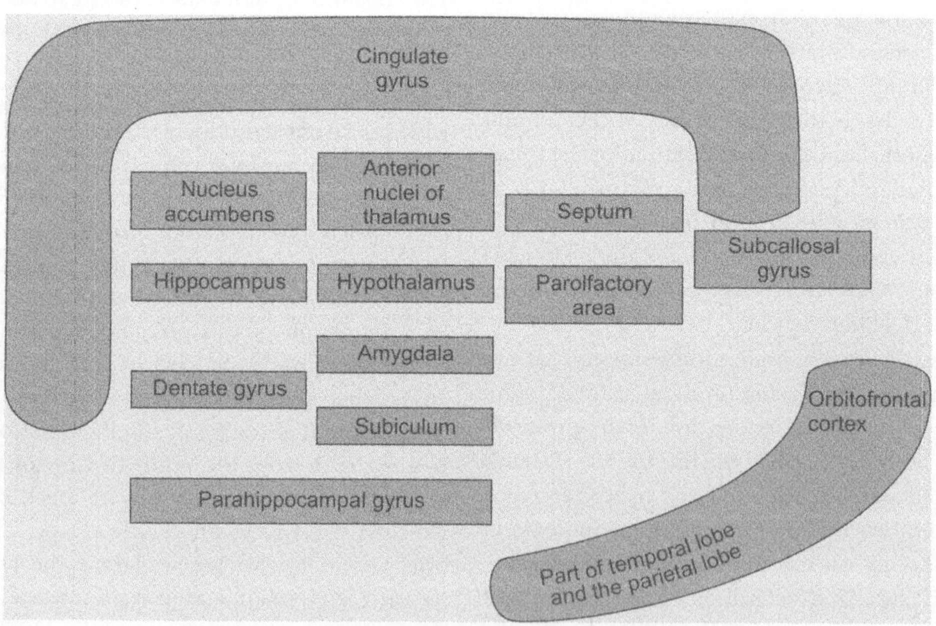

Fig. 17.5 Structures generally included in the limbic system

brain stem. Some of the better known pathways are described briefly below.

Papez Circuit: James Papez, an eminent neuroanatomist, described a classical circular pathway which is known after him (Fig. 17.6). By demonstrating the projections from the cortex to the limbic structures, he provided a structural basis for the influence of thoughts on emotions. The projections from the limbic structures back to the cortex explain how emotions reach consciousness.

Medial forebrain bundle: Medial forebrain bundle is a major efferent connection of the limbic system. It projects from a large number of limbic structures to the hypothalamus, and from there to the reticular formation. Through the medial forebrain bundle the limbic system can influence autonomic and endocrine activity.

Other connections: Amygdala projects to other regions of the limbic system by means of stria terminalis and the ventral amygdalofugal pathway. Amygdala receives inputs from limbic structures, olfactory pathways and other sensory pathways.

Amygdala and the hippocampal formation are extensively connected with the associated cortex, thus providing a link between the limbic system and the neocortex.

Subiculum is an interesting collection of gray matter interposed between the hippocampus and the neocortex. The subiculum provides extensive reciprocal connections between the limbic system and the neocortex.

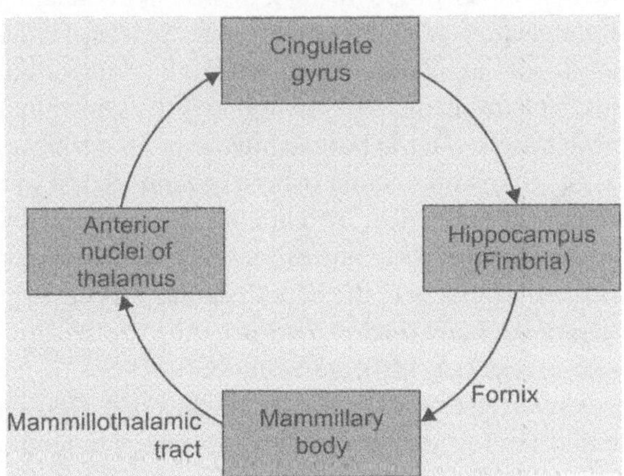

Fig. 17.6 The neural pathway described by Papez

The limbic cortex receives projections from the sensory cortex and sends efferents to various neocortical areas, including the prefrontal cortex.

Thus the limbic system has extensive reciprocal connections with either side of the neuraxis. The connections with the neocortex provide a synthesis of emotional and rational thought. The connections with the hypothalamus and reticular formation provide the structural basis of the endocrine, autonomic and motor (somatic) consequences of the limbic-neocortical interaction.

Functions

All functions of the limbic system primarily arise from its fundamental role in generating *emotions.* Limbic system adds feelings to sensory experiences, and then lets these feelings direct behavior.

Emotions: Experience and Expression

Limbic system adds an affective, or emotional component to sensory experience. The limbic system helps us interpret a sensory experience as pleasant or unpleasant. The neocortex interprets a pleasant experience as a reward, and an unpleasant experience as a punishment. Reward and punishment direct animal and human behavior to an amazing degree.

'Reward centers' have been localized in the septum and some regions of the hypothalamus. The most powerful 'punishment center' has been localized in the periventricular zone of the hypothalamus.

Hypothalamus and limbic projections to the reticular formation play an important role in producing the external manifestations of emotion. Exteriorization of emotions has endocrine components such as adrenaline secretion; autonomic components such as increase in heart rate, rise in blood pressure, piloerection, salivation and dilatation of pupils; and somatic components such as pacing up and down, frowning, baring of teeth and extension of claws. Stimulation of punishment centers in the brain can give rise to a rage reaction.

The animal is visibly angry and aggressive. On the other hand, there are also areas in the limbic cortex which can suppress the rage reaction. Stimulation of 'reward centers' makes an animal tame and docile.

Memory

Emotions and memory are closely linked. After having a pleasant or unpleasant experience, one would like to remember it so that the pleasant experiences can be repeated and unpleasant once can be avoided. Among the limbic structures, memory function has been localized to the hippocampus and the temporal limbic cortex.

Learning

Memory and learning are closely linked. Remembering does not ensure learning but some degree of remembering is essential for all types of learning.

Preservation of Self

Activities which aid preservation of self such as feeding, drinking and defence are associated with strong emotions. Limbic system not only generates these emotions, it also helps in performing the actions which satisfy these emotions. Absence of food or water creates an unpleasant feeling of deprivation, which in turn motivates the animal to find food. That the limbic system plays a part in the act of finding food (feeding behavior) is suggested by experiments in which stimulation of certain regions of the amygdala or hypothalamus induces eating, or chewing movements. Stimulation of some other regions induces drinking behavior or rage reaction.

Preservation of Species

Sexual deprivation can generate a drive almost as strong as food deprivation. As in case of other types of motivational behavior, limbic system plays a part in creating the sex urge and also in the execution of sex behavior. Stimulation of certain regions of the hypothalamus or amygdala induces some components of sex behavior. Thus the limbic system aids also the preservation of the species.

Kluver-Bucy Syndrome

Kluver, a psychologist, and Bucy, a neurosurgeon, observed in 1938 that if the anterior portion of temporal lobe cortex was removed in monkeys, they exhibited interesting changes in behavior. When the anterior temporal cortex is removed, invariably some other limbic structures, specially amygdala, are also damaged. The monkeys in whom such an operation is done show an abnormally exaggerated tendency to examine objects by putting them in the mouth and by sniffing at them. In spite of the obsession with examination of objects, they exhibit psychic blindness, i.e. they seem to see the object but fail to understand what it is. They may start eating inedible objects; the normally vegetarian monkey turns carnivorous. The animal shows reduced aggression, behaves like a tame animal, but loses fear. A characteristic feature of Kluver-Bucy syndrome is indiscriminate hypersexuality: a male monkey with the syndrome would readily have sex with a female of another species. Kluver-Bucy syndrome is interesting but neither throws much light on the function of specific limbic structures nor on human psychological disorders.

HYPOTHALAMUS

Hypothalamus is a tiny part of the brain, weighing only 10 g. It derives its name from being located under the thalamus. Although small in size, hypothalamus is a structure of major importance. It is the nodal point for regulation of almost all homeostatic mechanisms mediated by neural as well as hormonal mechanisms. The hypothalamus may be visualized as an integrating center where several neural and endocrine influences originating throughout the brain converge. After due processing, the neural and endocrine outputs of the hypothalamus diverge to all parts of the body (Fig. 17.7). Since the hypothalamus is so extensively involved in body functions, it has been referred to at several places in the book. Here we shall bring together at one place its major functions only.

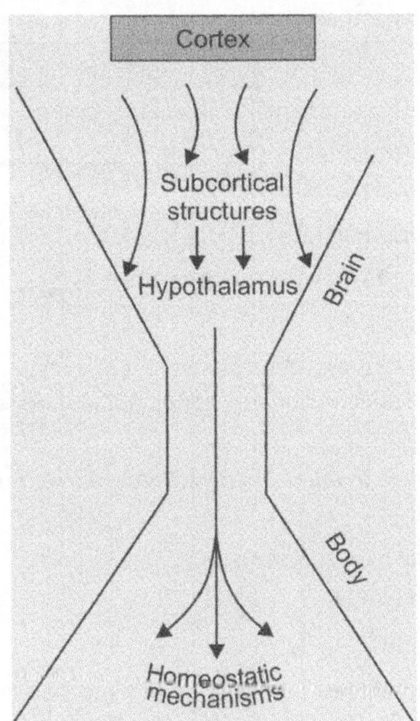

Fig. 17.7 The hypothalamus acts like a funnel which transmits the influences of the brain on several homeostatic mechanisms of the body

Functional Anatomy

The hypothalamus consists of a large number of nuclei (Fig. 17.8) and also fiber tracts.

Connections

The afferent and efferent connections of the hypothalamus have been summarized in Tables 17.4 and 17.5.

Hypothalamo-hypophysial Relationships

The hypothalamus is intimately related to both the anterior and posterior lobes of pituitary (hypophysis).

The supraoptic and paraventricular nuclei and some other neurons of the hypothalamus synthesize antidiuretic hormone (ADH) and oxytocin. These substances travel along the axons of these neurons, which terminate in the posterior pituitary. From the posterior pituitary, these hormones diffuse into the bloodstream (see Fig. 11.4).

Neurons in several nuclei of the hypothalamus also secrete various hypophysiotropic hormones

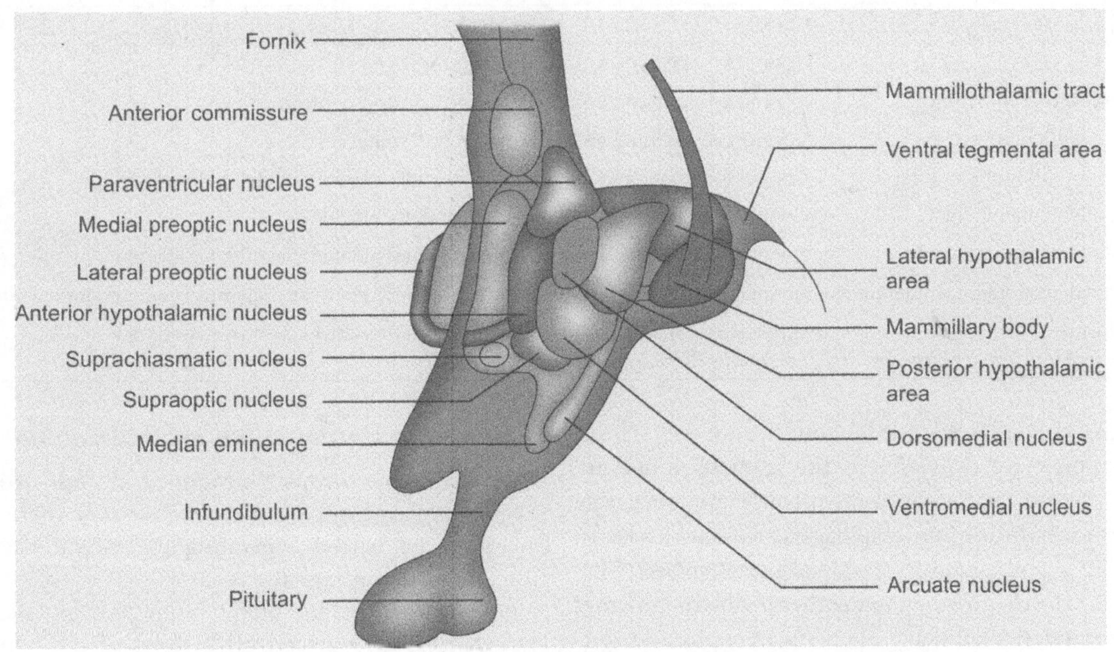

Fig. 17.8 Nuclei of the hypothalamus

Table 17.4 Afferent connections of the hypothalamus

Tract	*Connections*
Fornix*	Connects hippocampus to hypothalamus, mainly mamillary bodies
Amygdatohypothalamic fibers, principally stria terminalis	Connect amygdala to hypothalamus, mainly anterior hypothalamus, preoptic area and ventromedial nucleus
Medial forebrain bundle*	Connects limbic structures to hypothalamus
Periventricular system*	Connects midbrain and sensory pathways to hypothalamus
Ventral tegmental cholinergic bundle	Connects viscera to hypothalamus
Ventral tegmental noradrenergic bundle	Connects nucleus of tractus solitarius and ventrolateral medulla to paraventricular nuclei, periventricular nuclei, supraoptic nuclei, and lateral hypothalamic nuclei
Mesolimbic dopaminergic system	From the wall of the third ventricle to medial hypothalamic nuclei. From one region of hypothalamus to another
Dorsal noradrenergic bundle	Connects locus ceruleus to dorsal hypothalamus
Serotonergic neurons	Connect raphe nuclei to hypothalamus
Thalamohypothalamic fibers	Connect thalamus to hypothalamus
Retinohypothalamic fibers	Connect optic nerve fibers to suprachiasmatic nucleus of hypothalamus
Corticohypothalamic fibers	Connect cerebral cortex to hypothalamus directly, and indirectly via the thalamus

*Also contains efferent fibers

Table 17.5 Efferent connections of hypothalamus

Tract	*Connections*
Fornix	Connects hypothalamus to limbic system
Medial forebrain bundle	Connects hypothalamus to mesencephalic tegmentum
Periventricular system	Connects hypothalamus to midbrain and spinal cord
Tubero-infundibular tract	Connects arcuate and ventromedial nuclei of hypothalamus to infundibulum
Mamillothalamic tract	Connects mamillary bodies to anterior thalamic nuclei
Mamillotegmental tract	Connects mamillary bodies to tegmental reticular nuclei of the midbrain
Hypothalamohypophysial tracts	Connect supraoptic and paraventricular nuclei of hypothalamus to posterior pituitary
Neurons which secrete hypophysiotropic hormones	Originate in hypothalamic nuclei. Axons terminate in median eminence Secretions diffuse into the portal vessels

(releasing and release inhibiting hormones). These hormones are delivered by the axon terminals in the median eminence. In the median eminence, the hormones diffuse into a capillary network which leads to the hypothalamo-hypophysial portal vessels. The portal vessels give way to another capillary network in the anterior pituitary where the hypophysiotropic hormones are delivered (see Fig. 11.4).

Blood-brain Barrier in the Hypothalamus

Since hypophysiotropic hormones diffuse from the median eminence into portal vessels, there is obviously no barrier separating the neural tissue from blood in this region.

A weak or absent blood brain barrier (BBB) characterizes also several other areas of the hypothalamus, and has functional importance. For example, some regions of the hypothalamus detect changes in the temperature or osmolarity of blood. This is also possible only because of a weak BBB.

Functions of Hypothalamus

Functions of the hypothalamus touch almost every aspect of body function. Only some of the better studied functions will be discussed here.

Temperature Regulation

The hypothalamus has sensors which detect changes in the temperature of blood. It also receives information from temperature receptors in the skin. The information is matched with the set point for body temperature. Depending on the difference between the actual body temperature and the set point (normally 37° C), the hypothalamus initiates appropriate responses.

The anterior hypothalamus detects changes in body temperature by monitoring the temperature of blood. If the body temperature is higher than the set point, it initiates machanisms for heat loss, viz. vasodilatation in the skin, and sweating.

The posterior hypothalamus is responsible for initiating responses if the body temperature is lower than the set point. The responses are either for conservation of heat (vasoconstriction in the skin and piloerection), or for increasing heat production (shivering and release of adrenaline).

Thus the hypothalamus behaves like a thermostat. It initiates responses which tend to keep the body temperature constant at a level close to the set point.

Regulation of Food Intake

Regulation of food intake by the hypothalamus depends on the interaction of two areas. One of these areas is located medially, in the ventromedial nucleus (VMN) of the hypothalamus. This area has been called the satiety center because when an animal is full, it makes the animal stop eating. The other area is located in the lateral hypothalamus (LH). This area has been called the feeding or hunger center because it makes the animal look for food and eat.

The satiety center and hunger center were discovered by BK Anand, the renowned Indian physiologist, while working with JR Brobeck in Prof. JF Fulton's laboratory at Yale in 1951. He observed that if the VMN of rats was destroyed by passing a strong electric current through it (making an electrolytic lesion), the animals overate. They went on eating to the extent that they grew very fat. But if the lesion was made in the LH, the rats stopped eating. They preferred to die of starvation rather than eat. From this it was inferred that when it is intact, the VMN is responsible for satiety while LH activity induces feeding.

The mechanism by which hypothalamus regulates food intake seems to be through glucosensitive neurons in the VMN. These neurons are sensitive to the level of glucose utilization. When an animal is well fed, the blood glucose level is high, and these neurons utilize more glucose. That makes the neurons more active. Greater activity in VMN inhibits the feeding center in LH and thereby induces satiety. When the level of glucose utilization in VMN is low, LH is not inhibited. Therefore the animal eats. Subsequent work has suggested the neurotransmitters which may be involved in regulation of food intake, and also that intake of each macronutrient may be regulated separately (Table 17.6). It is interesting that

Table 17.6 Effects of neurotransmitters which stimulate food intake when applied locally in the hypothalamus

Neurotransmitter	*Area of application*	*Nutrient intake selectively stimulated*
Neuropeptide Y*	Perifornical area**	Carbohydrate
Norepinephrine	Paraventricular nucleus	Carbohydrate
Galanin	Paraventricular nucleus	Fat
Opiates	Paraventricular nucleus	Protein

* The most powerful stimulant of food intake known.
** The most sensitive site for stimulating feeding.
(Based on Kandel et al 1995).

cholecystokinin (CCK) is released after a meal by the gastrointestinal tract and also in the brain. Peripheral as well as central actions of CCK inhibit feeding and induce satiety. There may be other interactions also between gastrointestinal and central neural mechanisms regulating food intake. For example, distension of the stomach increases VMN activity, as demonstrated by KN Sharma in BK Anand's laboratory. Consequently, the animal feels satiated when the stomach is full.

The hypothalamic and other related mechanisms described above regulate only short-term food intake. There are further mechanisms which regulate long-term energy balance by controlling food intake as well as energy expenditure. Thus regulation of food intake by VMN and LH is only a small part of a comprehensive control system.

Regulation of Water Balance

Body maintains water balance by responding to changes in osmolarity and changes in fluid volume. The hypothalamus has mechanisms for responding to both. Body responds to disturbances in water balance by controlling either water intake or renal water loss. The hypothalaus plays an important role in controlling both.

Changes in osmolarity: Hypothalamic osmoreceptors are located in the anterior hypothalamus. Osmoreceptors are neurons, the activity of which is altered by changes in the osmolarity of plasma. When the osmolarity of plasma is high, the osmoreceptors induce thirst, which increases water intake, and also induce secretion of antidiuretic hormone (ADH), which reduces urinary loss of water. Both these responses lower the osmolarity and tend to bring it towards normal.

Changes in fluid volume: Changes in fluid volume are primarily detected by volume receptors in the right atrium, left atrium and pulmonary vessels. Large changes in volume also affect the activity of arterial baroreceptors in the carotid sinus and aortic arch. A decrease in fluid volume leads to the secretion of renin, which in turn eventually generates angiotensin II. Angiotensin II has several effects, such as vasoconstriction and release of aldosterone, both of which are beneficial when fluid volume is low. In addition, angiotensin II also has two effects on the hypothalamus. First, it stimulates release of ADH. Second, it stimulates thirst, or drinking behavior. It is interesting that circulating angiotensin II affects the activity of the subfornical organ (SFO). SFO sends a message to the preoptic area of the hypothalamus, employing an angiotensin-like molecule as a neurotransmitter. The preoptic area also receives information from baroreceptors. Information from the baroreceptors and the SFO is put together to determine the drinking behavior (Fig. 17.9).

Reproduction

First, as the source of gonadotropin releasing hormone (GnRH), the hypothalamus has an important role in reproduction (Chapter 12). Secondly, hypothalamus,

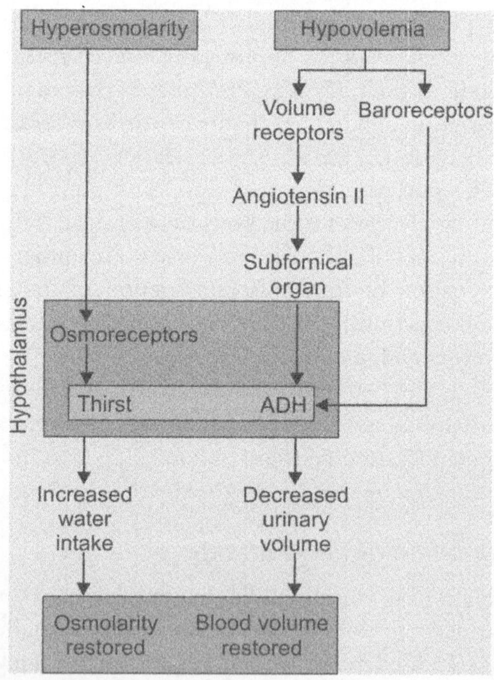

Fig. 17.9 Role of hypothalamus in regulation of water balance. Information about fluid osmolarity as well as fluid volume affects the thirst mechanism as well as ADH secretion. Changes in drinking behavior and urinary water loss act synergistically to restore fluid osmolarity and volume

along with other parts of the limbic system, affects sex behavior. The role of hypothalamus in sex behavior has been studied mainly in animals, and in them it appears to be significant. In human beings, basic sex behavior is concealed and complicated by social and psychological factors. But the underlying mechanisms at hypothalamic level are possibly similar to those in animals.

Emotions

As seen above, hypothalamus mediates the functions of the limbic system, including those related to emotions. Hypothalamus is concerned with emotional exteriorization. Both fear and rage reactions have been induced in animals by appropriate hypothalamic stimulation. Reward as well as punishment centers have been localized in the hypothalamus.

Putting together mechanisms for emotional experiences in the same region of the brain which also has centers for feeding, drinking and sex behavior makes sense. Food, water and mate are often sought for pleasure rather than to meet a physiological need. In contrast, food, water or sexual deprivation are associated with emotional distress.

Autonomic Control

Hypothalamus mediates the autonomic effects of the limbic system. In general, stimulation of the anterior hypothalamus gives parasympathetic responses while stimulation of the posterior hypothalamus gives sympathetic responses.

Endocrine Functions

As discussed above, hypothalamus is intimately related to anterior as well as posterior pituitary. It synthesizes various releasing and inhibiting hormones which are delivered to the anterior pituitary by the hypothalamo-hypophysial portal system. Through these hormones, the hypothalamus can influence a wide range of endocrine functions (Fig. 17.10). The hypothalamus

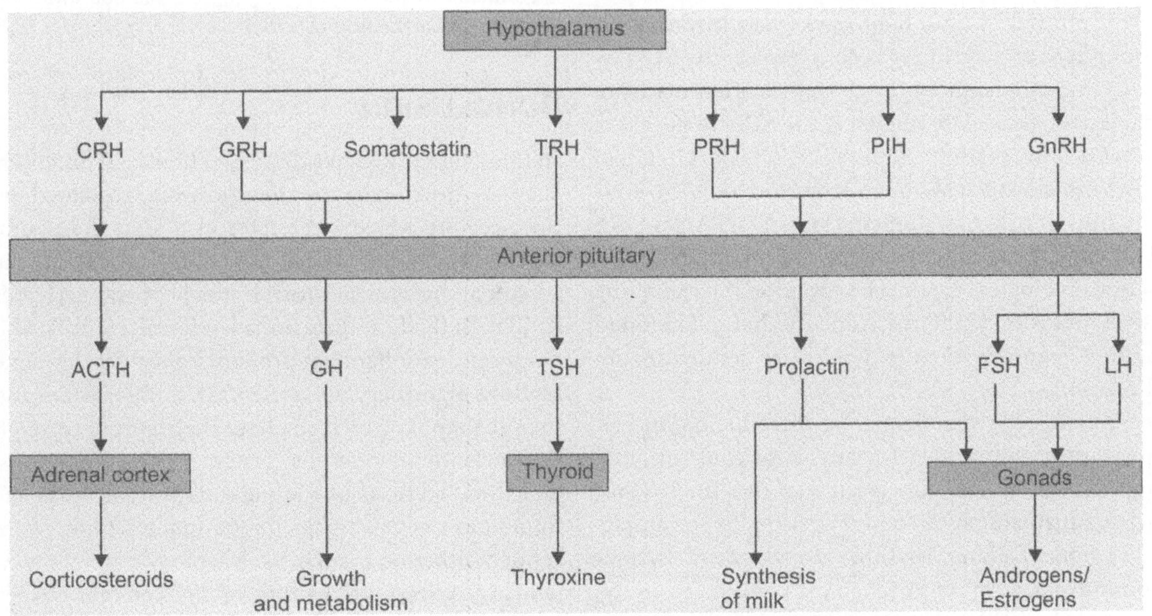

Fig. 17.10 The wide ranging endocrine influences of the hypothalamus mediated by its actions on the anterior pituitary

also synthesizes hormones of the posterior pituitary, viz. vasopressin or antidiuretic hormone (ADH) and oxytocin.

Sleep

Stimulation of suprachiasmatic nucleus (SCN) or preoptic area of the hypothalamus induces sleep in experimental animals. SCN has a major role in circadian rhythms (see below), of which sleep is one.

Circadian Rhythms

Several body functions show a circadian (24-hour) rhythm. These functions include feeding, drinking, locomotor activity, sleep, corticosteroid secretion, body temperature and melatonin secretion by the pineal. Most of these functions are regulated by the hypothalamus. Therefore it is only appropriate that a mechanism for maintaining the circadian rhythmicity of these functions is located in the suprachiasmatic nucleus (SCN) of the hypothalamus.

The rhythm of the endogenous clock is normally an exact 24-hour system. This precision is achieved by the normal 24-hour light-dark cycle. Information about light and darkness is conveyed to the SCN by retinohypothalamic fibers as well as afferents from the lateral geniculate nuclei. If the SCN is deprived of this information, the precision of circadian rhythms is disturbed but an approximately 24-hour rhythm is still maintained (Figs 17.11A and B). Therefore SCN has also been termed an endogenous biological clock. The functional basis of the clock seems to be the rhythmic discharge exhibited by SCN neurons even *in vitro* after removal from the brain.

What is the significance of introducing an element of rhythm in so many functions of vital importance? It has been speculated that the rhythm helps anticipate physiological deficits. For example, a 24-hour feeding rhythm introduces a certain compulsion, a certain mechanical periodicity, in the act of eating. The animal does not instead wait for a caloric deficit to signal the need for food.

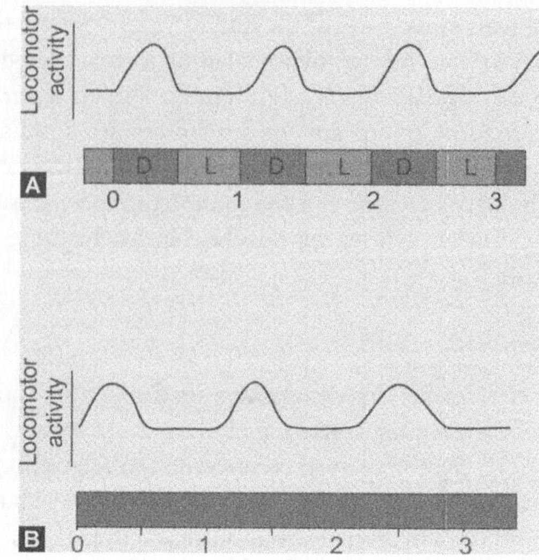

Figs 17.11A and B Circadian rhythm of locomotor activity in rats. (A) Rats exposed to a 12-h dark 'D' and 12-h light 'L' cycle resembling a normal day. Being nocturnal animals, rats show much more activity in dark than in light; (B) Rats exposed to continuous darkness. Locomotor activity still maintains circadian rhythmicity, although less precise than in A. The persistence of rhythmicity in the absence of an external cue indicates an endogenous biological clock

CONCLUSION

In this chapter we have discussed how vital functions such as heart beat or digestion are regulated by the nervous system. We have also seen the neural mechanisms underlying pain and pleasure, the basic emotions which drive much of the activities of life. Both these functions—visceral control, and emotions—are handled predominantly by the same sections of the nervous system, viz. limbic system and hypothalamus, which mediate their effects through the autonomic nervous system. These functions, and these sections of the nervous system, form the foundation of the higher forms of animal life. More refined functions, such as learning and memory, which require participation of the cerebral cortex, have been superimposed on this foundation. But that has not diminished the value of the functions which evolved earlier. No superstructure can stand without its foundation.

QUESTIONS

1. What is the significance of having dual control through sympathetic and parasympathetic innervation?
2. Explain the following observations :
   a. Adrenaline usually produces a rise in blood pressure. But if ergot is injected before adrenaline, adrenaline produces a fall in blood pressure.
   b. Acetylcholine usually produces a fall in blood pressure. But if atropine is injected before acetylcholine, a high dose of acetylcholine gives a rise in blood pressure.
   c. If a cat is exposed to a barking dog, its heart rate increases. The increase is less marked after denervation of the heart. A small increase in heart rate persists even after inactivation of adrenals.
3. List any four functions of the body which are partly voluntary and partly involuntary. What is the significance of mixed control in these functions?
4. Give in one word each the effect of the sympathetic nervous system on:
   1. Heart rate
   2. Respiratory rate
   3. Bronchi
   4. Skeletal muscle blood vessels
   5. Pupil of the eye
   6. Salivary secretion
   7. Gastrointestinal motility
   8. Musculature of the urinary bladder
   9. Internal urethral sphincter
   10. Liver glycogen
5. Give the site of action of curare, atropine and hexamethonium.

ANSWERS

1. It is quite true that modulation of activity in both directions may be achieved by single innervation as in case of blood vessels. Most blood vessels have only sympathetic vasoconstrictor innervation, and it has a certain basal tone. Increase in the activity of these fibers induces vasoconstriction and decrease in their activity induces vasodilatation. Thus both vasoconstriction and vasodilatation are achieved by a single set of nerve fibers. But many organs, such as the heart, have both sympathetic and parasympathetic supply. Dual innervation increases the efficiency of modulation. This fact may be understood by comparing the situation to an automobile. The speed of a vehicle may be increased or decreased by using only the accelerator. But even the best driver has sometimes got to use the brake in order to achieve more efficient slowing. Hence automobiles are provided with an accelerator as well as a brake. Dual innervation increases the efficiency of modulation in the same way as an accelerator and a brake.
2. a. Adrenaline has an affinity for both alpha and beta adrenergic receptors. Most vascular beds in the body have alpha receptors. When adrenaline combines with the alpha receptors it leads to vasoconstriction, and hence a rise in blood pressure. Ergot blocks alpha adrenergic receptors. Therefore, if adrenaline is preceded by ergot, adrenaline is able to give only beta adrenergic response. The blood vessels in skeletal muscle have beta receptors, and stimulation via these receptors produces vasodilatation. Hence beta adrenergic stimulation by adrenaline, in the absence of alpha stimulation, leads to a fall in blood pressure. This observation was first reported by Sir Henry Hallett Dale in 1913.
   b. Acetylcholine produces a fall in blood pressure through
   (i) vasodilatation and (ii) slowing of the heart. Both these actions are mediated by muscarinic receptors, and are blocked by

atropine. After administration of atropine, a high dose of acetylcholine is still able to stimulate autonomic ganglia and adrenal medulla because these actions of acetylcholine are mediated by nicotinic receptors. Stimulation of parasympathetic autonomic ganglia is ineffective because of atropinization. Stimulation of sympathetic autonomic ganglia releases noradrenaline which produces vasoconstriction. Stimulation of adrenal medulla releases adrenaline, the predominant effect of which is also vasoconstriction. Therefore, after atropinization, acetylcholine may induce a rise in blood pressure. This observation was also first reported by Sir H.H. Dale in 1914.

c. Exposure to a barking dog excites a cat, leading to sympathetic stimulation. Activation of sympathetic nerves supplying the heart increases the heart rate. Sympathetic activity also stimulates the adrenal medulla, releasing adrenaline, which also increases the heart rate. After denervation of the heart, increase in heart rate is mainly produced by the adrenaline released from the adrenal medulla. Therefore after adrenal inactivation much of the increase in heart rate disappears. However, the slight increase which still persists is due to the release of noradrenaline at extracardiac sympathetic nerve endings in the body. Part of this noradrenaline is absorbed into the circulation and may increase the heart rate. The slight increase in heart rate may also be due to incomplete denervation of the heart or incomplete inactivation of the adrenal medulla. These observations were first made by Walter Bradford Connon in 1927.

3. Respiration, swallowing, defecation and urination.

   Voluntary control of respiration makes activities like singing and swimming possible.

   Voluntary phase of swallowing ensures that we swallow food only after it has been chewed properly.

   Voluntary control of defecation and urination allows us some choice in determining the time and place for these functions.

   Involuntary control of all these functions relieves us of the necessity of paying too much attention to these activities. If conscious effort were required to breathe and swallow, we would have little time left to attend to anything else.

4. 1. Increases
   2. Increases
   3. Dilate/Relax
   4. Dilate
   5. Dilates
   6. Decreases
   7. Decreases
   8. Relaxes
   9. Contracts
   10. Breakdown/glycogenolysis

5. All the three are anticholinergic drugs. However, they block different categories of cholinergic receptors. Curare blocks the neuromuscular junction in skeletal muscle, atropine blocks the receptors for postganglionic cholinergic nerve endings, and hexamethonium blocks cholinergic receptors in autonomic ganglia.

CHAPTER

18 Nervous System: Sleep-wakefulness and Higher Functions

"Memory is a net; one finds it full of fish when he takes it from the brook; but a dozen miles of water have run through it without sticking."

OLIVER WENDELL HOLMES

Chapter Outline

- Reticular Formation
- Electroencephalography
- Sleep-wakefulness
- Speech
- Learning
- Memory

We have so far discussed neural functions which support the basic processes of life and aid survival by preservation of self and preservation of the species. Now we shall discuss the fascinating phenomenon of sleep, and some functions which are prominent only in highly evolved organisms.

Before we discuss sleep, a summary of reticular formation is in order. Reticular formation is involved in motor control (Chapter 16), autonomic control (Chapter 17) and also sleep.

RETICULAR FORMATION

Reticular formation (*reticulum*, little net) is a complex neural network in the core of the brain stem. It is called reticular because, under the microscope, it looks like a network of nerve fibers. The appearance is due to the richness of its connections. Although the network looks disorganized, in fact it has specific connections directed at accomplishing important functions. The reticular formation (RF) is extensively connected to the spinal cord, hypothalamus, other limbic structures, cerebellum, thalamus and cerebral cortex.

Anatomy

Anatomically, RF may be referred to as medullary, pontine and midbrain RF. Or, its neuronal groups (nuclei) may be classlified in terms of their distance from the midline. The midline nuclei are called the raphe nuclei (*raphe*, midline seam). Lateral to the raphe are the large celled nuclei, and still more laterally are the small celled nuclei.

Efferent Connections

The efferent connections of the reticular formation may be divided into ascending and descending projections.

Ascending projections: The large cholinergic neurons of midbrain and pontine RF project to the cerebral cortex via relays in the thalamus. The small adrenergic neurons which extend throughout the entire length of RF also project extensively to the cerebral cortex via relays in the intralaminar nuclei of the thalamus. The serotonergic neurons of raphe nucei in the lower pontine and medullary RF also project to the thalamus and cerebral cortex basides projecting to the hypothalamus and limbic structures.

Descending projections: The pontine and medullary reticulospinal tracts project to the spinal cord where they affect extensor muscle tone. Besides, motor function is also influenced by RF indirectly. Noradrenergic neurons from several areas of the RF project to the cerebellum, and dopaminergic neurons of midbrain RF and substantia nigra project ot the basal ganglia. The influence of cerebellum and basal ganglia on motor function has been discussed in previous chapters.

Serotonergic neurons in the raphe nuclei of medullary RF project to the substantia gelatinosa of spinal cord where they control transmission of pain impulses.

Neurons of the RF also project to the respiratory, vagal and sympathetic preganglionic neurons to control respiration, cardiac function and vasomotor function.

Afferent Connections

All sensory inputs, besides following well-defined specific pathways, also send collateral connections to the ascending RF. The fiber tracts conveying slow pain send the richest collateral connections to the ascending RF. In addition, all the structures to which RF projects send reciprocal connections to the RF.

Functions

Some functions of RF have been already discussed, and some will be discussed later in this chapter. But, the various functions have been enumerated below.

Modulation of Pain

Serotonergic neurons of the endogenous pain relief system belong to the raphe nuclei of medullary RF (Chapter 15).

Regulation of Tone and Posture

RF modulates the tone of extensor (antigravity) muscles. The pontine (medial) reticulospinal tract has an excitatory influence while the medullary (lateral) reticulospinal tract has an inhibitory influence on extensor muscle tone (Chapter 16).

Autonomic Control

RF carries the influences of the limbic system and hypothalamus to the spinal cord (Chapter 17). Respiratory, cardiovascular and other autonomic effects may be observed by electrical stimulation of discrete areas of RF.

Sleep-wakefulness

All ascending sensory tracts give collaterals to the RF (Chapter 15). These sensory inputs project to the midline and intralaminar thalamic muclei. From the thalamus, they project to the cerebral cortex in a diffuse manner.

Activation of this pathway leads to arousal. That is why all sensory stimuli have the capacity to keep us awake. This system which contributes to wakefulness has been called the ascending reticular activating system (ARAS).

Some areas of RF may induce sleep of a specific type. Serotonergic neurons of the raphe nuclei induce slow wave sleep. Some adrenergic and cholinergic neurons of RF influence rapid eye movement sleep (see below).

Before going into a discussion on sleep-wakefulness, we shall get introduced to electroencephalography, a technique indispensable for the study of sleep.

ELECTROENCEPHALOGRAPHY

Electroencephalography involves recording the electrical activity of the brain with the help of surface electrodes placed on the scalp. The record is called an electroencephalogram (EEG). To record an EEG, the electrodes are placed in the frontal, parietal, temporal and occipital regions according to a precisely defined system. These are called active electrodes. An indifferent electrode may be placed on the tip of the seventh cervical vertebral spine or may be attached to both ears and earthed. An EEG records the potential difference between two active electrodes (bipolar recording), or between an active and the indifferent electrode (monopolar recording). The EEG leads are named accordingly.

Physiological Basis of EEG

An EEG samples the summated activity of a very large number of cortical neurons close to the active electrode(s). The record depends on the summation of excitatory and inhibitory postsynaptic potentials (EPSPs and IPSPs). It is important to remember that an EEG does not originate in action potentials. The amplitude of EEG waves depends on how synchronous the activity of the neurons being sampled is. Synchronous activity gets summated to give large waves. On the other hand, asynchronous (or desynchronized) activity leads to simultaneous deflections in opposite directions, which cancel each other out. Therefore desynchronized activity is associated with small amplitude waves.

EEG Waveforms

Some of the common, well-categorized EEG waves have been described below. Although the postsynaptic potentials, which form the basis of EEG, are in millivolts, because of the manner of recording, EEG waves are in microvolts.

Alpha Waves

Alpha waves are typically recorded when a person is awake but inattentive. He is mentally relaxed, and not distracted by sensory stimuli. Therefore, alpha rhythm is best recorded in a silent room with the subject's eyes closed. Alpha rhythm is also called Berger rhythm, after Hans Berger, a pioneer in electroencephalography.

Alpha waves have an average amplitude of about 50 microvolts in adults, and a frequency of 8-13 per second. Their relatively high amplitude suggests synchronized activity. Alpha rhythm is best recorded from the parietal and occipital regions (Fig. 18.1).

Beta Waves

Beta waves are typically recorded when a person is awake and alert. He is mentally busy or tense. The alpha rhythm of an individual may be generally promptly replaced by beta rhythm by asking the person to open the eyes or by exposing the person to a sensory stimulus such as a clap, a bang, or a touch (Fig. 18.1).

An EEG rhythm, quite indistinguishable from beta rhythm, is also recorded when a person is in dream sleep.

Beta waves have an average amplitude of 20 microvolts, and a frequency of 13-30 per second. The brain is presumably highly active when beta waves are recorded, but the amplitude of the waves is low due to the activity being desynchronized. Beta rhythm is best recorded from the frontal and parietal regions.

Theta Waves

Theta waves may be recorded when a person is in light sleep, during emotional stress in adults, and sometimes quite normally in awake children.

Theta waves have an average amplitude of 10 microvolts in adults and a frequency of 4-7 per second.

Delta Waves

Delta waves are typically recorded when a person is in deep sleep (Stage 4 slow wave sleep).

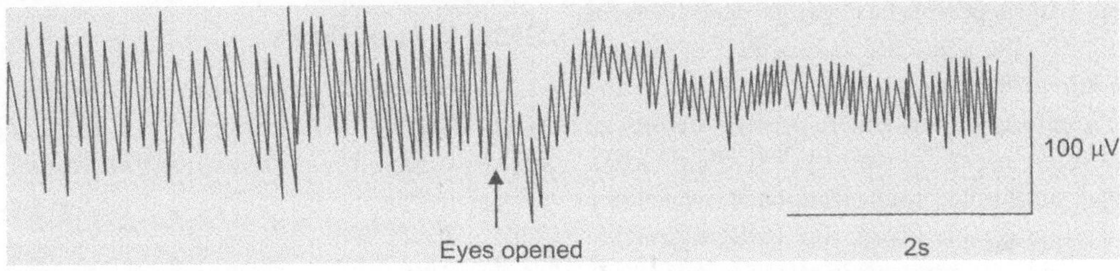

Fig. 18.1 An electroencephalographic tracing showing that alpha rhythm is replaced by beta rhythm upon opening the eyes. Right parieto-occipital lead (Based on a human EEG record. *Courtesy:* Department of Physiology, All India Institute of Medical Sciences, New Delhi)

Delta waves have an average amplitude of 100 microvolts and a frequency of 0.5-4 per second. Delta waves may be seen in an experimental animal after a subcortical transection which severes the thalamocortical fiber tracts. Thus delta rhythm seems to represent a highly synchronous inherent activity of cortical neurons when deprived of thalamic inputs.

SLEEP-WAKEFULNESS

Although poets have considered sleep a close cousin of death, the similarity is only superficial. Sleep is only an altered state of consciousness during which some of the body functions are depressed and some others activated. A person in sleep appears unconscious but can be easily aroused by a variety of stimuli. In contrast, a person in coma cannot be aroused even by painful stimuli.

Architecture of Sleep

During the 7-8 hours that we sleep, we go through a number of phases which repeat themselves in a predictable fashion. The architecture of sleep became clear for the first time when William Dement and Nathaniel Kleitman recorded whole-night electroencephalograms. As a person starts falling asleep, his alpha rhythm is gradually replaced by slower EEG waves of higher amplitude till he has a well-defined delta rhythm. The gradual transition has been arbitrarily divided into four phases : stage 1, 2, 3 and 4 (Fig. 18.2). Stage 4 is the phase of typical delta rhythm. Since the frequency of EEG waves during stage 3 and 4 is low, this phase is known as slow wave sleep (SWS). During stage 1 and 2, the person is in light sleep; stages 3 and 4 are stages of deep sleep. After a person has been in deep SWS for about an hour, the sequence is repeated in reverse order, i.e. the person passes from stage 4 to 3, 2 and 1. Then something remarkable happens : the person continues to be asleep but the EEG suddenly assumes a low amplitude high frequency waveform, quite indistinguishable from the beta rhythm of awake state. Since the person is asleep but the EEG resembles that of the awake state, this stage of sleep is also known as paradoxical sleep. Paradoxical sleep is associated with dreams and rapid eye movements (REM), and is often called REM sleep. After that, SWS and REM sleep alternate with each other throughout the night, the duration of SWS phases becoming gradually less and that of REM phases becoming longer. Also, the period of SWS is spent more in stages 1 and 2 than in stages 3 and 4 as the night progresses. The alternation of SWS and REM sleep is repeated 5-7 times every night.

Physiological Variation with Age

The duration and architecture of sleep show marked variation with age. The total duration of sleep declines steeply during childhood and youth till it reaches a plateau at the age of about 30. A further decline may take place in old age. However, there is marked individual variation in the 'normal' duration of sleep, and it possibly reflects a variation in requirement. SWS shows a change in character with age. The duration of stage 4 SWS declines steeply during childhood and youth, and somewhat slowly after the age of about 30. Stage 4 SWS may disappear completely after the age of 60 years. REM sleep declines sharply till puberty, and then rather slowly. It levels off in middle age, and shows a further sharp decline after the age of 60. In short, a person about 60 years of age spends most of the sleeping time in stage 1 and 2 SWS. Along with this, there is also a return to the childhood biphasic pattern of sleep, i.e. sleeping twice a day: a longer sleep during the night, and a shorter sleep during the afternoon. Barbiturates suppress stage 3 and 4 SWS and also REM sleep. Hence they give rise to a sleep pattern similar to that of old age even in a young person.

Slow Wave Sleep

As a person falls asleep, the EEG shows progressive changes. During stage 1 SWS, the EEG shows low voltage and high frequency thus resembling the awake and alert EEG as well as the REM sleep EEG. These waves are interspered with 'sleep spindles'. Sleep spindles are recurrent bursts of a waxing and waning pattern resembling alpha waves. Each spindle lasts 1-2 seconds. Sleep spindles are a characteristic

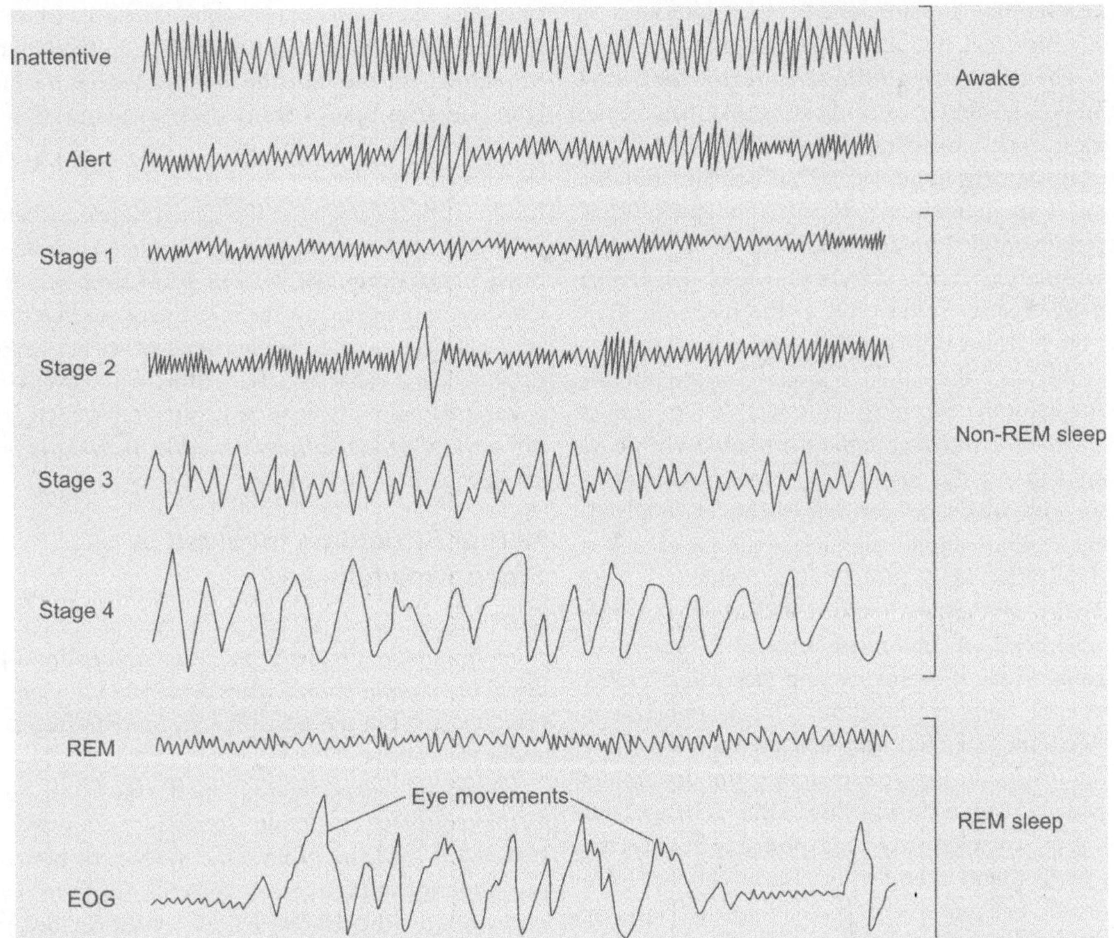

Fig. 18.2 Human EEG during the awake state and in different stages of sleep. The electrooculogram (EOG) has also been given under the REM sleep EEG because the presence of rapid eye movements distinguishes this state from the Stage 1 non-REM sleep

feature of stage 3 SWS. Stage 3 SWS shows high voltage low frequency EEG waves. In stage 4 SWS, the voltage of the EEG waves becomes still higher and the frequency still lower. Stages 3 and 4 of SWS are also referred to as 'delta sleep' because the EEG waves fall in the range of delta waves.

Besides the EEG correlates, there are other physiological changes also during SWS. Most of these changes are suggestive of increased parasympathetic activity. The respiratory rate and heart rate fall and the vasomotor tone is reduced. Consequently the blood pressure falls. The basal metabolic rate is reduced. Gastrointestinal motility is somewhat increased, and the pupil is markedly constricted. Skeletal muscle tone is low. Without generally being aware of it, there is a change of posture every 20 minutes.

REM Sleep

The REM phase is a very interesting phase of sleep for reasons more than one. It is the phase during which we dream. Everyone has REM sleep, and hence everyone dreams, every night, although so many claim that they get a very sound 'dreamless' sleep. The EEG during REM sleep resembles that of the awake and alert stage, indicating that the cerebral cortex is very active, and the metabolic rate of the brain is actually increased by 20 percent, but the person is apparently deep asleep. That is why REM sleep is also called paradoxical sleep. Some internal stimulus often results in spontaneous awakening from REM sleep some time in the morning. It is only those dreams during which we get up that we remember. All the other dreams of the night are forgotten by the morning. However, if a person is woken up by external stimuli during any REM phase at any time of the night, he generally recounts a dream with which he was 'busy'. That is what tells us that we all dream during each of the 5-7 phases of REM sleep that we go through each night.

The physiological correlates of REM sleep include irregular heart rate and respiratory rate, cessation of gastrointestinal movements and decreased ability to regulate body temperature. That is one reason why extremes of cold and hot weather are more uncomfortable at night than during the day. Males get penile erection during REM sleep. The eyeballs show rapid roving movements, probably because the eyes try to follow the moving objects being seen in the dream. Eye movements can be recorded by doing an electro-oculogram (EOG), which is nothing but an electromyogram of the extraocular muscles. The skeletal muscles are completely flaccid during REM sleep, the muscle tone being almost absent.

The duration of REM sleep varies with age. Its total duration forms 20-25 percent of the total sleeping time in young adults, 50 percent in full term newborn children, 60-65 percent in children born 2-4 wk prematurely, and 80 percent in children born 10 wk prematurely. From this data, one might speculate that in the uterus, most of the sleeping time of the fetus is occupied by REM sleep. Further, since a newborn spends about two-thirds of the day sleeping, chances are that the fetus sleeps most of the time. Thus the fetus is likely to be in REM sleep almost all 24 hours of the day. On the basis of these facts, one may draw two conclusions. First, REM sleep has some very important functions; and second, the importance of the functions of REM sleep declines with age. The role of REM sleep in maturation of neural function has been compared to that of physical exercise in the development of skeletal muscles. It has been postulated that the genetic code for some basic movements is decoded, or translated into actual movements, during REM sleep. REM sleep serves as a bedroom rehearsal for the movements so that there is no clumsiness when the movements are performed in the open.[1] That is why instinctive movements apparently do not have to be learnt. A newborn does not have to be taught how to suckle. It has probably already learnt it in REM sleep in the uterus.

Neural Structures Involved in Sleep-wakefulness

Our current understanding of neural structures predominantly involved in sleep-wakefulness is based on experimental studies performed during the last 60 years. But there is still a lot more to be learnt about the subject.

Bremer's experiments performed in the 1930s consisted of brain sections performed at two levels. If the brain was sectioned between the superior and inferior colliculi (*cerveau isole* preparation), the animal's EEG waveform became permanently synchronized, i.e. high in amplitude, low in frequency. With this EEG, the animal may be considered asleep. If the brain was sectioned between the medulla and spinal cord, i.e. in such a way as to separate the brain from the spinal cord (*encephale isole* preparation), the animal stayed awake and retained the sleep-wakefulness cycle. However, if in the *encephale isole* preparation, the cranial sensory nerves were cut, the animal went to sleep. From these observations, Bremer concluded that so long as some sensory stimuli continued to reach the higher levels of the brain, the animal remained awake. When

[1]Compare this with the bathroom rehearsal of aspiring singers.

the sensory inputs were withdrawn, the animal fell asleep.

Bremer's experiments were further extended by Moruzzi and Magoun in 1949. They found that if only specific ascending sensory tracts were severed by producing lateral tegmental lesions, the animal remained awake. However, if the nonspecific sensory pathways were interrupted by producing lesions in the reticular formation, the animal went to sleep. On the basis of these experiments, Moruzzi and Magoun postulated that the awake state is due to various sensory inputs sending collaterals from specific pathways to the reticular formation. The reticular formation projects to nonspecific nuclei of the thalamus which, in turn, project in a diffuse manner to the cerebral cortex. Activation of these diffuse projec-tions keeps the cortex in a state of arousal. Conversely, withdrawal of sensory stimuli makes these pathways silent, thereby sending the animal to sleep. Thus sleep was considered to be a passive phenomenon which depended on the absence of stimuli which keep us awake. This theory of sleep remained popular for long because of its simplicity, and because it is supported by common sense and some every day observations. Minimizing sensory stimuli by lying down (withdrawal of proprioceptive impulses) on a softbed (withdrawal of impulses from pressure receptors) in a dark, warm and silent room (withdrawal of inputs from visual, temperature and auditory receptors) is conducive to sleep. But there are some common observations which do not support the passive theory of sleep. A worried person may not be able to sleep even under the most comfortable conditions, whereas a tired carefree person may fall asleep on a railway platform.

Some experiments by Moruzzi and his other associates performed in the late 1950s did not support the above theory. For example, if they delivered barbiturates (a group of drugs which depress neuronal function) selectively to the rostral pons and cerebral cortex, the animal fell asleep. But if the barbiturates were delivered selectively to the caudal brain stem, the animal woke up even if it was already asleep. These experiments suggested that there is an area in the caudal brain stem which actively induces sleep. Seeing the contradictions between his later experiments and previous theory, Moruzzi revised his theory in the true scientific spirit.

Further work has localized the areas inducing sleep to the raphe nuclei, the nucleus of solitary tract, the suprachiasmatic nucleus and preoptic area of hypothalamus, and some nonspecific nuclei of the thalamus. There may be more such areas. The functional significance of induction of sleep by each of these areas is not clear but what it means is that sleep is at least partly an active process which is induced when something happens rather than being passively induced when nothing is happening.

Circadian Nature of the Sleep-wakefulness Cycle

The sleep-wakefulness cycle follows a 24 hours, or circadian (*circa*, about; *diem*, day) rhythm, and is related to the light-dark cycle. If the external cues in the form of light and darkness are removed, the sleep-wakefulness cycle still remains circadian although it has a tendency to lengthen to 25-30 hours. The biological clock for the sleep-wakefulness cycle is located in the suprachiasmatic nucleus (SCN) of the hypothalamus. SCN seems to have an inbuilt circuitry which results in circadian oscillations in neuronal activity. SCN also receives afferent fibers from the retina via the retinohypothalamic pathway. Thus it seems SCN itself is capable of introducing a circadian rhythmicity in sleep-wakefulness with a cycle length slightly longer than 24 hours. This endogenous rhythm is further entrained to the light-dark cycle by retino-hypothalamic fibers to become an exact 24-hour rhythm.

Neurotransmitters Involved in Sleep-wakefulness

Raphe nuclei, involved in induction of SWS, and the preoptic area, involved in induction of REM sleep, employ serotonin as the neurotransmitter. Some neurons in the pontine reticular formation which fire rapidly in a phasic manner during REM sleep employ acetylcholine as the neurotransmitter. Locus ceruleus, a region in the pontine reticular formation, the neurons of which show reduced activity during REM sleep, employ noradrenaline as the neurotransmitter. Cholinergic neurons of the pontine reticular formation and adrenergic neurons of locus ceruleus thus show reciprocal activity. There is also evidence for a non-locus ceruleus noradrenergic ascending fiber system which plays a hypnogenic role at the level of the preoptic area.

Sleep Producing Substances

The search for chemical agents which might be responsible for induction of sleep has been most fruitful in experiments on sleep-deprived animals. Sleep-deprivation presumably leads to a rise in the production of these substances through a negative feedback effect. The brain tissue, cerebrospinal fluid (CSF), blood, and even urine of sleep-deprived animals have substances which, when injected into the cerebral ventricular system of other animals, induces sleep. The first experiments of this type were performed by Henri Pieron in 1913 on dogs. He demonstrated that dogs receiving CSF from sleep-deprived donor dogs slept for hours, while the recipients of CSF from normal donors remained awake. Recent work has confirmed these observations and identified several candidate sleep producing substances (SPS). The best known SPS are muramyl dipeptide (MDP), delta sleep-inducing peptide (DSIP), arginine vasotocin (AVT), and interleukin-1 (IL-1). Most of the known sleep producing substances induce SWS. It is interesting that MDP is a component of bacterial cell walls whereas IL-1 is released in infections. MDP possibly acts via IL-1. The sleep-inducing effect of IL-1 explains why a person having an infection feels sleepy. IL-1 also induces fever, and is therefore also called endogenous pyrogen. Fever is possibly a beneficial response to infection, and so is sleep which perhaps helps recovery by compelling the patient to take rest. It is truly remarkable that these helpful responses have been so intimately woven with the classical immunological responses to infection.

Now we go to some higher functions of the nervous system, which are conspicuously better developed in man than in any other species.

SPEECH

Speech of the type seen in human beings is not seen in any other animal. Two well-known areas of speech are located on the left side of the brain in right-handed persons.

Broca's Area

Broca's area is located in the frontal cortex, anterior to the face area in the precentral gyrus, on the left side in right-handed persons. It receives information from Wernicke's area and sends it to the motor cortex. Broca's area is also called the motor speech area.

Wernicke's Area

Wernicke's area is located at the posterior end of the superior temporal gyrus on the left side. It is connected to Broca's area by a bundle of fibers known as the **arcuate fasciculus**. Wernicke's area is also called the sensory speech area.

Mechanism of Speech

Sounds that we hear are perceived by the auditory cortex. But if the sounds heard belong to a language we understand, the meaning is understood only when the information reaches Wernicke's area. It is interesting that Wernicke's area is located close to the auditory area and is connected to it. Thus Wernicke's area may be considered a special part of the auditory association cortex.

If a person has to say something, in response to what he has heard, or otherwise, the words are planned in Wernicke's area. The plan is passed on to Broca's area by the arcuate fasciculus. The sentence is formulated in Broca's area and transmitted to the motor cortex (precentral gyrus) for execution. It is interesting that Broca's area is situated close to the face area of the motor cortex because the muscles involved in execution of speech also belong to the face area.

The above account is based on a theory proposed by Wernicke more than a hundred years ago but is considered valid even today. However, it may be added that the function of speech cannot be sharply localized to a few areas. It involves virtually every part of the brain, although the participation of a few areas is more prominent. Secondly, speech, as commonly understood, may be restricted to human beings. But communication, as a general faculty is seen in animals too. Thus speech is not an add-on to the animal brain but merely an elaboration of a basic design worked out long before the evolution of the human brain. Among features which have helped the development of human speech are not only elaboration of the brain but also the increase in the mobility of the larynx. Finally, the basic mechanisms of spoken speech, written speech and even sign language (used by the deaf) are the same. For example, comprehension of written matter may need strengthening of some connections between the visual cortex and Wernicke's area. Similarly, expression of the written word may need strengthening of some connections between Broca's area and the hand region of the motor cortex. But the basic mechanism remains the same.

Aphasias

Aphasias are disorders of speech resulting from lesions in the brain. Much of what we know about the mechanism of speech has been learnt from observations made on patients having various types of aphasia. There are three basic types of aphasia.

Motor Aphasia

Lesions in Broca's area lead to a type of defect called motor aphasia. The patient understands what he hears but cannnot respond properly. His speech is not fluent, and he uses very few words in his speech. His language tends to the telegraphic in that the joining words such as conjunctions and prepositions may be missing.

Sensory Aphasia

Lesions in Wernicke's area lead to a type of defect called sensory aphasia. The patient does not understand what he hears or reads. Since comprehension is lacking but motor speech area is intact, he speaks very fluently but does not talk sense.

Conduction Aphasia

Lesions of the arcuate fasciulus lead to a type of defect called conduction aphasia. Since Wernicke's area is intact, the patient understands what he hears or reads. But because of the lesion in the arcuate fasciculus, he cannot use this understanding while speaking or writing. The result is that he produces fluent but faulty speech and makes plenty of mistakes in what he writes. Thus the patient may *seem to have* sensory aphasia. But the two can be distinguished by evaluating comprehension. In sensory aphasia, the patient cannot understand speech while in conduction aphasia, he understands spoken as well as written speech.

LEARNING

Learning is a sustained change in behavior or performance potential. The change is a result of some experience, which can threfore be called a learning experience. Most experiences have a teaching potential, but unfortunately we generally learn nothing from them. There are many types of learning but we shall focus here on two experimental paradigms which throw some light on the mechanisms of and motivation for learning.

Classical Conditioning

This is the type of learning studied extensively by Pavlov in dogs. If a dog is presented with food which it likes, its mouth starts watering as a result of increased secretion of saliva. Food is called the unconditioned stimulus (UCS) for the salivation reflex. Now a bell is rung near the dog. The sound of the bell *does not* lead to salivation. But if the bell is immediately followed by food a few hundred times, the dog *learns* to expect food after the bell. Therefore now the bell alone also leads to salivation. Sound of the bell is called the conditioned stimulus (CS) for the salivation reflex. The reflex response to a CS is called a conditioned reflex (Figs 18.3A to C).

The broader implication of classical conditioning is that it tells us how we *learn* about the relationship between associated events. We learn to identify

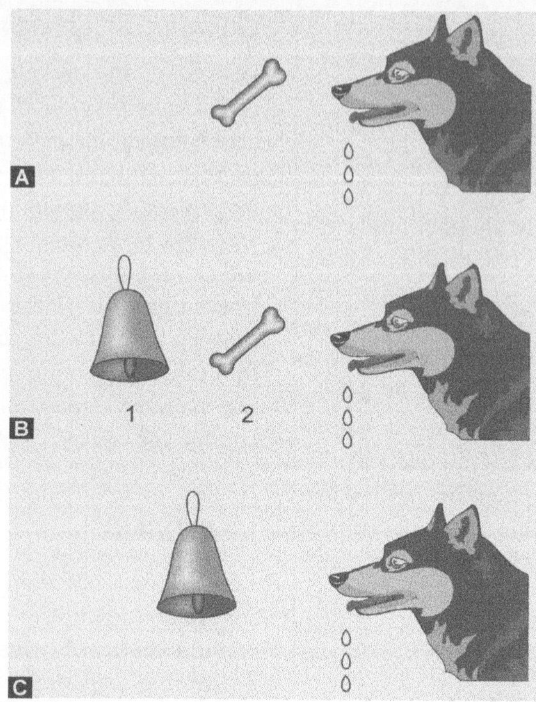

Figs 18.3A to C Conditioned reflex. A bone makes a dog's mouth water (A), if the ringing of a bell (1) precedes the presentation of a bone (2), and the sequence is repeated several times (B), the dog ultimately responds just to the bell by watering of the mouth (C)

events which occur together or in quick succession predictably and reliably. Then we try to look for a cause and effect relationship between the associated events, which leads to still more learning. For example, repeatedly observing that dark clouds are followed by rain leads us to predict rain whenever we see dark clouds. Next, we try to find whether the two are linked by cause and effect, and if so, how.

Operant Conditioning

Although operant conditioning was discovered by Thorndike, it was studied extensively by Skinner. Skinner used for his experiments a box which is now known as the Skinner box. Inside the box (Fig. 18.4) is a bar-shaped lever on one side, and just outside the box is a container full of food pellets. Pressing the bar releases one food pellet at a time into a food cup in the box. When a rat is placed in the box, it first explores its surroundings out of curiosity. In the process, sooner or later, it hits the bar. The action turns out to be a happy accident because it leads to a food pellet appearing in the cup. Soon the rat learns that pressing the bar leads to the appearance of the pellet. The rat now has a means of operating on the environment in a manner which is rewarding. That is why Skinner called the rat's behavior operant behavior. Pressing the bar may lead to a reward (reinforcement) or a punishment (e.g. an electric shock). If it leads to a reward, the rat presses it again and again. If it leads to a punishment, the rat avoids pressing the bar.

There are some essential differences and similarities between classical and operant conditioning. Now that you have learnt something about both, try to think what these are. Then look for them in Table 18.1. To put it succinctly, both involve conditioning.[2]

[2]Conditioning means learning to respond to a condition, e.g. a bell, or a lever.

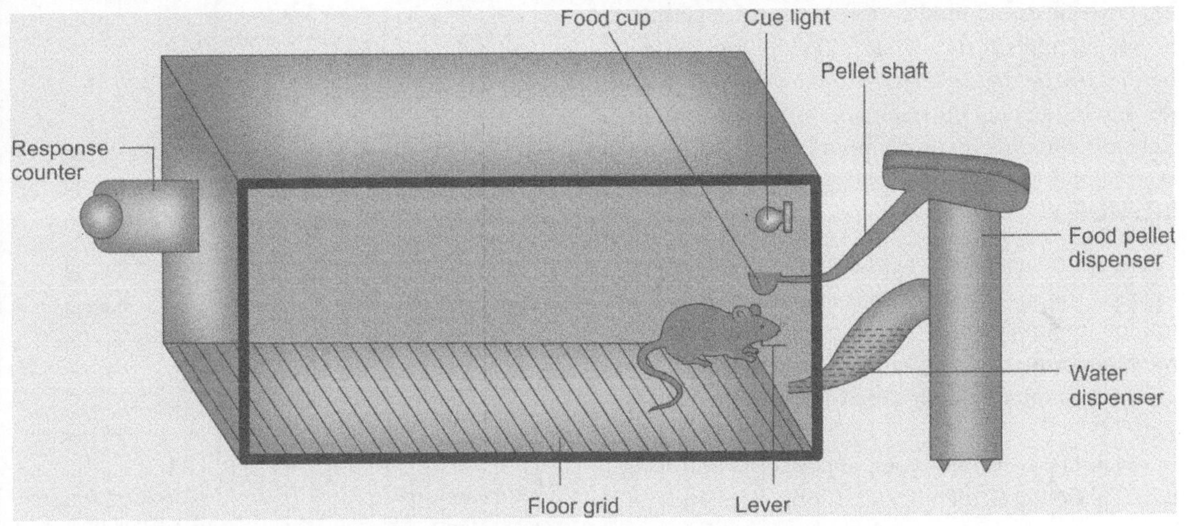

Fig. 18.4 The Skinner box

Table 18.1 Classical conditioning vs Operant conditioning

Classical conditioning	*Operant conditioning*
Similarity	
Organism learns to predict a sequence (e.g. bell will be followed by food)	Organism learns to predict a sequence (e.g. pressing the bar will be followed by food)
Differences	
Organism responds passively to changes in the environment (e.g. bell)	Organism actively operates on the environment (e.g. presses the bar)
Organism cannot control or trigger the sequence	Organism can trigger the sequence of events
The response is to the conditioned stimulus	The 'response' is to learning from past experience
The response (e.g. salivation) is a reflex action	The 'response' is a voluntary action (i.e. behavior is emitted)

Classical conditioning conditions a reflex, while operant conditioning conditions behavior.

The broader implication of operant conditioning is that it tells us how we *learn* to respond in a particular way on the basis of past experience. A behavior which consistently, or at least frequently, leads to a pleasant experience (reward), is repeated. On the other hand, a behavior which leads to an unpleasant experience (punishment) is not repeated. For example, married couples learn over the years which behavior pleases, and which annoys, the partner. Gradually each starts repeating the behavior which pleases the spouse, and starts avoiding actions which annoy him/her.

Biological Basis of Learning

There is ample evidence that learning is associated with considerable structural and functional changes in the brain. The changes involve formation of new synapses, and changes in the effectiveness of synapses. Change in effectiveness of synapses means facilitation or inhibition of the synapses, which in turn may be due to modulation of neurotransmitters or ion channels at the synapses. While formation of new synapses may be restricted to an early period in the development of the brain, modulation of synaptic transmission goes on throughout life.

MEMORY

Learning and memory are closely related. All learning involves remembering some past experience, but not all memory leads to learning. For example, remembering a *sloka* without understanding its meaning cannot be considered learning in the true sense.

Memory is of two types: **short-term** and **long-term**. Short-term memory and long term memory are not a single graded process. Short-term memory is generally confined to less than 12 items and lasts only a few minutes. For example, a telephone number may be found from the directory, used for making a call, and promptly forgotten. A special process seems to be necessary for transferring material from short-term to long-term memory.

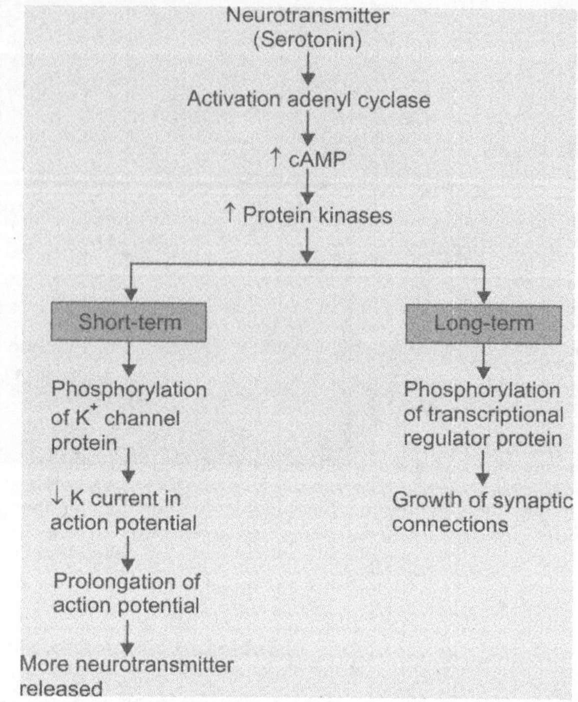

Fig. 18.5 Difference between the synaptic mechanisms of short-term and long-term memory

Neural Substrate of Memory

Several areas of the brain contribute to memory. There is something to be said for Lashley's hypothesis that memory is not a location specific process. He found that memory loss was proportional to the amount of cerebral cortex ablated rather than the area from which it was ablated. On the basis of experiments performed in the course of neurosurgery, Penfield localized memory primarily to the hippocampus and the temporal cortex. Several other experiments have also indicated a special place for the hippocampus and its to and fro connections with the cerebral cortex in the process of memory.

Cellular and Molecular Basis of Memory

The fundamental difference between short-term and long-term memory is that short term memory involves merely modulation of synaptic transmission by modification of pre-existing proteins (e.g. ion channel proteins). On the other hand, long-term memory involves formation of new synaptic connections and synthesis of new proteins. The link between short-term and long-term memory, at least in some cases, is cyclic AMP. cAMP can induce only modification of existing proteins in a short time. But if elevation of cAMP is persistent, it can phosphorylate transcriptional regulator proteins, and thereby influence synthesis of new proteins (Fig. 18.5).

Long-term Potentiation

Long-term potentiation (LTP) is a phenomenon observed in the hippocampus which may provide the electrophysiological basis for at least certain types of memory.

What is LTP?: There are three major excitatory pathways from the subiculum to CA1 region of hippocampus. High frequency stimulation of any of the three pathways leads to an increase in the magnitude of EPSP in hippocampus neurons. The change in EPSP may last for days or weeks, and is called LTP.

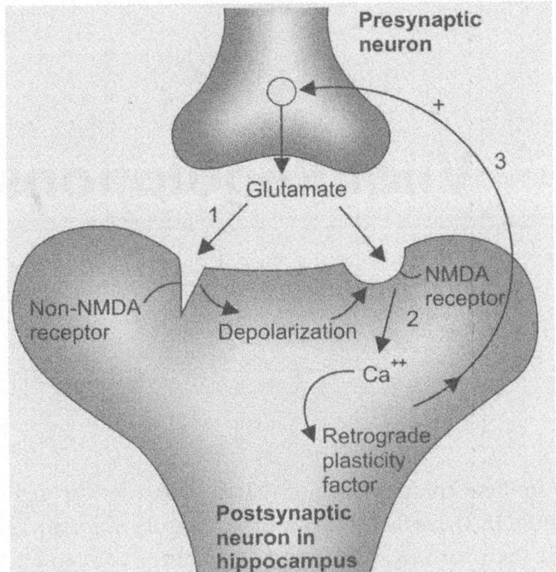

Fig. 18.6 The key steps in long-term potentiation (LTP). Stimulation of glutamate leads to depolarization (EPSP) via non-NMDA receptors (1). Depolarization removes the block from NMDA receptors so that now glutamate can act via NMDA receptors also. Activation of NMDA receptors leads to accumulation of calcium ions in the postsynaptic neurons (2). Calcium leads to the release of retrograde plasticity factor, which acts on the presynaptic neuron to bring about a long-term increase in the release of glutamate (3). Increased release of glutamate leads to a higher EPSP, which is called LTP

Mechanism of LTP: High frequency stimulation of nerve fibers projecting to the hippocampus would lead to release of excess transmitter. The neurotransmitter released is glutamate. Glutamate acts on hippocampal neurons via two type of receptors: non-NMDA and NMDA (n-methyl D-asparate) receptors. Normally transmission takes place via only the non-NMDA receptors because NMDA receptors are blocked. NMDA receptors are normally blocked because they are doubly gated: chemically and voltage gated. Only glutamate (a chemical) is not enough to occupy these receptors and initiate a biological effect. In addition, some depolarization (change of voltage) is also necessary. If excess glutamate is released by high frequency stimulation, non-NMDA receptors achieve enough membrane dopalarization to remove the block from NMDA receptors. Removal of the block leads to calcium ion influx into the postsynaptic neurons. Calcium influx leads to persistent activation of (a) calcium/calmodulin kinase, and (b) protein kinase C. Activation of these enzymes phosphorylates some ion channel proteins which, in turn, leads to an increase in EPSP. This may be the mechanism for induction of LTP. Maintenance of LTP involves another mechanism, which is also dependent on accumulation of calcium ions in postsynaptic neurons. Accumulation of calcium in the postsynaptic neurons leads to release of retrograde plasticity factor from dendritic spines of the postsynaptic cell. This factor diffuses into the presynaptic terminal and induces a long term increase in the release of neurotransmitter (glutamate). The essentials of the mechanism underlying LTP have been summarized in Figure 18.6.

CONCLUSION

Learning and memory are interesting but ill-understood subjects. Psychologists study them only at the surface level; neurobiologists have so far only managed to scratch the surface. Computer scientists have now started providing some insights into these mechanisms by copying some of the simpler accomplishments of the human brain. But the depths of these fascinating processes have yet to be explored.

QUESTION

1. Why is it more difficult to wake up:
   a. A young person than an elderly person, and
   b. A person during the first half of sleep than during the second half?

ANSWER

1. It is more difficult to wake up a person from stage 3 or 4 SWS than from stage 1 or 2 SWS. An elderly person spends very little time in stage 3 or 4 SWS, and also most of the SWS during the second half of sleep is stage 1 or 2.

CHAPTER

19 Vital Regulations

"I get my exercise acting as a pallbearer to my friends who exercise."

—CHAUNCEY DEPEW

Chapter Outline

- Physiology of Exercise
- Physiology of Fluid Balance
- Regulation of Acid-base Balance

In this chapter we shall discuss some vital functions of the body which require integrated activity of several systems of the body. Hence these functions can be best understood after you have studied all the systems of the body. On the other hand, studying these functions would help you revise your knowledge of various systems of the body.

PHYSIOLOGY OF EXERCISE

All of us have personal experience of exercise. Even those who do not jog, cycle or swim perform physical exercise because, in physiological terms, any physical activity which needs more energy than the resting state is physical exercise. Thus walking or doing household work is also exercise.

During exercise skeletal muscles consume additional energy. The additional energy is supplied by an increase in blood flow to the muscles. The blood flow increases due to local, neural and humoral factors. Irrespective of the cause of the increase in blood flow, it needs adjustments in cardiovascular system. The additional energy consumed during exercise ultimately comes from enhanced oxygen consumption, and also results in enhanced carbon dioxide production. The changes in internal environment brought about by these factors require respiratory adjustment. Further, cardiovascular and respiratory adjustments have to be coordinated with each other, and with the level of exercise.

Physiological responses to exercise have two aspects. One is the acute response to a single bout of exercise. The second is the long term adaptation of the body to regular exercise. The second aspect is called the effect of training.

Cardiovascular Responses to Exercise

In order to meet the increased expenditure of energy in exercising muscles, the blood flow through the skeletal muscles increases. This is partly due to redistribution of blood flow, i.e. more blood goes to skeletal muscles but less to some other parts of the body. But redistribution alone cannot explain the extent to which muscle blood flow increases during exercise. Much of the increase is due to an increase in cardiac output. The mechanisms underlying these interrelated responses to exercise have been described below briefly.

Increase in Skeletal Muscle Blood Flow

Skeletal muscle blood flow increases during exercise as a result of local as well as neural and humoral factors.

Local factors: Exercising muscles consume more oxygen and produce more carbon dioxide. As a result, PCO_2 in exercising muscles increases. Other substances such as hydrogen ions and potassium ions also accumulate in exercising muscles. Carbon dioxide, hydrogen ions and other metabolites which accumulate in exercising muscles are vasodilators. Vasodilatation increases blood flow. Regulation by local factors is the most important mechanism for increasing blood flow during exercise.

Neural factors: Exercise is a form of stress, and like most stresses, is accompanied by sympathetic overactivity. Skeletal muscles are unique in having sympathetic cholinergic vasodilator fibers. Activation of these fibers dilates the arterioles in muscles and thereby increases muscle blood flow.

How do the sympathetic nerve fibers supplying muscle blood vessels know when to get activated? One route is through the cerebral cortex down the hypothalamus and sympathetic nervous system. Cerebral cortex is the seat of thinking. That is how even the thought of exercise improves muscle blood flow. Thus blood flow increases in anticipation of the exercise. Besides this anticipatory mechanism, muscle blood flow also increases reflexly.

Humoral factors: Exercise stress, like other activators of the sympathetic nervous system, releases adrenaline from the adrenal medulla. Adrenaline brings about a beta receptor-mediated vasodilatation in skeletal muslces. This mechanism may contribute to the anticipatory vasodilatation as well as the increased blood flow seen later during exercise and also for a short while after the exercise.

Redistribution of Blood Flow

The enormous increase in muscle blood flow during exercise is primarily due to an increase in cardiac output. But some help is provided by the reduction in blood flow to some other regions such as kidneys and viscera (Fig. 19.1). The reduction is due to sympathetic nerve stimulation and release of adrenaline. Both these bring about vasoconstriction in renal and splanchnic circulation. The blood flow through the skin may increase because exercise tends to raise body temperature. Temperature regulatory mechanisms bring about vasodilatation in the skin, which helps in maintaining body temperature during exercise.

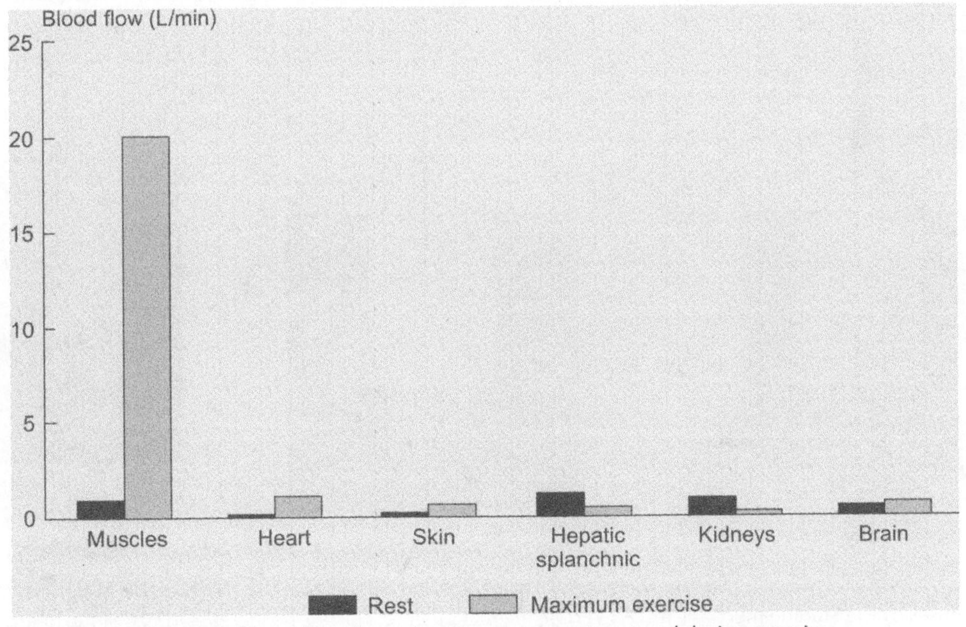

Fig. 19.1 Blood flow through various organs at rest and during exercise. Observe the redistribution of blood flow during exercise

Cardiac Output

During exercise, the heart rate (HR) increases and the stroke volume (SV) also increases. Since cardiac output is the product Tof HR and SV, the cardiac output increases markedly.

Heart rate: The HR increases even before the exercise begins (Fig. 19.2). the anticipatory tachycardia is mediated by the influence of the cerebral cortex on medullary cardiac centers. Some increase in HR is due to the release of adrenaline. The HR increases further as the exercise continues. An important factor contributing to the increase in HR during exercise is the increase in venous return. Increase in venous return stretches the right atrium, and consequently the sino-atrial node, leading to an increase in heart rate. This is known as the Bainbridge effect. Other factors contributing to the increase in HR during exercise are:

a. Reflexes originating in the exercising muscles and joints, and
b. Adrenaline released by the adrenal medulla.

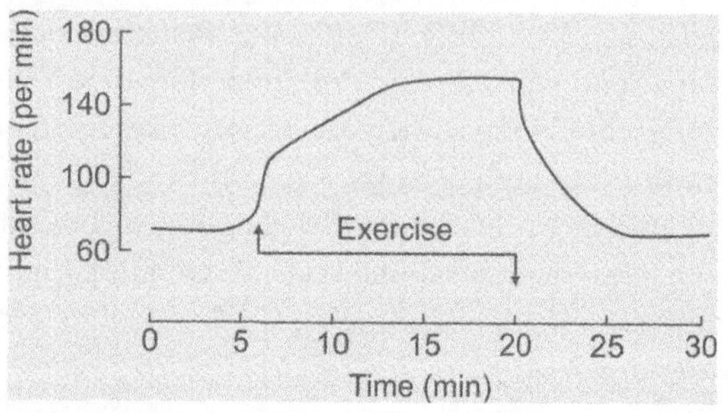

Fig.19.2 Heart rate response to moderate exercise

Stroke volume: The increase in venous return during exercise may also lead to an increase in SV. Increase in venous return stretches the right ventricle, leading to an increase in initial length of the muscle fibers. That, in turn, increases the SV. As you would recollect, this phenomenon is due to Starling's law of the heart (Chapter 5). This seems to be the mechanism for increase in SV during exercises performed in the flat posture, e.g. swimming.

But in exercises performed in the erect posture, the end-diastolic volume does not increase. Thus the Starling's mechanism cannot be responsible for increasing the SV during these exercises. In such cases the increase in SV is associated with a decrease in end-systolic volume (Fig. 19.3). The mechanism behind the increase in ejection without any stretching of

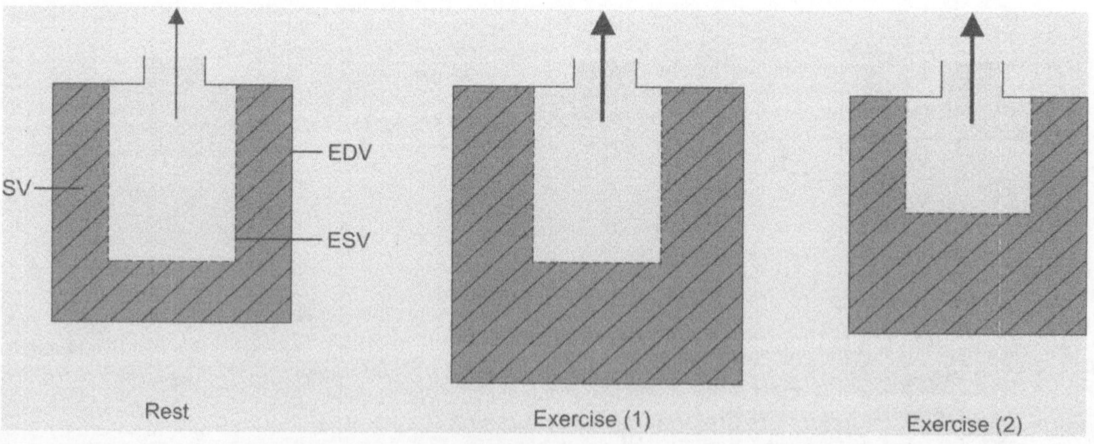

Fig. 19.3 Two alternative mechanisms for increase in stroke volume during exercise. (1) Exercise in flat posture: Stroke volume increases by the Starling mechanism. (2) Exercise in erect posture: There is no increase in size of the heart. The stroke volume increases by decreasing the volume left behind at the end of systole. SV, stroke volume; EDU, end diastolic volume; ESV, end systolic volume

the ventricles is the increased activity of sympathetic nervous system. You may recollect that sympathetic stimulation increases the force of contraction at any given muscle length.

Blood Pressure

The systolic blood pressure increases during exercise (Fig. 19.4) due to an increase in cardiac output. The diastolic pressure does not change much during exercise because it depends primarily on peripheral resistance (PR). During exercise, vasodilatation in exercising muscles tends to lower the PR while vasoconstriction in viscera tends to raise the PR. The change in diastolic pressure depends on the net change in PR. Since the net change is usually very small, the change in diastolic pressure is also very little.

Effect of Training on Cardiovascular Function

Cardiac output can increase to a much greater extent during exercise after physical training. Therefore much more intense exercise can be undertaken after training than before training. This happens because training affects both HR and SV.

The resting HR after training is generally low. This is thought to be due to an increase in vagal tone. Hence the magnitude of maximum increase in HR is greater in trained persons although the upper limit of the heart rate stays constant at about 180 per min.

The SV increases as a result of physical training. The increase is due to cardiac hypertrophy.

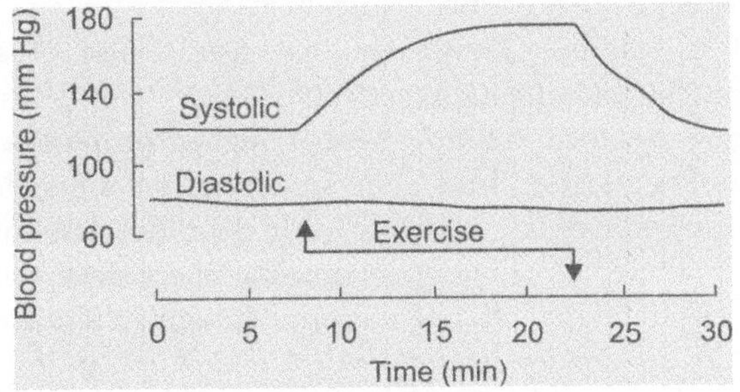

Fig.19.4 Systolic and diastolic blood pressure response to severe exercise

The effect of training on cardiac output has been illustrated using arbitrary but plausible figures in Table 19.1 and Figure 19.5.

Respiratory Responses to Exercise

During heavy exercise, there may be a 25-fold increase in oxygen consumption as well as carbon dioxide production. The respiratory responses to exercise meet this challenge by:

a. Increasing the ventilation (Fig. 19.6),
b. Increasing blood flow through the lungs so that perfusion matches the ventilation, and
c. Increase in diffusion capacity to make the best use of the opportunity created by the increased ventilation and perfusion during the short time available for exchange of gases.

Mechanism of Respiratory Responses to Exercise

The increase in pulmonary ventilation during exercise is due to a combination of chemical and neural mechanisms.

Chemical: During exercise there is an increased degree of oscillations in arterial PO_2 and PCO_2 synchronous with respiration. These oscillations stimulate the carotid body chemoreceptors and explain part of the increase in hyperventilation.

Neural: As in case of cardiovascular responses, hyperventilation also begins at the mere thought of exercise, i.e. before the exercise actually begins. This anticipatory increase is possibly mediated by the cerebral cortex. Part of the increase in pulmonary ventilation during exercise is mediated by reflexes originating in the joints and muscles involved in the exercise.

Table 19.1 Effect of training on cardiovascular function

	Before training		*After training*	
	Rest	*Maximal exercise*	*Rest*	*Maximal exercise*
Heart rate (beats/min)	80	180	60	180
Stroke volume (mL)	60	80	80	120
Cardiac output (L/min)	4.8	14.4	4.8	21.6

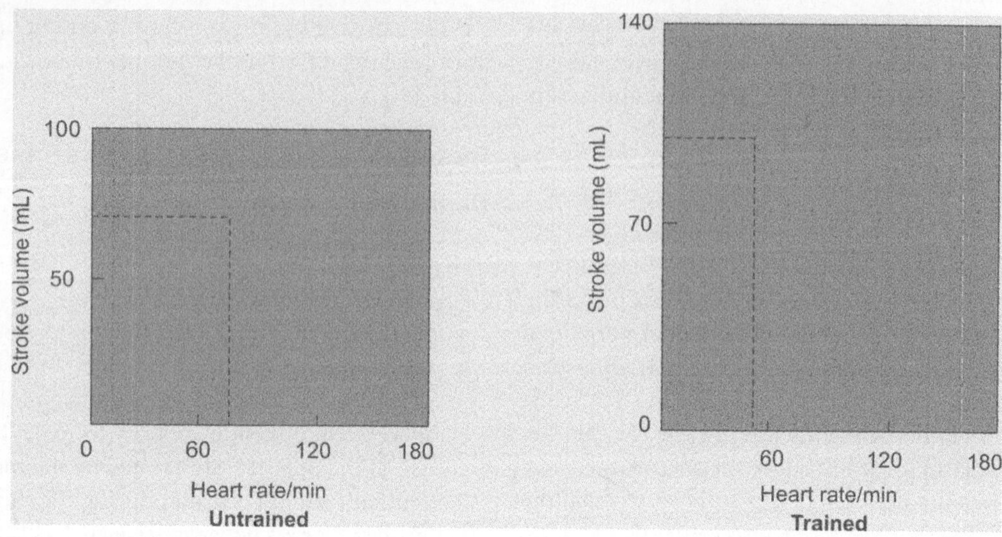

Fig.19.5 Effect of training on cardiac output. Since cardiac output is the product of heart rate and stroke volume, the rectangles in this figure represent the cardiac output. Dotted lines represent the situation at rest, and continuous lines that during maximal exercise. The resting cardiac output is the same in untrained and trained athletes, but in the trained athletes it is achieved at a lower heart rate by increasing the stroke volume. The upper limit for useful increase in heart rate is the same in both categories of athletes. But the trained athlete has a higher reserve because of a lower resting heart rate. Thus the trained athlete shows a greater increase in heart rate as well as stroke volume during maximal exercise, and is thus able to achieve a much higher cardiac output than an untrained athlete

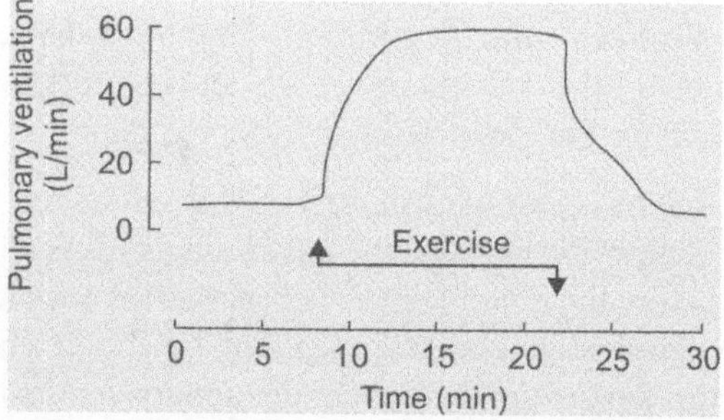

Fig. 19.6 Ventilatory response to mild exercise

The increase in pulmonary blood flow during exercise is due to an increase in the cardiac output, the mechanism of which has been discussed already.

The increase in pulmonary diffusion capacity during exercise is almost entirely due to the increase in pulmonary blood flow.

Effect of Training

There is no consistent effect of training on vital capacity or other measures of pulmonary function. What it implies is that in healthy individuals pulmonary function is usually not a limiting factor in determining the maximum intensity of exercise that they can undertake.

Response of Muscles to Exercise

It is common knowledge that regular use of a muscle leads to its hypertrophy. Apart from this, long distance runners have a higher proportion of slow muscle fibers while sprinters have a higher proportion of fast muscle fibers in their muscles. But the altered distribution of muscle fibers does not seem to be the effect of training.[1] It seems there are

[1]What else can it be due to? Think about the answer before you read further.

genetically determined differences in muscles fiber composition. Through a process of trial and error, an aspiring athlete finally selects the type of sporting event for which her muscles are best equipped.

Endurance Training

Endurance training (e.g. long distance running) does lead to an increase in mitochondrial activity of muscles. This improves the ability of muscle fibers to generate energy during exercise. Further, this type of training also improves the vascularity of muscles. This improves the ability of muscle fibers to extract oxygen from the blood. Finally, endurance training increases the glycogen content of muscles. This increases the reserve fuel available during exercise.

Strength Training

Strength training (e.g. short distance running) leads to muscular hypertrophy. Further, there is an increase in the synthesis of actin and myosin in the muscles. Finally, there is an increase in the efficiency with which muscles are used: there is a cutting down of that activity of muscles which is not required for the desired movements.

Endocrine Responses to Exercise

Several endocrine responses help the body adjust to the challenge of exercise. Some of these responses have been described below briefly.

The secretion of *ADH* and *aldosterone* increase during exercise. Exercise is often associated with excessive sweating (why)?[2] Sweating leads to fluid loss. ADH and aldosterone reduce fluid loss in the urine and thereby help maintain fluid balance.

Several *pituitary hormones* are secreted in response to exercise. These, together with the *adrenal hormones* and *glucagon* , help mobilize and utilize fuels which provide energy during exercise. The endocrine responses to exercise have been summarized in Table 19.2.

[2]To maintain body temperature.

Table 19.2 Endocrine responses to exercise

Hormone(s) secreted	*Functional significance in exercise*
ADH and Aldosterone	Fluid balance
ACTH and Glucocorticoids	Mobilization of fats and proteins
Adrenaline and Glucagon	Mobilization of carbohydrates and fats
Endorphins	Stimulation of food intake Relief from pain

Carbohydrates are mobilized by breaking down glycogen in muscles and liver. Fats are mobilized from adipose tissue in the form of free fatty acids. Proteins may also be mobilized as amino acids to serve as fuel.

Insulin secretion is, in fact, reduced during exercise. However, enough insulin is available in muscles for glucose utilization. Brain, for which glucose is spared in case of shortage, does not need insulin for utilizing it. Further, exercise leads to a sustained improvement in sensitivity of peripheral tissues to insulin. That is why exercise is helpful in diabetes mellitus.

Endorphins released during exercise not only stimulate food intake and relieve the discomfort of exercise, but also relieve mental stress and induce a sense of well being.

Metabolic Adjustments in Exercise

The mechanism and source of energy supply in exercise depends on the intensity and duration of exercise. For example, in a short bout of intense exercise such as a 100 meter sprint, all the energy comes from anaerobic metabolism *during* the exercise. *After* the exercise, the high energy compounds used (e.g. ATP) are replenished by aerobic metabolism. But in prolonged low intensity exercise such as a marathon race, much of the energy is derived from aerobic metabolism *during* the exercise itself. Secondly, during such exercise, after the initial use of ATP, creatine phosphate (CP) and glycogen, most of the energy comes from oxidation of fats.

Effect of Training

As a result of training, there is an increase in the size of energy stores, i.e. CP and glycogen, in the muscles. Secondly, there is an increase in the number and size of mitochondria in the muscle. Both these adaptations improve energy supply during exercise.

Fatigue

Fatigue is a word which is used in many different contexts. Fatigue may be acute or chronic, subjective or objective, physical or mental. Here we are concerned with muscle fatigue of the acute, objective, physical variety. We may define fatigue as a transient inability to maintain or repeat a task involving muscular contraction as a result of preceding performance of an identical or similar task.

Site of Fatigue

Logically, there can be four sites of fatigue (Fig. 19.7):

1. *Central nervous system:* Fatigue due to involvement of the central nervous system may be loosely considered 'psychological'. Although it does occur, and is an important cause of fatigue, there comes a point when even the best motivated subject is unable to continue the muscular effort.
2. *Motor nerve:* This is one site that has never been shown to be the site of fatigue.
3. *Neuromuscular junction:* In the isolated nerve-muscle preparation, neuromuscular junction is the site of fatigue. The underlying cause of junctional fatigue seems to be the exhaustion of acetylcholine. In the intact human being, only the fast twitch muscle fibers, which get fatigued early, are the ones which seem prone to fatigue at the neuromuscular junction.
4. *Muscle:* When even a well-motivated person cannot perform a muscular effort, muscle seems to be the site of fatigue. The muscle becomes fatigued due to depletion of energy reserves (CP and glycogen), accumulation of lactic acid, or some other factors, or a combination of several factors.

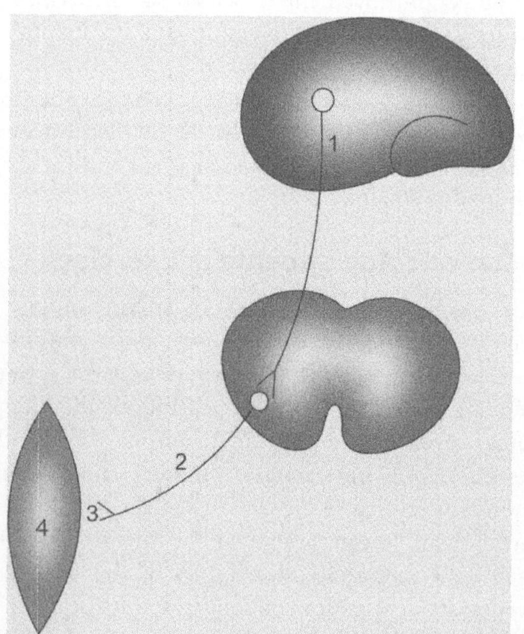

Fig. 19.7 Theoretical possible sites of fatigue. 1, central nervous system; 2, motor neuron; 3, neuromuscular junction; 4, muscle

We may conclude that in the intact organism the central nervous system and the muscle itself are the most probable sites of fatigue.

Other Factors Associated with Fatigue

Several factors influence the degree of effort needed to precipitate fatigue. One important factor is motivation. But there are also other more tangible factors which affect the onset of fatigue.

Diet: An appropriately timed high carbohydrate diet for sufficient duration can increase the glycogen stores of muscle. Diet-induced increase in muscle glycogen stores has been shown to delay the onset of fatigue in case of prolonged exercise.

Blood sugar: Prolonged exercise may lead to hypoglycemia. Hypoglycemia may precipitate fatigue. Hence sugar or glucose drinks during prolonged exercise may delay the onset of fatigue.

Pain: Pain anywhere in the body may accelerate the onset of fatigue. More specifically, an exercise such as hanging from a horizontal bar induces pain in the arms and hands. The pain compels the person to terminate the effort before true muscle fatigue has set in.

Body temperature: Exercising in hot environment, or prolonged exercise in any environment, tends to raise the body temperature. In such a situation, the skin blood flow increases as a part of the temperature regulatory mechanisms. Increase in skin blood flow reduces the maximum extent to which blood flow to skeletal muscles may increase. That is how a rise in body temperature accelerates the onset of fatigue.

Conclusion

Fatigue is a complex phenomenon affected by a very large number of factors, not all of which are known or properly understood.

PHYSIOLOGY OF FLUID BALANCE

The volume of blood and other body fluids is regulated accurately. The regulation is accomplished by regulating both fluid intake and fluid loss.

Fluid Compartments of the Body

About two-thirds of the body weight (range, 45-70%) is water (Fig. 19.8). This comes to about 40 L in an adult, and is called **total body water** (TBW).

About two-thirds of TBW is inside the cells, and is called **intracelluar fluid** (ICF). In an adult, ICF is about 25 L.

The remaining water, i.e. 15 L, is outside the cells, and is called **extracellular fluid** (ECF). The ECF constitutes the internal environment of the body, and is maintained constant with respect to temperature, pH, osmolarity, ionic composition, and oxygen and carbon dioxide tension. About one-fifth of ECF is plasma. The remaining ECF is almost entirely between cells, and is called interstitial fluid. A small quantity of ECF is also present as cerebrospinal fluid (CSF), aqueous humor, synovial fluid, gastrointestinal secretions, and fluid in the urinary tract.

Blood Volume

Blood is partly cells, and partly fluid. The fluid (plasma) is about 3 L, and the cells (mainly RBC) about 2 L. Thus the total blood volume in an adult is about 5 L.

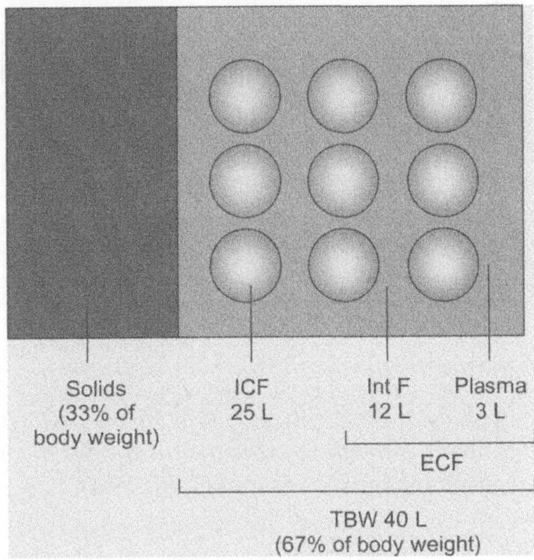

Fig. 19.8 Fluid compartments of the body. Water forms about two-thirds of the body weight. ICF, intracellular fluid; Int F, interstitial fluid; ECF, extracellular fluid; TBW, total body water

Regulation of Blood Volume and the Volume of Other Body Fluids

Mechanisms for regulation of blood volume overlap with those for regulation of fluid balance. But blood volume is regulated more accurately than the volume of fluid in other compartments.

Loss of body water is usually associated with an increase in osmotic pressure of body fluids. The body has mechanisms which respond to a rise in osmolarity of body fluids by retaining water. Thus these mechanisms help regulate both the osmolarity and the volume of body fluids.

Fluid balance depends on fluid intake and fluid loss. The major intake is in the form of water and other drinks. The major output is in the form of urine, and in hot weather, also as sweat. The average fluid intake and output in different forms is as given in Table 19.3. The fluid lost as sweat is dictated by the requirements of temperature regulation, not by those of fluid balance. Therefore the fluid balance is

Table 19.3 Fluid compartments of the body*

Compartment	Fraction of body weight	Volume
Total body water	60%	40 L
Intracellular fluid	40%	25 L
Extracellular fluid	20%	15 L
Plasma	4%	3 L
Interstitial fluid	16%	12 L

*Approximate values in a 70 kg adult.

achieved, in the long run, primarily by regulation of water intake through the mechanisms of thirst, and by regulation of urinary output (Table 19.4).

Table 19.4 Water balance

Intake	Volume (mL)		Loss	Volume (mL)	
	Cold weather	Hot weather		Cold weather	Hot weather
Water as drinks	1600	2400	Urine	1500	1000*
Water in food	1000	1000	Sweat	100	1500**
Oxidation	200	200	Skin	500	500
			Airways	400	300
			Feces	300	300
TOTAL	2800	3600		2800	3600

*Although urinary water loss can be reduced to even 500 mL, it is desirable for renal health that water intake be kept high so that urinary volume does not fall so low.

**May increase up to 5000 mL if heavy manual work is performed in hot weather. The water intake increases correspondingly to achieve water balance.

Short-term Regulation

Any acute change in blood volume is compensated within minutes by a redistribution of fluids between the blood and interstitial fluid. This happens because of a change in normal capillary hemodynamics. Normally, the pressure relationships are such that at the arterial end of capillaries, fluid is filtered out into the interstitial fluid, and at the venous end of capillaries almost an equal volume of fluid is reabsorbed so that blood volume is essentially constant (Fig. 19.9). However, if there is an acute fall in blood volume, the capillary hydrostatic pressure falls. As a result, the filtration at the arterial end becomes less than reabsorption at the venous end. This shift tends to restore the blood volume at the expense of the interstitial fluid. Capillary hemodynamics has been discussed in greater detail in Chapter 5.

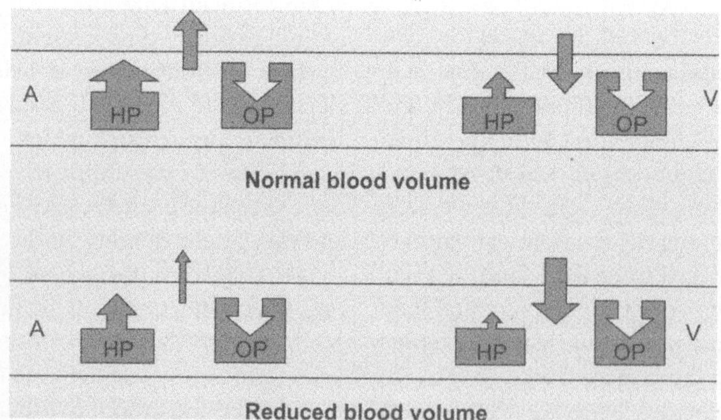

Fig.19.9 Capillary hemodynamics under normal and reduced blood volume. Capillary hydrostatic pressure (HP) favors filtration across the capillary into the interstitial fluid, and osmotic pressure (OP) favors reabsorption. Normally filtration at the arterial end (A) equals reabsorption at the venous end (V). When the blood volume is reduced, reabsorption exceeds filtration

Long-term Regulation

Long-term regulation of fluid balance is through the adjustment of water intake by the thirst mechanism, and of water output by adjustment of the urinary volume.

Thirst: Thirst is felt in the mouth but generated largely in the hypothalamus. The hypothalamus has some neurons which are specially sensitive to osmolarity. When the osmolarity of blood increases, osmoreceptors of hypothalamus stimulate the thirst mechanism. When we are thirsty, we take water. Addition of water to the body fluids reduces their osmolarity, bringing it back towards normal.

Since increase in osmolarity is generally the result of water loss from the body, the thirst mechanism helps in maintenance of water balance.

Urinary volume: Physical factors as well as several neurohumoral mechanisms adjust the rate of urine formation to suit the requirement of fluid balance.

1. *Physical mechanism:* A change in blood volume tends to change urine output through a physical mechanism (Fig. 19.10). Increase in blood volume increases urinary output. Increased water loss tends to reduce blood volume to normal. The same mechanism works in the opposite direction if the blood volume falls below normal.
2. *Antidiuretic hormone (ADH):* ADH is stimulated both in response to reduction in blood volume and increase in osmolarity (Fig. 19.11). ADH reduces urine output, and thus tends to restore fluid balance.
3. *Atrial natriuretic factor (ANF):* Natriuresis means increased urinary excretion of sodium. Hence ANF is the name that has been given to a hormone which increases urinary sodium excretion. If sodium excretion is increased, water excretion is also secondarily increased. Hence ANF increases not only sodium excretion but also urinary volume. ANF is released, as the name suggests, from the right atrium. Atrial volume receptors (Fig. 19.11) not only affect ADH secretion but also affect ANF secre-

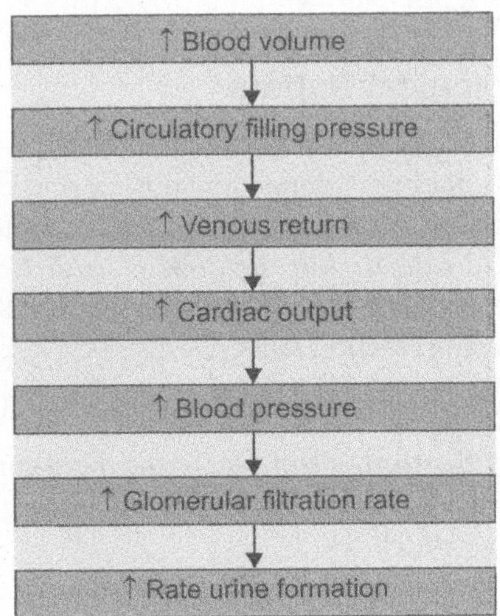

Fig. 19.10 Effect of blood volume on rate of urine formation. This physical mechanism contributes to regulation of blood volume

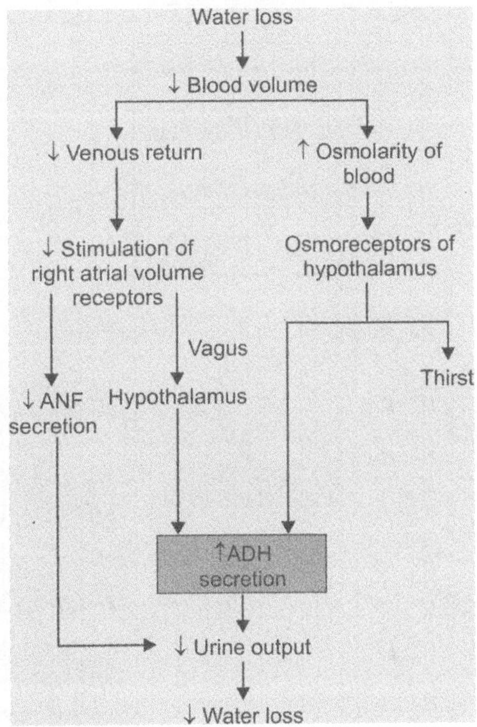

Fig. 19.11 Effect of fluid volume on rate of urine formation. This hormonal mechanism contributes to regulation of blood volume

tion. A decrease in blood volume inhibits ANF secretion. Reduced ANF secretion decreases urinary output and thereby tends to restore blood volume back to normal.

4. *Renin:* Renin is secreted by the kidneys in response to reduced renal blood flow. If there is a reduction in blood volume, the renal blood flow is reduced, leading to renin secretion (Fig. 19.12). Renin eventually leads to formation of angiotensin II. Angiotensin has at least two effects which help in a situation of low blood volume. First, angiotensin II is a powerful vasoconstrictor. Vasoconstriction raises the blood pressure which helps in overcoming, at least temporarily, the deliterious effect of low blood volume on tissue perfusion pressure. Second, angiotensin II releases aldosterone from the adrenal cortex, the effects of which are discussed below.

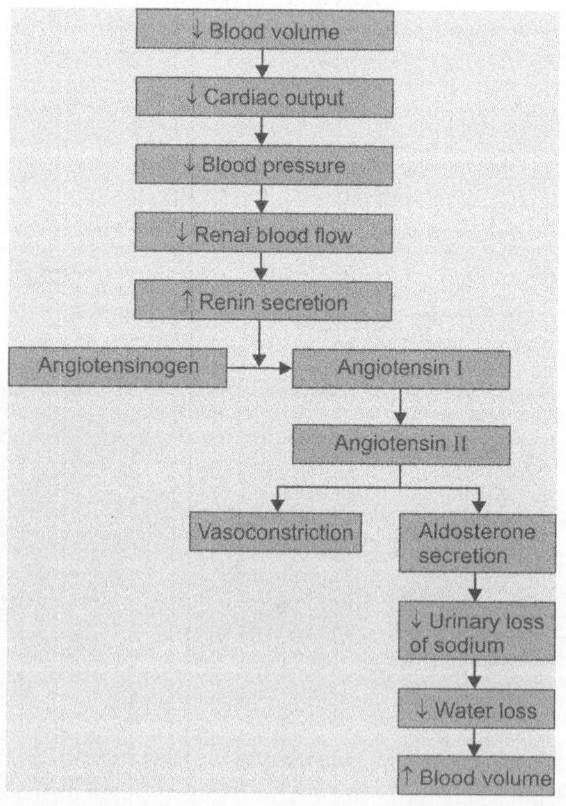

Fig. 19.12 Regulation of blood volume by the renin-angiotensin system

5. *Aldosterone:* Aldosterone secretion is stimulated by angiotensin II as well as some other stimuli associated with depletion of body fluids. Aldosterone acts mainly on the kidneys where it increases sodium reabsorption and potassium excretion, thereby promoting sodium retention and potassium loss. Sodium retention leads to water retention. Thus aldosterone helps restore the volume of extracellular fluids.

REGULATION OF ACID-BASE BALANCE

Cells can function normally only if the hydrogen ion concentration or pH inside and immediately outside the cell is maintained within a narrow range. The normal pH of extracellular fluids is 7.4.

The pH of body fluids is constantly challenged by normal metabolism because metabolic end products (e.g. carbon dioxide and lactic acid) are acidic. The acid (hydrogen ions) is ultimately removed from the body by the kidneys. But action by kidneys needs time. Immediate regulation of pH is due to various buffer systems in the body. Less quick, but still short-term, regulation of pH is brought about by the respiratory system. And, finally, long-term regulation of pH is brought about by the kidneys.

Physiological Buffers

A buffer is usually a mixture of substances, the pH of which does not change much if an acid or alkali is added to it. Common buffers are a mixture of a weak acid and its salt, e.g. H_2CO_3 and $NaHCO_3$. Suppose we add a strong alkali such as NaOH to it, the following reaction takes place:

$$H_2CO_3 + NaOH \longrightarrow NaHCO_3 + H_2O$$

Thus the strong alkali, NaOH, has been converted into $NaHCO_3$, a weak alkali. Therefore the pH does not change much.

Suppose we add a strong acid such as HCl to the same buffer, the following reaction takes place:

$$NaHCO_3 + HCl \longrightarrow NaCl + H_2CO_3$$

Thus the strong acid, HCl, has been converted into H_2CO_3, a weak acid. Therefore the pH does not change much.

Thus the acid component of the buffer (H_2CO_3 in the above example) buffers alkalies. The acids are buffered by the salt component ($NaHCO_3$ in the above example). Therefore, on the whole, a buffer is most effective when the salt and acid component are in equal concentration. The concentration of the salt and acid vary with the pH of the buffer. The pH at which the salt and acid concentration are equal is called the pK. This is often expressed as the Henderson- Hassellbalch equation:

$$pH = pK + \log \frac{[salt]}{[acid]}$$

If [salt] = [acid],

$$pH = pK + \log 1$$

or $pH = pK + 0$

or $pH = pK$

Thus pK of a buffer is the pH at which the salt and acid concentrations of the buffer are equal. Since this is the situation when the buffer is most effective, a buffer is most effective when the pH is equal to its pK.

There are three major buffers in the body fluids.

Bicarbonate Buffer

The bicarbonate buffer, which we have used as an example above, is a very important buffer in extracellular fluids. The pK of the bicarbonate buffer is 6.1. The pH of extracellular fluids is 7.4. Therefore, using Henderson-Hasselbalch equation,

$$7.4 = 6.1 + \log \frac{[bicarbonate]}{[carbonic\ acid]}$$

In body fluids, carbonic acid may be considered synonymous with carbon dioxide.

$$\text{Therefore, } \log \frac{[HCO_3^-]}{[CO_2]} = 7.4 - 6.1 = 1.3$$

$$\text{or } \frac{[HCO_3^-]}{[CO_2]} = \text{Antilog } 1.3$$

$$\text{or } \frac{[HCO_3^-]}{[CO_2]} = 20$$

Normally, the bicarbonate/carbon dioxide ratio in plasma and other extracellular fluids is 20. In acidosis or alkalosis, the ratio is altered. To restore normal pH, it is *not* necessary to restore normal concentrations of bicarbonate and carbon dioxide.[3] What is important is to restore the bicarbonate/carbon dioxide ratio to 20. For example, in metabolic acidosis, the bicarbonate concentration falls and the pH also falls. In such a situation, respiration is stimulated. Rapid and deep breathing washes off carbon dioxide. That reduces carbon dioxide concentration. Bicarbonate concentration is already low. Hence the ratio is restored to 20, and the pH of extracellular fluids returns to 7.4.

Repeating the example with figures might make it more clear.

Normal arterial plasma bicarbonate concentration = 24 mmol/L

Normal arterial plasma carbon dioxide concentration = 1.2 mmol/L

Normal bicarbonate/carbon dioxide ratio

= 24/1.2

= 20

Normal pH = 7.4

Suppose, in the arterial plasma of a patient having acidosis,

Bicarbonate concentration = 14.4 mmol/L

Carbon dioxide concentration = 1.2 mmol/L

$$pH = 6.1 + \log \frac{14.4}{1.2}$$

$$= 6.1 + \log 12$$

$$= 6.1 + 1.08$$

$$= 7.18$$

Hence the pH of arterial plasma in this patient will be 7.18.

As a result, his respiration is stimulated. He washes off carbon dioxide, and brings its concentration down to 0.72 mmol/L. After washing off carbon dioxide,

[3]Why not? If not, what should be restored to normal for correcting the pH of extracellular fluids? Think for yourself before reading further.

$$pH = 6.1 + \log \frac{14.4}{0.72}$$

$$= 6.1 + \log 20$$

$$= 6.1 + 1.3$$

$$= 7.4$$

Thus the pH of the plasma has been brought back to normal without any change in bicarbonate concentration. Such a situation is called compensated metabolic acidosis.

If pH is altered due to a respiratory disturbance, it is compensated by bringing about a change in bicarbonate concentration through an alteration in renal bicarbonate excretion.

The importance of the bicarbonate buffer lies in the fact that the concentrations of both components of the buffer can be altered by the body. Carbon dioxide concentration can be altered by the respiratory system, and bicarbonate concentration can be altered by the kidneys. If the acid-base disturbance is due to a respiratory abnormality, the kidneys can alter the bicarbonate excretion to compensate for the acid-base disturbance. If the acid-base disturbance is due to a renal abnormality, the respiratory system can alter the carbon dioxide elimination to compensate for the acid-base disturbance. If the acid-base disturbance is due to some other cause (e.g. diabetes for gastroenteritis), respiratory system can alter carbon dioxide elimination to provide quick, short-term compensation, and kidneys can alter bicarbonate excretion for long-term compensation.

Protein Buffer

Proteins act as buffers because of the amino acids which have free acid radicals, or because of histidine, which has an imidazole group. These features make it easy for proteins to accept or give up hydrogen ions without much change in pH. Among extracellular fluids, proteins are important as buffers in plasma, as plasma proteins, and also in red blood cells, as hemoglobin. Further, proteins are important as buffers also in intracellular fluids.

Phosphate Buffer

Phosphates can act as buffer because they can exist as dihydrogen phosphate or monohydrogen phosphate. Phosphates are important as buffers in the renal tubular fluid and in the intracellular fluids.

Limitations of Buffers

Buffers minimize the effect of addition of acid or alkali to a fluid on its pH. But buffers do nothing to the processes which add or remove acid or alkali to or from the body fluids. This can be done by the lungs and kidneys, and therefore these two organs make an important contribution to acid-base balance.

Respiration and Acid-base Balance

Respiratory activity affects acid-base balance of the body because it eliminates carbon dioxide from the body. Carbon dioxide is an acidic substance. Therefore an increase in respiratory activity reduces the acidity of body fluids. Pathological hyperventilation (e.g. hysterical) can eliminate so much carbon dioxide from the body as to lead to respiratory alkalosis. On the other hand, respiratory depression (as in barbiturate poisoning) leads to carbon dioxide retention, and consequently, respiratory acidosis.

Not only does change in respiratory activity affect acid-base balance, change of pH of extracellular fluids also affects respiratory activity. That is how respiratory activity can contribute to acid-base homeostasis. A fall in pH of extracellular fluids stimulates peripheral chemoreceptors in the carotid and aortic bodies, and also central chemoreceptors in the medulla oblongata. Stimulation of these chemoreceptors reflexly leads to an increase in the rate and depth of respiration. Increase in pulmonary ventilation washes off carbon dioxide leading to a rise in pH. Thus the original disturbance is corrected (Fig. 19.13). The same mechanism working in the opposite direction may correct a rise in pH to some extent. But since respiratory activity is meant primarily to meet the metabolic needs of the body, its contribution to acid-base balance is limited. More

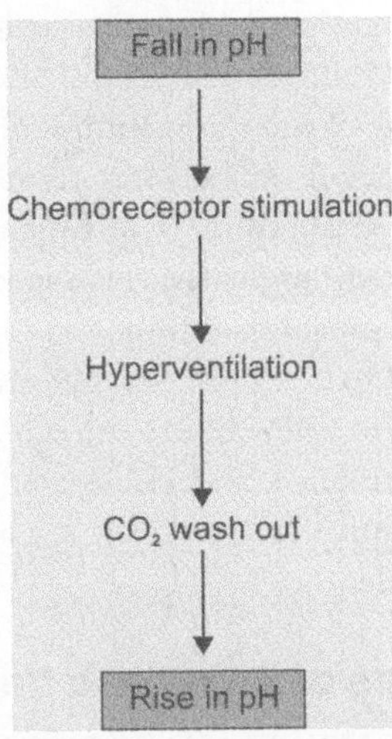

Fig. 19.13 Compensation for acidosis by the respiratory system

effective and relatively permanent measures for acid-base balance are taken by the kidneys.

Kidneys and Acid-base Balance

The byproducts of metabolism are mostly acidic. Kidneys provide the final mechanism for maintenance of the pH of body fluids in spite of the production of these acidic substances. They do so by:

a. *Reabsorption of bicarbonate*: Bicarbonate being an important buffer, it is retained by the kidneys by reabsorption.
b. *Generation of bicarbonate*: Kidneys generate also fresh bicarbonate for the body in order to replenish the bicarbonate used up in the process of buffering acids.
c. *Secretion of hydrogen ions*: Renal tubules secrete hydrogen ions into the urine, thereby removing some acid from the body.

Further, the above processes are subject to regulation depending on the needs of acid-base balance in the body. Let us study these processes in some detail.

Large segments of the nephron have carbonic anhydrase activity in the epithelium. Carbonic anhydrase dissolves carbon dioxide in water to form carbonic acid. Carbonic acid dissociates into

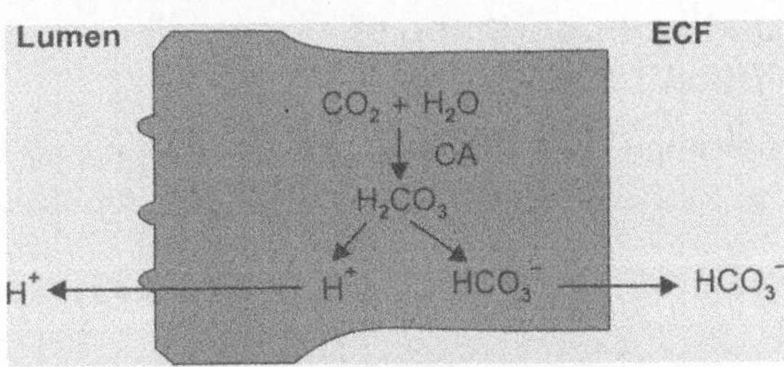

Fig. 19.14 Mechanism of reabsorption/generation of bicarbonate and secretion of hydrogen ions in the tubular cells of the nephron. The carbon dioxide may be derived from metabolism in the cell, or it may enter the cell from the bloodstream, or it may enter the cell from the lumen. CA, carbonic anhydrase

bicarbonate and hydrogen ions. Bicarbonate is reabsorbed whereas hydrogen ions are secreted into the lumen (Fig. 19.14).

Fate of Secreted Hydrogen Ions

The hydrogen ions secreted into the lumen are buffered in the tubular lumen (Why?).[4] The principal buffers available in the lumen are the ammonia buffer and the phosphate buffer.

Ammonia buffer: Ammonia can buffer H^+ as follows:

$$NH_3 + H^+ \longrightarrow NH_4^+$$

Ammonia required for this purpose is synthesized in tubular epithelium from amino acids. About 60 percent of the ammonia is synthesized from glutamine, and the remaining 40 percent from other amino acids.

The ammonia buffer helps in excreting H^+ as ammonium salts (Fig. 19.15), which are only weakly acidic.

Phosphate buffer: Phosphate can buffer H^+ as follows:

$$H^+ + HPO_4^{2-} \longrightarrow H_2PO_4^-$$

The phosphate buffer helps in excreting H^+ as dihydrogen phosphates (Fig. 19.16), which are only weakly acidic.

[4]The buffering is important to prevent corrosive injury to the tubular cells.

Relative Importance of Different Mechanisms

As mentioned earlier, buffers do not affect the acid-base balance in a radical way; they only minimize the impact of a change. Lungs also have a limited role because carbon dioxide elimination is basically linked up with oxygen consumption: its link with acid-base balance is only a short-term arrangement, not a long-term solution. The organ that is truly dedicated to acid-base balance is the kidney. But all the three mechanisms are important because of the time they need to act. Buffers act at once, lungs take a few minutes to a few hours to compensate for an acid-base disturbance, and kidneys take 3-5 days to do the maximum that they can in case of an acid-base disturbance.

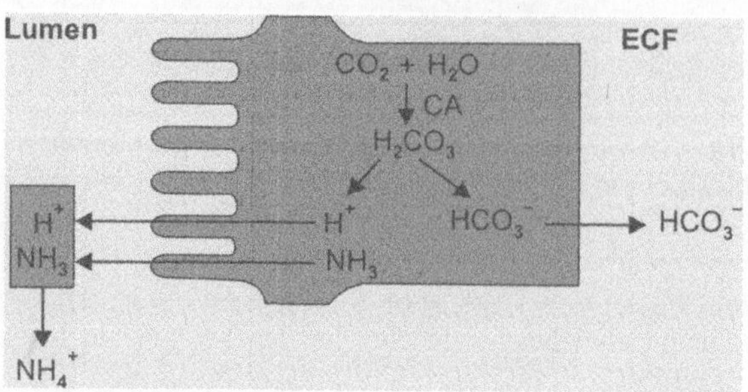

Fig. 19.15 Buffering action of ammonia in the renal tubules. CA, carbonic anhydrase

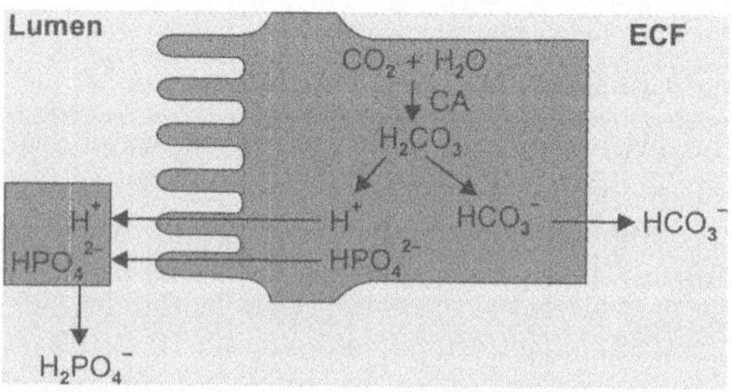

Fig. 19.16 Buffering action of the phosphate buffer in the renal tubules. The phosphate buffer is much more important in the distal nephron than in the proximal nephron

Disturbances of Acid-base Balance

Disturbances of acid-base balance are of two types: acidosis and alkalosis. Acidosis is due to accumulation of acids, or depletion of alkalies. Alkalosis is due to accumulation of alkalies, or depletion of acids. In response to acidosis or alkalosis, the body first compensates, and then tries to correct the disturbance. Compensation tends to restore the bicarbonate/carbon dioxide ratio to 20. This is achieved by either the kidneys changing the bicarbonate concentration, or the lungs changing the carbon dioxide concentration.

Depending on the cause of acidosis or alkalosis, it is termed respiratory or metabolic. The principal features of different types of acidosis and alkalosis have been summarized in Table 19.5.

Table 19.5 Acidosis and alkalosis

Disturbance	*Common causes*	*Abnormality*	*How compensated*
Respiratory acidosis	Diffusion defect in lungs Respiratory obstruction Paralysis of respiratory muscles Depression of respiratory centers in CNS	Accumulation of carbon dioxide	Renal retention of bicarbonate
Respiratory alkalosis	Hyperventilation following acute exposure to high altitude	Low carbon dioxide level	Excess urinary loss of bicarbonate
Metabolic acidosis	Diarrhea Diabetic ketoacidosis Renal failure	Low bicarbonate level	Hyperventilation to wash off carbon dioxide
Metabolic alkalosis	Vomiting of gastric contents	High bicarbonate level	Hypoventilation to retain carbon dioxide*

* Very limited compensation because hypoventilation leads to hypoxia, which stimulates respiration.

CONCLUSION

This chapter brings together at one place some of the most vital regulatory mechanisms of the body. Studying them after learning something about all systems of the body is an interesting way to revise many aspects of physiology. Further, these topics are also among the most clinically relevant in physiology.

QUESTION

1. A comatose patient with respiratory depression has the following blood chemistry:
   Arterial bicarbonate concentration = 24 mmol/L
   Arterial carbon dioxide concentration = 2.4 mmol/L
   a. Comment on the patient's condition.
   b. What will be the patient's blood pH?
   c. How will the patient's kidneys respond to the situation? How will the renal response help the patient?

ANSWER

1. a. The patient's bicarbonate concentration is normal but carbon dioxide concentration is high. Carbon dioxide concentration is high because of inefficient removal from the body due to respiratory depression. The patient has respiratory acidosis.

   b. The pH can be calculated using the Henderson-Hasselbalch equation.

   $$pH = pK + \log \frac{[salt]}{[acid]}$$

   pK of the bicarbonate buffer = 6.1

   $$\therefore pH = 6.1 + \log \frac{24}{2.4}$$
   $$= 6.1 + \log 10$$
   $$= 6.1 + 1$$
   $$= 7.1$$

   The calculation confirms that the patient has respiratory acidosis.

   c. The patient's kidneys will respond by excreting less bicarbonate. That will raise the blood bicarbonate concentration. As a result, the bicarbonate/carbon dioxide ratio will rise and the pH will also rise towards normal. Suppose the bicarbonate concentration rises to 48 mmol/L. then,

   $$pH = 6.1 + \log \frac{48}{2.4}$$
   $$= 6.1 + \log 20$$
   $$= 6.1 + 1.3$$
   $$= 7.4$$

   After the blood pH has become normal, the patient will have compensated respiratory acidosis.

CHAPTER

20 Yoga

"Yoga is a methodised effort towards self-perfection."

—SRI AUROBINDO

Chapter Outline

Why should yoga be included in a book on physiology? For reasons more than one. Physiology deals with normal function. A normal human being may be at rest or taking exercise, may be at sea level or at high altitude. In the process of coping up with these challenges, body functions undergo adaptive changes. But in spite of these changes, the human being remains normal. Therefore the altered function remains within the scope of physiology. That is why exercise physiology and high altitude physiology are included in books on physiology. Similarly, some normal human beings take to yoga. Yogic practices alter body function, but the function is still within the normal range. Therefore yoga, and the way it affects us, are within the scope of physiology. Secondly, yoga, or some distorted versions of it, are being increasingly used for the prevention and treatment of coronary heart disease, hypertension, diabetes and several other diseases. Therefore every health professional should be familiar with yoga. Thirdly, the patients now frequently ask their doctor or nurse whether yoga would help them. Finally, familiarity with yoga might inspire the reader to adopt it in her own life. That will be all the better for her and her patients.

WHAT IS YOGA

Yoga is a popular but commonly misunderstood word. It is frequently equated with asanas, pranayama and meditation. These are merely techniques which, if practiced with the right attitude, can help in the pursuit of yoga. But if these techniques are practiced mechanically, or as a ritual, without the right attitude it is impossible to make any progress on the yogic path. Having talked about what yoga is not, let us see what it is. In the words of Sri Aurobindo, yoga is a methodized effort towards self-perfection. The yogic techniques are a part of the methodized effort. The goal of yoga is self-perfection. It is commonly admitted that man is basically imperfect. Therefore, if a person pursuing yoga (called *sadhak*, if male, and *sadhika*, if female) reaches the goal of perfection (called *siddhi*), she has crossed, or transcended, the limitations of the human state. One might say that she has achieved union with the Divine. Thus, yoga is a methodized effort towards self-perfection with the ultimate aim of achieving union with the Divine (Fig. 20.1). That is the origin of the word yoga (*yuj*, union).

Perfection may be classified into perfection of the body, or the mind, or both. Accordingly, there are different schools of yoga (Fig. 20.2).

SCHOOLS OF YOGA

Although there are several schools of yoga, we shall discuss only four of the best known ones, which also illustrate best the principles outlined above.

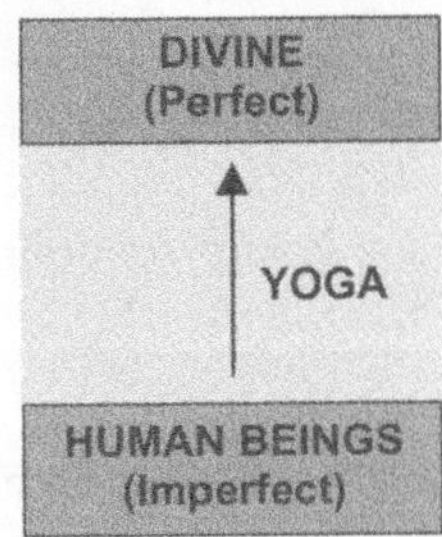

Fig. 20.1 Yoga is a journey towards perfection, or union with the divine

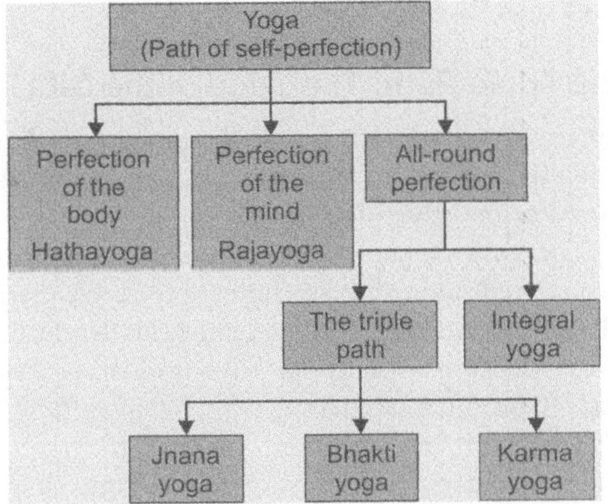

Fig. 20.2 The dominant emphasis of different schools of yoga

Hatha Yoga

Hatha yoga aims primarily at perfection of the body. A perfect body means a strong and healthy body. The techniques of hatha yoga include asanas, pranayama and kriyas. If carried to extremes, hatha yoga not only makes the body healthy, but can also enable the yogi to perform physical feats which resemble miracles. For example, he may be able to live in a confined space for a long time, or may be able to control his heart rate. These extremes also constitute a weakness of hatha yoga. In the process of pursuing physical perfection, the *sadhak* may spend all the time on yogic practices. Having achieved remarkable physical prowess, he may start exhibiting it. Thus, a noble task gets reduced to entertainment, and does not good either to the yogi, or to anybody else.

The basic book of hatha yoga is *Hatha Yoga pradipika* compiled by Svatmarama Yogindra in the 15th century.

Raja Yoga

Raja yoga aims primarily at perfection of the mind. A perfect mind is a calm, quiet and peaceful mind. The basic technique of raja yoga is meditation. But since only a healthy body can work towards a peaceful mind, some basic asanas and pranayama are also a part of raja yoga. Patanjali, the master of raja yoga, breaks the process into eight parts. That is why Patanjali's yoga is also called **ashtanga yoga**. The eight components of ashtanga yoga are:

Yama

Yama is essentially a set of five don'ts (Table 20.1):

a. *Ahimsa* (non-violence), i.e. do not cause injury.
b. *Satya* (truth), i.e. do not tell a lie.
c. *Asteya* (non-stealing), i.e. do not steal.
d. *Brahmcharya* (celibacy), i.e. do not indulge in sensory pleasures.
e. *Aparigraha* (non-receiving), i.e. do not accept gifts, or do not be greedy.

The yamas should be practiced in thought, word and deed.

Niyama

Niyama is essentially a set of five do's:

a. *Shaucha* (cleanliness), i.e. internal and external purification.
b. *Santosh* (contentment), i.e. being satisfied with what we are given.
c. *Tapas* (austerities), i.e. disciplining our movements, or concentrating of energies on our objective.
d. *Swadhyaya* (study), i.e. study of the scriptures.
e. *Ishwarpranidhan* (surrender to God), i.e. placing full trust in the will and wisdom of God.

Asana

Asana, i.e. postures which are steady and comfortable.[1]

[1]More details are given later in the section on yogic practices.

Table 20.1 Perennial truths

Yama (Raja yoga)	*Pancha shila (Buddha)*	*The ten commandments (Old Testament)*
Ahimsa	1. Abstain from killing	6. You shall not kill
Satya	4. Abstain from lying	9. You shall not bear false witness against your neighbor
Asteya	2. Abstain from stealing	8. You shall not steal
Brahmcharya	3. Abstain from adultery	7. You shall not commit adultery
Aparigraha		10. You shall not covet your neighbor's house...or anything that is your neighbor's
	5. Abstain from liquor	

The remarkable similarity between yama, pancha shila (five precepts) of the Buddha, and the last five of the ten commandments is obvious from the Table.

Pranayama

Pranayama, i.e. control of prana, usually interpreted as breath control.

Pratyahara

Pratyahara, (gathering towards, or bringing together), i.e. restraint of the senses so as to free the mind.

Dharana

Dharana (concentration). The object of concentration may be a part of the body, a sound or an idea.

Dhyana

Dhyana, (meditation), i.e. letting the mind flow towards the point(s) of concentration.

Samadhi

Samadhi, (superconsciousness), i.e. transcending ordinary consciousness based on perception of external objects.

The principal weakness of raja yoga is that it promotes aloofness and asceticism. *Yogasutras,* compiled by Patanjali between 300 and 500 AD, are the basic text of raja yoga. An English translation of the Yogasutras together with an excellent commentary by Swami Vivekananda is readily available as an inexpensive paperback of about 300 pages.

The Triple Path: The Yoga of the Gita

The triple path of work, knowledge and devotion is a synthesis, and yet leaves scope for greater emphasis on one or the other of its three components.

The path of knowledge, or *gyana yoga,* works through reflection and discrimination. As ordinarily followed, it resembles raja yoga, and leads to rejection of the world as an illusion. Thus, gyana yoga also tends to promote asceticism.

The path of devotion, or *bhakti yoga,* is characterized by intense adoration of the Divine. As ordinarily followed, this path also leads to such intense absorption in the object of worship that the *sadhika* cuts herself off from everyday activities.

The path of works, or *karma yoga,* is often considered the ideal path in today's action-oriented world. It is generally interpreted as the disinterested performance of one's duty. This is an oversimplification and a somewhat distorted interpretation of the Gita. A *sadhika* following karma yoga does not consider herself to be the doer, but only an instrument of the Divine. Therefore she seeks to know the Divine will. Having known that, she seeks to fulfill it through action, which is performed without any sense of egoism, without any desire, and without a sense of victory or defeat, success or failure.

The three streams of the triple path need not be pursued exclusively. In fact, Sri Aurobindo made the penetrating observation that starting with any one of them, one would eventually come to pursue also the other two. For example, Divine *love* leads to *knowledge* of the Beloved, and finally to Divine service (*work*). So also, *knowledge* leads to *love* of that which is known, and finally to His service (*work*). Dedicated *work* implies *love*, which in turn prompts the lover to know the Beloved (*knowledge*) (Fig. 20.3). The beauty of the triple path lies in relying on our three basic instruments—head, heart and hands—for achieving perfection. Use the head to know the Highest, use the heart to love the Best, and use the hands to serve the Greatest.

Although the triple path comes close to the ideal, its practice has been flawed by the exclusive practice of only one of the three paths in antagonism to the other two.

The basic book on the triple path is the Gita. The Gita has a universal appeal: just next to the Bible, it is the most translated book in the world. Its appeal lies in the guidance it provides in situations of conflict, in situations of moral crisis, when there are more than one alternative courses of action available, and there is some very valid justification for each. Arjuna's dilemma in the battle of Kurukshetra symbolizes such moments in life, and the solution outlined by Lord Krishna to resolve the dilemma can be generalized to resolve similar doubts in everyday life. The solution thus arrived at is ideal, and at the same time restores inner joy and peace.

Integral Yoga

Integral yoga is a very powerful synthesis of different schools of yoga formulated by Sri Aurobindo at the beginning of the twentieth century. It leans heavily on the yoga of the Gita but incorporates the central principles of other major schools of yoga as well. The uniqueness of integral yoga lies in emphasizing the following:

a. The world is a manifestation of the Divine. Since the Divine is real, the world is also real. It may not be the whole reality but it is not an illusion. Therefore, the Divine cannot be realized by rejecting the world. Thus, integral yoga actively discourages asceticism.
   Gita is also primarily a book of action in the world. But with the passage of time, spirituality has come to be equated with asceticism. Swami Vivekananda and Sri Aurobindo have made powerful pleas in the recent past for correcting this distortion.
b. The emphasis is on divinization of daily life. By emphasizing the possibility and necessity of transforming ordinary everyday work, yoga becomes a path open to all.
c. Integral yoga does not stop at the salvation of the individual. The *sadhika* should also work towards psychospiritual transformation of all those who come in contact with her.

Integral yoga is, thus, integral in ways more than one. First, it integrates several lines of yoga. Second, it integrates spiritual quest with worldly existence. Finally, it combines personal calm and delight with concern for universal psychospiritual transformation. The basic text of integral yoga is *The Synthesis of Yoga* by Sri Aurobindo.

THE YOGIC ATTITUDE

From the above description, specially that of *yama* and *niyama*, we already have some idea of the yogic

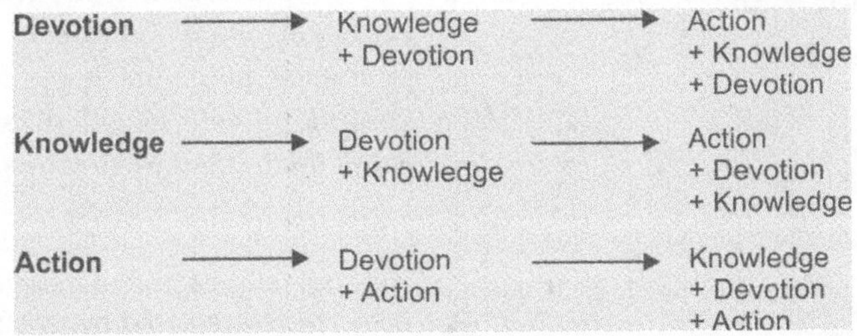

Fig. 20.3 Starting with the path of devotion, knowledge or action, one ultimately ends up following all three

THE HUMAN MACHINE

Using a gadget is great,
But making the machine is greater still.
Inventing the instrument, however,
Needs the greatest skill.

Life is a machine
Invented by the Divine.
Into matter He injects life
To make it a tool divine

The role of we mortals
Is the simplest of all.
To use the machine,
To fulfill His plans big and small.

To do His bidding
Is easier said than done.
The road to His plans
Is blocked by bullies more than one.

The first bully is ego,
A bloated balloon.
Puncture it as you may,
It fills itself soon.

The second bully is desire,
A multiplying tribe.
Oust one, and find two
Begging for a bribe.

Despair not,
For there are friends.
They can facilitate
The journey to His ends.

The first friend is surrender.
Silence your mind,
And you will hear
His voice, clear and kind.

Reason no more,
Do what he says.
Conflict only clouds the vision,
You anyway end up where He takes.

The second friend is merger.
There is after all,
The same divine spark,
In beings big and small.

If you are in pain,
I should weep as well.
Your moments of joy
Should make my heart swell.

Merger is easy to preach
But difficult to practice.
That my needs come first,
Is very easy to establish.

To fit into His plans,
There are thus dictums four.
No ego, no desire,
Total surrender, merge more.

attitude. It has been broken into five components and summarized below in a less dogmatic tone.

Dealing with the Ego

Ego is the awareness of an individual as a distinct entity. Since this awareness separates the individual from everybody else, it is referred to as the separative ego. In yoga, separative ego is not considered to be a deep or lasting truth because all creation is a manifestation of the same Divine. If this basic truth is grasped, the individual is overcome by a new sense of unity with the rest of creation. Control, and ultimately elimination, of the separative ego is an important part of the yogic attitude. With this change of attitude, the person loses her feeling as the doer of her actions. She considers herself merely as an instrument of the Divine. We are often advised 'not to show off' or 'not to think too much of ourselves'. The yogic attitude carries this standard advice to its idealistic extreme. Elimination of the separative ego is the most vital part of the yogic attitude. If this part can be accomplished, the other components outlined below follow[2] automatically as a matter of course.

Dealing with Desires

Man is a creature with endless desires. He learns repeatedly that fulfillment of desires does not guarantee perpetual happiness. But still he keeps coming up with new desires and tries frantically to fulfill them. He always seems to be under the illusion

[2]One has to be careful so that the 'normal' separative ego does not get replaced by its still more deadly form, the spiritual pride.

that fulfillment of the latest desire is sure to bring lasting happiness. Reduction, and finally elimination, of desires is also an essential part of the yogic attitude. Most desires are aimed primarily at boosting the ego. Therefore, controlling the ego also controls desires. As Sri Aurobindo points out, desires starve in the absence of support from the ego.

Surrender

Surrender requires faith in a superior force that runs the world in accordance with His designs which are perfect. Accepting whatever happens happily in a spirit of surrender brings deep and lasting inner peace. A person with the ego under control finds total surrender convenient.

Universal Love

Pure love is extended to all without reservation and without any expectation. Further, this love is full of concern but devoid of attachment.

Sincerity

In practice, sincerity is the most important virtue. We generally know what to do, but lack the will to do it. Sincerity makes us do the right thing even at the expense of risk or inconvenience.

THE YOGIC PRACTICES

The yogic attitude forms the necessary background and accompaniment of all yogic practices. We shall discuss briefly the more visible and relatively popular forms of yogic practices.

Asanas

Asana, literally, means a posture. Asanas may be classified into three groups depending on their primary purpose: relaxation, physical exercise or meditation.

Asanas for Relaxation

These asanas provide physical relaxation, and if properly performed, also mental relaxation. Shavasana is the principal asana in this category (Fig. 20.4). It is performed at the beginning and end of a session of asanas, and also sandwiched between other asanas which provide physical exercise. Another common relaxing posture is makarasana (Fig. 20.5).

Shavasana relaxes the body because the muscles are completely relaxed voluntarily.[3] It also relaxes the mind through deep and conscious breathing, and autosuggestion. Shavasana is an extremely useful asana, specially for busy people under stress. Shavasana is the one asana recommended to them if they do not have time for any more.

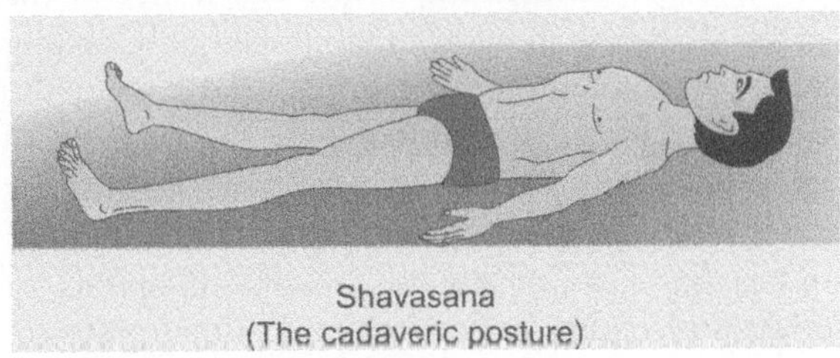

Shavasana
(The cadaveric posture)

Fig. 20.4 Shavasana, a relaxing posture. One should lie down with feet apart, hands away from the body, palms facing upwards, with the eyes closed, and breathe slowly and deeply. As the air goes in, the abdomen goes up, and as the air is breathed out, the abdomen comes down. The whole body should be relaxed completely and the mind should be at peace

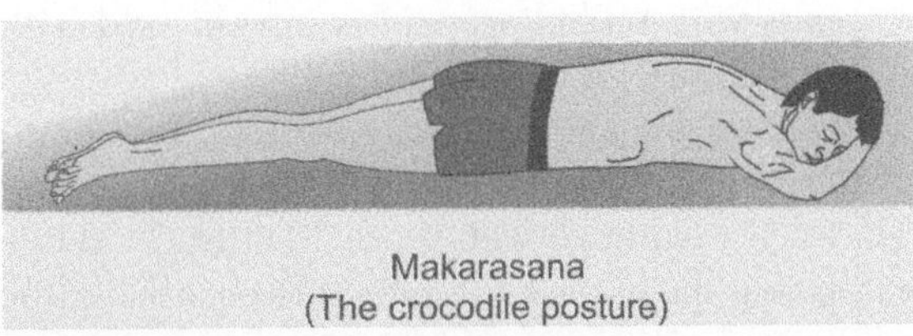

Makarasana
(The crocodile posture)

Fig. 20.5 Makarasana, a posture particularly suitable for relaxing between asanas which are performed with the belly touching the ground, such as bhujangasana and dhanurasana

[3]Simply lying down supine does not relax the muscles completely. Afterlying down, further muscle relaxation can be achieved by voluntary effort. As the muscle tone gets abolished, one gets a feeling of sinking into the ground.

Asanas for Physical Exercise

These asanas are the best known part of yoga. A sequence of 10-15 asanas which would take 30-45 minutes to perform can provide good exercise to all parts of the body. A typical asana starts with an initial position *(sthiti)*. From that position a slow and graceful movement is performed till the final position of the asana is reached. The final position commonly imposes severe stretch on some parts of the body. In the final position, the pose is held for some time (usually 10-30 seconds). The duration of the holding time depends on the endurance of the person. The pose should be maintained only as long as the person is comfortable in it, and can enjoy the stretch. After the posture has been held for some time, the person returns to a relaxing posture by performing a slow and graceful movement. Several studies have shown the superiority of asanas to ordinary physical exercises in terms of their physical benefits, and even more their psychological benefits and therapeutic effects. Therefore, it is natural to ask how these asanas are different from other physical exercises. The special features of asanas are:

1. The movements are slow, gentle and graceful.
2. Stretching alternates with relaxation.
3. Every pose is followed by a counterpose.
4. The session of asanas begins with relaxation, ends with relaxation, and is interspersed with relaxation.

But even the above features are not enough to call the asanas yogasanas. Asanas become yogasanas only when performed with the right attitude. While performing the asanas, the thoughts occupying the *sadhika's* mind should be that she is working towards physical perfection so that her body can be a fit temple for the Divine that resides within, and can be an efficient instrument of the Divine will.

A reasonable sequence of asanas is given in the accompanying box, and many of the asanas have been illustrated in Figures 20.6 to 20.10.

Asanas for Meditation

Three asanas are generally considered suitable for meditation: *padmasana*, *sukhasana* and *vajrasana* (Fig. 20.11). During padmasana or sukhasana, the hands may be placed in one of the three positions illustrated in Figure 20.12.

The description of asanas here is meant only to illustrate the general principles. Much more details are necessary for actually performing the asanas. Detailed guidance is readily available in books and CDs, but the best option probably still is to begin under the supervision of a good teacher. In any case, it is important to bear in mind that the final pose of some asanas may be impossible to achieve for many persons. In such cases it may be harmful to exceed the limits of flexibility of the body. It is enough to make a movement in the right direction with the right attitude although the final pose may not be perfect. Further, persons with an ailment should start appropriate asanas only under professional guidance. Finally, there is only one basic rule for asanas. They are postures which are steady and comfortable. An unsteady or painful posture is not an asana. Therefore such postures should not be attempted, even if a book illustrates them. Everything cannot be done by everybody in the world.

Pranayama

Pranayama, literally, means control of *prana*. *Prana*, in Indian philosophy, refers to all forms of energy in the universe. Life force is one part of this energy. Life force, in an individual, is symbolized by breathing. That is why *pranayama* is generally considered to mean regulated breathing. But an advanced yogi can control many other manifestations of *prana* as well.

The essence of the practice of *pranayama* is slow and deep breathing. Such breathing is economical because it reduces dead space ventilation. It also renews air throughout the lungs in contrast with shallow breathing which renews air only at the base of the lungs.

Meditation

We have talked about the rules of conduct which comprise *yama* and *niyama*, and also something about asanas and *pranayama*. These are the first four steps in raja yoga. The next four steps, viz. *pratyahara*, *dharana*, *dhyana* and *samadhi* may be

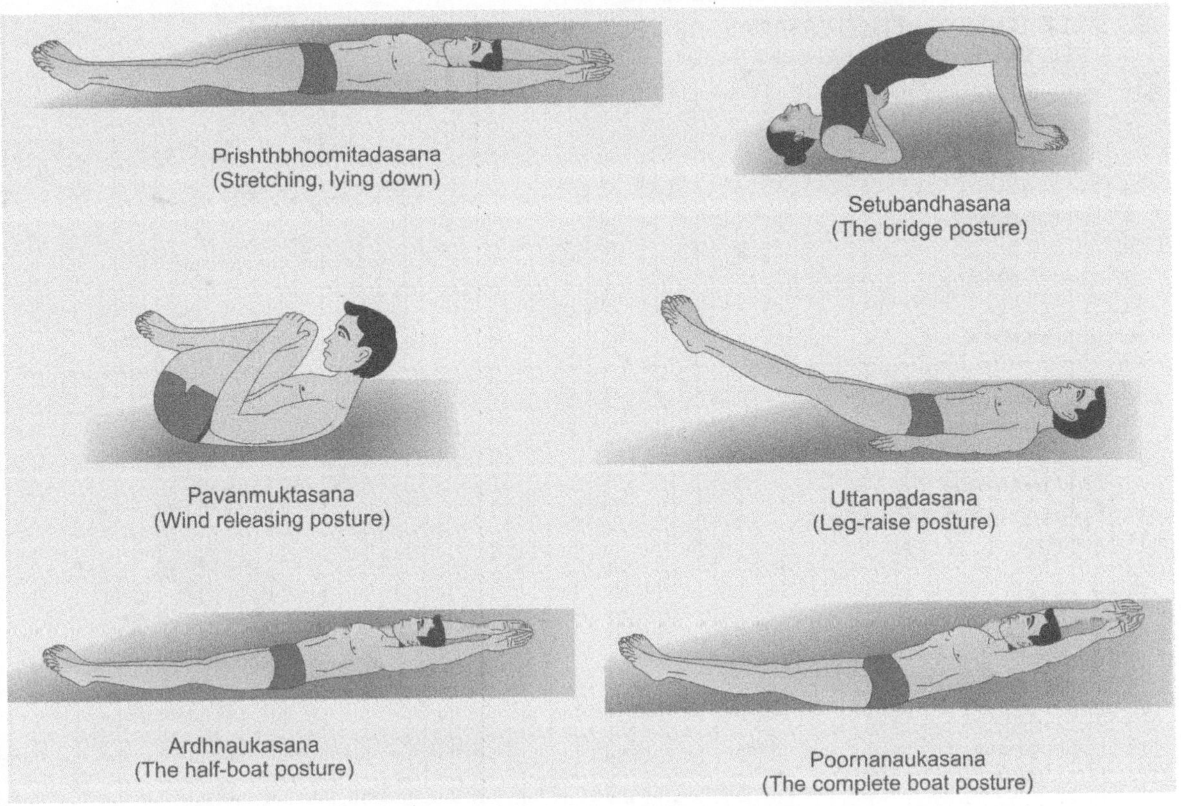

Fig. 20.6 A set of asanas performed lying down

collectively, although somewhat incorrectly, called meditation.

Although meditation can be performed at any time and at any place, it is preferable to do it at nearly the same time and at a fixed place everyday. It may be done once or twice a day, about 20 minutes each time. The best timings are dawn and dusk. The place should be a quiet and clean corner. It may help create the right mood and atmosphere if an altar is set up as a focal point in the chosen corner. The altar may have a picture of some representation of God, or the guru, or some neutral object(s) such as flowers or a candle.

Meditation proper should be preceded by a proper posture or *asana*. As discussed earlier, the recommended postures are *padmasana*, *sukhasana* or *vajrasana* (Fig. 20.11). If sitting on a chair is more convenient, that is also acceptable. The basic principle of the posture of meditation is that it should be steady and comfortable. The abdomen, chest, neck and head should be in one straight line, i.e. the spine should be erect. Lying down is *not* a suitable posture for meditation because it is too passive, and may induce sleep.

After assuming the right posture (asana), the next step is to attend to the breathing. Take four or five deep and very slow breaths. Slow and deep breathing has a calming effect on the mind and facilitates meditation proper. A deep inspiration, followed by a brief period of breath holding and then a very slow expiration is a simple form of *pranayama*.

The next step is *pratyahara*, which literally means 'bringing together' or 'gathering towards'. The mind is normally very restless. It is always crowded with

A SEQUENCE OF KEEP FIT ASANAS FOR BEGINNERS (Duration: About 1 Hour)

1. Warming up
2. Shavasana
3. Prishthbhoomitadasana

3a. *

4. Setubandhasana

4a. *

5. Pavanmuktasana

5a. *

6. Uttanpadasana

6a. *

7. Ardhnaukasana
8. Poornanaukasana

8a. *

9. Baddhakonasana
10. Pashchimottanasana
11. Konasana

11a. *

12. Vajrasana
13. Shashankasana
14. Ushtrasana
15. Parvatasana
16. Makarasana
17. Bhujangasana

17a. Makarasana

18. Dhanurasana

18a. *

19. Sarvangasana

19a. *

20. Matsyasana

20a. *

21. Tadasana
22. Padahastana

22a. Tadasana

23. Trikonasana
24. Katichakrasana
25. Utkatasana

25a. *

* Shavasana
(*Courtesy:* Sri Aurobindo Ashram, Delhi Branch)
An audio CD providing instructions for these asanas is available from Sri Aurobindo Ashram (Delhi Branch), New Delhi 110 016.

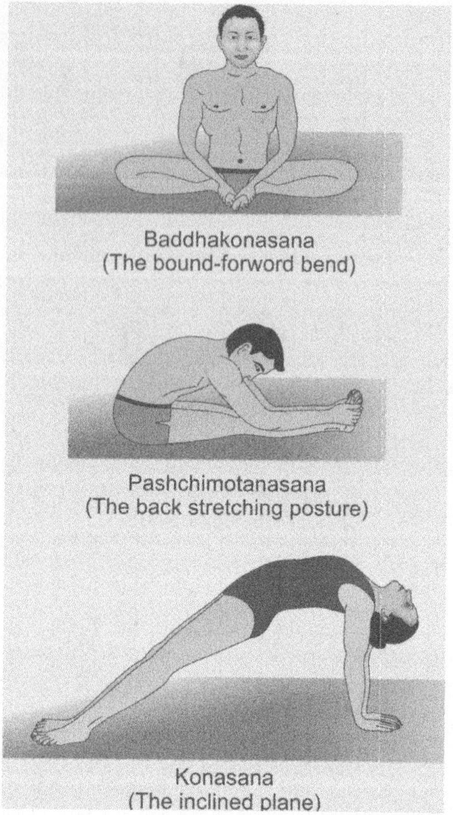

Baddhakonasana
(The bound-forword bend)

Pashchimotanasana
(The back stretching posture)

Konasana
(The inclined plane)

Fig. 20.7 A set of asanas performed sitting up. The arrows in baddhakonasana indicate that after assuming the posture shown, the person bends forward

thoughts. Most of these thoughts relate to objects as perceived by the senses. By minimizing and ignoring sensory input, the thoughts can be reduced. One way to reduce sensory input is to close the eyes. But that is far from enough. It needs conscious effort to reduce the density of thoughts. As the density of thoughts decreases, they can be given a certain direction. That is what is meant by 'bringing the thoughts together' or 'gathering them towards' a desired point. Concentrating the thought on a point is called *dharana*, which is the next step.

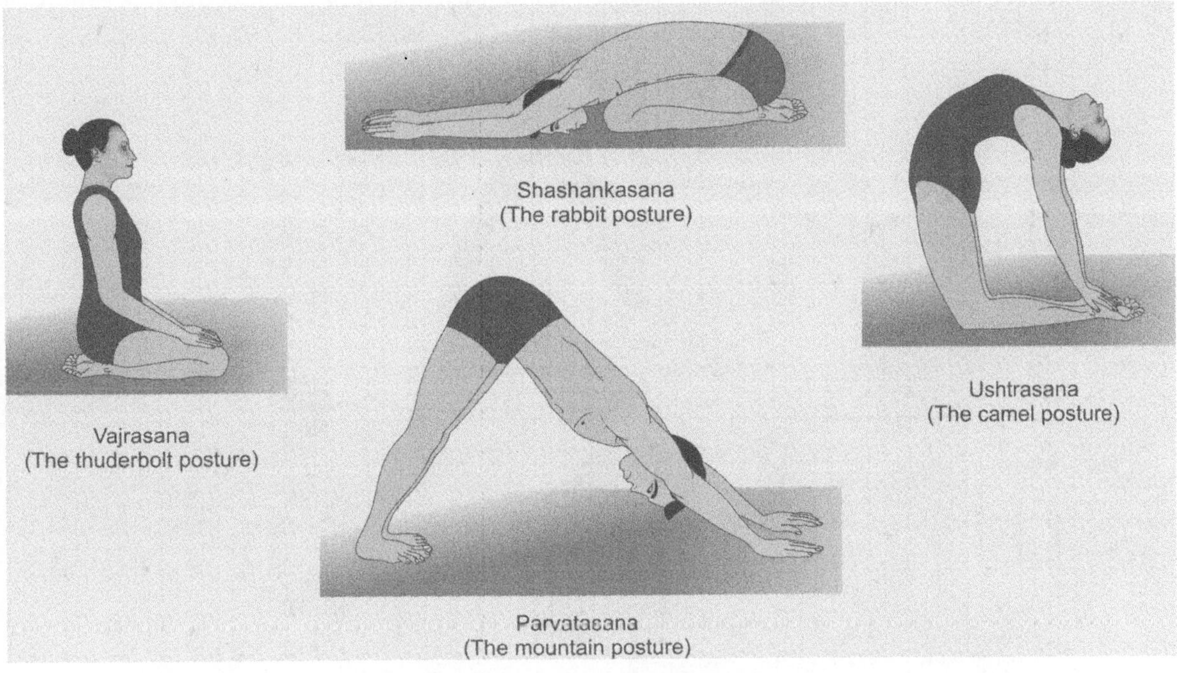

Fig. 20.8 A set of asanas performed sitting up

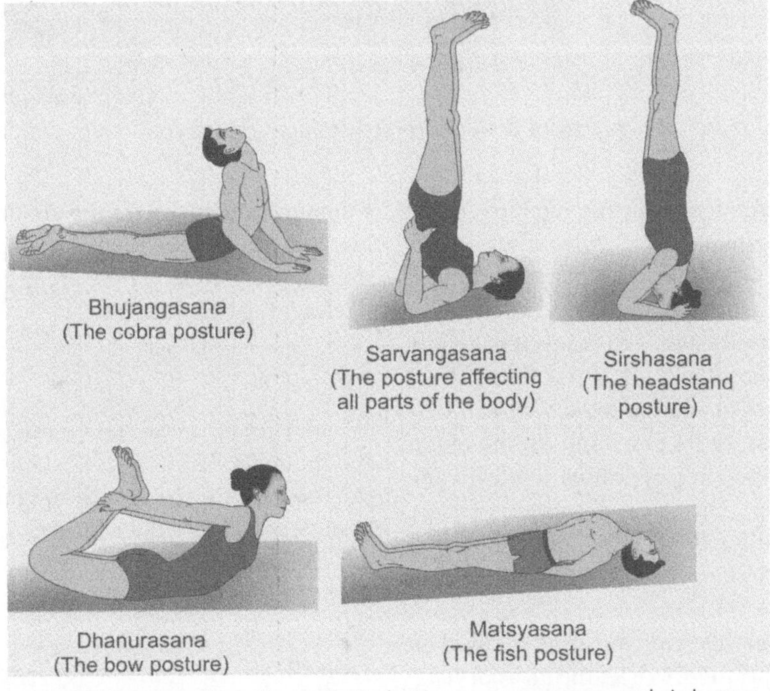

Fig. 20.9 A set of very popular asanas. Note the similarity between sarvangasana and sirshasana. Both provide similar benefits but sarvangasana is much easier and safer. Sirshasana is a risky posture which should not be attempted by beginners. Sarvangasana is a safe alternative to sirshasana

Trikonasana
(The triangular posture)
Tasasana
(The 'tad' tree posture
–stretching, standing)
Padahastasana
(Touching the toes)
Utkatasana
(The chair posture)

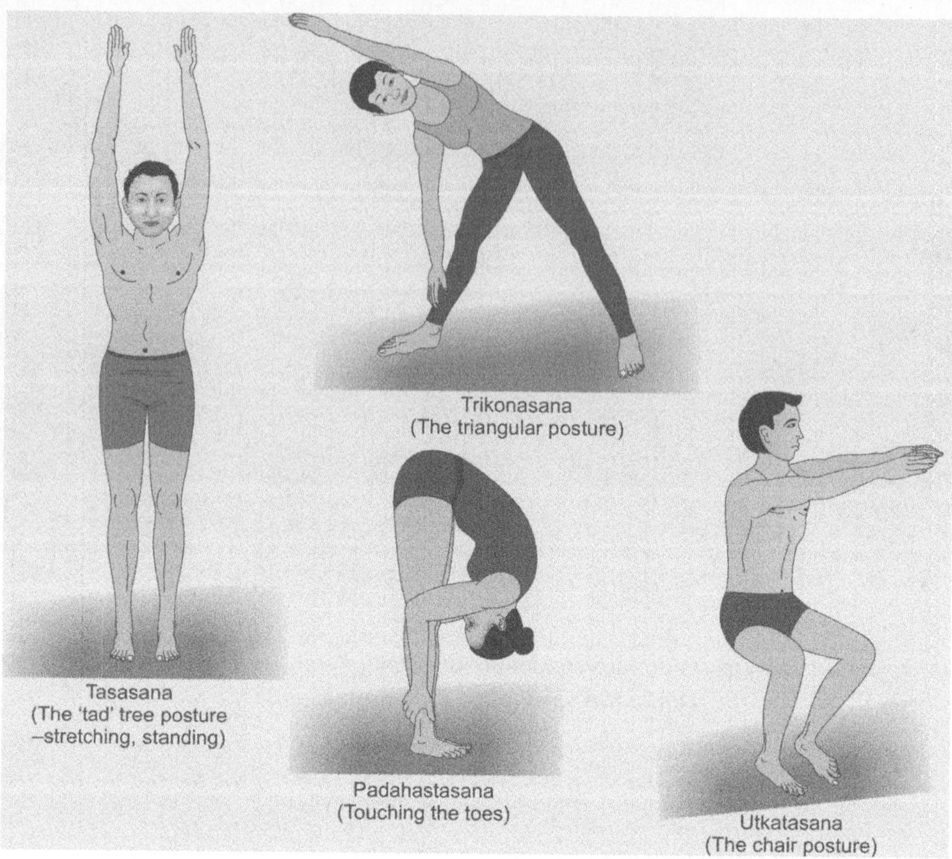

Fig. 20.10 A set of asanas performed standing up

The next question is, during dharana, what should we concentrate on? The choice is unlimited. It may be a form of God, a sound, a mantra, a flower, a flame, an idea or a thought. Although the choice is unlimited, once a choice has been made, it is helpful to maintain some constancy. It is not desirable to shift from one choice to another too often.

During dharana, we fix our mind on the object or sound or idea of choice, repeating it slowly and calmly to ourselves. This is a strenuous process, and cannot be continued for long. Therefore, after fixing our attention for a while, we enter *dhyana*, or meditation proper.

Meditation means allowing the mind to dwell on the object of concentration. We let the ideas develop systematically, step by step (Fig. 20.13). While we are enlarging on the chosen idea or object, other random thoughts again invade the mind. Thoughts are the greatest and the most common difficulty during meditation. There are at least three ways of overcoming this difficulty.

Ignore

We may let the mind run on but pay no attention to the thoughts. For example, when we are walking on the road, we see so many things but pay no attention to most of them. In the same way, unwanted thoughts can also be ignored. If the thoughts are ignored, they tend to fade away.

Reject

This is a more active, more aggressive, method of dealing with thoughts. The thoughts are actively

Pasmasana
(The lotus posture)
Sukhasana
(The comfortable posture)
Vajrasana
(The thunderbolt posture)

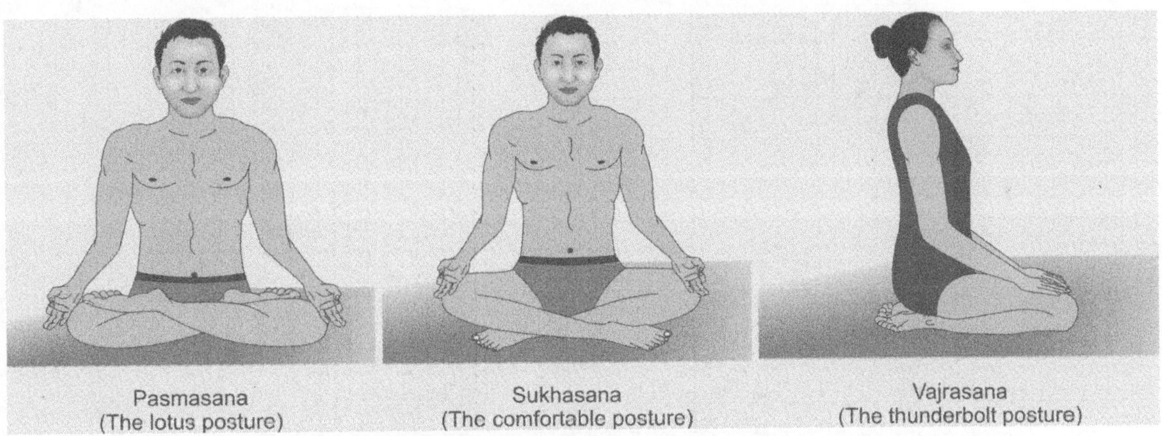

Fig. 20.11 Asanas suitable for meditation

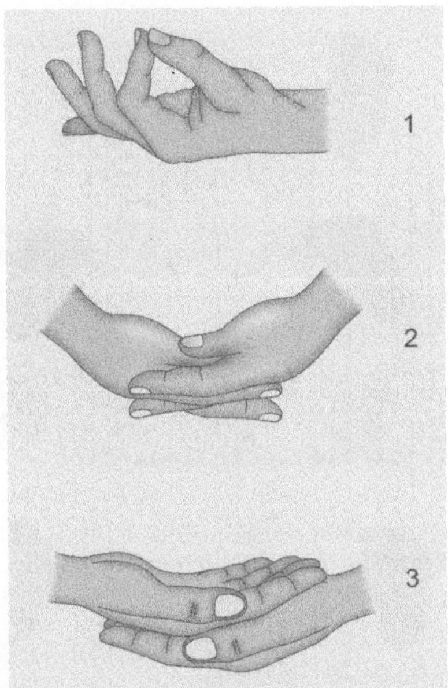

Fig. 20.12 Three alternative hand positions during meditation. 1. Chin mudra. 2. Interlocked fingers. 3. One hand cupping the other (anjali mudra)

stopped before they enter the mind, or cut short ruthlessly at the earliest possible stage. Active rejection of thoughts gradually builds up a vacant mind in which only the higher consciousness can settle.

Record

One may keep a few small pieces of paper and a pencil handy during meditation. This method is most useful for handling thoughts concerning 'things to be done'. Once such thoughts have been jotted down, they are less likely to recur because now we know that the tasks will not be forgotten.

By meditating regularly, one may reach a stage when the mind or consciousness identifies itself with the object of meditation. At this stage one forgets that one is meditating. This is the beginning of samadhi. A person in samadhi achieves a superconscious state. Such a person acquires knowledge which cannot be acquired by the reasoning mind. By going beyond reason and sensory perception, the consciousness can overcome, or transcend, the limitations of the ordinary mind. Since meditation takes us in the direction of transcendence, it is a transcendental process.

Long before *samadhi* is achieved, one or two sessions of meditation a day lead to a meditative attitude towards all our daily activities. Everything that we do is accompanied by a feeling of inner peace and calm.

The process of meditation may be summarized as follows:

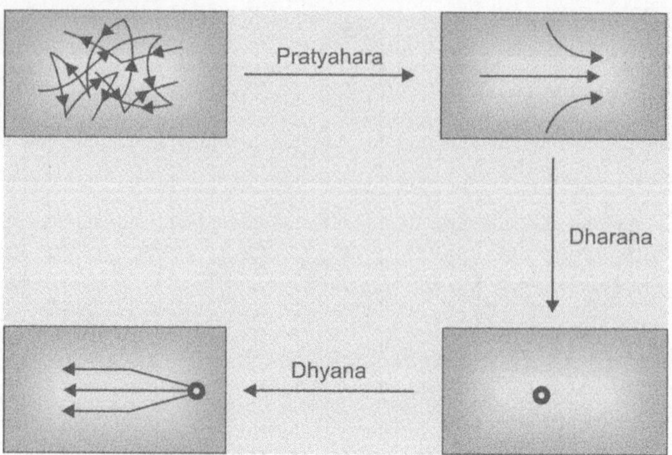

Fig. 20.13 Progressive steps in meditation

1. Assume the right posture at a fixed time and place. Close your eyes.
2. Breathe slowly and deeply.
3. Gather your thoughts.
4. Concentrate on a chosen object or sound or idea.
5. Let the mind dwell on the object of attention.

PHYSIOLOGICAL EFFECTS OF YOGA

Scientific studies on yoga generally suffer from major defects. Some of them have been done on highly accomplished yogis, but the number of subjects is very small. Others have been done on students, soldiers or patients after a few weeks or months of practice of a few yogic techniques. In such cases the pursuit of yoga has obviously been very half-hearted. But in spite of these limitations, considerable data is available on the physiological effects of yoga (Fig. 20.14).

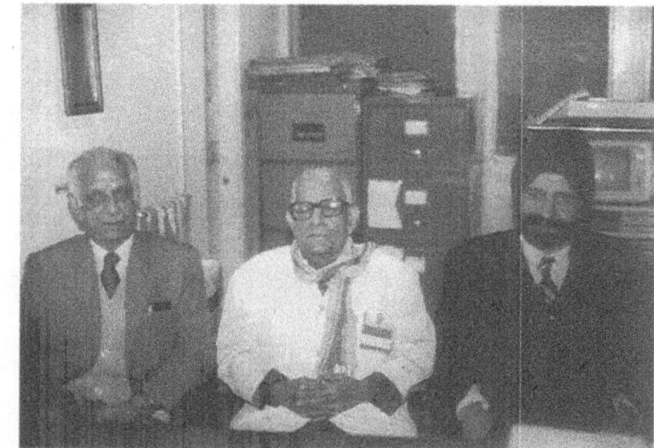

Fig. 20.14 Three pioneers in research on physiological effects of yoga. From left to right: Professor BK Anand, Professor Baldev Singh and Professor GS Chhina

Physical Endurance

Yogic exercises and meditation have been shown to improve athletic performance and increase hand grip strength. Further, yogic practices enable the athlete to turn out a given level of performance with a smaller rise in heart rate and respiratory rate. Studies in which yogic practices have been compared with other physical exercises have generally shown yogic practices to be superior in this respect.

Cardiovascular Effects

Yogic practices generally lead to a decrease in resting heart rate and blood pressure. The effects may, however, not be sustained for too long after the yogic practices have been discontinued.

Respiratory Effects

Yogic exercises lead to an improvement in respiratory function as shown by a decrease in resting respiratory rate but an increase in vital capacity, timed vital capacity, maximum voluntary ventilation, and maximal inspiratory and expiratory pressures. Transcendental meditation alone leads to a decrease in resting respiratory rate and tidal volume suggesting a decrease in oxygen consumption.

Metabolic Rate

As indicated above, there may be a decrease in oxygen consumption as a result of yogic practices. Accomplished yogis can reduce their basal metabolic rate so much that their oxygen consumption may come down to only about half the 'normal' value.

Effects on the Nervous System

Studies on meditation have shown that it leads to an increase in the time spent by the person in the alpha rhythm of the EEG. Since alpha rhythm is associated with a peaceful mind, it provides objective evidence for a reduction in restlessness. Further, sensory stimuli do not block the alpha rhythm during meditation (Fig. 20.15). Consistent with this is the general tendency of yogic practices to shift the autonomic balance in favor of the parasympathetic division. There are also reports indicating that yogic practices lead to an improvement in fine coordinated movements, reduction in reaction time and better auditory discrimination.

Endocrine Changes

Yogic practices have been reported to reduce the baseline and average levels of glucocorticoids. But the glucocorticoid response to an acute challenge is enhanced by these practices. These observations may be interpreted to mean that although the long-term stress level is reduced, the capacity to cope up with an acute challenge improves.

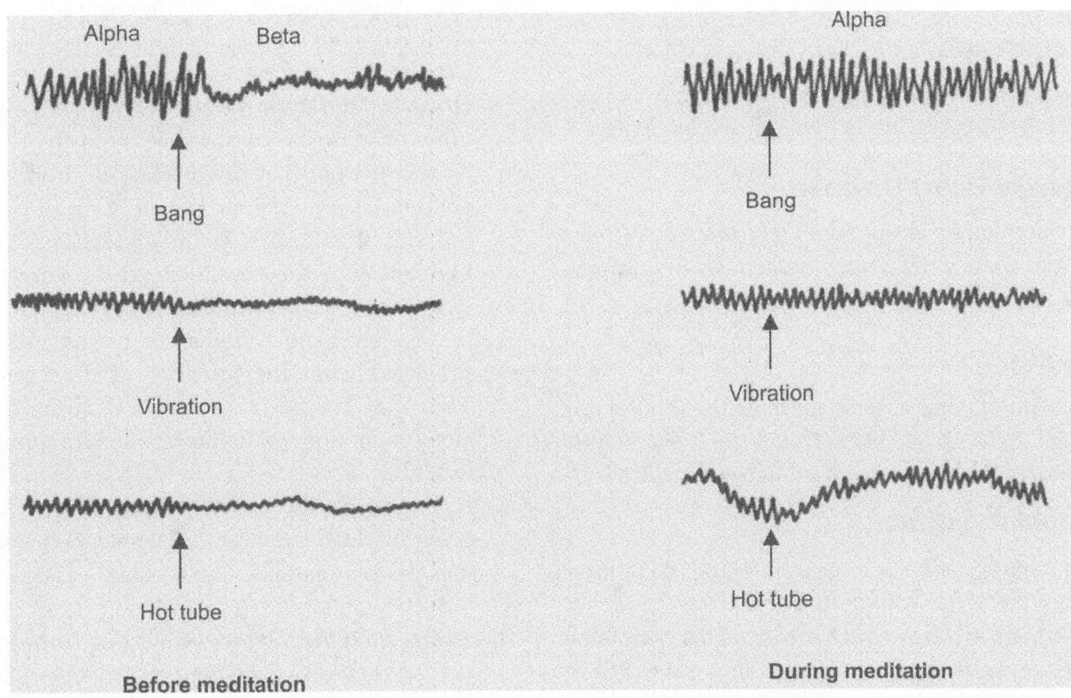

Fig. 20.15 EEG of a yogi before meditation and during meditation. Auditory, vibratory and thermal stimuli block the alpha rhythm when he is not in meditation. No blockage of the alpha rhythm occurs when he is in meditation. (*Courtesy:* Department of Physiology, All India Institute of Medical Sciences (AIIMS), New Delhi, India)

Other Biochemical Changes

Meditation and asanas have been shown to reduce the fasting blood glucose level and the total serum cholesterol level. These changes are likely to reduce the risk of diabetes and atherosclerosis.

YOGA IN HEALTH AND DISEASE

Yoga attracts the modern man as an easy way to good health. But as the foregoing discussion shows, yoga is neither easy nor is its goal good health. The fact that it also leads to good health is incidental. However, some selected yogic practices have been used in a variety of diseases with reasonable success as discussed below.

Orthopedic Problems

Yogic asanas have been found helpful for backache, cervical spondylosis and some forms of arthritis.

Hypertension

Regular meditation brings down the systolic and diastolic blood pressure in hypertensive patients.

Coronary Heart Disease

Lifestyle changes along the yogic lines have been shown to reduce the degree of stenosis in coronary arteries.

Diabetes

A selection of yogic asanas, specially those involving a spinal twist, have been found to be a helpful component in the treatment of diabetes mellitus.

Bronchial Asthma

A combination of yogic exercises and devotional sessions has been found to reduce the frequency and severity of asthmatic attacks. This treatment also changes the peak expiratory flow rate (PEFR) towards normal.

Psychological Problems

The philosophy of yoga has been used for enabling patients to see their psychological problems from a different point of view. This promotes a change in attitude which helps psychological problems.

MECHANISMS UNDERLYING EFFECTS OF YOGA

The mechanisms underlying the physiological effects of yoga and its beneficial effects in several diseases are heterogeneous. Some of the mechanisms are obvious and simple, while others are either complex or unknown. Some plausible mechanisms have been enumerated below:

1. Since yogic asanas, besides everything else, are also physical exercises, their effects on muscle strength and flexibility of the body are easy to understand. Besides, they also improve the posture and relieve muscle spasm. All these effects have obvious value in orthopedic problems.
2. The improvement in cardiorespiratory efficiency can also be explained on the basis of the effects of yogic asanas as physical exercise. However, the improvement is more than with other exercises of comparable intensity. It may be pointed out that the increase in thoracic or abdominal pressure, or the duration of breath holding, involved in some yogasanas is quite high although the exercise is gentle. Therefore, stimulation of cardiorespiratory reflexes may be at a level much higher than what may be predicted from the intensity of the exercise. That may be the reason for a disproportionately high improvement in cardiorespiratory function.
3. As pointed out earlier, yogic practices, in general, shift autonomic balance in favor of the parasympathetic. This may explain the reduction in heart rate and blood pressure.
4. The reduction in body weight due to physical exercise may also contribute to beneficial effects in arthritis, diabetes, hypertension and coronary heart disease.
5. Change in diet and mental relaxation may also contribute to beneficial effects in diabetes, hypertension and coronary heart disease.

CONCLUSION

We have discussed the most basic principles of yoga. Even this elementary discussion shows that yoga is not primarily a system of medicine. It is a simple and humane way of life open to all. It has potential for individual salvation as well as collective upliftment of the human race. As a by product, it can also promote health and prevent disease.

QUESTIONS

1. Who is fit to pursue yoga?
2. Which type of yoga is easy?
3. If the whole lifetime may not be sufficient to reach perfection *(siddhi)*, why embark on yoga at all?
4. What is the minimum time per day required for yoga?
5. Is it incorrect to start asanas before achieving perfection in *yama and niyama*?
6. What time of the day is best for asanas?
7. What dress is best for asanas?
8. Can *sirshasana* be dangerous?
9. What type of diet is suitable for yoga?

ANSWERS

1. The answer is: everyone. The path of yoga is open to all. Anyone who feels a call to it should embark on it in all sincerity.
2. The answer is: none. Sincere pursuit of yoga is an uphill and apparently never-ending quest.
3. Fortunately the outcome of yoga is not an all or none phenomenon. Every bit of progress brings commensurate inner peace and joy. The graded nature of the process makes it easy to adopt the dictum, enjoy the journey and forget about the destination.
4. This is a common question which should not be asked. The question reflects popular misconceptions about yoga. Yoga is not a part time activity. It should influence, transform and divinize every activity of the day.
5. No, that would effectively exclude most of us from the practice of asanas. While perfection in yama and niyama is not necessary, a conscious effort to enforce them in daily life is highly desirable before embarking on asanas.
6. Early morning, after emptying the bowels, and on empty stomach, is the best time for asanas. If that is inconvenient, the asanas should be performed more than 4 hours after the previous meal. For example, if lunch is over at 2 pm, asanas may be performed after 6 pm.
7. Any loose and comfortable dress is satisfactory The dress should not reduce the flexibility of the body. Cotton is better than synthetic fabrics because it lets the sweat evaporate.
8. Yes, sirshasana is potentially dangerous because it may twist the neck. It is an asana only for experts. Non-experts can derive the benefits of sirshasana from the much simpler and safer sarvangasana.
9. Yogic diet is not a rigid diet. A simple but wholesome vegetarian diet, free from stimulants, is considered the best. However, along with several other desires, the desire for rich food is also likely to disappear gradually during the practice of yoga. It is better to change the diet in keeping with the change of heart rather than impose a drastic change abruptly.

Index

Page numbers followed by *f* refer to figures and those followed by *t* refer to tables

O

P

R

S

T

U

V

W

Y

Z